ESSENTIALS OF CONTEMPORARY CHINESE ACUPUNCTURISTS' CLINICAL EXPERIENCES

Chief Editors Chen Youbang & Deng Liangyue
Chief English Editor Zhang Kai

FOREIGN LANGUAGES PRESS BEIJING

First Edition 1989

ISBN 0-8351-2267-0
ISBN 7-119-01042-5

Published by Foreign Languages Press
24 Baiwanzhuang Road, Beijing, China

Printed by Foreign Languages Printing House
19 West Chegongzhuang Road, Beijing, China

Distributed by China International Book Trading Corporation
(Guoji Shudian), P.O. Box 399, Beijing, China

Printed in the People's Republic of China

THE EDITORS' WORDS

Acupuncture and moxibustion are important components of traditional Chinese medicine. Clinical experiences are essential in the science of acupuncture and moxibustion. Developing clinical advantages and increasing therapeutic effects are considered the key points for the promotion and development of acupuncture and moxibustion as well as of traditional Chinese clinical medicine. This book features the essentials of clinical experiences and provides information and reference materials to readers. As the editors, we hope our readers will share its benefits in their clinical practice and study.

The book consists of sixty-nine articles, each of which is the clinical speciality of a professor, an associate professor, or a research fellow. Every article is composed of three parts. Part One gives a brief introduction to the author's background, his or her major achievements, representative works, working unit and current professional titles. Part Two deals with the academic characteristics and medical specialties; it covers the theory, technique, prescription, acupoints, acupuncture and moxibustion treatment and other treatment methods such as qigong and massage, and the instruments of acupuncture and moxibustion. Part Three is a consideration of the case records, in which some typical cases are analyzed as proof to the theory under discussion, and some difficult cases, although not strictly related to the topic being discussed, are adopted when deemed necessary. Not every article mentions all these items. There are a total of 293 cases collected in the book.

We are indebted to China Association of Acupuncture and Moxibustion, the Acupuncture Institute of the China Academy of Traditional Chinese Medicine, the First Affiliated Hospital of the Tianjin College of Traditional Chinese Medicine, and other seniors in the field of acupuncture and moxibustion for their great help and support in completing this work.

Cui Yueli, former Minister of Public Health and President of the China Association of Traditional Chinese Medicine, autographed the title of the book; Hu Ximing, Vice-Minister of Public Health, Director of the State Administration of Traditional Chinese Medicine and President of the China Association of Acupuncture and Moxibustion, wrote the foreword; and Lu Zhijun, Honorary President of the China Association of Acupuncture and Moxibustion and Executive Chairman of the Preparatory Committee of the World Federation of Acupuncture and Moxibustion, inscribed the book.

A number of people have been of great help in completing this work. We would like to thank Shi Yuguang, Wu Xuezhang, Gu Li, Bai Yongpo, Li Weiheng, He Shuhuai, Zheng Qiwei, Shan Shujian, Qin Wenguang, Gao Zhenwu, Fu Xingguo and Xue Ligong for their valuable editorial assistance.

We are indebted to Fang Tingyu, Wang Yici, Huang Guoqi, Ye Huan, Xu Yao, Wang Huizhu, Chen Fang, Tao Jinwen, Jin Huide, Tu Tianying, Wang Zhaolong, Ding

Xiaoping, You Benlin, Li Lianyu, Du Wei, Tian Hong and Zhang Kai for their translation work.

Thanks are also due to Dale Campbell, Kuang Peihua and other staff editors of the Foreign Languages Press for the great pains they have taken to check and improve the typescript and proofs.

We sincerely hope that our readers will offer their comments and suggestions with a view to revision and improvement for the second edition.

The Editorial Committee
January, 1989

FOREWORD

The field of Chinese acupuncture and moxibustion has a long history, dating back thousands of years to the ancient past. *The Internal Classic*, written during the Warring States Period (484-221 B.C.), makes up 70 to 80 percent of the coverage on acupuncture and moxibustion.

A Classic of Acupuncture and Moxibustion, compiled by Huang Fumi (215-282) during the Jin Dynasty on the basis of *The Internal Classic, The Illustrated Chart of Acupoints* and *Therapeutic Importance of Acupuncture and Moxibustion,* is regarded as an authoritative monograph in China and has become an important book to be shared with the world.

Following the publication of this classic, there appeared a number of famous acupuncturists in different dynasties, such as Sun Simiao (581-682) during the Tang Dynasty, Wang Weiyi (987-1067) during the Song Dynasty, Hua Boren (the fourteenth century) during the Yuan Dynasty and Gao Wu and Yang Jizhou (the sixteenth century) during the Ming Dynasty. They all made brilliant contributions to the development of acupuncture and moxibustion.

After the founding of the People's Republic of China, the field of acupuncture and moxibustion was rejuvenated with the formulation of the policy to develop traditional Chinese medicine. In the subsequent decades, following the essentials of *The Internal Classic* and *Classic on Medical Problems,* we have created many new acupuncture methods, thus inheriting and developing the science of acupuncture and moxibustion. Now, great importance has been attached to the therapy of acupuncture and moxibustion, which has already become an important component of world medicine.

To carry forward the science of acupuncture and moxibustion, Chen Youbang, Deng Liangyue and other specialists and professors compiled the present book, *Essentials of Contemporary Chinese Acupuncturists' Clinical Experiences,* in which the works are full of new ideas that will not only help popularize the subject but also stimulate its academic development. I highly recommend this book. Looking back through history and forward to the future, I am happy to promote the cause of acupuncture and moxibustion. Therefore, I offer this foreword herewith.

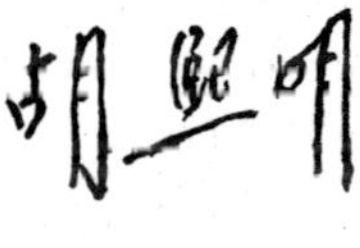

Hu Ximing*
January, 1989, Beijing

*Vice-Minister of the Public Health, Director of the State Administration of Traditional Chinese Medicine, and President of China Association of Acupuncture and Moxibustion

CONTENTS

FULL UNDERSTANDING OF A DISEASE AND SIGNIFICANCE OF ARRIVAL OF QI

—Yu Shuzhuang's Clinical Experience

Yu Shuzhuang, born in 1924 and a native of Anci County, Hebei Province, was determined to become a medical doctor since his childhood, and he was enthusiastic about acupuncture. He went to Beijing at the age of eighteen to study traditional medicine for ten years under the instruction of Feng Jiqing, Zhao Xiwu and Zhang Wenxiang. In 1951 he started his practice and in 1953 he became a teacher at the Beijing College of Traditional Chinese Medicine. Then he changed his job and worked in the Beijing Municipal Hospital of Traditional Chinese Medicine in 1968 in clinical work and researching acupuncture. Yu thinks that the most important thing in treatment of diseases by acupuncture is to have different needling sensations, the intensity of which is based on the depth of needling to treat various conditions.

For any case he asks five questions. In his research of the meridian system he has discovered the method of conducting qi by a patient himself, and in collaboration with the Academia Sinica in 1976, he also discovered the recessive transmission of acupuncture reaction. His six research achievements won the first and second prizes awarded by the Ministry of Public Health and the Beijing Municipal Commission of Science and Technology. In addition, about seventy papers written by him were published. Now he is an associate professor in the Acupuncture Department, Beijing Municipal Hospital of Traditional Chinese Medicine and director of the Standing Committee of the China Acupuncture Association.

I. Academic Characteristics and Clinical Specialities

1. Awareness of a disease

During his long clinical practice he has learned that five principles of awareness are essential to improve the curative effect of acupuncture, i.e. 1) awareness of the problem; 2) awareness of the syndrome the disease attributes to; 3) awareness of the affected meridians; 4) awareness of the meridians to be treated and point selected; and 5) awareness of the methods of treatment

1) *Awareness of the problem* There is no universal therapy and the same is true of acupuncture, which is markedly effective for some conditions, yet not good for other conditions. Therefore inquiry about the nature of the disease ensures that one knows exactly how things stand, e.g. low back pain—a common ailment that has different causes. Some are organic problems (such as pain caused by tuberculosis of the lumbar vertebrae, bone tumour or by visceral disorders), and some are functional disorders (such as pain caused by cold, trauma, strain, etc.). Without knowing the nature of a disease the

acupuncturist does not understand why the former has no response to acupuncture treatments and the latter is cured by only one needling of Kunlun (B 60). Another example is wind-stroke (cerebro-vascular disease), which can be divided into two categories (hemorrhagic and ischemic ones) the treatment for the two types in the acute stage varies greatly. For the former hemostasis is necessary, and for the latter it is advisable to invigorate blood circulation. In this case how could you fail to distinguish the two syndromes. Since the development of modern tests, it is important to know a disease by its modern medical term, and to differentiate the syndrome according to the rules and theory of traditional Chinese medicine.

2) *Awareness of the syndrome* Acupuncture treatment cannot be separated from the theory of treatment based on differentiation of syndromes. A syndrome represents the nature of a disease, and the interrelation between many factors which influence the onset and development of a disease. Because differentiation of syndromes is the prerequisite for treatment, only by knowing the characteristics of the disease can one decide what principles and methods of treatment may be used. For instance, in cases of deficiency the reinforcing method is applied, in cases of excess the reducing method is used, in cases of too much heat, the heat-removing method is applied, and in cases of too much cold, the warming method is used. Disease cause must be found out in differentiation of syndromes, for it can tell the true from false manifestations of the case (e.g. a case of cold showing pseudo-heat symptoms, or a case of excess in reality showing sham symptoms of insufficiency). The above is the guiding ideology of traditional Chinese medicine in "differentiation of syndromes to seek disease cause and treatment." If there are such symptoms as eating much yet feeling constantly hungry, lassitude, haggardness, dizziness, shortness of breath, palpitation, much perspiration, insomnia, dream-disturbed sleep, several bowel movements a day, yellow-white complexion, reddish tongue with a thin, white coating, fast pulse and a basal metabolic rate of +98, the case is diagnosed as thyroidism. You can not say this is a case of insufficient qi and blood owing to the symptoms of yellow-white complexion, lassitude, etc. The cause of insufficient qi and blood must be found out. Eating much yet feeling hungry indicates presence of excessive fire, which is verified by the teaching in medical classics that "abundant fire consumes qi." From this it can be seen that the deficiency is brought about by qi consumption due to too much fire. Deficiency is a pseudo-phenomenon, or symptom, whereas fire is the root cause. If the latter fails to be dealt with and attention is only paid to deficiency, how can the disease be cured? Thus, Yu thinks a. Finding out the cause is the only way to make a correct differentiation, and b. That the old saying—reinforcing method cannot be applied to deficiency cases—is not true, for real deficiency cases should be treated by the reinforcing method, but pseudo-deficiency is an exception.

3) *Awareness of the affected meridians* In acupuncture therapy, differentiation of the affected meridians is more significant than that of syndromes, which indicates that in addition to differentiation of pathological conditions in accordance with the eight principal syndromes, the state of the zang-fu organs, qi and blood and etiological factors, it is essential to know what meridians are affected. This is the basis for point selection. If one does not understand the affected meridians and only knows Zusanli (S 36) for relief of gastric pain, Neiguan (P 6) for pectoral pain with stuffiness, Weizhong (B 40)

for low back pain, it is merely a method of selecting points for symptoms. For example, practice shows that Hegu (LI 4) is very effective in the treatment of toothaches, but not all toothaches can be removed by needling Hegu (LI 4). Because it is the Yuan-(Source) point of the Large Intestine Meridian of Hand-Yangming, it is natural that toothaches due to afflictions of the Yangming Meridian can be relieved by needling this point. But for toothaches due to other causes there is no response from this point. In short, differentiation of the affected meridians is believed the way to seek the cause before treatment. Here are some methods to know the affected meridians. First, one should be familiar with meridians and syndromes, then one is able to find out the problems of the meridians and decide the points to be used. In related medical examination, one should examine the painful areas, the presence of bloody meridians, subcutaneous tubercles, cords, swelling, depression, skin temperature, and whether the pulse condition is strong or weak, tenderness of certain points, etc. Without examination and only by listening to the patient's complaints it is difficult to know the particular painful spots and the meridian afflicted. When a patient complains he has a pain in the shoulder and arm, and the examination tells that it is a pain in the anterior part of the shoulder, this is a case in which the Yangming Meridian has been afflicted, points of this meridian should be used (including Tiaokou (S 38)). When the pain is at the posterior of the shoulder and elbow, the Hand-Taiyang Meridian has been afflicted, then points of this meridian should be selected. If there is a pain in the shoulder and arm, it indicates the Hand-Shaoyang Meridian has been afflicted, and points of this meridian are to be used. If the pain spreads to the nape and costal region when the arm is being raised, it suggests the Yangqiao Meridian has been afflicted and the Shu-points of it should be selected. When a patient complains of low back pain, the doctor must examine the painful spots and see if the muscle of this part is stiff. If there are congestive vessels in the lower limbs where Foot-Taiyang and Foot-Shaoyang Meridians pass, and a fullness feeling of the collaterals near Weizhong (B 40), the collateral should be pricked until it bleeds, then immediate good results can be seen. Now let's go back to the example of the toothache. It is stated in the *Treatise of Meridians* and *Miraculous Pivot* that "when pathological changes occur in the Large Intestine Meridian of Hand-Yangming, a toothache arises. But the cause of pathological changes varies, so one should be cautious in differentiation of syndromes. If it is a severe toothache with a full feeling at Daying (S 5) it proves the existence of strong pathogenic factors, showing pathological changes in the Large Intestine Meridian of Hand-Yangming due to excessive stomach fire, and the Stomach Meridian of Foot-Yangming Meridian has been afflicted. In this case triple puncture technique is applied to Daying (S 5) and Neiting (S 44). If there is tenderness in Ermen (SJ 21), Sizhukong (SJ 23) or in Qubin (G 7), Fubai (G 10), Wangu (SI 4), it indicates pathological changes have occurred in the Large Intestine Meridian of Hand-Yangming due to abundant wind and fire in the Sanjiao Meridian of Hand-Shaoyang. It is advisable to select Ermen (SJ 21), Sizhukong (SJ 23) or Fubai (G 10) and Wangu (SI 4). If the above signs are not present and there is a full feeling at Yangxi (LI 5), it means the Large Intestine Meridian of Hand-Yangming has been afflicted, then Hegu (LI 4) is to be used. A dull toothache with a loose tooth and without the above signs indicates pathological changes in the Large Intestine Meridian due to flaming up of fire in the Kidney Meridian of Foot-Shaoyin. It is advisable to select Taixi (K 3). This shows selecting points of the corresponding meridian.

4) *Awareness of the meridians to be treated and points selected* The above concerns the afflicted meridians, where the question is which meridian should be treated and what points selected. This is because traditional Chinese medicine emphasizes holistic treatment, e.g. the kidney must be taken into consideration in treating the heart problem (cardiac pain); when phlegm is expected to be removed, the spleen should be taken care of at the same time; qi-stimulation is the prerequisite to phlegm-expulsion; the blood system is dealt with first in wind-relief, for wind interrupts smooth circulation of blood; when pathogenic factors are to be dispelled it is important to strengthen the patient's resistance; treat the yang aspect for diseases of yin nature; treat the yin aspect for diseases of yang nature; and when the zang-fu organs are in a state of excessiveness, it is necessary to treat the fu-organs. Another example is rheumatic or rheumatoid arthritis, manifested by generally painful joints, severe pain in the knee joints, aversion to wind, cold, pale complexion, puffy tongue with white coating and weak pulse. This is a case due to pathogenic cold and damp, showing lower body resistance. The yang meridian is diseased because a preponderance of yin impairs yang. Naturally the yang aspect should be dealt with first, however, it is proper to select Zhongwan (Ren 12), Qihai (Ren 6), Zusanli (S 36), Dazhui (Du 14) with the reinforcing method instead of points of the yang meridians. It seems it does not follow the principle of selecting points of the corresponding meridian, but in fact the patient's resistance is low, and is not able to get rid of pathogenic factors by itself. Therefore the priority is to improve the body's resistance. This is the approach that treats the root cause of a disease. Some regard the reacting place as the points. Others believe points are not necessarily the reacting places. Yu thinks the latter have a better understanding than the former in terms of meridian and point selection. For instance, cardiac pain is often accompanied by tenderness of Tanzhong (Ren 17), Shenfeng (K 23), Lingxu (K 24), Rugen (S 18), Yingchuang (S 16), Yuanye (G 22), Xinshu (B 15) and Zhiyang (Du 9) (in mild cases, pain and tenderness is only found on points, in severe cases, tenderness is found in the chest and back). Tenderness also found on the distant points, such as Tongli (H 5), Lingdao (H 4) (in mild and severe cases, there is tenderness along the meridian, and in most severe cases a conscious pain appears along the meridian), Neiguan (P 6), Jianshi (P 5), Fuliu (K 7), Jiexi (S 41), Taibai (Sp 3), Gongsun (Sp 4), Qiuxu (G 40) and Kunlun (B 60). It doesn't mean all the symptoms appear simultaneously in the same person. An oppressed feeling in the chest, shortness of breath and cardiac pain must be associated with tenderness on Tongli (H 5) and Lingdao (H 4) —a key symptom of the heart problem. When tenderness appears on Rugen (S 18) you would find tenderness on Jiexi (S 41), or when tenderness appears on Yuanye (G 22) tenderness of Qiuxu (G 40) is often seen. It is true of other meridians. For example, a patient suffering from stuffiness in the chest, shortness of breath, aggravated by cold and stress, frequent cardiac pain, white-coated tongue and a deep and thready pulse is diagnosed as having a deficiency in the spleen and kidney, obstruction of yang in the chest. Meridian examination shows there is a tenderness on Yuanye (G 22), Qiuxu (G 40) (++)~(+++), a sign of pathological changes in the Heart and Gallbladder Meridians. Treatment: Tonifying the spleen and kidney, removing retardation of qi and blood

travelling in the chest to reinforce vital function. Point selection: Zhongwan (Ren 12), Qihai (Ren 6), Zusanli (S 36), Guanyuan (Ren 4) (moxibustion applied), Tongli (H 5), Qiuxu (G 40). Method: The reinforcing method is applied. The points selected are located at the four meridians of the Heart, Gallbladder, Du and Stomach.

5) *Awareness of treating methods to be used* Treating methods include acupuncture, moxibustion, fire needling, bloodletting and manipulations. The methods employed depend on the disease condition—deficiency, excess, cold or heat, combining consideration of the function of the approaches and manipulations. Acupuncture has been wildly used in treatment because it has the function to reinforce the deficiency syndrome, reduce the excess condition, remove heat and cold, send useful elements up and bring wastes down, activate blood circulation to eliminate stasis. Bloodletting is the first alternate method in relieving heat, fire and blood stasis, so acupuncture is usually used to treat mild cases. If there are manifestations of abundant fire, heat due to toxity, summer heat, stirring-up of wind or coma due to heat or excessive emotional activities and upward invasion of fire (known as fire symptoms caused by abundant pathogenic factors), the condition is treated by bloodletting and acupuncture to eliminate fire and stasis. In conditions of deficiency, it is unwise to employ bloodletting, acupuncture alone is used. The function of acupuncture in activating yang qi and relieving cold is second to moxibustion and fire needling, therefore in treatment of mild cases of deficiency and cold, acupuncture is used only. As to stasis due to protracted cold, yang diminishing or perishing, it is necessary to apply acupuncture and moxibustion. Fire needling is one of the warming methods, but it is different from moxibustion, for the latter can be employed to treat not only rheumatic or rheumatoid arthritis due to cold, but deficiency and cold in the internal organs. We usually use moxibustion instead of fire needling to restore yang from collapse. Moxibustion is helpful in reinforcement, breaking up obstruction and removing stasis. It is considered as an auxiliary hand. Acupuncture, moxibustion and bloodletting sometimes are used together for prolonged pain of the lower back and legs due to stasis caused by accumulation of cold. If there are congestive vessels in the lower limbs and fullness of the vessel near Weizhong (B 40), prick the vessel until it bleeds; moxibustion is applied to Shenshu (B 23), etc. to activate yang; or needling is given to Huantiao (B 30), Yanglingquan (B 34) to promote smooth flow of qi in the meridians. Sometimes fire needling, bloodletting and acupuncture are used together to treat pain and motor impairment of the shoulders, fire needling disapplied locally. In cases of numbness and distending pain, puncture the Jing-(Well) point until it bleeds to remove stasis through activating the blood circulation.

2. Aiming at arrival of qi

In accordance with his study of the ancient medical classics, and his own experience, Yu says various sensations of qi, the intensity of needling reaction and the depth of the needles inserted are the basis to get a good response in treatment. It is said in *Miraculous Pivot*, the earliest book on acupuncture, that "the chief purpose of acupuncture is to bring about the arrival of qi and good effect." Practice has shown that when the needle is inserted to a certain depth the patient may have a feeling of either distention or pain, numbness, electric shock, tic, coolness or heat. Any needling reaction has its own indication. For this reason, proper needling reaction and intensity is used in light of the nature of the disease—deficiency, excess, cold or heat, the duration of a disease, the condition of the patient's health, sensitivity to acupuncture and stages of a disease. If one is able to make the patient feel any needling reaction he desires, he is truely a good acupuncturist.

1) *Different needling reactions and their indications*

a. Distention and sore feeling: It is commonly seen clinically, often appearing at the same time. Mild reaction of soreness and distension is especially helpful to patients of the deficiency syndrome (deficiency of qi, blood, yin or yang), of chronic problems and a weak build. Patients after treatment often feel free from suffering.

b. Numbness, electric shock-like feeling: This is a stronger reaction, helpful to the excess syndrome, such as acute diseases, and to patients of strong constitution. For example, puncture Huantiao (G 30) with an electric shock-like feeling spreading to the foot to treat stem sciatica, hysterical paralysis, hemiplegia and poliomyelitis. But in sciatica when the sharp pain is removed and only slight pain remains or there is a numb sensation in the lateral part of the foot this needling reaction does not help. It is also helpful to renal colic or amenia when the electric shock-like feeling conducts to the lower abdomen.

c. Hot sensation: It is conducive to the cold syndromes (cold, deficiency syndrome, cold-damp syndrome and cold-wind syndrome), such as rheumatism or rheumatoid arthritis and diarrhoea due to cold-damp, low back pain due to deficiency in the kidney, facial paralysis, palsy, atrophy of muscles.

d. Cool sensation: It is helpful to the heat syndromes (wind-heat syndrome, fire-heat syndrome, heat syndrome due to toxity, heat-dry syndrome), such as the common cold due to affliction of wind and heat, sore throat, toothache due to affliction of wind and fire, or to stomach fire, hypertensive headache due to liver fire, migraine due to fire.

e. Tic feeling: It is helpful to gastroptosis, prolapse of uterus.

f. Painful feeling: Pain is not the intended reaction the operator seeks for when acupuncture is applied to the points of the four limbs and trunk. But a painful feeling is desired when you needle the Jing-(Well) points of the foot, such as Shixuan (Extra 30), Yongquan (K 1), Renzhong (Du 26), ear points and Changqiang (Du 1). In this sense, a painful feeling is one of the normal needling reactions. In addition, the curative effect is influenced by the conducting direction of the painful reaction. Two conducting directions are seen clinically, concentric and eccentric. The latter is easier to attain and the former is reached by special manipulations. Although the eccentric needling reaction is helpful to various diseases, the concentric needling reaction (known as leading qi to the diseased part) may strengthen the curative effect, which has been proved in treatment of persistent facial spasm, thyroid adenoma.

2) *Intensity of the needling reaction and indications* Intensity of the needling reaction is decided by the finger force on insertion of the needle, the depth of insertion, the duration of manipulation and the reaction of the individual to acupuncture. Generally speaking, strong finger force brings about intense needling reaction. Yet an individual sensitive to acupuncture may have a strong reaction with light finger force. It is

important for the operator to carefully observe the sensitivity of the individual and exert the proper finger force to gain the appropriate intensity to cure the ailment.

Strong needling intensity is good for acute diseases, excess syndromes and patients of a strong build. Mild needling intensity is helpful to chronic diseases, deficiency syndromes and patients of weak build. But the quality of deficiency and excess varies the intensity of the needling reaction. For instance, a temporary relief seen after acupuncture therapy suggests intensity of the needling reaction is not enough. Then exert more finger force on insertion of the needle or prolong the duration of the operation to obtain a cure. On the contrary, when the disease worsens several hours or one or two days after the acupuncture therapy, it indicates the needling reaction is too strong and should be reduced, i.e. to exercise less finger force or shorten the duration of treatment.

3) *Depth of needling and indications* It is pointed out in *Miraculous Pivot* that "the seventh is shallow puncture (one of the nine needling techniques to puncture the skin superficially with a short filiform needle in treatment of dermatoneuritis)," and "the fifth is 'Shu-point puncture' (one of the five needling techniques to treat osteal pain, e.g. cervical ossificans, by thrusting the needle deeply to the bone)." This is proof of the depth of the needle according to the location of the disease. Practice shows the function of the meridians is generated by the needle tip, and the deeper the needle is inserted the more the reaction is felt in general.

4) *Factors influencing the needling reaction*

a. The needling reaction and the condition: It has been proved by practice that patients of the cold-deficiency syndrome tend to have hot sensation; and patients of heat-excess syndrome are likely to have a cool feeling.

b. The needling reaction and the depth of a needle inserted: Soreness is often seen at any portion of the body. But when the needle tip reaches the deepest place, obvious soreness presents and when it touches the motor point, tic sensation is felt. Tic sensation also appears when the needle is being rotated. Numbness and an electric shock-like feeling is felt when the needle touches the nerve-trunk or nerve branches. Arrival of qi at the diseased part is brought about by the meridian itself punctured.

c. The needling reaction and manipulations: After qi arrives slowly and lightly press the needle for one or two minutes, then push the needle to the required depth, now a hot sensation is often present; or puncture the needle to the required depth until the arrival of qi, then pull it to the shallow part and retain the needle for one or two minutes, then a cool feeling will appear.

5) *The needling reaction and individual variations* Persons sensitive to acupuncture have needling reactions readily, but for those insensitive it is difficult to have hot or cool sensations. For the insensitive patients a hot needling reaction is gained with the help of warm needling, a cool reaction is had by bloodletting.

In short, "proper needling brings about the arrival of qi and curative effects," which is essential in treating diseases with acupuncture. But the significance of manipulations lies in the nature of conditions—cold, heat, deficiency and excess, a particular patient, different stages of a disease, varied intensity of needling reaction and the desired depth of needling.

3. Qi flow method

Qi flow method is a kind of manipulation in which the qi stimulated from the points below the elbow and knee arrives at the diseased part.

1) *Twirling and vibrating* After the qi arrives, slightly twirl and vibrate the needle to further induce the qi arrival. The successful qi flow rate was 90.81 percent in an experiment of 1,558 cases, and the rate of qi arriving at the diseased part is 56.4 percent.

2) *Pressing-needling* After the arrival of qi, the operator holds the needle towards the diseased part, and gives force to the handle. Meanwhile, percussion is applied along the course of the related meridian. In 516 cases under experiment, the successful qi flow rate is 99.68 percent, and the rate of qi arriving at the diseased part is 55.10 percent.

3) *Pressing-needling by the patient* After arrival of qi the patient holds the needle towards the diseased part. Under experiment using 304 patients, the successful qi flow rate is 89 percent, and the rate of qi arriving at the diseased part is 51.6 percent. This approach is only applicable to the points of the upper limbs. As to the lower limbs the pressing manipulation may be done by others.

4) *Aspects to be concerned*

a. Selection of needles: Needles of 1 to 1.5 cun are usually selected as the operative duration is longer. The needle should be straight with a smooth sharp tip.

b. The patient should lie down and the operator should be in a sitting position. The belt of the patient should be loose to allow the free flow of qi.

c. Ask the patient to close his eyes and regulate his breath, to relax and concentrate on the needling sensation. Answer the questions the operator asks. The environment should be quiet.

d. Arrival of qi: Twirling and vibrating follow the insertion of the needle to induce the arrival of qi. There are three kinds of arrival of qi (mild, moderate, and strong). The appropriate one is moderate. Strong arrival of qi is inappropriate. When a patient has a feeling of soreness, numbness and distension under the needle tip, and the operator doesn't feel tenseness around the needle tip, it is the mild arrival of qi. If a patient has obvious soreness, numbness and distension and the operator feels tenseness around the needle tip, it is the moderate arrival of qi. If a patient has an obvious soreness, numbness and distension, and tic presents around the point, the operator only has tenseness around the needle tip but found the contraction of the muscles in the vicinity, it is the strong arrival of qi.

e. Observation of the arrival of qi: After qi arrival it is necessary to observe the spread of the needling reaction. For example, when Hegu (LI 4) is punctured, the patient would have a painful feeling, or the needling sensation conducts to the index finger, thumb, palm or little finger. In this case the depth and direction of the needle inserted should be adjusted, until there is a sore, numb, distending, hot feeling under the needle tip, or when the needling sensation goes upward along the meridian, one should continue to twirl and vibrate the needle to conduct qi flow.

f. Activating qi flow: In this approach two things should be noted. One is the time of the presence of qi flow, usually in three to five minutes after stimulation. The other is that when qi cannot pass through the joints, first wait for a short time, and then press along the meridian to induce qi travel through the joints.

g. Duration of stimulation of qi flow: When the qi reaches the diseased part, stimulation ceases. If the qi fails to arrive at the diseased part or no qi flows at all, qi stimulation stops within fifteen to twenty minutes.

II. Case Analysis

Case 1: Rubella.

Name, Hou x x; sex, female; age, 11; date of the first visit, August 18, 1981.

Complaints General rubella presented for nearly three and half years. One evening in the spring of 1978 large patches of rubella appeared on the back. On that day she had had shrimps and done some exercises and was caught in wind after sweating. She went to see a doctor and after treatment the rubella was relieved but reoccurred constantly. The rubella, pale red in colour, spread to the whole body from the back. Each time when she ate Chinese chive, beef or lamb, fish or shrimp there presented large patches of rubella, which caused the mouth and lip to swell and abdominal pain. Tested for allergies, she was found to be allergic to fifteen kinds of foods, such as rice, millet, corn, and others. In the winter of 1980, she had loose stools. When she ate anything difficult to digest she felt unable to control her feces. About twenty doses of herbal extracts and thirty ampules of histamine were administered. There was no response to the drugs. Clinical examination showed yellow and pale complexion, thin body build, a pale tongue with a white coating and soft pulse.

Differentiation Interior and exterior deficiency syndrome, weak defensive qi due to exterior deficiency. Pathogenic cold and wind retained in the skin when they attacked the body. Failure of transportation of nutrients and water in the spleen and stomach was caused by interior deficiency. The Spleen Meridian of the Foot-Taiyin and Stomach Meridian of Foot-Yangming were affected.

Method Replenishing qi to strengthen superficial resistance, tonifying the spleen and stomach.

Prescription Group 1: Dazhui (Du 14), Dachangshu (B 25) and Weizhong (B 40).

Group 2: Tianshu (S 25), Zusanli (S 36) and Quchi (LI 11).

Treatment procedure Warm reinforcement was applied to the above points. After arrival of qi, mild soreness and distension was desirable. The two groups of points were alternately used and treatment was given every other day. Ten treatments constituted a course. No herbs were administered at the same time. After the first course of treatment rubella disappeared. After that the second course followed to strengthen the effect. Then the therapy ceased. Five months later (in the summer of 1982) there was no relapse.

Remarks Dazhui (Du 14) replenishes qi to strengthen superficial resistance. Dachangshu (B 25), Tianshu (S 25) and Zusanli (S 36) tonify the spleen and stomach. Quchi (LI 11) disperses the wind and cold. Weizhong (B 40) harmonizes the blood system when the defensive qi becomes strong and the spleen and stomach's function turns to normal. From this we can see that rubella is not caused by allergy, but by insufficient defensive qi and lowered function of the spleen and stomach.

Case 2: Toothache (Pulpitis)

Name, Feng x x; sex, female; age, 32; date of the first visit, September 16, 1975.

Complaints The patient complained of toothache on the left side for a month. The attack was induced by exposure to cold, hot or sour and sweet stuffs. Pain was aggravated at night. On the initiative stage acupuncture was applied to Xiaguan (S 7), Jiache (S 6) and Hegu (LI 4). Analgesic was administered with success. But in the previous two days intolerable pain occurred in the molar teeth. There was no response to analgesic. Physical examination showed yellow tongue coating, slippery and rapid pulse.

Differentiation Pathogenic wind and fire attacking the Gallbladder Meridian of Foot-Shaoyang.

Method Dispelling wind and fire from the Gallbladder Meridian of Foot-Shaoyang.

Prescription Hegu (LI 4), Jiache (S 6), Jianjing (G 21), Fubai (G 10), Wangu (G 12).

Treatment procedure Hegu (LI 4) was needled first for ten minutes, then Jiache (S 6) followed. The pain remained and tenderness was found at Jianjing (G 21), Wangu (G 12), Fubai (G 10), Tianchong (G 9) and Qubin (G 7), worse at the first two points. When left Jianjing (G 21) was needled for ten minutes, the toothache was relieved for a while. Then Fubai (G 10) and Wangu (G 12) were punctured and the toothache stopped. Another five treatments were given successively. Ten days later a follow-up study showed no relapse.

Remarks The toothache was due to pathological changes in the Large Intestine Meridian of Hand-Yangming caused by pathogenic wind and fire in the Gallbladder Meridian of Foot-Shaoyang. Hegu (LI 4) and Jiache (S 6) failed to respond to treatment. Clinical examination showed it was a Shaoyang syndrome and Fubai (G 10), Wangu (G 12) were effective in killing pain. This case shows that one should not only know the affected area, but also the diseased meridian.

Case 3: Mouth and eye awry

Name, Wang x x; sex, male; age, 74; date of the first visit, September 8, 1983; case No. 1486.

Complaints The patient complained of migraine on the right side nine years before while sleeping at night with the window open. Four and five days later mouth and eye awry occurred with no response to any treatment.

Physical examination showed a frequent tic in the right side of the face, aggravated on cloudy days. When he read, ate or faced the wind, the eyes teared. He often heard drum-beating sound in the ears. The philtrum bent to the right. There was often headache and the right side of the face was averse to cold. He had red tongue proper with white coating, floating and string-taut pulse. There was a tenderness at Yifeng (SJ 17).

Differentiation Retention of pathogenic cold and wind in the Stomach Meridian of Foot-Yangming and Sanjiao Meridian of Hand-Shaoyang.

Method Dispersing the pathogenic wind and cold to remove tic.

Prescription Sibai (S 2), Juliao (S 3), Dicang (S 4), Daying (S 5), Yifeng (SJ 17),

Wangu (G 12), Fengchi (G 20), Jiache (S 6), Zusanli (S 36), Zhongwan (Ren 12), Qihai (Ren 6), Waiguan (SJ 5), Hegu (LI 4) (selected alternately).

Treatment procedure First fire needling was applied to Sibai (S 2), Juliao (S 3), Dicang (S 4), Yifeng (SJ 17), Wangu (G 12) and Jiache (S 6), five to seven of which were employed each time to remove cold. Second, Zusanli (S 36), Zhongwan (Ren 12) and Qihai (Ren 6) were needled with the reinforcing method to strengthen the body resistance. Waiguan (SJ 5) and Hegu (LI 4) were selected alternately. When the induced qi conducted to the diseased part there would be a hot sensation in the face, then cold could be dispersed. Fire needling was given six times and in the second course three times were given, after which the frequency of the tic decreased by nearly half. But aversion to wind and cold on the face still remained. One of Wangu (G 12), Fengchi (G 20) and Yifeng (SJ 17) (of the diseased part) were used alone in the second course of treatment to dispel cold. Hegu (LI 4), Waiguan (SJ 5) (selected alternately) and Yanglao (SI 6) were used, and the induced qi was led to the diseased part. Sibai (S 2) and Yangbai (G 14) were selected to treat the eye trouble. After fourteen treatments the tic was greatly relieved. In the third course bloodletting was done in either Yifeng (SJ 17) or Wangu (G 12), then fresh crushed ginger was applied. Either Hegu (LI 4) or Waiguan (SJ 5) was needled each time. Sibai (S 2) and Juliao (S 3) on the diseased side and Zusanli (S 36) on both sides were used with the reinforcing method. After five treatments tenderness was no longer found at Yifeng (SJ 17) and ear ringing disappeared. After thirteen treatments tic was nearly controlled. When tenderness at Yifeng (SJ 17) was gone, there was a tenderness at Juliao (S 3). Wangu (G 12) and both Zusanli (S 36) were needled with the reinforcing method and the qi at Lieque (L 7) was conducted to the diseased site. Juliao (S 3) was pricked and applied with fresh crushed ginger. This time the tic was removed, then the acupuncture therapy was ended. In total 44 treatments were given for this case. A follow-up in December 1985 showed no relapse except the occasional onset of a tic.

Remarks It was a protracted condition lasting for nine years. There had been no response to any treatment because of persisting pathogenic cold in the body, which brought about the symptoms described above. The warming method was employed to dispel cold and alleviate the suffering.

Case 4: Dizziness (insufficient supply of blood in the vertebral arteria basilaris)

Name, Wang x x; sex, male; age, 63; date of the first visit, April 13, 1985; case No. 18451.

Complaints Eight days before he suddenly had dizziness, nausea, and vomited once, and the blood pressure was 180/110 mm Hg. Two days ago there was severe dizziness, blurred vision, incoherent speech, weak lower limbs, thirst without desire to drink and dry stools. He took Bezoar Resurrection Bolus by himself. Then he was hospitalized as an emergency case. He said he had had hypertension for more than twenty years and coronary heart disease for about ten years. Physical examination showed flushed face, obesity, yellow, thick-coated tongue, lack of saliva, string-taut and slippery pulse, blood pressure 150/110 mm Hg. Babinski's sign (+), right finger to nose test (+), horizontal flickering of eyeballs.

Differentiation Preponderance of fire turned from liver yang, upward invasion of pathogenic wind and fire.

Prescription Baihui (Du 20), Hand 12-Jing-(Well) (Extra) and Taiyang (Extra 2).

Treatment procedure Bloodletting was applied to Baihui (Du 20) and Hand-12-Jing-(Well). A day later dizziness was relieved markedly and he slept soundly. On the second day he was found to have yellow dry coating, string-taut and slippery pulse. Blood pressure was 170/110 mm Hg. Taiyang (Extra 2) and Hand Shixuan (Extra 30) were pricked and then blood pressure lowered to 150/100 mm Hg. *Powder of Rhubarb and Glycyrrhizae* uralensis Fisch, Dried Glauber's Salt (10 g each) were given twice a day. He was able to move the bowels, which suggested the fu-organ obstruction had been removed. The above treatment controlled the acute condition. Then from April 18, the method of subduing exuberance of yang in the liver, invigorating the blood circulation and nourishing yin were adopted. In one month's time all the symptoms disappeared.

Remarks Bloodletting of the Jing-(Well) (Extra) and Shixuan (Extra 30) had a marked effect on the severe type of wind-stroke, i.e. the zang-fu organs and meridians being attacked. From February to June, 1985, fifty-one cases were admitted to the acupuncture wards of our hospital. Among them thirty-one cases were treated with this procedure and the acute condition was controlled in two or three days, the maximum being seven days. But the procedure was only suitable to the excess syndrome.

Case 5: Lumbago (prolapse of uterus)

Name, Hao x x; sex, female; age, 46; date of the first visit, September 4, 1975.

Complaints The patient had suffered low back pain for years, more severe on the right side. Marked pain occurred on standing and movement. The pain prevented her from lying flat. Other symptoms included poor appetite, dizziness, dream-disturbed sleep, fidgets, pale red tongue with dry coating. Acupuncture had been applied to Kunlun (B 60) and Houxi (SI 3) without success. Then she told the doctor that she had a prolapsed uterus (II) for three years and there was a bearing-down sensation in the lower abdomen.

Differentiation Hypofunction of the spleen and kidney and sinking of qi.

Method Tonifying the kidney and spleen to strengthen qi.

Prescription Guanyuan (Ren 4), Zigong (Extra 19), Sanyinjiao (Sp 6) and Qugu (Ren 2).

Treatment procedure The needles were inserted into Guanyuan (Ren 4) and Zigong (Ren 19) towards Qugu (Ren 2). After arrival of qi the patient felt an upward contraction of the uterus. The reinforcing method was applied to Sanyinjiao (Sp 6). One treatment alleviated the pain. The above points and Qugu (Ren 2) were used to lift the uterus to its normal position. Six treatments cured the prolapse of the uterus and alleviated the low back pain.

TECHNIQUE OF SUPERFICIAL INSERTION WITH FREQUENT ROTATION

—Ma Shiming's Clinical Experience

Ma Shiming, male, born in 1918 in Hangzhou, and a native of Wuxi, Jiangsu Province, was apprenticed to his uncle to learn traditional Chinese medicine (TCM) when he was twelve. He entered the Zhejiang Special School of Traditional Chinese Medicine at the age of fourteen. Two years later, he was transferred to Shanghai New China Medical College. After graduation he started his own private medical practice in Shanghai in the same year. He then entered the Tokyo Acupuncture School in Japan and stayed there for two years. In 1937, he came back and has practised in Wuxi, Shanghai and Hangzhou since then. He worked in the Central Clinic of Hangzhou from 1953 to 1956. From 1956, he worked in Hangzhou United Hospital of Traditional Chinese Medicine (now the Municipal Traditional Chinese Medicine Hospital in Hangzhou). Dr. Ma has much experience in the treatment of the sequela of encephalitis, infantile poliomyelitis, facial paralysis, enuresis, infantile diarrhoea and dysmenorrhea. He has published some academic papers, such as *On the Techniques of Superficial Insertion with Frequent Rotation*. Now he is an associate professor in the Acupuncture Department of Hangzhou Municipal Hospital of Traditional Chinese Medicine.

I. Academic Characteristics and Medical Specialities

1. Technique of superficial insertion with frequent rotation

Handed down in his family for generations, Ma has been applying this technique successfully in clinical treatment for many years.

A 1 to 1.5 cun-long needle is inserted into the skin helped with the finger pressure and rotated to 0.2 to 0.3 cun deep, and then rotated rapidly ten times. The rapid rotation of the needle with proper pressure is required until the patient feels the needling sensation at the local area. As *The Internal Classic* says: "When qi comes, keep it well with great care." The methods of either reducing or reinforcing can be applied according to the disease following the principles of reinforcement in the case of deficiency and reduction in the case of excess. The needles may be withdrawn after the methods of dredging the meridians and activating the qi and blood circulation are manipulated. Since the needle is inserted only 0.2 to 0.3 cun deep, even at the facial area or the area around the eye, the needle can still be manipulated with rapid rotation. Dr. Ma thinks that the therapeutic effect of acupuncture is achieved by qi arrival, qi promotion, and regulating the mental spirit. Yang Jizhou (1522-1620) of the Ming Dynasty said that, "the onset of all kinds of diseases always happens in Rongwei layers, then further attack either the skin, muscle, tendons or vessels. Once acupuncture is given, usually Rongwei layers are needled with either the reinforcing or the reducing method, and the disease of skin, muscle, tendons or vessels would be removed. So needles should go neither too shallow nor deep though sometimes the diseases are of different depth." This quotation is taken as the guiding principle by Dr. Ma for his technique of superficial insertion with high frequent rotation. Clinically he manipulates needles by puncturing shallowly and undertakes the reinforcing or the reducing method. For example, a patient during an asthma attack might have the symptoms of shortness of breath and difficulty lying down. For treatment, needling both chest points and back points is not suitable. Dr. Ma would select only one point, Suliao (Du 25), to be needled about 0.2 to 0.3 cun deep with rapid rotation, the patient at the same time felt soreness. Thus the qi of the lung is dispersed and the symptoms of heaviness of the chest and shortness of breath stopped immediately.

The records of the technique of superficial insertion date back to the days when *Miraculous Pivot* was written. The techniques of skin puncture, extremely shallow puncture, perpendicular puncture and superficial puncture noted in the *Miraculous Pivot* are all included in today's superficial insertion. Cutaneous needle acupuncture, wrist-ankle acupuncture or scalp acupuncture are also a development of superficial insertion. Physically, the corresponding superficial areas of the body reflected by the functional activities of the twelve regular meridians are the places where the qi of the meridians is distributed, so the acupuncture treatment must be carefully administered and follow the essential principles of needling. Dr. Ma has developed this traditional technique of superficial insertion by combining shallow puncture with high frequent rotation. The main characteristics are gentle and even with rapid rotation in a small application. Generally a one-cun needle, No. 32, is used. Even for needling Huantiao (G 30), Dr. Ma still uses a short needle about 1.5 cun at most to make the needling sensation radiate down to the foot. In this way the therapeutic effect seems higher than using a long needle to cause an electric shock-like sensation down to the heel from this point. Clinically, he often uses this technique in the treatment of facial paralysis, sequela of windstroke, dermatopruritus; infantile enuresis, infantile diarrhoea, infantile poilia, sequela of encephalitis or gynecological and obstetrical disorders. During treatment he selects the different points by following the course of the meridians which are involved in the disease with either the reinforcing or reducing method according to the pathological condition.

II. Case Analysis

Case 1: Infantile poliomyelitis

Name, Jin x x; sex, male; age, 4.

Complaints Two months before he had chills, fever, headache, nausea, vomiting and restlessness for one week; then followed by paralysis of the right leg with difficulty in standing and motor impairment. Examination showed a decrease of muscle tension, disappearance of tendon reflex and muscular atrophy; skin temperature of the diseased leg was lower than that of the healthy side and there was weakness of the lower back in a sitting posture. The patient was diagnosed as sequelar of poliomyelitis in the Children's Hospital. Before he came to see Dr. Ma the child had been treated with acupuncture in some other hospitals many times, but little result was obtained.

Prescription Shenshu (B 23), Zhibian (B 54), Baohuang (B 53), Huantiao (G 30), Chengfu (B 36), Biguan (S 31), Fengshi (G 31), Futu (S 32), Jiexi (S 41), Qiuxu (G 40), Zhongfeng (Liv 4), Taichong (Liv 3), Neiting (S 44), Bafeng (Extra), Yongquan (K 1), Inner-Neiting (Extra) and Zusanli (S 36).

Treatment procedure He was treated once a day by selecting six to seven points from the above prescription. The superficial insertion was used for all the selected points with high frequency of rotation. One week after the treatment the patient felt some needling sensation, and he continued to receive both acupuncture and massage treatment for about two months. After that the patient could flex and extend his diseased leg, but still could not walk normally. After four months of treatment, his symptoms disappeared completely.

Explanation Dr. Ma always uses the technique of superficial insertion with frequent rotation in the treatment of infantile poliomyelitis, and good result can be obtained through the regulation of qi and activating the blood circulation and muscles and promoting the meridians. But he prefers to give acupuncture treatment as early as possible after the onset of the disease. During the treatment, the patient should do some exercises such as massaging the diseased limbs, or flexing, stretching and abduction movement. At the same time, supply more nutrients to the patient, for instance, bone soup, fish liver and cow milk, in order to strengthen the body's antipathogenic factors.

Case 2: Facial paralysis

Name, Jin x x; sex, male; age, 59.

Complaints The patient suddenly noticed a numb sensation on the right side of the face when he got up in the morning. A week later, he came to the hospital. An examination showed a disappearance of the right forehead crease, an inability to frown, unclear speech, a twisted mouth, shallow nasolabia groove, slight swelling of the face, a twisted tongue, salivation, dropping fluid when drinking, auricular pain on the affected side, irritability, foul smell and constipation.

Prescription On the affected side: Yangbai (G 14), Taiyang (Extra), Touwei (S 8), Yintang (Extra), Zanzhu (B 2), Yuyao (Extra), Sizhukong (SJ 23), Jingming (B 1), Sibai (S 2), Xiaguan (S 7), Jiache (S 6), Daying (S 5), Yingxiang (LI 20), Heliao (LI 19), Dicang (S 4), Chengjiang (Ren 24), Jiachengjiang (Extra), Jinjin, Yuye (Extra), Fengchi (G 20), Yifeng (SJ 17), Baihui (Du 20), Renzhong (Du 26) and Hegu (LI 4). Hegu (LI 4) and 7-8 points from the above prescription are selected for each treatment with moderate stimulation and even movement.

Treatment procedure Dr. Ma applied the superficial insertion technique with high frequency of rotation. Treatment was given daily and after seven treatments all the symptoms improved, but the patient still could not close the eye completely and was unable to frown. After fifteen treatments, the symptoms became much better. The patient completely recovered after twenty-five treatments.

Explanation Acupuncture therapy has very good therapeutic effect in the treatment of peripheral facial paralysis. If the clinical result is not so effective after two weeks treatment, we can suggest the patient take some Powder for Treating Wry-mouths, composed by the prepared giant typhonium tuber, scorpion, earthworm, and arisaema with bile. The daily dosage varies according to the individual condition. During treatment, the patient is advised not to take strongly acidic, hot food, pungent food or drink alcohol. The patient is also asked to sleep more, speak and read less, be careful to avoid exposure to wind and cold, and should put on masks over the face in case of going out on cold days. Dr. Ma prefers to give acupuncture treatment as early as possible after the onset of the disease; otherwise, when there appears the sequela, acupuncture treatment is usually of little help. For some cases, delayed treatment may cause a life-long problem.

APPLICATION OF QI CONDUCTING AND MERIDIAN REGULATING MANIPULATION

—Ma Ruilin's Clinical Experience

Ma Ruilin, a native of Beizhen County, Liaoning Province, was born in 1922. Influenced by his uncle Ma Yudian, a famous veteran TCM doctor, and his cousin Ma Zuoquan, he became interested in traditional Chinese medicine when he was young, then he began to learn medicine from Wang Huimin, a famous local TCM doctor. He started his private clinic in 1941, and attended the advanced TCM training course for teachers affiliated with the Ministry of Public Health in 1952. He followed his studies with Yue Meizhong, Gao Fengtong and Sun Huiqing respectively from 1955 to 1958. He started teaching at the Liaoning College of Traditional Chinese Medicine in 1958. Dr. Ma advocates that doctors should be good at conducting qi under the needle to achieve the treatment's purpose by regulating the flow of the meridian qi. His works include *Acupuncture and Moxibustion, The Plum-Blossom Needle Therapy,* and *Brief Account on Treatment of Deafness and Muteness.* He has also published more than twenty academic papers. Now, he is the standing member of Liaoning Association of Traditional Chinese Medicine, the standing member of China Acupuncture Society, and the president of Liaoning Acupuncture Society.

I. Academic Characteristics and Medical Specialities

1. Conducting qi and regulating meridians—the key points for acupuncture

Conducting qi is to keep the free flow of the meridian qi in order to regulate and restore the normal physiological functions. During treatment, the needling sensation should be controlled by rotating, lifting and thrusting, and vibrating in combination with massage along the meridians, or against the meridians or pressing along the meridians, which are used independently or in combination. In addition, the accurate selection of acupoints with indefinite depth is significant for qi arrival.

1) *Migraine* This is mostly due to accumulation of the pathogenic heat in the Shaoyang Meridian, going upward to attack the head. The remote points are mainly selected from the Shaoyang Meridian. Needle Zhigou (SJ 6) of Hand-Shaoyang first, if the pain can not be checked immediately, Guangming (G 37), and Zulinqi (G 4) are added. In severe cases, in addition to the above points, Fengchi (G 20) can be combined to promote the flow of local meridian qi. The reducing method with lifting, thrusting and rotating are used in combination with the auxiliary manipulations such as massage along or against the meridian, or pressing along the meridian.

2) *Nephroptosis* The frequently used points are Shenshu (B 23), Qihaishu (B 24) and Sanyinjiao (Sp 6) with lifting, thrusting and rotating manipulation. Needle Shenshu

(B 23) and Qihaishu (B 24) obliquely with the needle 69° to 70° directed to the vertebrae until the needling sensation appears. Needling Sanyinjiao (Sp 6) should radiate the needling sensation along the meridian to the heart. Since the nephroptosis is mostly due to deficiency of Kidney Yang, Shenshu (B 23) and Qihaishu (B 24) may tonify the kidney and reinforce qi and Sanyinjiao (Sp 6) is able to activate the meridian qi to restore the organic functions.

3) *Tinnitus and deafness* Tinggong (SI 19), Tinghui (G 2) and Yifeng (SJ 17) are selected as the main points, in combination with Zhongzhu (SJ 3) or Zuqiaoyin (G 44) or Taixi (K 3) in case of kidney deficiency. The three main points may be needled 0.8 to 1.5 cun deep to keep the needling sensation radiating to antrum auris. The remote points Zhongzhu (SJ 3) and Zuqiaoyin (G 44) are manipulated based on the appearance of the needling sensation travelling along the meridian to the heart.

4) *Hairline boils* This is an excess syndrome due to damp and heat. The treatment should reduce the heat, activate the blood circulation, remove the stagnation and dispel wind. Dazhui (Du 14), Fengchi (G 20), Quchi (LI 11) and Hegu (LI 4) are selected as the main points, in combination with surrounding puncture on the affected area. Dazhui (Du 14) is perpendicularly needled 0.5 to 1.0 cun deep, Fengchi (G 20) is punctured 1.0 to 1.5 cun deep towards the opposite canthus, Quchi (LI 11) and Hegu (LI 4) are perpendicularly needled. The surrounding puncture is performed 1 cm around the boils. Reducing is applied, retaining the needle for twenty to thirty minutes. The success rate was 100 percent.

2. Treatment of hiccup by regulating the stomach and qi flow

The depth of insertion is based on the individual and the nature of the disease. Different depths of insertion on the same point may achieve the same curative effect. The disease may be cured if acupuncture is able to free the meridians, promote the circulation of qi and blood, and regulate yin and yang. Therefore, the depth of insertion is not the most important in acupuncture treatment.

Case examples: 1) In the spring of 1983, Dr. Ma was invited to treat a patient who had sudden hiccups, difficulty in swallowing food and insomnia after his coronary heart disease was treated. The examination showed: Clear mind, flushed complexion, pale red tongue with white and slightly brown coating, string-taut forceful pulse. The case resulted from anger after eating. Neiting (S 44) was needled with rotating method. As soon as the needling sensation reached the abdomen, the hiccups stopped immediately. 2) On March 5, 1983, a male patient with hiccups for one month came for treatment. Hiccups came during the day, and were relieved after sleep. The examination showed: clear mind, sallow complexion, normal speech, free of odor, a purplish red tongue with scanty white coating, liver pulse string-taut, stomach pulse weak. Differentiation: Dysfunction of the stomach in descending, perversion of qi due to deficiency. Zhongwan (Ren 12) and Taichong (Liv 3) were needled with manipulation of qi conducting and meridian regulating, the hiccup stopped immediately. 3) A male patient aged sixty-eight suffered from paralysis due to cerebral hemorrage for eight years. The examination showed: Mental confusion, slightly red complexion, aphasia, continuous belching, red tongue proper with slight yellow coating, superficial and full pulse. Differentiation: Deficiency of stomach yin, and retention of heat in the stomach leading to dysfunction of the stomach in descending. Zusanli (S 36) was perpendicularly needled 1.5 cun deep with thrusting and rotating manipulation. Two treatments cured the case. Among these three cases, one was treated with shallow insertion on the local point, one with shallow insertion on a distal point, the third with deep insertion on the distal point. The locations of the points and the depth of insertion are different, but the effects were the same, because the stomach and qi were both regulated.

3. Clinical experience in point selection

For inflammation, swelling and pain due to trauma or closed fracture, Dr. Ma has two combining methods of the points.

1) *Selecting the point from the two points* First, try to find out the most sensitive point by pressing the affected area. Second, find out the most sensitive point when the affected limb is in active or passive movement. Reducing is applied by lifting, thrusting and rotating after the needling sensation is obtained. Retain the needles for twenty minutes. For instance, a male patient aged thirty-six was unable to flex, stretch and lift his right arm. His shoulder joints could only move when the body moved. After the first treatment based on the method mentioned above, the motor ability of the arm was restored with flexion of 40°-50°, stretching of 15°-20° and abduction of 15°-20°. He was treated seven times in all, and restored to normal.

2) *Selecting the point from one end* This is used for the patients with closed fracture of the limbs with local feverish sensation, swelling and distension. Select the points on the meridians 20 to 30 cm away from the paracentral end of the swelling and distension. If the swelling and distension are located on the three Yin Meridians, points are selected from the yin meridians; if they are on the three Yang Meridians, select the points from the yang meridians. But if the swelling and distension occur on the whole area of the fracture, select the points from all the Yin and Yang Meridians. Reducing is applied after the appearance of needling sensation, and retain the needles for twenty minutes. Dr. Ma once treated a male patient with a fracture of the right tibia with swelling, distension and pain on the affected area, the affected leg 4.5 cm thicker than the healthy one. The body temperature 38° to 40°C, white blood cells 18900/m^3, neutrality 89. After retaining the needles for thirty minutes, the body temperature was reduced to 36.5°C, and the white blood cells to 8800/m^3, and the neutrality was 81.

II. Case Analysis

Case 1: Gastroptosis

Name, Tian x x; sex, male; age, 45; case No. 1396.

Complaints Stomach pain for seven years, accompanied by borborygmus, constipation, loss of appetite, thin body, absence of thirst, normal sleep. The examination showed:

Sallow complexion, emaciation, red tongue proper, white coating, retarded pulse, soft and flat abdomen without obvious tenderness, but with intestinal gurgling. Barium meal examination: The lowest part of the stomach 10 cm below the intercristal line. Differentiation: Deficiency of the spleen qi, deficiency of the spleen and stomach yang. Principle of treatment: Reinforce the stomach qi and strengthen the spleen.

Prescription Zusanli (S 36), Zhongwan (Ren 12), Gongsun (Sp 4) and Tianshu (S 25).

Treatment procedure Perpendicular insertion was used at Zhongwan (Ren 12) 0.8 to 1.2 cun deep, Zusanli (S 36), 0.1 to 1.5 cun deep, Gongsun (Sp 4) Tianshu (S 25), 0.8 to 1.2 cun deep with reinforcing method. When the qi conducting and meridian regulating manipulation used at Zusanli (S 36), the patient felt the numbness going upward along the lateral aspect of the leg to the epigastric region, and then the abdominal vibration could be found. The symptoms were greatly improved after acupuncture. After seven treatments the barium examination showed the stomach 6 cm above the original place.

Explanation Gastroptosis is mainly due to constitutional weakness, deficiency of the spleen and stomach qi, failing to support the stomach. Treatment is given to reinforce qi of the middle jiao and regulate the spleen and stomach. Zusanli (S 36) is an important point of the Foot Yangming Meridian for gastric disorder, Zhongwan (Ren 12) is the Front-Mu point of the stomach, where the qi is infused, Gongsun (Sp 4) can strengthen the spleen and Tianshu (S 25) is the Front-Mu point of the Large Intestine Meridian.

Case 2: Facial pain (trigeminal neuralgia)

Name, Liu x x; sex, male; age, 55; date of the first visit, March 25, 1983.

Complaints The patient suffered from paroxysmal facial pain on the right side for three months, ten to twenty times a day. In severe attacks, cutting pain appeared. He was diagnosed in a hospital as having trigeminal neuralgia, but the hospital failed in the treatment. The examination showed: Suffering appearance with sallow complexion, red tongue proper with yellow coating, string-taut rapid pulse. Differentiation: Heat of the three yang meridians attacking the head and stagnation of the meridian qi, leading to unbearable pain. Principle of treatment: Reduce heat and eliminate the depression.

Prescription Neiting (S 44).

Treatment procedure Oblique insertion at the angle of 45° was applied, 0.5 to 0.8 cun deep with rotating manipulation. During the manipulation of qi conducting and meridian regulating, the patient felt the cool sensation going upward along the lateral aspect to the abdomen, stomach and cheek, then he felt coolness in the mouth, and pain was relieved immediately. After three treatments, the condition was greatly improved. He had mild attacks two or three times only a day. He was cured after seven treatments.

Explanation Facial pain is due to excess heat in the Stomach Meridian, which goes upward to the face and the head. Excessive stomach fire with obstruction of the qi causes pain. In this case, reduce fire and activate the meridian qi in combination with the corresponding manipulations.

Case 3: Anoxic encephalopathy

Name, Chen x x; sex, female; age, 2; date of the first visit, August, 1976.

Complaints On July 28, 1976, the patient had convulsions, stiff neck, blindness, deafness and facial paralysis. Examination: Dull sight, retarded light reaction, foaming mouth, clear respiratory sound without rale, weak arms failing to hold objects, inability to sit, flaccid paralysed, deafness, blindness, hemochrome 10.4 g, white blood cell 12900/mm^3, lobocyte 62 percent, lymph 30 percent, acidophilia 8 percent, and potassium 1.16 mg equivalent/liter.

Differentiation Obstruction of the meridians due to deficiency of yang qi. Principle of treatment: Activate the flow of the meridian qi and induce resuscitation.

Prescription Dazhui (Du 14), Fengchi (G 20), Yamen (Du 15), Tinghui (G 2), Neiguan (S 44), Hegu (LI 4), Guangming (G 37) and Juegu (G 39).

Treatment procedure After ten treatments, the vision and hearing ability were somewhat improved, and after twenty treatments, the movement of the upper limbs improved, and after twenty-eight treatments, speech was restored, and she could see 10 to 20 cm. After forty treatments, hearing, eyesight and speech were completely restored.

Explanation The sudden attack of deafness and blindness is caused by trauma, which gives rise to obstruction of the meridian qi to stop qi and blood from going upward to the head. Acupuncture may dredge the meridians, promote qi and blood circulation, and regulate yin and yang. Dazhui (Du 14) and Yamen (Du 15), the points of the Du Meridian, are able to activate yang qi and dredge the meridians. Guangming (G 37) is an important point for eye problems. Juegu (G 39), one of the Eight Influential Points, is able to treat flaccid limbs. Scalp acupuncture is added to clear the mind and improve the hearing.

DEEP INSERTION OF ZHONGWAN (REN 12), HEAVY MOXIBUSTION AT GUANYUAN (REN 4), BLOODLETTING AT WEIZHONG (B 40), AND VENOUS CUPPING THERAPIES

—Wang Fengyi's Clinical Experience

Wang Fengyi, a native of Ninghe County, Hebei Province, was born in 1925. When he was very young, he acknowledged Ji Tianshu and Zhao Shijin, the two well-known TCM doctors in Heilongjiang as his teachers. After graduation, he started his teaching work in the Teaching and Researching Group of Traditional Chinese Medicine of the First Department of Medical Therapy in Harbin Medical University. Having practised for more than thirty years, he has studied acupuncture, moxibustion, cupping and selection of the points according to "Zi Wu Liu Zhu" noted in *Internal Classic.* He has published twenty-five papers and nine works. He is now the director of the Acupuncture Department of the First Affiliated Hospital to Harbin Medical University, deputy chief physician, the standing member and secretary-general of Heilongjiang Society of Acupuncture and Moxibustion.

I. Academic Characteristics and Medical Specialities

1. Deep insertion of Zhongwan (Ren 12)

This method is selected according to the patient's constitution, body build, age, and the pathological condition. For adults, the depth is about 4 to 5 cun (proportional measurement), with the needle slowly inserted along with respiration, by which the needle penetrates the abdominal wall to peritoneum, then to the anterior gastric wall with the needle tip touching the posterior gastric wall. Apply reinforcing for deficiency and reducing for excess. It is often used in clinic for acute and chronic gastritis, gastric spasm, gastriptosis, and volvulus of stomach with immediate effect. For instance, a patient with acute gastritis accompanied by severe abdominal pain and vomiting was treated by deep insertion of Zhongwan (Ren 12) with reducing method. Abdominal pain and vomiting stopped immediately after treatment. (It is dangerous to puncture deep at Zhongwan (Ren 12), so it is advised that beginners should be careful with this point.)

2. Heavy moxibustion at Guanyuan (Ren 4)

Dr. Wang regards Guanyuan (Ren 4) as the storehouse of the essence for men and blood for women, and the reservoir of the primary qi. Moxibustion can warm Dantian and strengthen the Kidney Yang, nourish the kidney to benefit the essence and marrow. It is frequently employed to treat impotence, anuresis, amenorrhea and wei syndrome. For instance, a patient, who had been married for six months and who was impotent, was treated successfully by moxibustion at Guanyuan (Ren 4) three times with 150 cones each time. The next year, he had a son. Another patient was paralysed in the lower limbs and he was incontinent for a month. He was first treated with acupuncture on points from Yangming Meridian but this failed, and then he was treated by moxibustion at Guanyuan (Ren 4) once every ten days, with a hundred cones each time. After three treatments he was cured.

3. Bloodletting at Weizhong (B 40)

The patient is asked to stand with both Weizhong (B 40) points exposed for sterilization. Prick the veins at Weizhong (B 40) for bleeding. It is often used for acute lumbar sprain, acute vomiting and diarrhoea, lumbago, leg pain and multiple furuncle and swelling. For instance, a male patient sprained his back when doing physical labour, the pain was so severe that he could not lie on his back and his breathing was limited. Bleeding at Weizhong (B 40) for 2 ml of blood, and immediately relieved the pain, and his motility was restored. Another male patient was diagnosed as having febrile vomiting and diarrhoea (acute gastroenteritis). All the symptoms were checked after bleeding at Weizhong (B 40).

4. Venous cupping

Dr. Wang holds that many diseases are related to blood heat and stagnation. Venous cupping can remove the blood stagnation, and activate the blood circulation, dispel the pathogenic factors and smooth the meridians. Therefore, it is often used in the clinic to treat inflammations, high fevers and pain syndrome. For instance, a patient with flu had high fever, headache and general lassitude, had venous cupping at Dazhui (Du 14), Feishu (B 13), and Xinshu (B 15). He felt relieved and all the symptoms disappeared. Another female patient aged forty-four had fever for two days, accompanied by abdominal pain, diarrhoea with pus and bloody stools, ten times a day and thirst without the desire to drink. Microscopy: bacillary dysentery. She was treated twice with venous cupping at Dazhui (Du 14), Pishu (B 20), and Dachangshu (B 25), and recovered completely. Microscopy: stools (-). Another male patient fifty-eight years old suffered from angina pectoris and coronary heart disease. He suddenly felt precordial pressing pain with shortness of breath. The pain was gradually relieved after one treatment by venous cupping at Shenzhu (B 23), Xinshu (B 15) and Jueyinshu (B 14).

II. Case Analysis

Case 1: Diabetes insipidus
Name, An x x; sex, male; age, 25; case No. 54.

Complaints The patient had excessive thirst and urination, accompanied by nocturnal emission, general lassitude, listlessness, insomnia, dizziness and headache. The examination showed: Emaciation, malnutrition, a red tongue with a thin yellow coating, deep and retarded pulse. Differentiation: General deficiency of yin, damaged by emotional factors and overstrain, consumption of kidney yin leading to deficient-fire steaming the lung and stomach, fire, with lack of water, getting fierce and water, with strong fire, getting drained, thus excessive drinking and excessive urination occur. Principle of treatment: Nourish yin and reinforce the kidney.

Prescription 1. Guanyuan (Ren 4), Sanyinjiao (Sp 6); 2. Shenshu (B 23), Sanjiaoshu (B 22); and 3. Neiguan (P 6), Taixi (K 3).

Treatment procedure Apply reinforcing method with filiform needles on all the above mentioned points. Retain the needles for thirty minutes. The three groups of points are used alternately. Treat once a day. Ten treatments constitute a course. Rest for one week between the courses. After the third course of treatment, the general symptoms disappeared, the amount of drinking and urination became normal.

Case 2: Chronic nephritis

Name, Wang x x; sex, male; age, 13.

Complaints The patient started coughing four months before, associated with palpebral edema and scanty urine, which was diagnosed in a hospital as nephritis. After being treated for two weeks, edema disappeared, but attacked again one week later, starting from the eyelids to the whole body, scanty urine in dark yellow colour, for the last two weeks, edema became aggravated and patient was mentally confused. He was further diagnosed as having chronic nephritis and psendouremia. Examination: General severe edema, irritability, mental confusion, incoherent speech, short breath, tongue with sticky yellow coating, dry and lustrous skin, subcutaneous cracks and capillary congestion, the heart sounds not clear, severe edema on head and nape, the marked depression of the limbs on pressure, marked edema on abdomen with shifting dullness, liver and spleen not felt, severe edema of testis, nervous system positive, deep thready and rapid pulse, red blood cell 3690,000/mm^3, urinary albumin (+++), specific gravity 1.05, red cell 1 to 2, white cell 5 to 6, epithelial cell 3 to 4, non-protein nitrogen 33.3 mg percent, plasma protein 2.79 percent.

Differentiation Cough with shortness of breath at the very beginning is due to an attack on the lung by pathogenic wind, causing dysfunction and dispersing of lung qi. Scanty urine and edema are due to dysfunction of the lung qi failing to regulate the water passage and send the water down to the urinary bladder. The wind is yang and characterized by upward movement, thus edema started from the eyelids. Long-standing accumulation of water and dampness is transformed into fire, and burn the humour into phlegm, the internal disturbance of phlegm-fire mists the clear yang, leading to mental confusion, irritability and incoherent speech. Flabby tongue with yellow coating, deep and rapid pulse are the signs showing accumulation of water and dampness turning into heat. Principle of treatment: Induce the resuscitation, reduce heat and eliminate water.

Prescription Renzhong (Du 26), Yongquan (K 1), Shixuan (Extra).

Treatment procedure Reducing is applied at Renzhong (Du 26), Yongquan (K 1) with lifting-thrusting and rotation. Prick Shixuan (Extra) with a three-edged needle to bleeding. After treatment, the patient felt clearer mentally, and urine increased. For the second visit, reduce Daling (P 7), and reinforce Taixi (K 3). For the third visit, reinforce Shenshu (B 23) and Sanyinjiao (Sp 6) with lifting, thrusting and rotating. For the fourth visit, reduce Shuifen (Ren 9) and Neiguan (P 6), and reinforce Yinlingquan (Sp 9). After that, urine was greatly increased. For the fifth visit, reduce Quchi (LI 4) and Zusanli (S 36). General edema disappeared and mental clearness was restored to normal after one week of treatment. After another two weeks of treatment to consolidate the effect, routine urine examination was also restored to normal. The follow-up visit for seven years showed no relapse.

Explanation Renzhong (Du 26) and Shixuan (Extra) function to restore the mental clearness. Renzhong (Du 26) is able to promote resuscitation, while Yongquan (Sp 9) is able to restore the mind, and reinforce the kidney to promote urination. The combination of the three points will double the effects.

TREATMENT OF SCROFULA, WINDSTROKE AND PARAPLEGIA

—Wang Leting's Clinical Experience

Wang Leting (1896-1984), born in Xianghe County, Hebei Province, was enthusiastic about acupuncture since his childhood, and was apprenticed to a well-known acupuncturist, Chen Suqing. He had undertaken clinical acupuncture treatment for more than fifty years. Since 1929, in clinic, he advocated, treating radically, the stomach is the base, in treating paralysis, take Du Meridian first, and regulating qi first in case of affection by wind, qi circulates then the wind will be gone. Shu points of the five zang organs used in combination with Geshu, Wang's Jiaji prescription, Du Meridian thirteen needles prescription, and old ten points prescription were his experienced prescriptions and his exploration in the treatment of windstroke, traumatic paraplegia and gastro-intestinal diseases. He was a professor and chief of the Acupuncture Department of Beijing Municipal Hospital of Traditional Chinese Medicine.

I. Academic Characteristics and Clinical Specialities

1. Point penetration with a golden needle in the treatment of scrofula

Scrofula refers to tuberculosis of the cervical lymph nodes, which mostly occurs in childhood, and adolescence, and is frequently seen over the neck, thoracic wall, supraclavicular fossa, axillary fossa and groin, but in clinic, mostly found at the neck and axillary fossa. It has a long chronic course, and pus flows out on rupture, and is hard to cure it. The disease is mainly due to stagnation of liver qi, accumulation of phlegm, coagulation of phlegm-fire or due to yin deficiency resulting in deficiency of lungs and kidneys, and of deficiency-fire burning inside. Dr. Wang accorded that the region below the neck and subclavicle is the place where the Large Intestine Meridian of Hand-Yangming and Gallbladder Meridian of Foot-Shaoyang pass. Good results were obtained by penetrating Quchi (LI 11) towards Binao (LI 14) with a six-inch gold needle in treating scrofula. According to Dr. Wang's experience for many decades and in treatment of several hundred cases, a six-inch golden needle is not only effective for cervical lymph node tuberculosis, but also effective for tuberculosis on the axillary, supraclavicular fossa and grain. In light of Wang's experience, one needle penetrating three points functions to treat scrofula—Quchi (LI 11), Wuli (LI 13) and Binao (LI 14) are the points of Hand Yangming Meridian, which originates from the radial aspect of the index finger and travels along the external aspect of the upper limb through the shoulder, scapular, neck to the side of the nose. According to the principle—the region where the meridian passes is the place of indications—needling of the region is able to facilitate the circulation of qi and blood in the obstructed meridians, and to dissipate the masses. In addition, Hand-Yangming and Hand-Taiyin are externally and internally related, needling of Hand-Yangming is therefore able to regulate indirectly qi of the lung, which dominates qi, distributes essence, and faces all the blood vessels. Therefore penetrating Quchi (LI 11) towards Binao (LI 14) can regulate both the Lung and Large Intestine Meridians. The functions: Regulate qi and blood circulation, dredge the meridians, eliminate stasis, disperse swelling, and promote muscle regeneration. The treatment of scrofula through the regulation of the function of the lung and large intestine is done by regulating the function of zang organs, qi, blood and the whole body. The manipulation is as follows:

1) *Preparation before needling* a. Pressing along the meridian: Before needling, the doctor has to press the skin and muscle along the joining line from Quchi (LI 11) and Binao (LI 14) in order to relax the meridians. b. Locating the points: The patient, who is in sitting position, flexes both forearms and arches the chest while the doctor uses his thumb to press a "+" at the end of transverse crease of the elbow with the centre of the marking of Quchi (LI 11) point. c. Local sterilization: Sterilize the points and the operator's hands with routine iodine and alcohol. d. Inspecting the needles.

2) *Needling procedures* a. Penetrating the skin: The tip of the needle is dipped in glycerine. Pick up the needle handle with the middle and index fingers of the doctor's right hand and press the needle tail with the thumb, then touch Quchi (LI 11) point with the needle tip. The needle is 45° inclined to the extension line of the upper arm. The doctor's left hand holds the needle body lightly, then penetrates it quickly into 0.5 to 1 cm in depth subcutaneously. b. Inserting the needle stably and quickly: The doctor holds the needle with the thumb and index finger, rotates and gradually withdraws the needle to the subcutaneous space, lying down the needle, then penetrates along the subcutaneous tissue forward quickly and backward slowly to facilitate the penetration. c. Subcutaneously penetrating: Direct the needle tip towards Binao (LI 14) point without any deviation, and let the needle body touch the subcutaneous tissue moderately. d. Penetrating Binao (LI 14): Penetrate the needle tip into Binao (LI 14) point. The patient should have distension and a heavy feeling.

3) *Strengthening the stimulation* a. Scraping the needle: Press the skin of Quchi (LI 11) with the doctor's left hand, and scrape the needle handle with the thumb nail backwardly six to eight times for women, seven to nine times for men to induce and promote qi. The patient feels hot distension. During the process (about 15 minutes), scrape the needle once more. b. Twisting and twirling the needle: Reducing method is applied to those who had local red, swelling and pain, while reinforcing is used for those who had local hard masses, but free of redness or swelling. The needle should be turned round about 180°, and twisted once more after fifteen minutes.

4) *Withdrawing the needle* a. After needling for thirty minutes, a sterilized cotton ball is pressed on the Quchi (LI 11) point. b. Withdraw the needle slowly by the right hand. c. Ask the patient to massage the needled spot with the cotton ball.

5) *Auxillary treatment* a. Fire needle: For chronic cases, the hard masses of tuberculosis or small hard nodes after treatment, a fire needle may be applied (It is also used to discharge the pus). The hard nucleus is fixed by the doctor's left thumb and index finger, hold the needle with the right hand and burn it on an alcohol burner until it gets

red, then immediately penetrate the center of the hard nucleus, followed the circumference of the hard nucleus for three or four needles, in a depth of two thirds of the needle body. If it is used for extraction of the pus, press the nucleus gently by hand after penetration to help discharge the pus. b. Application of moxa cones at the tip of the elbow: Apply five to seven cones each time, frequently used for those in auxillary or failed in long-standing treatment.

2. Thirteen methods in treating windstroke

For windstroke, Dr. Wang accorded basically to the classification of *Synopsis of the Golden Chamber*, i.e. external wind invading the body, the pathogenic factors deeply affected. The degree of the disease is divided into invading the collaterals, invading meridians, invading fu organs and invading zang organs. He classified windstroke into three categories according to his experience: a. Invading zang-fu organs: chiefly mental illness, suddenly falling down and coma, which is again divided into tense and flaccid syndrome, hemiplegia left after regaining the consciousness. b. Invading the meridians: absence of coma, sudden onset, numbness of hands and feet, hemiplegia, aphasia, facial paralysis, and salivation from the corner of the mouth after recovery of consciousness. c. Sequelae: a long course hemiplegia, deviation of the mouth and eyes, aphasia, deficiency of qi and blood, and weakness of the spleen and stomach. The guiding idea in treating windstroke is to treat the qi first, windstroke can be cured after promoting the circulation of qi. He always said that careful, clinical examination was needed. The obstruction of the meridian was usually due to pathogenic wind internally and externally fighting against phlegm, heat, damp and stagnation, resulting in a loss of nutrition of the muscles and tendons. Therefore, the chief principle was to treat the meridian qi, actually it referred to dredging the meridians and activating the collaterals. When blood circulates freely, the blood vessels are free of obstruction. Thus, the muscles and tendons are nourished.

Through the whole schedule of his treatment of windstroke, he also emphasized regulation of qi, blood and zang-fu. For example, among the thirteen methods in treating windstroke, twelve needles on the hands and feet, thirteen needles on Du Meridian method, Back-Shu point method, old ten needles method, treating six fu method and penetrating Mu method are all the products of this viewpoint.

1) *Needling to correct facial paralysis* It is suitable for external wind invading the collaterals, the disease is mild, and the course is short, only half of the facial muscle is paralysed, deviation of the mouth and flaccid eyelids, salivation from the corner of the mouth, tears and difficulty chewing. Prescription: Renzhong (Du 26), Chengjiang (Ren 24), Dicang (S 4), Jiache (S 6), Quanliao (SI 18), Yangbai (G 14), Sibai (S 2), Daying (S 5), Hegu (LI 4). Function: Dispel wind and correct the paralysed facial muscle, clear and activate the meridians.

2) *Penetrating to correct the paralysed facial muscle* It is suitable for chronic sequelae due to invasion of wind in order to strengthen the therapeutic action, so it is called penetrating in correction of the facial paralysis method. Prescription: Yangbai (G 14) towards Yuyao (Extra 3), Zanzhu (B 2) towards Sizhukong (SJ 23), Sibai (S 2)

towards Chengqi (S 1), Fengchi (G 20) towards Fengfu (Du 16), Taiyang (Extra 2) towards Quanliao (SI 18), Heliao (LI 19) towards Juliao (S 3), Dicang (S 4) towards Jiache (S 6), Quchi (LI 11), Hegu (LI 4). Function: Clear and activate the meridians, dispel wind and correct deviation. (Note: The purpose of penetration is to strengthen the therapeutic effect.)

3) *Twelve needles on hands and feet* This prescription is formed by carefully selecting five Shu points on the hand and foot. It is the first choice in treating hemiplegia. Prescription: Quchi (LI 11), Hegu (LI 4), Neiguan (P 6), Yanglingquan (G 34), Zusanli (S 36), Sanyinjiao (Sp 6). Function: Clear and activate the meridians, regulate qi and blood. (Note: This prescription is not only the first choice in treating hemiplegia, but also in treating hypertension, paraplegia, Bi-syndrome and other asthenic syndrome.)

4) *Check hemiplegic method* It is suitable for hemiplegia, wind obstructing the meridian. The group of points on the affected area is applied to regulate qi and blood, and to disperse wind and activate collaterals. Prescription: Baihui (Du 20), Fengfu (Du 16), Fengchi (G 20), Jianyu (LI 15), Quchi (LI 11), Hegu (LI 4), Huantiao (G 30), Weizhong (B 40), Yanglingquan (G 34), Xuanzhong (G 39), Taichong (Liv 3). Function: Clear the meridians and activate collaterals, relax the tendons and facilitate the joints. (Note: Baihui (Du 20) and Fengfu (Du 16) of the Du Meridian are used to dispel the wind and clear the meridians. Fengchi (G 20), Huantiao (G 30), Yanglingquan (G 34) and Xuanzhong (G 39) of Gallbladder Meridian, Jianyu (LI 15), Quchi (LI 11) and Hegu (LI 4) of Yangming Meridian, Weizhong (B 40) of the Bladder Meridian, Taichong (Liv 3) of the Liver Meridian are used to coordinate yin and yang, balance the interior and exterior, communicate superior and inferior, regulate qi and blood, dredge the meridian, and promote the recovery of the function of the affected limbs.)

5) *Twelve penetrating methods* It is suitable for chronic hemiplegia with dystrophy. Prescription: Jianyu (LI 15) towards Binao (LI 14), Yifeng (SJ 17) towards Jiafeng (Extra), Quchi (LI 11) towards Shaohai (H 3), Waiguan (SJ 5) towards Neiguan (P 6), Hegu (LI 11) towards Laogong (P 8), Yangchi (SJ 4) towards Daling (P 7), Huantiao (G 30) towards Fengshi (G 31), Yangguan (Du 3) towards Ququan (Liv 8), Yanglingquan (G 34) towards Yinlingquan (Sp 9), Juegu (G 39) towards Sanyinjiao (Sp 6), Qiuxu (G 40) towards Shenmai (B 62), Taichong (Liv 3) towards Yongquan (K 1). Function: Clear the meridians and activate collaterals, relax tendons and joints.

6) *Inducing resuscitation method* It is suitable for windstroke with coma, corresponding to the apoplectic stage of a cerebral vascular accident. Induce resuscitation to recover from coma. Prescription: First penetrate with a three-edged needle Baihui (Du 20), and Sishenchong (Extra 6) for bloodletting or twelve Jing-Well points of hand and foot to bleeding, and then needle Renzhong (Du 26), Chengjiang (Ren 24), Fengchi (G 20), Fengfu (Du 16), Hegu (LI 4), Laogong (P 8), Taichong (Liv 3) and Yongquan (K 1). Function: Induce resuscitation. It is indicated in sudden syncope, coma, facial paralysis, hemiplegia, twisting of the mouth, flushed face, spasm of the hand, retention of urine and feces, coarse breathing and profuse sputum, falling into the tense syndrome in traditional Chinese medicine. For acute cases, bleeding therapy is chiefly used by Dr. Wang. There are two bleeding methods, by a three edged needle or by a filiform needle. The former bleeds a lot, suitable for excess syndrome and heat syndrome, while the latter

bleeds less, suitable for deficiency syndrome and syndrome due to stagnation. A three-edged needle for bleeding is chiefly used in windstroke of tense syndrome, coma due to excessive heat, syncope, blood stasis and pain. The function of bleeding at Baihui (Du 20) and Sishenchong (Extra) in this prescription is for resuscitation; the function of bleeding at twelve Jing-Well points is for reducing heat, smoothing the liver and resolving phlegm. The former prescription is for first aid, while the latter for resuscitation. The function is stable and sustained. These two prescriptions are special for unconsciousness, functioning in nourishing the kidney-water, reducing heat-fire of the heart and inducing resuscitation. Dr. Wang realized that the combination of Laogong (P 8) and Yongquan (K 1) points is able to clear the mind, dispel heat and calm the mind. Its effect is similar to Niuhuang Qingxin Wan (Bezoar Sedative Bolus).

7) *Method for restoring yang from collapse* This method is suitable for coma and syncope, opening the eyes and mouth, pallor, flaccid hands and retention of urine, snoring and rale due to excessive phlegm, coldness of the four extremities, weak pulse, and exhaustion syndrome. Prescription: Shenque (Ren 8) (moxibustion), Qihai (Ren 6), Guanyuan (Ren 4) (moxibustion), Baihui (Du 20), Neiguan (P 6) and Zusanli (S 36), Yongquan (K 1). Fill flat the umbilicus with dry salt, and cover with a piece of ginger, apply moxibustion with several dozen large moxa sticks and moxibustion at Qihai (Ren 6) and Guanyuan (Ren 4), then needle Baihui (Du 20), Neiguan (P 6), Zusanli (S 36) and Yongquan (K 1). Function: Restore yang from collapse.

8) *Du Meridian thirteen needles method* Du Meridian can govern the yang of the whole body. For hemiplegia, both yin and yang are weak, both qi and blood deficient. Needling Du Meridian activates the yang, promotes the balance of yin and yang, and facilitates recovery of hemiplegia and regulates the whole organism. Prescription: Baihui (Du 20), Fengfu (Ren 16), Dazhui (Du 14), Taodao (Du 13), Shenzhu (Du 12), Shendao (Du 11), Zhiyang (Du 9), Jinsuo (Du 8), Jizhong (Du 6), Xuanzhong (G 39), Mingmen (Du 4), Yaoyangguan (Du 3) and Changqiang (Du 1). Function: Strengthen yang and benefit qi, fulfil the marrow and tonify the brain. (Note: Du Meridian thirteen needles prescription is not only suitable for windstroke and hemiplegia, but also for paralysis and dystrophy, depressive and manic state, epilepsy, Bi-syndrome, etc.)

9) *Treating Back-Shu points method* It is suitable for sequelae of windstroke with long duration, weakness of the five zang organs and deficiency of both qi and blood, yin and yang, fatigue, and atrophy of limbs. Prescription: Geshu (B 17), Feishu (B 13), Xinshu (B 15), Ganshu (B 18), Pishu (B 20) and Shenshu (B 23). Function: Regulate qi and blood, yin and yang. (Note: It is not only used for hemiplegia, but also for deficiency, insomnia, seminal emission, depression and mania, irregular menstruation, hysteria, hemoptysis and bloody stool.)

10) *Old ten needles method* It is suitable for hemiplegia, gastro-intestinal tract disturbance, loss of appetite, epigastric distension and fullness, belching, regurgitation of acid and hiccup. Prescription: Shangwan (Ren 13), Zhongwan (Ren 12), Xiawan (Ren 10), Qihai (Ren 6), Tianshu (S 25), Neiguan (P 6) and Zusanli (S 36). Function: Regulate the middle jiao and strengthen the stomach, regulate qi and blood, ascend the clarity and descend the turbidity, and regulate the gastro-intestinal tract. (Note: This prescription is emphasized in regulating the stomach, and is widely used.)

11) *Treating Ren Meridian method* Ren Meridian is the sea of the yin meridians. Its significance is to nourish yin and reinforce yang, to dredge qi, facilitate breathing, ascend the clarity and descend the turbidity, and regulate the gastro-intestinal tract. It is indicated in hemiplegia and has a function in regulating yin and yang, and promoting gastro-intestinal function, suitable for treating hemiplegia, disharmony between spleen and stomach, accumulation of dampness and phlegm and abundance of sputum. Prescription: Ren Meridian twelve needles (Chengjiang (Ren 24), Lianquan (Ren 23), Tiantu (Ren 22), Zigong (Ren 19), Tanzhong (Ren 17), Jiuwei (Ren 15), Shangwan (Ren 13), Zhongwan (Ren 12), Xiawan (Ren 10), Qihai (Ren 6), Guanyuan (Ren 4), and Zhongji (Ren 3)). Function: Tonify yin and support yang, and regulate the gastro-intestinal tract.

12) *Treating six fu points method* The selection of six fu points is similar to the five zang points plus Geshu (B17). The six fu organs belong to yang, and function well in case of descending. It is discharging, but not storing. The functions are receiving, transportation and digesting the food into chyme, discharging the wastes, regulating the three jiao, facilitating urination and defecation. Obstruction of six fu organs will cause qi stagnation, hiccup occurs in mild cases, while pain, vomiting, distension and obstruction in severe cases. After windstroke, sequelae of hemiplegia remain in the chronic cases, especially dysfunction of the gastro-intestinal tract, nutritional deficiency, difficulty with urination and defecation, declining of the function of qi and zang-fu organs. So, the selection of the Shu points of the six fu organs in combination with the Front-Mu points will give evident results. Prescription: Back-Shu points of the six fu organs, (Danshu (B 19), Weishu (B 21), Sanjiaoshu (B 22), Dachangshu (B 25), Xiaochangshu (B 27) and Pangguangshu (B 28)). Function: Transport water and food, regulate the six fu organs. (Note: The function of the six Back-Shu points is quite broad, in addition to the treatment of hemiplegia, dysfunction of the gastro-intestinal tract, disturbance of urination and defecation, also for the treatment of cold deficiency of spleen and stomach, retention of water and food, pain around the stomach, damp, heat, diarrhoea, vomiting and hiccup.)

13) *Needling the Front-Mu points* It refers to the needling zang-fu Front-Mu points, which are defined according to the interior essence qi which converges in the chest and abdomen. The Front-Mu points are distributed on the chest and abdomen, and named according to the location of zang-fu organs, but not limited to one meridian. The Front-Mu points are close to the zang-fu organs. Prescription: Zhangfu (L 1), Tanzhong (Ren 17), Juque (Ren 14), Qimen (Liv 14), Zhongmen (Liv 13), Tianshu (S 25), Zhongwan (Ren 12), Guanyuan (Ren 4), and Zhongji (Ren 3). Function: Regulate zang-fu, supplement qi and regulate yin. (Note: It is not only used in the sequelae of windstroke, hemiplegia, but also in paraplegia. It is suitable for the chronic case, weakness of the function of zang-fu organs, abnormal rising of liver qi, hiccup, hypochondriac pain, abdominal distension, prolonged diarrhoea due to dysfunction of the stomach, yang deficiency of spleen and kidney, derangement of transportation, urinary and fecal incontinence. The aim is to warm the kidney and spleen, consolidate the function of the intestine and stop diarrhoea, reduce damp-heat of the liver and gallbladder, treat hysteria, and improve deficiency symptoms.)

3. Eleven methods in treating paralysis

Muscle atrophy and contraction of the four limbs are due to disuse after paralysis. Traumatic paraplegia is due to injury of the spinal column by direct or indirect external forces caused either by fracture of the bone or by dislocation of the spinal column, by complete or incomplete injury of the spinal cord or by cauda equina (below the level of injury of the spinal cord), causing paresthesia of the limbs, complete or incomplete loss of motor function and incontinence of both sphincters. Since 1965, much clinical experience research has been done on paraplegia. New advances have been made based on theories from ancient medical books. "Taking Du Meridian first in treating paralysis" is Dr. Wang's new development. He realized that paraplegia corresponds to the injury of Du Meridian in traditional Chinese medicine, so in the treatment of paralysis, the Du Meridian should be chosen. Dr. Wang always said that treating paralysis is not limited to one point. It should use the twelve meridians of the body, extra points and eight collaterals and the function of their zang-fu organs, then we should care for the injury, recover and improve the functional state of the organism. Therefore, in treating paraplegia, we should emphasize the whole body. The injury of Du Meridian is at different levels. The degree of injury and the clinical manifestations vary from ordinary paralysis. Through clinical experiences the eleven methods of treating paraplegia evolved.

1) *Treating Du Meridian method* a. Prescription: Baihui (Du 20), Fengfu (Du 16), Dazhui (Du 14), Taodao (Du 13), Shenzhu (Du 12), Shendao (Du 11), Zhiyang (Du 9), Jinsuo (Du 8), Jizhong (Du 6), Xuanshu (Du 5), Mingmen (Du 4), Yangguan (Du 3), Changqiang (Du 1). b. Function: Dredge Du Meridian, tonify marrow and strengthen the brain.

2) *Treating Jiaji method* a. Prescription: 3 mm lateral to the both sides of the lower border from T2, one point every other vertebra, down to L 4, sixteen points in all. b. Function: Dredge yang qi and regulate zang-fu organs.

3) *Treating Back Shu method* a. Prescription: Feishu (B 13), Xinshu (B 15), Geshu (B 17), Pishu (B 20), Ganshu (B 18), Shenshu (B 23). b. Function: Tonify five zang organs and benefit qi and blood.

4) *Treating bladder method* a. Prescription: Baliao, Huantiao (G 30), Chengfu (B 36), Yinmen (B 37), Weizhong (B 40), Chengshan (B 57), Kunlun (B 60), Yongquan (K 1). b. Function: Regulate stagnation, strengthen tendons to facilitate walking.

5) *Treating Ren Meridian method* a. Prescription: Juque (Ren 14), Zhongwan (Ren 12), Xiawan (Ren 10), Qihai (Ren 6), Guanyuan (Ren 4), Zhongji (Ren 3), Liangmen (S 21), Tianshu (S 25), Shuidao (S 28), Zhangmen (Liv 13). b. Function: Nourish vital essence, soothe the liver and normalize the functions of the stomach.

6) *Treating spleen and stomach method* a. Prescription: Qichong (S 30), Biguan (S 31), Futu (S 32), Dubi (S 35), Zusanli (S 36), Shangjuxu (S 37), Xiajuxu (S 39), Jiexi (S 41), Xiangu (S 43), Neiting (S 44), Sanyinjiao (Sp 6). b. Function: Regulate the spleen and strengthen the stomach, nourish the blood and tendons.

7) *Treating the liver and bladder method* a. Prescription: Daimai (G 26), Juliao (G 29), Fengshi (G 20), Yanglingquan (G 34), Yangjiao (G 35), Guangming (G 37), Xuanzhong (G 39), Qiuxu (G 40), Zulinqi (G 41), Xiaxi (G 43), Taichong (Liv 3).

b. Function: Tonify the tendons, strengthen the bone, relax the liver and facilitate joints.

8) *Treating foot three yin method* a. Prescription: Qichong (S 30), Yinlian (Liv 11), Qimen (Liv 14), Yinlingquan (Sp 9), Sanyinjiao (Sp 6), Zhaohai (K 6), Taichong (Liv 3). b. Function: Nourish yin and blood, relax spasm and diminish the wind.

9) *Treating hand three yang method* a. Prescription: Jianyu (LI 15), Jianzhen (SI 9), Quchi (LI 11), Sanyangluo (SJ 8), Ximen (P 4), Hegu (LI 4), Yangchi (SJ 4), Zhongzhu (SJ 3). b. Function: Dredge yang qi, regulate blood circulation.

10) *Treating hand three yin method* a. Prescription: Jugu (LI 16), Yifeng (SJ 17), Xiabai (L 4), Chize (L 5), Zhigou (SJ 6), Shenmen (H 7), Daling (P 7). b. Function: Tranquilize the mind by nourishing blood, softening the tendons and dredging the meridians.

11) *Regulating yin and yang method* a. Prescription: Quchi (LI 11), Neiguan (P 6), Hegu (LI 4), Yanglingquan (G 34), Zusanli (S 36), Sanyinjiao (Sp 6). b. Function: Dredge the meridians and balance yin and yang.

II. Case Analysis

Case 1: Scrofula (tuberculosis of the lymph node of the neck)

Name, Xie x x; sex, female; age, 17; case No. 470843; date of the first visit, April 21, 1975.

Complaints Two hard nodules were found at the back of her right ear two years ago. Scrofula was diagnosed in another hospital, which was improved by taking Chinese herbs and injections of streptomycin. The nodules became swollen and hard for two months, but free from tenderness, accompanied by weakness of the limbs, occasional headache and easily angered. Appetite, sleep, urine, feces and menstruation normal. Her face was flushed, the tongue proper thin white with red tip. The pulse was deep, thready and slow. Examination: The tuberculosis of the neck was 6 x 6 cm, that of the axillary was 3 x 3 cm, normal fluoroscopy of the chest. The skin was not red, the nodule was hard, free of pain when pressed and immovable. Differentiation: Stagnation of qi and blood and accumulation of phlegm-dampness. Principle of treatment: Regulate qi and blood, dissipate swelling and disperse the mass.

Prescription Quchi (LI 11) towards Binao (LI 14).

Treatment procedure Six-cun needles were selected with reducing method, three times a week. After five treatments the lymph node shrunk to 2 x 2 cm in size. The cervical nodule became soft and divided into three nuclei. On May 18, the nodule was the size of a bean. On May 22, the nodules at the neck and axillary basically disappeared. No relapse was found after a follow-up visit two months later.

Case 2: Windstroke

Name, Zhao x x; sex, female; age, 65; date of the first visit, October 6, 1965.

Complaints Two years ago, she suffered from hypertension and left side hemiplegia. The motor function was restored after acupuncture treatment. She fell into a coma suddenly in the afternoon with hemiplegia of the right side. She had irritability, normal appetite and sleep, frequent constipation, normal urine. The tongue coating was thin, the pulse was superficial and string-taut. Differentiation: Deficiency of blood and heat in the liver, internal stirring up of deficiency-wind. Principle of treatment: Soothe the liver fire and diminish the wind, nourish qi and blood.

Prescription Twelve Jing-Well points, Baihui (Du 20), Renzhong (Du 26), and twelve needles on hands and feet.

Treatment procedure Needle the twelve Jing-Well points until bleeding appears, then needle Baihui (Du 20), Renzhong (Du 26) and the twelve needles on hands and feet with reducing method. Retain the needles for thirty minutes. She woke up after four treatments, gradually regained speech, defecation and normal movement of the limbs.

Explanation Since the case was acute and the coma happened suddenly, the twelve Jing-Well points were needled for bloodletting to pacify the liver-fire and diminish the pathogenic wind and tranquilize the mind. Baihui (Du 20) and Renzhong (Du 26) were used for resuscitation. The twelve needles on hands and feet were applied for dredging the meridians, regulating qi and blood. The mind was clear and movement of the limbs was recovered after four treatments.

Case 3: Sequela of windstroke

Name, Hou x x; sex, male; age, 60; case No. 605533; date of the first visit, August 7, 1976.

Complaints He suffered from hemiplegia on the left side for seven months. His left arm had pain and contracture, and he could only lift it to the level of his chest. He couldn't flex and extend his fingers and had difficulty in the left lower limb. He walked by leaning on someone. His appetite, urine and feces were normal. His blood pressure was 160/90 mmHg. His tongue proper was thin white, his pulse deep and thready. Differentiation: Deficiency of both qi and blood, loss of nourishment of the tendons and blood vessels. Principle of treatment: Reinforce qi and blood, relax muscles and tendons and activate the flow of qi and the blood.

Prescription Twelve penetrating points.

Treatment procedure Treat three times a week with reinforcing first then reducing. The pain on the upper limbs stopped after five treatments, the contracted arm relieved. The strength of the lower limbs increased, and lifting his leg improved. His tongue was thin and white. The pulse was string-taut. His blood pressure was 150/90 mmHg. After more than ten treatments with the above prescription, he could walk with a stick in the room. The flexion and extension of his fingers somewhat recovered. He could walk several meters, lift his arm to the level of his shoulder, and manage his daily life by himself after another ten treatments.

Explanation This case is deficiency of both qi and blood, loss of nutrition of the tendons, muscles and blood vessels. He was treated by nourishing qi and the blood, relaxing the tendons and muscles and activating qi flow. Twelve penetrating points were used with reinforcing first, then reducing to promote meridians and activate collaterals, relax tendons and muscles, and facilitate joints. After more than ten treatments he could walk with a stick, and the function of the fingers somewhat recovered. The function of the limbs were recovered after another ten treatments.

Case 4: Paraplegia

Name, Ge x x; sex, male; age, 31; date of the first visit, November, 1968.

Complaints He was injured in a car accident nine months ago. He lost consciousness followed by paraplegia and disturbance of both sphincters when he woke up. An X-ray revealed comminuted fracture of the scapular, fracture of right rib and compressive fracture of the lumbar vertebra. The fractures were healed after treatment with combined traditional Chinese medicine and Western medicine. But his legs were still paralyzed, associated with muscular atrophy, poor appetite, insomnia, incontinence of urine, and constipation. Examination: The muscle strength of the lower limbs was grade 0, the strength of musculi quadratus lumborum was grade II. The pain and tactile sensation were lost beneath T12, loss of abdominal, anal, crimasteric, knee and ankle reflexes. Sallow complexion, clear mind, pale red tongue with thin white coating, deep thready pulse, blood pressure 120/80 mmHg, and bedsore of 3 x 2 cm at the saclio-coccyxal region. Differentiation: Blood stagnation due to trauma, obstructing the meridians and muscles. Principle of treatment: Activate blood circulation to remove stagnation, nourish the muscles and tendons.

Prescription 1) Baihui (Du 20), Fengfu (Du 16), Dazhui (Du 14), Taodao (Du 13), Shenzhu (Du 12), Shendao (Du 11), Zhiyang (Du 9), Jinsuo (Du 8), Jizhong (Du 6), Xuanshu (Du 5), Mingmen (Du 4), Yangguan (Du 3), Changqiang (Du 1). 2) 3 mm lateral to both sides of the lower border from T2 to L4, one point every other vertebra, 16 in all. 3) Baliao, Huantiao (G 30), Chengfu (B 36), Yinmen (B 37), Weizhong (B 40), Chengshan (B 57), Kunlun (B 60), Yongquan (K 1). 4) Qichong (S 30), Biguan (S 31), Futu (S 32), Dubi (S 35), Zusanli (S 36), Shangjuxu (S 37), Xiajuxu (S 39), Jiexi (S 41), Xiangu (S 43), Neiting (S 44), Sanyinjiao (Sp 6). 5) Daimai (G 26), Juliao (S 3), Fengchi (G 20), Yanglingquan (G 34), Yangjiao (G 35), Guangming (G 37), Xuanzhong (G 39), Qiuxu (G 40), Zulinqi (G 41), Xiaxi (G 43), Taichong (Liv 3). These five groups of points were applied alternately.

Treatment procedure The reinforcing method was used. After the first course, he could stand by the wall with two crutches, and helped by others at both knees, he could sit up by himself. In the second course, the first, second, third, and fourth prescriptions and Shenshu (B 23), Dachangshu (B 25), Zhongwan (Ren 12), Qihai (Ren 6) and Guanyuan (Ren 4) were added. He could walk a few steps on crutches and guided by others. He had reflex bladder and defecation at a definite time, the bedsore was healed. After the third course, the third, fourth and fifth prescriptions were selected plus Guanyuan (Ren 4), Zhongji (Ren 3) and Shenshu (B 23). He could walk with one stick, the sensation was restored, but the muscle was still atrophied with bowl movements two to three times a day and with reflex bladder. After the fourth course, with the same method, he could walk with a stick more freely than before, normal bladder function, but with an urgent sensation, normal defecation, but incontinence during loose stool. After the fifth course, the first, third and fourth prescriptions were used in addition of Qihai (Ren 6), Guanyuan (Ren 4), Mingmen (Du 4) and Shenshu (B 23), he could walk by a stick, with normal sphincters. For consolidation of the result, several months' needling was added. He was clinically recovered, and he could undertake his original work.

Explanation He had paraplegia and disturbance of two sphincters. His syndrome was due to traumatic blood stagnation and obstruction of the meridians. The principle of treatment is to activate the blood circulation and dispel the stasis, and nourish the muscles and collaterals. The first, second, fourth, sixth and seventh prescriptions of "eleven methods" were repeatedly applied in addition to Shenshu (B 23), Dachangshu (B 25), Zhongwan (Ren 12), Qihai (Ren 6), Guanyuan (Ren 4), Zhongji (Ren 3) and Mingmen (Du 4) for regulating qi of the congenital kedney and acquired qi of the spleen, dredging the meridians so as to regulate the function of gastro-intestinal tract. Through the six months' treatment, he completely recovered his sensory, motor function and both sphincters and could do his original work.

THE APPLICATION OF THE DIFFERENTIATION OF THE MERIDIAN REACTION POINTS

—Dr. Wang Pinshan's Clinical Experience

Dr. Wang Pinshan was born in a family well-known for traditional Chinese medicine in Haicheng County, Liaoning Province in December, 1920. From his childhood, he began to learn traditional Chinese medicine from his father and to learn acupuncture from Dr. Liu Rentang. He has been engaged in clinical and teaching work for several decades and had a book *Simplified Manual for Acupuncture* and more than twenty academic papers published. With modern scientific technology, he has discovered the acoustic information transmitted along the meridians, confirming the objective existence of the running course of the twelve regular meridians on the body surface and the four extremities. His work *Studies on the Propagated Lines of Fourteen Meridians* was awarded the second prize by the Ministry of Public Health. He is now an associate professor and deputy chief doctor of the Acupuncture Department of the Affiliated Hospital of Liaoning College of Traditional Chinese Medicine.

I. Academic Characteristics and Medical Specialities

1. The abnormal change of the Shu points is an objective indication of the meridian diseases

Meridians, which have the specific properties to connect the zang-fu, including the extraordinary fu organs internally and the extremities externally, are a complete auto-regulating and auto-controlling system to maintain the normal life of the body. When the balance of the meridians is disturbed, the corresponding information reaction of the meridians will occur, such as allergic tenderness, soreness, numbness and subcutaneous nodules on the Shu points which are located on the body surface by the meridian anatomy. It is very helpful in clinical acupuncture treatment that these can be used as the indications for the meridian differentiation and point-selection along the meridians.

Under the premise of the four diagnostic methods and the eight principles, as well as the diagnosis and treatment based on differentiation, it is very important in acupuncture treatment to find out the mechanism of the disease and to judge its location. Based on the four diagnostic methods, including the physiochemical examination, the meridians should be palpated by the palmar fingers with the same strength to find out the changes on the Shu points (the potential changes of the Yuan-Source points of the twelve regular meridians and the hot-feeling degree of the Jing-Well points on the tips of the fingers and toes can also be examined as a reference). This can be used to judge the mechanism of the disease, and determine whether the disease is localized in the zang or fu organ or on the related areas.

The practice has proved that diseases of the brain, marrow, bones, vessels or mental disorders are closely related to the eight extraordinary meridians. For example, the common reaction points for epilepsy lie on Changqiang (Du 1) and Dazhui (Du 14) of the Du Meridian; the reaction point for disorder of qi is at Tanzhong (Ren 17) of the Ren Meridian; that for incontinence of urine at Qugu (Ren 2); that for the day disease at Shenmai (B 62) of the Yangqiao Meridian and that for the night disease at Zhaohai (K 6) of the Yinqiao Meridian; the reaction points for zang-fu diseases lie on the twelve regular meridians, such as Zusanli (S 36) for stomach disease, Yanglingquan (G 34) for gallbladder disease, Neiguan (P 6) for heart and chest diseases, Taichong (Liv 3) for liver disease, Yanglingquan (G 34) and Diji (Sp 8) for diarrhoea, and Gongsun (Sp 4) for dysmenorrhea. All these points reflect the information reaction of the meridians. The reaction points for the diseases of the head are mainly located on the hands and feet. Hegu (LI 4), Taichong (Liv 3), Neiting (S 44), Waiting (Extra) (the midpoint of the connecting line between Neiting (S 44) and Zulinqi (G 41)), Zulinqi (G 41), Diwuhui (G 42) and Shenmai (B 62) are the points which dominate head diseases. The reaction points for the diseases of the four extremities can be found in the abdomen. For example, there is a reaction point at Huangshu (K 16) at the side of the navel for rheumatic arthritis. Despite individual differences and different reactions, the characteristics of the body surface, internal organs and the local areas are clearly indicated. Therefore, in clinical diagnosis and acupuncture treatment, there are still objective indications to follow. Just as recorded in *Plain Questions* that "when low back pain is caused by Jueyin Meridian, the patient will feel a sensation across the loins as tight as the string of a bow from which the arrow is about to be shot. Needle Jueyin Meridian in the region on the lateral side of calf and above the heel, and insert the needle in the region where numerous tiny blood vessels may be felt." On the contrary, if we look for the mechanism of the disease according to the reaction points, we can also find out the fact that the mechanism of the disease is in the Jueyin Meridian, but the location of the disease is in the lumbar region, showing the guiding significance of the meridian theory in the acupuncture treatment.

To find out the objective indications of the objective changes on the Shu points, in addition to the fingers pressing with the same strength, the "pressure meter for meridian point," i.e. the spring pressure rod, can also be used. For example, 0.5 kg is marked (+++), 1 kg (++) and 1.5 kg (+). After comparison, the degree of the allergic reaction may be distinguished, whether the allergic reaction is alleviated during the treatment or subsides after treatment. Generally, if both the subjective symptoms and the allergic reaction disappear, it is considered that the disease is cured. If the subjective symptoms disappear, but the allergic reaction still remains, there will be the possibility of recurrence. If the subjective symptoms still exist, but the allergic reaction disappears, it shows that the disease has been transformed and the reaction has been displaced, so new reaction points should be detected and the therapeutic method should be altered accordingly. Therefore, the quantitation of the Shu point reaction based on the palpitation of the meridians makes the palpitation more objective and scientific and is of great help in the studies on the clinical treatment of the diseases.

2. The acoustic information transmitted along the meridian is a way to investigate the essence of the meridians

The studies on the propagated sensation along the meridians suggest that propagation must be accompanied by certain biophysical phenomena. With modern technology recording the acoustic information as the objective index, the microscopic changes in the process of propagation along the meridian should be detected, and the objective indications and the recording methods of the propagation should be investigated. An observation on forty-eight cases showed that the positive rate of the examination along the meridians was 84 percent and that for the control was 21.5 percent. Statistically the difference was very significant ($p < 0.01$). The acoustic information propagated along the meridian has confirmed the phenomenon of the propagated sensation along the meridians, and the objective existence of the running course of the twelve regular meridians on the body surface and on the four limbs.

Discernment: The local anaesthesia of the point and nerve block anaesthesia on brachial plexus can both be used to test the acoustic information along the meridian. It was found that the acoustic information for the patient with paraplegia was very low. In animal tests, it was found that acoustic information along the meridian could also be tested when the sciatic nerve, femoral nerve, peroneal nerve, the femoral artery and vein and popiteal artery and vein were cut off. When the muscle relaxant was injected into experimental animals, the acoustic information became very low and had nothing to do with the myoelectric control. Cutting the skin had no influence on the acoustic information, but cutting the soft tissue made it lower. When the animal was killed, the acoustic information became extremely low and even reached 0, indicating that the acoustic information along the meridians is a microscopic dynamic change inside the body. Biological acoustic information resulted from the extra energy released by the stress waveforms.

II. Case Analysis

Case 1: Hemiplegia (sequelae of meningoma of the left parietal lobe)

Name, Hu x x; sex, female; age, 50; date of the first visit, August 28, 1986.

Complaints The patient had had right hemiplegia for nine months and she had an operation of the meningoma of the left parietal lobe on November 19, 1985. After she was discharged from the hospital in December she began to suffer from headache, dizziness aggravated by coughing, aversion to cold and wind, numbness of the right upper limb, soreness and weakness of the right lower limb, difficulty in walking. There was no response after she took Chinese and Western medicine. Examination: Deep and thready pulse, pale red tongue proper, pallor, sound healing of the wound, inability to lift the right upper limb, functional disturbance of the fingers, and difficulty in walking. Tender points appeared at Tanzhong (Ren 17), Changqiang (Du 1), Gongsun (Sp 4), Shenmai (B 62), Zhaohai (K 6) and Hegu (LI 4), which showed the functional disturbance of the meridians after the brain operation. The position of the disease was in the head and on the Yangqiao and Yinqiao Meridians. The treatment should adjust the function of the Du, Ren, Yinqiao and Yangqiao Meridians.

Prescription 1. Tanzhong (Ren 17), Changqiang (Du 1) with the intradermal needles.

2. Shenmai (B 62), Zhaohai (K 6), Gongsun (Sp 4) and Waiting (Extra).

Treatment procedure Needling was performed on the above points in order. Spot needling was given on the points of the right side and the needles retained for thirty minutes on the left side. The patient was advised to practise Qigong. After ten treatments, headache and dizziness disappeared. No pain was reported even in coughing. The patient was no longer afraid of cold and wind and she could lift her right arm and carry objects with her hand. She could also walk steadily. Though the tenderness on the points did not vanish completely, the general conditions of the patient became much better after being treated for one month.

Case 2: Diarrhoea (duodenal ulcer)

Name, Wen x x; sex, male; age, 41; date of the first visit, July 11, 1986.

Complaints He had had three massive haemorrhages since 1971 when he suffered from a duodenal ulcer. He often had stomach pain, abdominal distension, and diarrhoea which became aggravated at night, anorexia and fatigue. After being treated for a long time, the patient showed no improvement. Examination: Deep, thready and tense pulse, pale tongue proper, thin coating, listlessness, sallow complexion, soreness and pain reactions and subcutaneous nodules at Diji (Sp 8), soreness and pain at Gongsun (Sp 4) and Yanglingquan (G 34) and tenderness at Hegu (LI 4), Zusanli (S 36), Waiting (Extra), Zhongwan (Ren 12), Guanyuan (Ren 4) and Taichong (Liv 3). Because of the long course of the disease, the patient had both qi and blood deficiency, blocking of the middle jiao and stagnation of meridian qi. This was the reason for the stomach pain. As well, dysfunction of the spleen resulted in abdominal distention and diarrhoea. The pathogenesis was mainly in the Spleen Meridian and the position was in the fu. The treatment should replenish the qi and nourish the blood, activate the flow of qi of the meridian and adjust the spleen and stomach.

Prescription 1. Zhongwan (Ren 12), Hegu (LI 4), Taichong (Liv 3), Zusanli (S 36) and Gongsun (Sp 4)

2. Guanyuan (Ren 4), Waiting (Extra), Yinlingquan (Sp 9), Diji (Sp 8) with the intradermal needles.

Treatment procedure Needling was performed on the above points in order to reinforce the Spleen Meridian and reduce the Stomach Meridian. The two groups of points were needled in turn every other day, the needles retained for fifteen minutes each time and ten treatments constitute one course. When the patient was examined after one course, it was found that his pulse was deep and fine and his tongue proper was red with a thin coating. His face was ruddy and he was in good spirits. His sleep and appetite improved greatly and the tenderness reaction was reduced. After the second course, all of the tenderness reactions disappeared. Clinically he was cured. The patient was advised to practise Qigong in order to consolidate the therapeutic effect.

Case 3: Bi-syndrome (rheumatic arthralgia)

Name, Hou x x; sex, female; age, 48; date of the first visit, August 7, 1986.

Complaints The patient suffered from joint pain since 1958. The symptoms varied with changes of weather. Both her ASO and ESR were normal. Though she visited many hospitals, she could not be cured. She had an operation on her right knee, but in vain. In June, she had sudden pain and swelling and rigidity of the knee joints and she could not walk. No response was found after she was treated with Chinese and Western medicine, plaster, acupuncture and physiotherapy. Examination: Soft and rapid pulse, red tongue proper, greasy coating, no fever, redness, swelling and tenderness on the knee joints. Meridian reaction: Allergic tenderness at Huangshu (K 16) of the Kidney Meridian, Hegu (LI 4) and Quchi (LI 11), Zusanli (S 36) and Waiting (Extra) of the Hand and Foot Yangming Meridians, Yinlingquan (Sp 9) and Gongsun (Sp 4) of the Spleen Meridian and Taichong (Liv 3) of the Liver Meridian. It showed that wind, cold and dampness had been retained for a long time and the attack occurred again because of the summer dampness and heat, which transformed into heat. The pathogenesis was mainly in the Kidney Meridian and the position of the disease was on the knees. The treatment was to remove the heat and dampness, activate the qi flow of the meridians and reinforce the body resistance to eliminate the pathogenic factors.

Prescriptions 1. Huangshu (K 16), Hegu (LI 4), Taichong (Liv 3), Yinlingquan (Sp 9), Zusanli (S 36).

2. Huangshu (K 16), Quchi (LI 11), Waiting (Extra), Gongsun (Sp 4).

Treatment procedure Needling was given according to the above order of the points with reinforcing of the Kidney Meridian and reducing of the Spleen Meridian. The two groups of points were needled in turn every other day. Waixiyan (Extra) was first needled with pricking method and the needles were retained for fifteen minutes. After five treatments the swelling was subsided and the tenderness was reduced. After ten treatments, the patient could walk normally free from pain at the knees. Since there was slight tenderness at Huangshu (K 16), the intradermal needles were used. No relapse was found according to the observation till September of the same year.

Case 4: Shaoyang headache (nervous headache)

Name, Wang x x; sex, female; age, 34; date of the first visit, July 12, 1986.

Complaints She had suffered from right side headaches for four years. Sometimes it was mild and sometimes severe. The patient felt dazed all day. According to the rheoencephalogram she was diagnosed as having elevated blood vessel tonicity. Her EEG and blood pressure were normal and her appetite was good. She also had polyuria and constipation. The headache was found to have nothing to do with her menstruation. There was no response to Chinese and Western medicine and acupuncture. Examination: String-taut and thready pulse, red tongue proper, thin and greasy coating, pink face, fluent speaking, tenderness at Zulinqi (G 41), Taichong (Liv 3), Hegu (LI 4) and Waiting (Extra). Differentiation: Fire of the liver and gallbladder disturbing the head, thus headache, when it affects the stomach and intestines, constipation appears. The pathogenesis lies mainly in the Gallbladder Meridian and the location of the disease is in the head. The treatment should soothe the liver and normalize the functions of the gallbladder, reduce the fire and dredge the meridians.

Prescription Zulinqi (G 41), Taichong (Liv 3), Hegu (LI 4) and Waiting (Extra).

Treatment procedure The Liver and Gallbladder Meridians were needled with the reducing method and the points were needled with the order listed above. Pricking method was performed on the right side while retaining the needle for fifteen minutes on the left side. Twirling and rotating were carried out every five minutes. After the second treatment, the headache and dizziness were alleviated. After the third treatment, the headache disappeared. After the fourth treatment, bowel movements became normal. After the fifth treatment, she felt comfortable. After another five treatments, the tenderness reaction vanished and the patient was cured. The follow-up visit two months later showed no relapse.

Case 5: Lumbago

Name, Shu x x; sex, female; age, 38; date of the first visit, August 14, 1986.

Complaints The patient had suffered from low back pain for five years since the delivery of her baby. The disease was treated as pathogenic wind-dampness, strain, deficiency of the kidney and trauma with no effect. After working for one hour, she had to lie down and have a rest. Her appetite, urination and bowel movement were normal. Menstruation was normal and the amount of the leucorrhoea was abundant. Examination: Deep and slow pulse, pale-red tongue proper, thin coating, sallow complexion, clear speech, tenderness at Zulinqi (G 41) and Mingmen (Du 4) points. According to the differentiation, if the Dai Meridian is affected and the meridian qi is stagnated, there will be lumbar pain. If the dampness-heat invades downwards, there will be plenty of leucorrhoea. The pathogenesis is in the Dai Meridian, and the position of the disease is on the lumbar region. Treatment should dredge the meridians and activate the flow of qi.

Prescription 1. Mingmen (Du 4) with the intradermal needling.

2. Zulinqi (G 41).

Treatment procedure After the needling, the needles were retained for fifteen minutes. Every five minutes, the needles on both sides were twirled and rotated for one minute. After the treatment, the pain in the lumbar region stopped immediately and the patient could move her waist freely, but there was still tenderness. After the second treatment, the patient was tired. After the third treatment, the amount of leucorrhoea was greatly reduced, and there was still a tenderness reaction after the fourth treatment. The tenderness disappeared when two more treatments were given and the patient was cured. For over a month, no attack of lumbago was found.

Explanation The key point in the acupuncture clinic is to master the pathogenesis, to find out the exact position of the disease and to perform a proper manipulation. These three points are so important that none of them can be missed. When we say "to master the pathogenesis," it means that we should judge the disease according to the following diagnostic factors as the physical conditions of the patient, the predisposing cause of the disease, the duration of the disease, the transformation of the syndrome and the meridian information. "To find out or to localize the position of the disease" refers to the localization of pathogenic position, the diseased area and the corresponding needling points. Manipulation includes the order of the needling, the intensity of the stimulation, and both the reinforcing and reducing applied only after the arrival of qi. Besides, the needling should vary with different patients. For a strong build, the needling should be deep and retention of the needle is preferable. For the patient who is thin, the needling should be shallow and quick. For babies, the needling should be shallow with quick insertion. Therefore, the strength of the stimulation should correspond to the syndrome complex. In a word, without the four diagnostic methods, the eight principles, the differentiation, the manipulation and the point selection, the acupuncture clinic will lose the TCM theoretical guidance, and without the meridian information and the meridian differentiation, the acupuncture clinic will lose the guidance of the meridian doctrine.

ACUPUNCTURE AND MOXIBUSTION CORRESPONDING TO THE SYNDROMES AND COMBINATION OF POINTS ACCORDING TO ITS RULES

—Dr. Wang Xuetai's Clinical Experience

Dr. Wang Xuetai was born at Yixian County, Liaoning Province in 1925. He was admitted in Jinzhou Medical College in 1944. After the victory of the Anti-Japanese War, the College merged with Shenyang Medical College where he continued his education. He was appointed as a physiology and anatomy teacher in the North China Medical School in October of 1948. Since then, he has researched acupuncture teaching and clinical work, as well as studied the literature, history and future of traditional Chinese medicine. He was one of the founders of the Acupuncture Training Course for postgraduates, the Acupuncture College, and the Journal of Chinese Acupuncture and Moxibustion. He was also active in setting up the World Federation of Acupuncture and Moxibustion Societies. He is now a standing member of the All-China Association of Traditional Chinese Medicine and deputy director of the China Association of Acupuncture and Moxibustion.

I. Academic Characteristics and Medical Specialities

1. The manipulation must be in accordance with the syndromes

In manipulation, Dr. Wang insists that the manipulation for the reinforcing method should be heavy insertion and light withdrawal of the needle and for the reducing method, light insertion and heavy withdrawal, which can be used respectively to treat the deficiency and excess syndromes. If the syndrome is neither deficiency nor excess, or both deficiency and excess, an even movement can be applied, that is, the insertion and withdrawal of the needle should be performed evenly and the strength exerted should be moderate. As to the needling strength, the intensity should be light for weak stimulation and heavy for strong stimulation. In practice, this should be performed according to the patient's reactions. So long as the needling depth is concerned, shallow needling, that is, the subcutaneous needling, should be applied for the exterior-heat syndromes, and the cold syndromes or some zang-fu diseases should be treated by deep penetration of the muscles, because these diseases are yin. For the moderate depth, it is required that the needle should be inserted into the muscles. As to the needling duration, coma and the heat syndromes should be treated with quick needling, that is, quick insertion and quick withdrawal, while the cold syndrome, severe pain or spasm treated by retaining the needles. Generally, the chronic and febrile diseases lie internally and slow needling method is used. Sometimes needling and retaining of the needle may be used alternatively.

Dr. Wang also emphasizes moxibustion. According to the temperature exerted on the points of the patient's skin and the effects produced, it is divided into three kinds: warm-heat moxibustion, in which the temperature given is mild, and the skin is not burned; blistering moxibustion, in which the temperature is high and the skin is burned; and the festering moxibustion, in which the temperature exerted is very high and a severe burn is produced on the local skin of the point. The warm-heat moxibustion is used to treat the cold syndrome and those febrile diseases without fever, the blistering moxibustion is for shock, collapse and hysteria, and festering moxibustion is for deficiency and cold syndromes. To sum up, all of the events, such as the needling intensity, needling depth or moxibustion, must correspond to the syndromes.

2. Rules for the selection of points

1) *Selection of points along the meridian in accordance with the method described in Treatise on Febrile Diseases and the theory related to the febrile diseases and the hand meridians*

a. The diseases of the three yang meridians belong to excess-heat syndrome. The Du Meridian is the crossing place of all the yang meridians. Then Baihui (Du 20), Fengfu (Du 16) and Dazhui (Du 14) can be selected to reduce the heat from all the yang meridians. Such diseases as fever, aversion to cold, headache, rigid neck, tense of the spine and back, general pain, nasal obstruction or running nose belong to the diseases of the Taiyang Meridian. In addition to the points of the Du Meridian, the Back-Shu points of the Bladder Meridian of Foot-Taiyang such as Dazhu (B 11), Fengmen (B 12), Feishu (B 13) and Fengchi (G 20) can be selected. Especially Fengchi (G 20) and Fengfu (Du 16) are effective to treat the disease caused by external wind-cold. For wind-heat and febrile diseases, the Shu points of the Lung Meridian of Hand-Taiyin and the Large Intestine Meridian of Hand-Yangming, such as Shaoshang (L 11), Shangyang (LI 1), Hegu (LI 4) and Quchi (LI 11) are selected. For high fever accompanied with sweating, not aversion to cold but aversion to heat, pain of the eyes, dry mouth and nose, and thirst, which belong to the syndrome of the Yangming Meridian, the Shu points of the Stomach Meridian of Foot-Yangming and the Large Intestine Meridian of Hand-Yangming, such as Zusanli (S 36), Lidui (S 45), Hegu (LI 4) and Quchi (LI 11) are selected. If the symptoms include bitter mouth, dryness of the throat, dizziness, alternating attack of cold and heat, fullness of the chest and hypochondrium, they are the syndromes of Hand-Shaoyang Meridian which are treated by needling the Shu points of the Sanjiao Meridian of Hand-Shaoyang and the Gallbladder Meridians of Foot-Shaoyang, such as Zhongzhu (SJ 3), Yemen (SJ 2), Guanchong (SJ 1), Waiguan (SJ 5), Yanglingquan (G 34) and Fengchi (G 20).

b. The diseases of the three yin meridians are deficiency and cold syndromes, which are treated with the points of the Ren Meridian, such as Zhongwan (Ren 12), Shenque (Ren 8), Guanyuan (Ren 4) and Qihai (Ren 6). For the diseases of the Taiyin Meridian, the points of the Spleen Meridian of Foot-Taiyin and the Stomach Meridians of Foot-Yangming, such as Yinbai (Sp 1), Gongsun (Sp 4), Sanyinjiao (Sp 6), Yinlingquan (Sp 9), Neiting (S 44), Zusanli (S 36) and Tianshu (S 25) are added. In case of cold limbs and weak pulse, lassitude and preference for sleep, it is the Shaoyin Meridian syndrome, which are treated with the Shu points of the Kidney Meridian of Foot-Shaoyin, such as Yongquan (K 1), Rangu (K 2), Taixi (K 3) and Fuliu (K 7). For chest discomfort, acid regurgitation, vomiting, diarrhoea with purulent blood, tenesmus; or cold limbs and clonic convulsion, they all belong to the diseases of the Jueyin Meridian. So the Shu points of the Hand and Foot Jueyin Meridians such as Laogong (P 8), Neiguan (P 6), Jianshi (P 5), Taichong (Liv 3), Zhongfeng (Liv 4) and Qimen (Liv 14) should be needled.

2) *Selection of points along the meridian is applicable to all the diseases of different systems*

a. Disease of the respiratory system

The Shu points of the Lung Meridian of Hand-Taiyin and the Large Intestine Meridian of Hand-Yangming, such as Taiyuan (L 9), Lieque (L 7), Chize (L 5), Zhongfu (L 1), Hegu (LI 4), Quchi (LI 11) and Feishu (B 13).

b. Cardiovascular diseases and diseases of the nervous system

The Shu points of the Heart Meridian of Hand-Shaoyin, the Pericardium Meridian of Hand-Jueyin and the Kidney Meridian of Foot-Shaoyin, such as Shenmen (H 7), Tongli (H 5), Lingdao (H 4), Neiguan (P 6), Jianshi (P 5), Yongquan (K 1), Taixi (K 3) and Rangu (K 2) are selected.

c. Hemopathic and hematopoietic diseases

Besides the Back-Shu points of the heart, liver, spleen, stomach and the Shu points of the Foot-Taiyin Spleen Meridian of Foot-Taiyin and the Stomach Meridian of Foot-Yangming, such as Sanyinjiao (Sp 6), Xuehai (Sp 10), Neiting (S 44), Zusanli (S 36) and Zhongwan (Ren 12) of the Ren Meridian are selected.

d. Diseases of the digestive system

The points of the Stomach Meridian of Foot-Yangming should be selected as the main points, such as Neiting (S 44), Xiangu (S 43), Jiexi (S 41), Xiajuxu (S 39), Shangjuxu (S 37), Fenglong (S 40), Zusanli (S 36), Tianshu (S 25) and Rugen (S 18). Besides, the Back-Shu points of the stomach and large intestine and Zhongwan (Ren 12) (the Front-Mu point) are also selected.

e. Diseases of the urogenital and reproductive systems

The Shu points of the Foot-Taiyin, Foot-Shaoyin and Foot-Jueyin Meridians and the Ren Meridian, such as Sanyinjiao (Sp 6), Fuliu (K 7), Taixi (K 3), Yinlingquan (Sp 9), Zhongwan (Ren 12), Shuifen (Ren 9) and Qihai (Ren 6) are selected.

f. Gynecological and obstetrical diseases

The treatment usually starts from the Chong and Ren Meridians and is often related to the Kidney Meridian of Foot-Shaoyin, the Liver Meridian of Foot-Jueyin and the Spleen Meridian of Foot-Taiyin. The points selected are Qihai (Ren 6), Guanyuan (Ren 4), Zhongji (Ren 3), Qugu (Ren 2), Rangu (K 2), Zhaohai (K 6), Yingu (K 10), Yinbai (Sp 1), Sanyinjiao (Sp 6), Diji (Sp 8), Yinlingquan (Sp 9) and Xuehai (Sp 10).

g. Eye diseases

Points are often selected from the yang meridians for eye diseases of a yang-heat nature. Points of the Stomach Meridian of Foot-Yangming are selected for diseases of the eyelid, points of the Large Intestine Meridian of Hand-Yangming for diseases of the white of the eye and those of the Gallbladder Meridian of Foot-Shaoyin and the Liver Meridian of Foot-Jueyin for diseases of the iris and the Shu points of the Kidney Meridian of Foot-Shaoyin for diseases of the pupil.

3) *Selection and combination of the points* Dr. Wang often selects a lot of points in combination. The method for combining the points is as follows:

a. The combination of the Back-Shu points and the Front-Mu points

Most of the points on the back are the Back-Shu points, while most of the points on the chest and abdomen are the Front-Mu points. One method is to select the Back-Shu point and the corresponding Front-Mu point. For example, Feishu (B 13) combined with Zhongfu (L 1) can be used to treat respiratory diseases; Jueyinshu (B 14) with Tanzhong (Ren 17) to treat diseases of heart and chest; Ganshu (B 18) with Qimen (Liv 13) to treat diseases of the liver, stomach and costal regions; Xinshu (B 15) with Juque (Ren 14) to treat cardiac and nervous diseases: Pishu (B 20) with Zhangmen (Liv 14) to treat diseases of the liver and spleen; Weishu (B 21) with Zhongwan (Ren 12) to treat diseases of the stomach and intestines; Sanjiaoshu (B 22) with Shimen (Ren 5) to treat disorders of water metabolism; Shenshu (B 23) with Jingmen (G 25) to treat diseases of the kidney and the reproductive system; Dachangshu (B 25) with Tianshu (S 25) to treat diseases of the intestines and abdominal pain; Xiaochangshu (B 27) with Guanyuan (Ren 4) to treat diseases of the small intestines, bladder and the reproductive system; Pangguangshu (B 28) with Zhongji (Ren 3) to treat diseases of the bladder and the reproductive system. The other method is to select the Shu point with the uncorresponding Front-Mu point. For example, Feishu (B 13) with Tanzhong (R 17) to treat cough due to deficiency of qi; Shenshu (B 23) with Guanyuan (Ren 4) to treat impotence and swelling of vulva; Mingmen (Du 4) with Zhongji (Ren 3) to treat enuresis; Xinshu (B 15) with Tanzhong (Ren 17) to treat pain of the cardiac region; Pishu (B 23) with Zhongwan (Ren 12) to treat stomach pain; Shenshu (B 23) with Tianshu (S 25) to treat abdominal pain due to deficiency and cold, and Ganshu (B 18) with Zhongwan (Ren 12) to treat pain due to disorder of the qi of the liver and stomach.

b. The combination of yin and yang points

This is the combination of the points of the externally-internally related meridians of the zang-fu organs. One method is to combine the points of the exterior meridian with those of the interior meridian. For example, Zusanli (S 36) with Sanyinjiao (Sp 6) for dyspepsia and impotence; Hegu (LI 4) with Lieque (L 7) for cold and headache; Waiguan (SJ 5) with Neiguan (P 6) for headache and chest pain; Hegu (LI 4) with Taiyuan (L 9) for nasal obstruction. The other method is the combination of non-externally and internally-related meridians. For example, Hegu (LI 4) and Shenmen (H 7) may be combined to treat insomnia, Xingjian (Liv 2) and Jiexi (G 41) to treat pain of the lower abdomen and ankles; Hegu (LI 4) and Neiguan (P 6) to treat acute tonsillitis; Zusanli (S 36) and Taichong (Liv 3) to treat stomatitis; Yinlingquan (Sp 9) and Yanglingquan (G 34) to treat pain of the lower abdomen and knees; and Yemen (SJ 2) and Shaoshang (L 11) to treat pharyngodynia.

c. The combination of the distant points and adjacent points

Points close to the location of the disease are called adjacent points, while those on the four extremities are referred to as the distant points. The adjacent points function directly on the disease and the distant points can be selected to dredge the meridians. When the meridian qi travels properly, yin and yang may be regulated, the deficiency can be replenished and the stagnancy removed. For example, Tiantu (Ren 22) and Hegu (LI 4) for asthma, Zhongwan (Ren 12) and Zusanli (S 36) for stomach pain, Guanyuan (Ren 4) and Taichong (Liv 3) for dysmenorrhea, Feishu (B 13) and Lieque (L 7) for coughing, Zhangmen (Liv 13) and Taichong (Liv 3) for chest pain, Jueyinshu (B 14) and Neiguan (P 6) for pain of the chest and ribs, Tanzhong (Ren 17) and Neiguan (P 6) for chest pain due to obstruction of qi, Guanyuan (Ren 4) and Sanyinjiao (Sp 6) for abdominal pain, Tianshu (S 25) and Zusanli (S 36) for abdominal pain and diarrhoea, Tianshu (S 25) and Shangjuxu (S 37) for irritable colon, and Qihai (Ren 6) and Taichong (Liv 3) for functional uterine bleeding.

d. The combination of the points on the upper part and the lower part

The yang meridians of the hands and feet cross at the head and the yin meridians of the hands and feet cross at the chest and abdomen. Therefore, chest and abdominal diseases can be treated by combining the points on the hands and feet. For example, Neiguan (P 6) and Gongsun (Sp 4) for stomach pain, Zhigou (SJ 6) and Zhaohai (K 6) for constipation, Hegu (LI 4) and Neiting (S 44) for toothache and sore throat, Quchi (LI 11) and Zusanli (S 36) for heat of the body, Shenmen (H 7) and Sanyinjiao (Sp 6) for insomnia, Hegu (LI 4) and Sanyinjiao (Sp 6) for prolonged labour, Hegu (LI 4) and Fuliu (K 7) for night sweating, Neiguan (P 6) and Zusanli (S 36) for stomach pain, Hegu (LI 4) and Jiexi (S 41) for dizziness, Tongli (H 5) and Yongquan (K 1) for palpitations.

4) *Selecting the points according to the symptoms* For fever (the elevation of the body temperature), needling Dazhui (Du 14), Dazhu (B 11), Fengmen (B 12), Feishu (B 13), Quchi (LI 11), Hegu (LI 4) and Zusanli (S 36) has a definite antipyretic action. According to the different conditions of the disease, the following points are added: For acute high fever without sweating, add Shangyang (LI 1), Shaoshang (L 11), Zhongchong (P 9), Lidui (S 45), or prick Shixuan (Extra 24) and the twelve Jing-Well points, reinforce Hegu (LI 4) and reduce Fuliu (K 7); for sweating, add Fengfu (Du 16), Fengchi (G 20), Neiting (S 44) and Taibai (Sp 3), reduce Hegu (LI 4) and reinforce Fuliu (K 7); for intermittent fever, add Fengfu (Du 16), Fengchi (G 20), Yemen (SJ 2), Yangchi (SJ 4), Waiguan (SJ 5), Xiaxi (G 43) and Chongyang (S 42); for chronic low fever, add Yuji (L 10), Jianshi (P 5), Fuliu (K 7), Rangu (K 2), Yongquan (K 1) and moxibustion at Zusanli (S 36); for hypothermia, moxibustion at Dazhui (Du 14), Gaohuang (B 43), Shenque (Ren 8) and Zusanli (S 36); for general soreness and weakness, needle Quchi (LI 11), Zusanli (S 36) and Yangfu (G 38) or moxibustion at Dazhui (Du 14), Shenzhu (Du 12), Tanzhong (Ren 17), Dabao (Sp 21) and Qihai (Ren 6); for profuse sweating, needle Daheng (Sp 15) or reduce Hegu (LI 4) and Yuji (L 10) and reinforce Fuliu (K 7) and Neiting (S 44); for sweating without stopping and lowered body temperature, moxibustion at Shenque (Ren 8); for night sweating, needle Jianshi (P 5), reduce Hegu (LI 4) and Yuji (L 10) and reinforce Fuliu (K 7); for headache (including dizziness), points can be selected according to the diseased position on the head and properties of the disease. For example, Shangxing (Du 23), Yintang (Extra 2) (Yintang penetrating Zanzhu is better) are combined with Hegu (LI 4), Lieque (L 7), Zusanli (S 36) and Neiting (S 44) for frontal headache, Qianding (Du 21), Baihui (Du 20) for parietal

headache, the combination with Taichong (Liv 3) and Sanyinjiao (Sp 6) for posterior parietal headache, needle Houding (Du 19), Fengchi (G 20), Tianzhu (B 10) combined with Wangu (SI 4) and Kunlun (B 60); for occipital headache, needle Taiyang (Extra 2), Touwei (S 8), Qubin (G 7) combined with Waiquan (SJ 5) and Yangfu (G 38) for migraine, and then according to the causes of the disease, the following points can be added. For headache due to fever, needle Quchi (LI 11), Zusanli (S 36) and prick Shaoshang (L 11), Shangyang (LI 1) or Shixuan (Extra 24); for hyperemic headache, needle Jianjing (G 21), Xingjian (Liv 2) or prick Baihui (Du 20), Taiyang (Extra 2), Lidui (S 45) and Zhiyin (B 67); for anemic headache, needle Dazhui (Du 14), Mingmen (Du 4), Quchi (LI 11), Zusanli (S 36) and Sanyinjiao (Sp 6) with more moxibustion; for headache due to dyshormonism, needle Mingmen (Du 4) and Sanyinjiao (Sp 6); for headache due to eye diseases, needle Fengchi (G 20) and Hegu (LI 4); for headache caused by ear, nose and throat diseases, needle Hegu (LI 4) and Neiting (S 44); for nervous headache, needle Hegu (LI 4) and Xingjian (Liv 2); for dizziness, needle Fengchi (G 20), Yifeng (SJ 17), Yintang (Extra 1), Hegu (LI 4), Fenglong (S 40), Jiexi (S 41), Shenmai (H 7) and Shenshu (B 23); for coma, needle Yintang (Extra 1), Shuigou (Du 26), Duiduan (Du 27), Chengjiang (Ren 24), Hegu (LI 4), Laogong (P 8), Zusanli (S 36), Lidui (S 45), and Yongquan (K 1). According to the different conditions of the diseases, the following points can be added. Prick Shixuan (Extra 30) and the twelve Jing-Well points for coma due to high fever, moxibustion on Baihui (Du 20), Shenque (Ren 8), Qihai (Ren 6) and needle Neiguan (P 6) for collapse and shock; for mental disorders, add Shuigou (Du 26), Chengjiang (Ren 24), Shangxing (Du 23), Jiache (S 6), Fengfu (Du 16), Xinshu (B 15), Jiuwei (Ren 15), Shaoshang (L 11), Hegu (LI 4), Laogong (P 8), Daling (P 7), Jianshi (P 5), Shenmen (H 7), Fenglong (S 40), Lidui (S 45), Yinbai (Sp 1), Shenmai (B 62), Zhaohai (K 6), Yongquan (K 1). For mania, the points should be mainly selected from the Yang Meridians; while for depression, the points should be selected from the Yin Meridians. For excessive dreaming, Xinshu (B 15), Shenmen (H 7), Neiting (S 44), Zuqiaoyin (G 44) and Taichong (Liv 3) should be treated by acupuncture and moxibustion. For amnesia, Baihui (Du 20), Dazhui (Du 14), Xinshu (B 15), Shenmen (H 7) and Zusanli (S 36) should be needled with moxibustion. For insomnia, it is best to give the needling before the patient goes to sleep and to retain the needles. For insomnia due to neurosis, Yintang (Extra 1), Shenmen (H 7), Quchi (LI 11), Sanyinjiao (Sp 6), Zhaohai (H 6), and Yongquan (K 1) are needled. For insomnia due to dyshormonism, add Mingmen (Du 4), Shenshu (B 23), Diji (Sp 8), Sanyinjiao (Sp 6), and Zhaohai (H 6). For insomnia due to tuberculosis, add Feishu (B 13), Quchi (LI 11), Hegu (LI 4), Taiyuan (L 9), Zusanli (S 36), and Yongquan (K 1). For insomnia due to gastro-intestinal diseases, add Weishu (B 21), Zusanli (S 36), and Sanyinjiao (Sp 6). For insomnia due to heart disease, add Neiguan (P 6), Taiyuan (L 9), Shenmen (H 7), and Zusanli (S 36). For lethargy, the points can be selected according to whether the case is deficient or excess. For excess cases, needle Shuigou (Du 26), Fengchi (G 20), Hegu (LI 4), Guanchong (SJ 1), Zusanli (S 36), and Fenglong (S 40). For deficiency cases, needle Quchi (LI 11), Neiguan (P 6), Zusanli (S 36) and moxibustion at Baihui (Du 20), Dazhui (Du 14) and Tanzhong (Ren 17). For chest pain, in addition to the points on the chest and the corresponding points on the back, the following points can also be selected. For example, if the pain occurs in the anterior aspect of the chest, Daling (P 7), Neiguan (P 6), Quchi (LI 11) and Taiyuan (L 9) are needled; if the pain occurs at the lateral aspect of the chest or at the hypochondrium, Zhangmen (Liv 13), Waiguan (SJ 5), Zhigou (SJ 6), Yangfu (G 38) and Taichong (Liv 3) are needled; for fullness and oppressed feeling of the chest, Tanzhong (Ren 17), Zhongfu (L 1) and Juque (Ren 14) should be needled in combination with Chize (L 5), Zhigou (SJ 6), Jianshi (P 5), Yanglingquan (G 34) and Xingjian (Liv 2). Needling is often applied for dry coughs without sputum or with purulent sputum and both needling and moxibustion are applied for coughs with white sputum or frothy sputum. For coughs due to acute respiratory tract infection, Fengchi (G 20), Dazhui (Du 14), Fengmen (B 12), Feishu (B 13) and Hegu (LI 4) are selected; for coughs due to chronic diseases, Feishu (B 13), Gaohuang (B 43), Tiantu (Ren 22), Zhongfu (L 1), Hegu (LI 4), Taiyuan (L 9), Chize (L 5) and Taixi (K 3) selected; for dry cough, Yongquan (K 1) is added; and for coughs with plenty of sputum, Fenglong (S 40) is added. For hemoptysis, Dazhui (Du 14), Jianzhongshu (SI 15), Jugu (LI 16), Tanzhong (Ren 17), Rugen (S 18), Daling (P 7) and Yongquan (K 1) are needled. For dyspnea, except respiratory tract obstruction, the points can be selected as follows: Dazhui (Du 14), Feishu (B 13), Qihai (Ren 6), Lieque (L 7), Taiyuan (L 9), Tongli (H 5), Fenglong (S 40), Zusanli (S 36) and Rangu (K 2) are selected with both needling and moxibustion for inspiratory dyspnea. Tanzhong (Ren 17), Zhongfu (L 1), Chize (L 5), Jianshi (P 5), Xingjian (Liv 2) and Taichong (Liv 3) are needled for expiratory dyspnea. For dyspnea with cyanosis, needle Shuigou (Du 26) and Shaoshang (L 11); for phrenospasm, needle Geshu (B 17), Jiuwei (Ren 15), Juque (Ren 14), Qimen (Liv 14), Zhangmen (Liv 13), Hegu (LI 4), Taiyuan (L 9), Taixi (K 3), Taichong (Liv 3) and moxibustion at Rugen (S 18). For pain in the cardiac region, Fengchi (G 20), Jueyinshu (B 14), Xinshu (B 15), Taiyuan (L 9), Jingqu (L 8), Shaochong (H 9), Jianshi (P 5), Jinggu (B 64), Kunlun (B 60) and Rangu (K 2) are needled. For palpitation, Fengchi (G 20), Shendao (Du 11), Juque (Ren 14), Daling (P 7), Shenmen (H 7), Tongli (H 5), Shaofu (H 8), Zusanli (S 36), Rangu (K 2) and Yongquan (K 1) are needled. For arrhythmia, Fengchi (G 20), Xinshu (B 15), Neiguan (P 6), Shenmen (H 7), Tongli (H 5) and Zusanli (S 36) are needled. For heart failure, needling should be performed on Neiguan (P 6), Taiyuan (L 9), Tongli (H 5) and Zusanli (S 36) and moxibustion at Tanzhong (Ren 17). For the severe cases, needling of Shuigou (Du 26) and Zhongchong (P 9) are added. For hypotension, Shuigou (Du 26) and Neiguan (P 6) are needled and moxibustion applied at Baihui (Du 20), Shangxing (Du 23) and Qihai (Ren 6). For local congestion, prick the adjacent points and the Jing-Well points of the related meridians. For local blood stasis, the adjacent points are needled and warm moxibustion is performed locally. For difficulty in swallowing, Geshu (B 17), Tiantu (Ren 22), Xuanji (Ren 21), Tanzhong (Ren 17), Juque (Ren 14), Neiguan (P 6), Hegu (LI 4), Shangqiu (Sp 5) and Dazhong (K 4) are needled. For upper abdominal pain, Weishu (B 21), Juque (Ren 14), Zhongwan (Ren 12), Qimen (Liv 14), Neiguan (P 6), Gongsun (Sp 4), Zusanli (S 36) and Taichong (Liv 3) are needled. For absence of fever, local warm-moxibustion may be performed. For nausea and vomiting, Zhongwan (Ren 12) and Neiguan (P 6) are mainly needled in combination with the following points: Pricking of Jinjing (Extra 10) and Yuye (Extra 10) if caused by acute infectious disease, pricking of Quze (P 3) and Weizhong (B 40) in case of continuous vomiting, Fengchi (G 20), Hegu (LI 4) and Taichong (Liv 3) and pricking of Shaoshang (L 11), Shangyang (LI 1) and Lidui (S 45) if caused by intracranial hypertension, Fengchi (G 20), Yinfeng (SJ 17), Hegu (LI 4) and Shenmai (B 62) if caused by inner ear disorders, Danshu (B 19), Qimen (Liv 14), Youmen (K 21), Zusanli (S 36) and moxibustion at Tanzhong (Ren 17) and Rugen (S 18) if caused by gastro-intestinal disease, Shenshu (B 23), Qimen (Liv 14), Sanyinjiao (Sp 6), and Zhaohai (K 6) if caused by gynecological disease, Zusanli (S 36) instead of Shenshu (B 23) and Sanyinjiao (Sp 6) for vomiting during pregnancy, Fengchi (G 20), Dazhu (B 11), Ganshu (B 18), Qimen (Liv 14), Xiajuxu (S 39), and Taichong (Liv 3) for acid regurgitation, Juque (Ren 14), Zhongwan (Ren 12), Qimen (Liv 14), Hegu (LI 4), Zusanli (S 36) and Neiting (S 44) for gastric acid and belching, Zhongwan (Ren 12), Pishu (B 20), Zusanli (S 36) and Rangu (K 2) for anorexia, Zhongwan (Ren 12), Qihai (Ren 6), Qichong (S 30), Hegu (LI 4), Yuji (L 20), and Zusanli (S 36) and moxibustion at Rugen (S 18), Tanzhong (Ren 17) and Daling (P 7) for hematemesis, Tianshu (S 25), Xiawan (Ren 10), Qihai (Ren 6), Zhangmen (Liv 13), Zusanli (S 36), Xiajuxu (S 39), Sanyinjiao (Sp 6), Xingjian (Liv 2) for pain in the middle abdomen, moxibustion at Shenque (Ren 8) for nausea and vomiting without fever, Pishu (B 20), Weishu (B 21), Zhongwan (Ren 12), Zusanli (S 36), Yinlingquan (Sp 9), Sanyinjiao (Sp 6), Taibai (Sp 3) and Dadu (Sp 2) and moxibustion at Shenque (Ren 8) for indigestion, Zhongwan (Ren 12), Qihai (Ren 6), Zusanli (S 36), Neiting (S 44), Sanyinjiao (Sp 6) and Gongsun (Sp 4) for abdominal distension, moxibustion with onion at Shenque (Ren 8) is also very effective. For acute diarrhoea, Shuifen (Ren 9), Tianshu (S 25), Qihai (Ren 6), Dachangshu (B 25), Zusanli (S 36), Yinlingquan (Sp 9), Sanyinjiao (Sp 6), Yinbai (Sp 1) are needled. Needling is preferable to the heat syndromes while moxibustion to the cold syndromes. For chronic diarrhoea, Mingmen (Du 4), Shenshu (B 23), Dachangshu (B 25), Tianshu (S 25), Shenque (Ren 8), Qihai (Ren 6), Zusanli (S 36), Sanyinjiao (Sp 6) and Fuliu (K 7) are selected and moxibustion is preferable. For constipation, Dachangshu (B 25), Tianshu (S 25), Qihai (Ren 6), Daling (P 7), Zhigou (SJ 6), Zhaohai (K 6), Fenglong (S 40), Yinlingquan (Sp 9) are needled. For hematochezia, if the colour of the blood is bright-red, needling should be used, if the colour is dark red, both needling and moxibustion should be used or moxibustion should be mainly used. For intestinal hemorrhage, Pishu (B 20), Mingmen (Du 4), Zhishi (B 52), Tianshu (S 25), Qihai (Ren 6), Neiting (S 44), Taichong (Liv 3) and Yinbai (Sp 1) are selected. For rectal and anal hemorrhage, Mingmen (Du 4), Changqiang (Du 1), Weizhong (B 40), Chengshan (B 57), Kunlun (B 60) and Fuliu (K 7) are selected. For diarrhoea, Dachangshu (B 25), Shangliao (B 31), Ciliao (B 32), Zhongliao (B 33), Xialiao (B 34), Changqiang (Du 1), Qihai (Ren 6), Guanyuan (Ren 4), Chengshan (B 57), Kunlun (B 60), Zutonggu (B 66) are needled. For pain in the hypochondrium, Qimen (Liv 14), Zhangmen (Liv 13), Waiguan (SJ 5), Ligou (Liv 5), Taichong (Liv 3), Yangfu (G 38) and Zulinqi (G 41) are needled. For hepatosplenomegaly, acupuncture and moxibustion are applied at Pishu (B 20), Juque (Ren 14), Zhangmen (Liv 3), Zusanli (S 36), Xingjian (Liv 2), Sanyinjiao (Sp 6) and festering moxibustion at Zhongwan (Ren 12), and Pishu (B 20). For jaundice, acupuncture and moxibustion are performed at Dazhui (Du 14), Feishu (B 13), Zhiyang (Du 9), Danshu (B 19), Pishu (B 20), Zhongwan (Ren 12), Shimen (Ren 5), Zusanli (S

36), Yinlingquan (Sp 9), Yongquan (K 1), especially more moxibustion should be given at Zhongwan (Ren 12). For ascites, Sanjiaoshu (B 22), Shenshu (B 23), Shuifen (Ren 9), Qihai (Ren 6), Zhigou (SJ 6), Yinlingquan (Sp 9), Sanyinjiao (Sp 6), Yingu (K 10) and Fuliu (K 7) are needled and more moxibustion at Shuifen (Ren 9), Shenque (Ren 8) and Qihai (Ren 6). For lower abdominal pain, if it is caused by intestinal diseases, Dachangshu (B 25), Tianshu (S 25), Qihai (Ren 6), Zusanli (S 36), Shangjuxu (S 37) and Sanyinjiao (Sp 6) are needled; if it is caused by bladder diseases, Xiaochangshu (B 27), Pangguangshu (B 28), Zhongji (Ren 3), Waiguan (SJ 5), Zhigou (SJ 6), Yinlingquan (Sp 9), Sanyinjiao (Sp 6) and Zhongfeng (Liv 4) are needled; if it is caused by disorders of the uterus and appendix, Shenshu (B 23), Guanyuan (Ren 4), Zhongji (Ren 3), Shuidao (S 28), Guilai (S 29), Daimai (G 26), Ququan (Liv 8), Taichong (Liv 3), Sanyinjiao (Sp 6) and Zhaohai (K 6) are needled. For hernia, Guanyuan (Ren 4), Guilai (S 29), Ququan (Liv 8), Ligou (Liv 5), Zhongfeng (Liv 4), Taichong (Liv 3), Dadun (Liv 1) are needled. In case the lower abdominal pain pertains to cold syndrome, moxibustion can be applied on the abdominal region. For anuria, Sanjiaoshu (B 22), Shenshu (B 23), Jingmen (G 25), Yinlingquan (Sp 9), and Sanyinjiao (Sp 6) are needled and Tianshu (S 25) and Qihai (Ren 6) with moxibustion. For anuresis, Duiduan (Du 27), Shuidao (S 28), Zhongji (Ren 3), Qugu (Ren 2), Shaofu (H 8), Yinlingquan (Sp 9), Sanyinjiao (Sp 6), Fuliu (K 7), Dazhong (K 4) and Xingjian (Liv 2) are needled and moxibustion is performed at Qihai (Ren 6). For hematuria, Xiawan (Ren 10), Guanyuan (Ren 4), Qichong (S 30), Daling (P 7), Yinlingquan (Sp 9) are needled. For frequency of micturition, moxibustion is given at Huangmen (B 51), Shenshu (B 23), Qihai (Ren 6) and Zhongji (Ren 3), and needling at Yinlingquan (Sp 9), Zusanli (S 36) and Sanyinjiao (Sp 6). For incontinence of urine, Chengjiang (Ren 24), Qugu (Ren 2), Pangguangshu (B 28), Yinlingquan (Sp 9), Taichong (Liv 3) are needled and Qugu (Ren 2) and Dadun (Liv 1) with moxibustion. For styma, Qugu (Ren 2), Shaofu (H 8), Sanyinjiao (Sp 6), Zhaohai (K 6) and Ligou (Liv 5) are needled. For penis pain, Zhongji (Ren 3), Sanyinjiao (Sp 6), Taixi (K 3), Ququan (Liv 8), Xingjian (Liv 2) and Dadun (Liv 1) are needled. For leukorrhagia with thick red or yellow excretions, needling is preferable, and for that with thin white secretions, acupuncture and moxibustion should be used together. The points selected are Mingmen (Du 4), Daimai (G 26), Qihai (Ren 6), Guanyuan (Ren 4), Yinlian (Liv 11), Sanyinjiao (Sp 6). For lochiorrhea after labour, acupuncture and moxibustion are given at Shenshu (B 23), Qihai (Ren 6), Guanyuan (Ren 4), Sanyinjiao (Sp 6) and Yinbai (Sp 1). For infantile vomiting of milk, Tanzhong (Ren 17) and Juque (Ren 14) are needled. For infantile night crying, Jianshi (P 5) is needled and Baihui (Du 20) applied with moxibustion. For infantile convulsion, Yintang (Extra 1), Shuigou (Du 26), Dazhui (Du 14), Shendao (Du 11), Hegu (LI 4), Shaoshang (L 11), Wangu (SI 4), Kunlun (B 60), Xingjian (Liv 2), Yinbai (Sp 1) and Yongquan (K 1) are needled. For pain of the eyes, Fengchi (G 20), Shangxing (Du 23), Jingming (B 1), Hegu (LI 4), Sanjian (LI 3), Daling (P 7), Tongli (H 5), Neiting (S 44), Kunlun (B 60), Shenmai (B 62), Zhiyin (B 67) and Zuqiaoyin (G 44) are needled. For itching of the eyes, Jianming (B 1), Taiyang (Extra 2), Fengchi (G 20), Hegu (LI 4), Guangming (G 37), Xiaxi (G 43), Ganshu (B 18) are needled. For congestion of the eyes due to acute inflammation, needle Jingming (B 1), Shangxing (Du 23), Taiyang (Extra 2) (bleeding), Hegu (LI 4), Zulinqi (G 41) and Zuqiaoyin (G 44) (bleeding). For congestion of the eyes due to chronic eye diseases, Jingming (B 1), Hegu (LI 4), Daling (P 7), Ganshu (B 18) and Xingjian (Liv 2) are needled. For photophobia, Zanzhu (B 2), Jingming (B 1), Taiyang (Extra 2), Hegu (LI 4), Erjian (LI 2), Guangming (G 37) and Taixi (K 3) are needled. For lacrimation, Jingming (B 1), Zanzhu (B 2), Fengchi (G 20), Hegu (LI 4), Wangu (G 12) and Jinggu (L 8) are needled. For pain in the ears, Ermen (SJ 21), Tinghui (G 2), Yifeng (SJ 17), Wangu (SI 4), Jiache (S 6), Hegu (LI 4) and Zusanli (S 36) are needled. For tinnitus, Tinghui (G 2), Yifeng (SJ 17), Shenshu (B 23), Mingmen (Du 4), Yangxi (LI 5), Wangu (G 12), Zhongchong (P 9), Taixi (K 3) and Zusanli (S 36) are needled. For an echo in the ears, Ermen (SJ 21), Tinggong (SJ 19), Tinghui (G 2) and Yifeng (SJ 17) are mainly needled and combined with the different points according to the different conditions. For example, if the echo is caused by high fever and acute inflammation, Yemen (SJ 2), Pianli (LI 6) and Xiaxi (G 43) are added or Shaoshang (L 11) and Zuqiaoyin (G 44) are pricked to bleeding; if the echo is caused by chronic diseases of the ear, Shenshu (B 23), Hegu (LI 4), Zhongzhu (SJ 3) and Waiguan (SJ 5) are added. For nasal obstruction, Fengchi (G 20), Fengfu (Du 16), Shangxing (Du 23), Shuigou (Du 26), Yingxiang (LI 20), Hegu (LI 4), Lidui (S 45) and Zhiyin (B 67) are needled. For a runny nose, Fengfu (Du 16), Fengchi (G 20), Shangxing (Du 23), Shuigou (Du 26), Yingxiang (LI 20) and Hegu (LI 4) are needled; if free from fever, Xiaxing (G 43) can be added for moxibustion. For dysosmia, Fengfu (Du 16), Fengchi (G 20), Dazhui (Du 14), Shangxing (Du 23), Yingxiang (LI 20), Hegu (LI 4), Taiyuan (L 9) and Zusanli (S 36) are needled. For epistaxis, Fengfu (Du 16), Fengchi (G 20), Shangxing (Du 23), Yintang (Extra 1), Dazhui (Du 14), Jianjing (G 21), Hegu (LI 4), Weizhong (B 40), Neiting (S 44) and Lidui (S 45) are needled. For sore throat, Fengfu (Du 16), Yamen (Du 15), Tianzhu (B 18), Hegu (LI 4), Daling (P 7), Neiguan (P 6) and Neiting (S 44) are needled. For laryngemphraxis, Hegu (LI 4) and Yongquan (K 1) are needled and Shaoshang (L 11) and Guanchong (SJ 1) are pricked to bleeding. For severe cases, Jinjing (Extra 10) and Yuye (Extra 10) are added. For hoarseness and aphonia, Yamen (Du 15), Lianquan (Ren 23), Hegu (LI 4), Lingdao (H 4), Jianshi (P 5), Zhigou (SJ 6) and Yongquan (K 1) are needled. For swelling of the tongue, Fengfu (Du 16), Lianquan (Ren 23), Hegu (LI 4), Shaoshang (L 11) and Laogong (P 8) are needled and Jinjing (Extra 10) and Yuye (Extra 10) are pricked to bleeding. For dyscinesia of the tongue muscles, Yamen (Du 15), Lianquan (Ren 23), Hegu (LI 4), Tongli (H 5), Zhongchong (P 9), Rangu (K 2) and Sanyinjiao (Sp 6) are needled. For salivation, Dicang (S 4), Jiache (S 6), Zhongwan (Ren 12), Youmen (K 21), Daling (P 7), Xiajuxu (S 39) and Rangu (K 2) are needled. For swollen upper lip, Yingxiang (LI 20), Shuigou (D 26) and Hegu (LI 4) are needled and for swollen lower lip, Chengjiang (Ren 24), Zusanli (S 36), and Neiting (S 44) are needled. For upper toothache, Xiaguan (S 7), Taiyang (Extra 2), Hegu (LI 4), Neiting (S 44) and Taixi (K 3) are needled. If the pain is located anterior, Heliao (LI 19) is added. For lower oothache, Jiache (S 6), Daying (S 5) and Hegu (LI 4) are needled. If the pain is located anterior, Chengjiang (Ren 24) is added. If the pain can not be cured, Fengchi (G 20) and Xingjian (Liv 2) are added. For masticatory atonia, needling and moxibustion are performed at Touwei (S 8), Qubin (G 7), Xiaguan (S 7), Jiache (S 6) and Hegu (LI 4). For masticatory spasm, Xiaguan (S 7), Jiache (S 6), Hegu (LI 4) and Waiguan (SJ 5) are needled and the needling retained a long time. For a stiff neck, Renzhong (Du 26) of the Du Meridian, Yintang (Extra 1), Baihui (Du 20), Fengfu (Du 16), Dazhui (Du 14), Mingmen (Du 4) and Changqiang (Du 1) are needled. For difficult flexion and extension of the four major joints, Quchi (LI 11), Hegu (LI 4), Yanglingquan (G 34), Zusanli (S 36) and Weizhong (B 40) are needled, retaining the needle for a long time. For finger spasm, Quchi (LI 11), Shousanli (LI 10), Hegu (LI 4), Yangchi (SJ 4) and Wangu (G 12) are needled. For systremma, Weizhong (B 40), Chengshan (B 57) and Kunlun (B 60) are needled. If it is caused by cold, moxibustion is used at Chengshan (B 57). For esthesiodermia, the treatment should start from needling the distance points along the meridian, then the adjacent and local points can be selected gradually, or the points on the healthy side can be selected. For skin dysesthesia or anesthetic, local points and the distant points on the upper portion of the related meridian can be selected and the affected part can be treated with warm moxibustion. For paralysis, if the local sensation is normal, local points and the distant points of the related meridian can be taken. If there is sensory disturbance in the affected area, the distant points of the related meridian or the points on the healthy side should be needled first, then treat the affected side. Warm moxibustion can be added on the affected area as well. For neck pain, needling and moxibustion can be given at Fengchi (G 20), Tianshu (S 25), Dazhui (Du 14), Houxi (SI 3), Jugu (LI 16), Kunlun (B 60) and Shenmai (B 62). For pain in the scapular region, both acupuncture and moxibustion can be applied to Jianjing (G 21), Jianzhongshu (SI 15), Jianwaishu (SI 14), Bingfeng (LI 12), Tianzong (SI 11), Zhigou (SJ 6), Houxi (SI 3) and Wangu (SI 4). For pain of the upper limbs and joints, the adjacent points are selected. For neuralgia, in addition to the points selected along the meridian, Yunmen (L 2) and Jiquan (H 1) are added for pain in the palm, Jianjing (G 21) added for pain of the radial aspect, and Jianzhen (SI 9) and Tianzong (SI 11) added for pain of the back. For pain in the armpit, needling and moxibustion are used at Jiquan (H 1), Jianzhen (SI 9), Shaohai (H 3), Neiguan (P 6), Yangfu (G 38) and Qiuxu (G 40). For backpain, besides the local points, Houxi (SI 3), Jingqu (L 8), Weizhong (B 40), Kunlun (B 60) and Shenmai (B 62) are added. For pain in the lumbosacral region, besides the local points, Shuigou (Du 26), Tianjing (G 21), Weizhong (B 40), Kunlun (B 60) and Shenmai (B 62) are selected. For pain of the lower limbs and joints, the adjacent points can be selected. For neuralgia, in addition to the points selected along the meridian, the points on the lumbosacral area can be added. For cold hands and feet, acupuncture and moxibustion can be performed at Quchi (LI 11), Hegu (LI 4), Fengshi (G 31), Neiting (S 44), Zusanli (S 36) and moxibustion at Dazhui (Du 14), Gaohuang (B 43) and Qihai (Ren 6). For facial edema, Shuigou (Du 26), Zhigou (SJ 6), Yemen (SJ 2), Jiexi (S 41) and Gongsun (Sp 4) are needled. For edema of the lower limbs, Sanjiaoshu (B 22), Shenshu (B 23), Zusanli (S 36), Xiajuxu (S 39), Yinlingquan (Sp 9), Sanyinjiao (Sp 6) and Fuliu (K 7) are needled and Shuifen (Ren 9) and Qihai (Ren 6) for moxibustion. For cutaneous pruritus, Fengchi (G 20), Dazhui (Du 14), Fengmen (B 12), Feishu (B 13), Jiuwei (Ren 15), Quchi (LI 11), Hegu (LI 4), Zhigou (SJ 6), Fengshi (G 31), Xuanzhong (G 39), Weizhong (B 40), Sanyinjiao (Sp 6), Xuehai (Sp 10) and Ligou (Liv 5) can be selected according to the conditions of the disease.

THE THEORETICAL RESEARCH AND APPLICATION OF SCALP ACUPUNCTURE

—Fang Yunpeng's Clinical Experience

Fang Yunpeng was born in Huaiyang County, Henan Province, in 1909. He graduated from Henan Medical College in 1936. In his early period, he did Western surgery. Since 1948, he studied traditional Chinese acupuncture by himself. He attended a refresher course of acupuncture held by the Ministry of Public Health of the Central Government in 1952. In October, 1958, the paper *The Trial Use of Acupuncture Instead of Analgesics and Cardiotonic* was published in the journal *Health Communication* in Xi'an, and *The Perpetual Calender of Acupuncture, Acupuncture Calender, Ziwuliuzhu, Linggui Eight Methods Circular Clock Table and Its Applications* were printed afterwards. *The Perpetual Calender of Acupuncture* was edited into BASIC II Programme, and put into the microcomputer. Dr. Fang treated diseases by combining traditional Chinese medicine with Western medicine. He has researched a new acupuncture method—"Scalp Acupuncture," and published a book on it. Now he is a professor of the Acupuncture Department of Xi'an Municipal Hospital of Traditional Chinese Medicine, and deputy president of the Acupuncture Association of Shaanxi Province.

I. Academic Characteristics and Medical Specialities

During his clinical practice, Dr. Fang discovered some areas which can be needled but have not been explained by the meridians and nervous theory on the scalp. Through the treatment of thousands of patients and the observations on 150 kinds of diseases, the acupuncture areas were gradually developed, including seven areas, and twenty-one projective areas for treating cerebral diseases.

1. Locations and indications of the points

1) *Hidden pictography* The point area looks like the auto-miniature of the human body on the coronary, sagittal and lamboid sutures. a. Head and neck region: Three cm long and 2 cm wide for the anterior aspect of the coronary point, in which the head is 2 cm long and wide, and the neck is 1 cm long and wide. b. Upper limbs: The area from the coronary-sagittal joint along the coronary suture to the sphenoid-parietal suture (sphenoidal point) is 11 cm, in which the area from the coronary point to the shoulder of hidden pictography is 2 cm, from the shoulder to the elbow is 3.5 cm, from the elbow to the wrist 3.5 cm, and from the wrist to the tip of the finger is 2 cm (the same bilaterally). c. Trunk: The total length is 14 cm from the coronary-sagittal point to the

tip of lamboid suture, and is divided into back, waist and buttock, in which the back is 6 cm long and 3 cm wide (it is divided into upper, middle and lower parts, 2 cm each); the waist is 4 cm long and 2 cm wide (it is divided into the upper and lower waist, 2 cm long each); and the buttock is 4 cm long and 3 cm wide (it is divided into upper and lower portions, 2 cm each). d. The lower limbs: The length from the tip of the lamboid suture along the lamboid suture downward to the star point is 9 cm, and is divided into the hip, knee and ankle. The length from the tip of the lamboid suture to the hip is 1.5 cm, from the hip to the knee is 3 cm, from the knee to the ankle is 3 cm, and from ankle to the tip of the toe is 1.5 cm.

Indications of the hidden pictography: Diseases of the nervous system, vascular system and motor system, such as nervous headache, trigeminal neuralgia, migraine, deafness, tinnitus, intercostal neuralgia, sciatica, polyneuritis, sequelae of encephalitis, concussion, neurasthenia, epilepsy, aphasia, disorder of vegetative nervous system, hemiplegia, hypertension, hypotension, coronary heart disease, cardiac dysrhythmia, sprain of the lumbar muscle, mastitis and vertigo.

2) *Hidden zang organs* It refers to the hemilateral miniature of the human viscera and skin which lies transversely at the anterior hairline. The head faces the midline of the forehead; the foot faces the frontal corner, and it is divided into upper, middle and lower jiao, 6.5 cm in total length. a. The upper jiao: It includes the viscera of the chest above the diaphragm, upper limbs, the skin sense and cerebral thinking, 3 cm in total. The anterior 2 cm of the upper jiao is the head and neck area, the width is 1 cm above the hairline, and 0.5 cm below the hairline. Take 2 cm lateral to the frontal midline, and 2 cm above the anterior hairline as one point, 1 cm lateral to the midline of the frontal hairline, and 3.5 cm above it as another point, the connecting line of these two points is the position of the upper limbs of hidden zang organs, and is divided into forearm, upper arm and hand, 0.5 cm each, 1 cm behind the upper jiao, 2 cm above the hairline, and 0.5 cm wide below it is the chest area. b. Middle jiao: The viscerae above the umbilicus and below the diaphragm and the skin sensation of the trunk are 1.5 cm long, 1.5 cm wide above the hairline, and 0.5 cm wide below it. c. Lower jiao: The skin sensation of the viscera below the umbilicus and the genital system is 2 cm long in total. One and a half cm anterior to the lower jiao, 1.5 cm above the hairline, and 0.5 cm below the hairline are the lower abdomen, buttock and hip respectively. Half cm posterior to the lower jiao, 1 cm below the hairline is the area from the knee to the ankle, 1 cm below the hairline, and 0.5 cm below it is the foot area (the same bilaterally).

Indications of hidden zang organs: Abnormal sensation of the viscera and the skin, especially to pain, touch, cold, hot, numbness, itching, and a tense sensation, such as gastric spasm, cholecystitis, diarrhoea, menorrhalgia, entero-cholic pain, irregular menstruation, trigeminal neuralgia, spontaneous sweating, palpitation, disorders of the vegetative nervous system, endocrine disorders, pruritus, urticaria, neurodermatitis, rosacea, psoriasis, eczema, and allergic rhinitis.

3) *Reverse zang organs and pictography* They are located at the projective area of the cerebral cortex sensory and motor centre on the surface of the scalp, i.e. the functional locating area on the surface of the scalp of precentral and postcentral gyri, and indicated in dysfunctions of the sensory and motor centre.

4) *Twenty-one points* Referring to the projective area of the cerebral cortex function locating area on the scalp surface. a. Speech projective area of motor speech centre: Indications: Motor aphasia, dysphonia, stuttering, paralysis of the tongue muscle, pseudo-bulbar paralysis, paralysis of the lip muscle, underdevelopment of the brain, and tremor of the tongue. b. Thinking: Situated between the prominence of the bilateral frontal bone. Indications: Mental retardation, dementia, hysteria, hallucination, schizophrenia, nerous headache, hypertension, ataxia, loss of consciousness, neurosis, and peptic ulcer. c. Writing-projective area of the writing centre: Indications: Chorea, tremor, paralysis, aphasia, agraphia, hypertension, hypotension, emphysema, and cortical edema. d. Memory-projective area of the reading centre: Indications: Alexia, hypomnesia headache, vertigo, tinnitus, palpitation, soreness and pain of the lower back and the leg, seminal emission, insomnia, dizziness, edema, shortness of breath, delayed development of the brain, and sequelae of encephalitis. e. Signal—projective area of the signal centre: Indications: Sensory aphasia, epilepsy, insomnia, nervous headache, hysteria, psychosis, retardation of comprehension, amnestic aphasia, and delayed development of the brain. f. Motor-Balance—projective area of the motor balance centre: Indications: Aphasia, polyneuritis, parkinsonism, cerebrovascular accident, ataxia, acromelalgia, and rheumatic arthritis. g. Vision—projective area of the visual centre: Indications: Disturbance of visual acuity, hallucination, defect of the visual field, retinitis, clouded of cornea, glaucoma, papilloedema, turbidity of vitreous body, acute and chronic conjunctivitis, cataract, spasm of the eyelid, headache, dizziness, vertigo, and epistaxis. h. Balance—projective area of the balance centre: Indications: Hemiplegia, vertigo, general ataxia, nystagmus, parkinson's disease and disturbance of speech. i. Respiration and circulation—projective area of the respiratory and circulatory centre: Indications: Cough, asthma, palpitation, shortness of breath, tachycardia, arrhythmia, rheumatic heart disease, hypertension, coronary heart disease, and emphysema. j. Auditory—projective area of the auditory centre: Indications: Nervous deafness, tinnitus, dizziness, epilepsy, hallucination, homonymous hemianopsia, hypertension, pain of the eye, hysteria, and abdominal distension. k. Olfactory and gastric—projective area of the olfactory and gastric centre: Indications: Smelling and tasting retardation, smelling and tasting disturbance, acute and chronic rhinitis, epilepsy, hypomnesia, dizziness, migraine, salivation, cold, eczema and psoriasis.

Note: The above points, except "Thinking," are all bilateral.

2. Selection and combination of points

1) *Selecting corresponding points* Take the points of hidden pictography, hidden zang organ, reverse zang organ, and reverse pictography corresponding to the affected portion: e.g. leg disease is treated by selecting the corresponding point on hidden pictography or hidden zang organ of the lower limbs.

2) *Selecting mimic body points* Mimic selection of body points is made according to differentiation on the theories of meridians, organ picture, Yin-Yang and Five Elements. Carefully select the points from the "hidden pictography," "hidden zang organ," "reverse pictography" and "reverse zang organ." For example: In the case of

gastric pain and vomiting, points can be selected from the stomach at the middle jiao of the hidden zang organ, or at the place corresponding to the Zhongwan point of hidden pictography.

3) *Selecting points according to the special functions* According to the indications, the central points, such as auditory point, are used in tinnitus and deafness.

4) *Selecting the crossing points* Select the points at the bilateral and symmetrical limbs of hidden pictography or hidden zang organ, or select the overlapping or crossing points.

5) *Combination of the points* Combine the points a. at the corresponding hidden pictography and hidden zang organ; b. at the corresponding reverse pictography and reverse zang organ; c. at the corresponding hidden and reverse pictography; d. at the corresponding hidden and reverse zang organs; e. with those on the hidden pictography and zang organs; and f. scalp points and other points.

II. Case Analysis

Case 1: Wei syndrome (sequela of myelitis)

Name, Zhang x x; sex, female; age, 32; date of the first visit, September 12, 1972.

Complaints In February, 1972, Zhang had fever, cough and general pain, especially pain of the four extremities. She felt cold in the lower limbs three months later, then she got paraplegia in the right lower limb more severe than the left, and she couldn't get up. She also lost her appetite, and became thin. Sequela of myelitis and spinal arachnoiditis were diagnosed. She was given dibazol and vitamin B, but with no response. When she was treated by acupuncture, she was thin, cold and flaccid in the lower limbs, and she couldn't stand without help.

Prescriptions Lower limbs of the hidden pictography (bilaterally), lower part of the reverse pictography (bilaterally).

Treatment procedure The flying needling method was adopted, and the needles were retained for forty-five minutes to one hour. The symptoms were gradually relieved, and she could come to the clinic herself after eight treatments. She basically recovered after nine treatments. She could work normally on April 14, 1973.

Explanation Sequela of myelitis falls into the aspect of wei syndrome in traditional Chinese medicine, which is characterized clinically by flaccid atrophy of muscle and bones, paresthesia of the skin, and impairment of the hands and feet. This case was caused by invasion of pathogenic heat, burning of yin essence obstruction of Yangming Meridian, and loosening the muscles, resulting in wei syndrome. For scalp acupuncture, needle the hidden pictography. Clinical practice proved that it has good effect to diseases of motor system and vascular system. In the Department of Physiology of Shandong University, the experimental observation proved that acupuncture can elevate the excitement of the anterior horn motor cells of the spinal cord. So in treating that disease, good results can be obtained in needling the hidden pictography of its corresponding position in combination with reverse pictography.

Case 2: Tremor (sequela of encephalitis)

Name, Pan x; sex, female; age, 4; date of the first visit, September 3, 1972.

Complaints She suffered from pneumonia at the end of June of 1972, and was admitted to a hospital and treated for one month. A sequela remained after discharge, and she had convulsions, tremors, protrusion of the tongue, and straight eyes, aphasia, and difficulty in swallowing. She did not respond to traditional Chinese medicine or Western drugs.

Prescriptions Treated by scalp needles at the head portion of hidden pictography, upper jiao of hidden zang organ and points for speech.

Treatment procedure Apply direct flying needle penetrating method, retaining the needle for thirty minutes. She could cry after the first treatment, the sound of crying became soft after second treatment at the mouth area of reverse pictography, upper and lower limb points were added on the hidden pictography in the third treatment. Rest for four days after nine treatments. The child could run, and take food by herself. All the symptoms were gone except unclear speaking. After another five treatments, she could call her parents. She was basically recovered.

Explanation Hidden pictography is an effective area in treating motor disease. Hidden zang organ is more effective for sensory diseases. For this case, the disease is situated at the cerebrum, the corresponding points on the head and the speech points were selected as the projective area on the scalp surface of the speech centre of the cerebral cortex, and motor aphasia chiefly treated. The combination of the above points can promote the restoration of the sequela of encephalitis.

Case 3: Chest pain (coronary heart disease)

Name, Chen x x; sex, female; age, 38; date of the first visit, November 9, 1981.

Complaints She began suffering chest pain and a depressed feeling of the chest in summer of 1980, which gradually became worse, especially after hard labour, accompanied with palpitation dyspnea, general fatigue, thin body, sighing, pallor, dark purple tongue, thin white coating, deep and thready pulse.

Examination ECG suggested: 1) Myocardial strain, 2) Insufficiency of blood supply to the coronary artery. Blood lipid: Cholesterol 200 mg%, triglyceride 113 mg%. REG: Increasing of the tension of all the cerebral arteries, poor elasticity. Fundus: Arteriosclerosis II stage. BP: 90/60 mmHg.

Prescription Scalp acupuncture at heart and chest part of hidden zang organ, corresponding to the middle jiao of reverse zang organ in combination with the corresponding hidden and reverse pictography, and points of respiration and circulation.

Treatment procedure Treat once daily, ten treatments as a course. Retain the needle for thirty minutes, and a rest for two days after five treatments, four courses in all. Result of follow-up examination: ECG: Essentially normal. Blood lipid: Normal. Function of left heart: Essentially normal. The heart function had evidently improved from the examination on October 30, 1981. BP: 120/80 mmHg. REG: Fluoroscopy of the chest and fundi had no evident changes. The chest pain and depressed feeling disappeared, she felt short of breath only during walking upstairs, she was in good spirits, appetite, urination and bowel movement normal.

Explanation Chest pain is due to stagnation of qi and blood, obstructing the meridians, and insufficient nourishment of the heart. In Western medicine, it is called coronary heart disease. The treatment is to promote the blood circulation of the meridians. The experiments have proved that scalp points of hidden zang organ and reverse zang organ had the function of lowering blood lipid, and lowering the excitement of the sympathetic nerve, slowing down the heart rate, decreasing the myocardial oxygen consumption, increasing the output per beat of the coronary arteries thus improving the myocardial ischaemic condition. In 1982, forty patients with coronary heart disease were treated by this method, the total effective rate for disappearance and alleviation of the symptoms was 96.5 percent. The effective rate of improvement of ECG was 87.5 percent. Blood lipid had decreased evidently ($P < 0.01$). The difference was significant ($P < 0.01$) for 6 indices of the left cardiac functions before and after needling.

Case 4: Vertigo (hypertension)

Name, Yang x x; sex, male; age, 47; date of the first visit, May 2, 1982.

Complaints He felt dizzy frequently and had headaches for one year, accompanied by insomnia, amnesia, excessive dreaming and tinnitus. Recently, because of stress, the symptoms became aggravated, constipation, yellow and reddish urine, red tongue, thin yellow coating, thready and string-taut pulse. He had a past history of hypertension. Examination: BP: 160/100 mmHg, heart and lung(-), heart rate 76/min., regular rhythm, absence of murmur, liver and spleen (-), kidney (-). ECG: Normal. Fluoroscopy of the chest (-). Fundus: Arteriosclerosis, stage I. Blood cholesterol: 189 mg%, triglyceride 89.2 mg%. REG: Slight increasing of the tonicity of cerebral arteries, decreasing of elasticity.

Prescriptions Scalp needling method, coronary sagittal point, writing point (bilateral), respiratory and circulatory points (bilateral) in combination with corresponding liver and kidney area of hidden zang organ, waist area of hidden pictography.

Treatment procedure Apply flying needle method, treat once daily, ten treatments as a course, rest for two days after five treatments, no medication during treatment, retain the needles for forty-five minutes. Blood pressure lowered after first treatment. Symptoms disappeared after one course. Results of follow-up visit: BP: 120/80 mmHg. Cardiac beat: 70/min., chest fluoroscopy (-). ECG: Normal, fundus normal. REG: The elasticity of all arteries were improved. Blood cholesterol 126 mg%, triglyceride 64 mg%. His tongue was pale red, thin white coating. The pulse was slow. After follow-up examination, his blood pressure maintained at 120/80 mmHg, others were all normal.

Explanation This case, according to pulse, belongs to vertigo of yin deficiency and yang excess. It is called hypertension in Western medicine. The scalp needle of coronary sagittal point, writing, respiratory and circulatory points are all good for lowering pressure. The animal physiological experimental observations proved that they can calm the sympathetic nervous function and maintain the circulatory function; diminish or lower the irritability of the vascular tonicity, and lower blood pressure. Blood pressure was lowered after needling the above points five minutes later, in general, the best effect obtained within fifteen minutes. Six hundred and thirty hypertension patients have been treated since 1983. The effective rate was 96 percent; markedly improved, 75.77 percent, the average from $172.5 \pm 18.59/102.6 \pm 9{,}64$ mmHg to $141.0 \pm 17.89/85.1 \pm 9.14$ mmHg. The statistic difference is significant ($P < 0.01$).

The following points should be noticed during application of scalp acupuncture:

1) *The depth of scalp needling* Quick and perpendicular penetrating (fly needling) is applied and the needle should reach to the periosteum. Dr. Fang thinks that the periosteum tissue of the head is a pressure receptor, and is sensitive to the pressure. The pressure can produce an action as an "impulsive wave," and is easy to induce the point effect, concentrate and strengthen the energy effects and transformation, and change the pathological state of the local cortex, thus exerting the therapeutic effects. However, this method is suitable for those who are strong and not afraid of needling.

2) *Attaching importance to the needling time* The needling time is closely related to therapeutic effect. Needling before the onset of the illness for the disease which has evident regular onset can achieve preventive action or alleviate the symptoms. For example, the best result for treatment of malaria can be obtained two hours before the onset of disease. For the paroxysmal disease with evident aura, marked effects can be obtained if needled at the beginning of appearance of the aura, such as epilepsy, hysteria, and periodical paralysis. For bronchial asthma, needle at the beginning of the depressed feeling of the chest and urgency of the breath. For chronic peptic ulcer, needle at the beginning of the uncomfortable symptoms of the GI tract. If the patient has periodical attacks, needle half an hour before sleep for insomnia and enuresis. For the sequelae of poliomyelitis, the earlier the treatment, the better the results. For treating hemiplegia, Dr. Fang thinks that needling may start immediately after coma. At that time the pyramidal tract is still in a shock stage, and needling can stimulate it and promote its recovery. The result will gradually decrease after the pyramidal tract enters the recovery period.

3) *Application of the points at the affected side* Dr. Fang compared the results on needling the affected side and needling on the opposite side in clinic. The results proved that needling the affected side is better than needling the opposite side.

4) *Points and manipulation with special therapeutic effects* a. The tip of lamboid suture of a scalp needle is indicated in prostatitis, and the effect is better than with drugs. Manipulation: Penetrate quickly and perpendicularly (flying needling) into the periosteum, and retain the needle for thirty to sixty minutes. b. Needling the head portion of hidden pictography and hidden zang organ can achieve better effect in the treatment of nervous headache. c. Balance, balance and motor and writing points are good for vertigo and hypertension with a success rate of 75 percent (637 cases). d. Selection of the corresponding visceral portion of lower jiao of the hidden zang organ of scalp needle is effective for dysmenorrhia, appendicitis (except necrosis type), cholecystitis and cholelithiasis. The flying needle method is used for the above manipulations, with the needle deeply touching the periosteum or penetrating slowly, with heavy manipulation, deep into the periosteum.

5) *Different layer and depth on the points treat different diseases* a. Skin layer —skin disorders such as itching. b. Muscular layer—gastric spasm, numbness and soreness of muscular lesions. c. Periosteum layer—acute and severe diseases and various kinds of pain.

REFRESHMENT OF THE MIND, QUANTITATION OF THE MANIPULATION, ZANG-FU DIFFERENTIATION AND THE PRICKING METHOD OF BLOODLETTING

—Dr. Shi Xuemin's Clinical Experience

Dr. Shi Xuemin was born in the western suburb of Tianjin in 1938. He graduated from the Tianjin College of Traditional Chinese Medicine in 1962. In 1965 he attended the research course of acupuncture and moxibustion sponsored by the Ministry of Public Health. From 1968 to 1972, he served as a doctor on a medical team working in Algeria. Soon after he returned home, he organized an acupuncture department in the No. 1 Hospital Affiliated with the Tianjin College of Traditional Chinese Medicine. The small acupuncture department which consisted only of three medical workers soon developed into a medical teaching and research centre with a hundred acupuncturists, a hundred beds, a daily outpatient rate of a thousand and ten departments with modern equipment.

Dr. Shi is systematized the experience of past acupuncturists and combined it with his own clinical knowledge to raise the academic level of acupuncture. He has had success in treating such acute and severe diseases as windstroke, colic pain of the gallbladder, and pulseless diseases. Acupuncture Treatment of Windstroke by Refreshing the Mind of Resuscitation that he designed, was awarded the second prize of the scientific and technological achievements by the Tianjin municipal government in 1986. The Four Major Factors in the quantitation of the needling manipulation that he put forward was chosen as a scientific research achievement by the Scientific and Technological Commission of Tianjin in 1986 and by the TCM circles in China. His main works include the book *The Practical Acupuncture and Moxibustion* and the theses *The Clinical Application of the Reinforcing and Reducing Methods by Twirling and Rotating the Needle and the Conception of Quantitation of the Manipulation* and *The Clinical Observations on 617 Cases of Cerebral Infarction Treated with the Method of Refreshing the Mind for Resuscitation.* He is now the president of the No. 1 Hospital Affiliated with the Tianjin College of the Traditional Chinese Medicine, director of the Acupuncture Department, chief acupuncturist and professor.

I. Academic Characteristics and Medical Specialities

1. Advocating the method of "refreshing the mind, regulating the mind and calming the mind"

1) *The needling method of refreshing the mind for resuscitation* For twenty years, Dr. Shi has been making a study on the physiology, pathology, diagnostics and therapeutics of the mind. He put forward the following four points: Location of the mind—the heart houses the mind and the brain is the residence of the mind; principles of the mind

—the mind dominates all the external life activities; disease of the mind—it is the starting point of various diseases; treatment of the mind—the needling must, first of all, refresh the mind. He advocates the needling method of refreshing the mind for resuscitation, which is divided into two submethods—the method of "major regulation of the mind" and the method of "minor regulation of the mind."

a. The method of major regulation of the mind: Neiguan (P 6) of the Pericardium Meridian of the Hand-Jueyin and Renzhong (Du 26) of the Du Meridian are selected mainly to treat mental confusion and loss of consciousness such as tense and flaccid windstroke, palpitation due to fright, hysteria, epilepsy, mania and coma due to sunstroke or poisoning, and the long-standing diseases which cannot be cured such as lumbocrural pain, tinnitus, deafness and convulsions. Usually Neiguan (P 6) and Renzhong (Du 26) are selected as the main points and certain supplementary points can be added symptomatically.

b. The method of the minor regulation of the mind: Shangxing (Du 23) and Yintang (Extra 1) of the Du Meridian and Neiguan (P 6) of the Pericardium Meridian of the Hand-Jueyin are selected mainly to treat inorganic palpitation, pain, enuresis, impotence, and seminal emission.

2) *New explorations on windstroke* Since 1972, Dr. Shi has made a new study on windstroke from the following three fields:

a. The pathogenesis: Acupuncturists in the past had different opinions on the pathogenesis of windstroke, such as deficiency of qi leading to the invasion of the body by the pathogenic factors, the external wind invading the internal organs, sudden hyperactivity of the heart fire, the phlegm and dampness causing heat, and water failing to nourish wood. According to the saying—if the mind is affected, the twelve organs will be diseased—recorded in *Internal Classic*, Dr. Shi has made a thorough analysis of the two major symptoms of windstroke—mental disturbance and motor disturbance of the extremities. He holds that the main pathogenesis of windstroke is the dysfunction of the mind, which fails to direct the qi and failure of the extremities in motor function.

b. Treatment principle and point prescription: As there were different opinions about the pathogenesis of the windstroke on the part of the ancient acupuncturists, the methods of treatment were also different. These included: Expelling the wind and dredging the meridians, clearing away the heat and eliminating the phlegm, soothing the liver to stop the wind, supplementing qi and nourishing the blood. The points selected were often those Shu points on the yang meridians according to the theory of treating flaccidity syndromes with Yangming points in order to dredge the meridians and collaterals. However, Dr. Shi opened a new way, that is, he took "refreshing the mind for resuscitation" as the main method according to "the mind be diseased in case of failure in inducing resuscitation." In the treatment, he tried to refresh the mind for resuscitation and improve the residence of mind—the physiological function of the brain. In the selection of points, the points from the yin meridians were mainly applied. The main points are Neiguan (P 6), Renzhong (Du 26) and Sanyinjiao (Sp 6); and the secondary points are Jiquan (H 1), Chize (L 5), Weizhong (B 40) and Hegu (LI 4). Renzhong (Du 26) is the crossing point of the Du Meridian and the Hand and Foot Yangming Meridians. Needling it can adjust the Du Meridian, refresh the mind and strengthen the brain because the Du Meridian originates from the uterus and goes up to the brain. Neiguan (P 6), one of the Eight Confluent Points, connects with Yinwei Meridian and belongs to the Luo-Connecting point of the Pericardium Meridian of Jueyin, and is able to nourish the heart, calm the mind and activate the qi and blood circulation. Sanyinjiao (Sp 6), a crossing point of the Foot-Taiyin, Foot-Jueyin and Foot-Shaoyin Meridians, is able to tonify the kidney and promote the marrow. The kidney stores the essence and the essence produces the marrow. The brain is the sea of marrow. If the sea of marrow is rich, the restoration of the physiological function of the brain may be promoted. It has been proved through microcirculatory, blood-rheological and animal tests that Renzhong (Du 26) and Sanyinjiao (Sp 6) can greatly improve the blood circulation in the brain, increase the brain perfusion and strengthen the elasticity of the blood vessels. Neiguan (P 6) can not only improve the function of the heart, enhance the contraction of the cardiac muscle and increase the cardiac output, but also increase the brain perfusion. The combined use of the three points can promote the metabolism and renovation of the brain tissues and improve the physiological functions of the brain. The remaining four points on the limbs can be used to dredge the meridians and collaterals.

c. The manipulations: As windstroke was often explained by ancient acupuncturists as deficiency of the body resistance leading to the invasion of the wind and treated with the method of dredging the meridians and points selected from the three Yang Meridians, the reinforcing method was always adopted. Based on the pathogenesis of windstroke and the establishment of the needling method of refreshing the mind for resuscitation, Dr. Shi suggested that the manipulation should be the reducing method. Through the repeated experiments, he has specified the concrete manipulating methods of each point which are explained as follows: First the bilateral Neiguan (P 6) point is needled perpendicularly to 1.5 cun deep with reducing method by twirling, rotating, lifting and thrusting the needle for one minute, then Renzhong (Du 26) is pricked with the sparrow-pecking method until lacrimation appears or the eyes are full of tears. Then Sanyinjiao (Sp 6) is needled 1 to 1.5 cun deep along the posterior aspect of the tibia with the needle tip directed posteriorly and obliquely forming an angle of 45° between the needle and the skin. The reinforcing method is adopted by lifting and thrusting the needle to make the affected lower limb jerking continuously three times. Jiquan (H 1) point is inserted 0.5 to 1 cun deep and 1 cun away from the point along the meridian. The reducing method should be used by lifting and thrusting the needle until the affected upper limb continuously jerks three times. Weizhong (B 40) is taken at the supine position with the legs lifted. The needle is inserted 1 to 1.5 cun deep with the reducing method by lifting and thrusting the needle until the affected lower limb jerks three times. When Hegu (LI 4) is needled, the needle tip should be directed to Sanjian (LI 3) point with the reducing method by lifting and thrusting the needle until the affected index finger jerks three times.

Six hundred and seventeen cases of cerebral infarction and 113 cases of cerebral hemorrhage diagnosed by CT scans were treated with the above method. The clinical curative rate were 67.12 percent and 49.56 percent respectively. The effective rate was 96.46 percent.

3) *Intractable headache treated with the method of regulating mind* The intractable

headache can be seen in many kinds of diseases. Dr. Shi believes that the pathogenesis of the pain is due to obstructed circulation of qi and blood. The circulation of qi and blood is closely related to the heart and mind. The mind could lead the qi. When qi circulates smoothly, the meridian is free, and if the meridian is dredged, it will be free of pain. Therefore, the method of regulating the mind is used by needling Neiguan (P 6) and Renzhong (Du 26) points to regulate the qi and mind. Thus, analgesia often results.

4) *Infantile enuresis treated with the method of calming the mind* This disease, in the past, was ascribed to insufficient kidney qi, deficiency cold in the upper part of the body and deficiency of the spleen and lungs leading to failure of constraining. The treatment usually includes nourishing the primary qi and supplementing the kidney, invigorating the spleen and replenishing the qi and astringing the lungs and reducing the urination. However, according to Dr. Shi's observation, the main predisposing factors for infantile enuresis are mental stress and fatigue. The treatment should regulate the heart and mind. The points selected should be those which can nourish the brain and tranquilize the mind. So Renzhong (Du 26), Yintang (Extra 1) and Baihui (Du 20) are often used with satisfactory results.

5) *Tinnitus and deafness treated with the method of refreshing the mind to eliminate the disturbance* This is a commonly and frequently encountered disease among the elderly. Nervous tinnitus and deafness can last for a life time. Long-term tinnitus and deafness can cause mental confusion and lassitude of the patients. Until now there is no good therapeutic method both at home and abroad. According to the saying of "the insufficiency of marrow producing vertigo and tinnitus" recorded in *Internal Classic,* Dr. Shi put forward that the pathogenesis of the disease was due to the confusion of the mind, and disturbance of the heart. Therefore, the treatment should strengthen the brain and invigorate the ears, refresh the mind to eliminate the disturbance. Clinically Neiguan (P 6), Renzhong (Du 26) and Baihui (Du 20) combined with Yifeng (SJ 17), Tinggong (SJ 19) and Tinghui (G 2) are used with satisfactory results.

6) *Hiccup treated with the method of calming the mind and regulating the flow of qi* Though being a mild disease, hiccup is a kind of stubborn disease with its long and repeated attacks. There have been reported hiccup cases which lasted continuously for seven to ten days without being cured. Dr. Shi believes that the pathogenesis of the disease is due to the failure of descending the stomach qi, and the emotional instability and mental irritability are the common predisposing causes. According to the principle of controlling the mind to make qi travel freely, Neiguan (P 6) and Renzhong (Du 26) are often selected as the main points and Tiantu (Ren 22) and Tanzhong (Ren 17) as the secondary points. Good therapeutic effects are often obtained with this method.

In addition, the method of refreshing the mind for resuscitation is also used to treat hysteria including hysterical blindness, aphasia, auditory and visual hallucination, convulsion, spasm, tremor and paralysis. Usually the diseases can be cured after the needling.

2. The quantitative study on the needling manipulation

Dr. Shi thinks that the acupuncture should have its own theory of quantitation since it belongs to the catalogue of natural science. In order to explore the standard needling manipulation, he takes the basic manipulations, such as twirling and rotating, lifting and thrusting, and has made a study on the direction of insertion, the depth of needling, the time of retention and the time of interval between two needlings. After ten years of painstaking work, he has achieved the satisfactory results.

1) *The theoretical study* Dr. Shi put forward four major factors for the manipulation of reinforcing and reducing by twirling and rotating the needle. a. The relation between the reinforcing and the reducing by twirling and rotating the needle and the direction of the action force: With the Ren and Du Meridians as the centre, the action force by twirling and rotating the needle to the left side and to the right side directed centripetally is reinforcing and that to centrifugally is reducing. (The direction of the action force on the left side is clockwise and that on the right is counterclockwise. On manipulation, add the action force and let the needle twirl back naturally. The continuous twirling and rotating forms the reinforcing method; for the reducing method, the left side is counterclockwise and the right side is the clockwise.) For the Ren and Du Meridians, the methods reinforcing and reducing by puncturing along or against the running course of the meridians respectively, reinforcing or reducing by manipulating the needle in cooperation with the patient's respiration and even reinforcing and even reducing are used. This clinical study is more specific and more standardized than the statements "to rotate the needle to the left is the cold-reducing and to the right is the heat-reinforcing" by the ancient acupuncturists and "the thumb going forward is reinforcing and the thumb going backward is reducing" by the modern acupuncturists. b. The relation between the reinforcing and reducing by twirling and rotating the needle and the degree of the action force: In twirling and rotating the needle, if the amplitude is small and the frequency is high (the limitation is 1/2 revolution and the frequency is over 120 times/min.), it is reinforcing. In twirling and rotating the needle, if the amplitude is large and the frequency is low (the limitation is over one revolution and the frequency is 50 to 60 times/min.), it is reducing. This viewpoint has made the statement "small amplitude and light force is reinforcing and large amplitude and heavy force is reducing" going from macroscopic to the quantitative category in which there are data to follow. c. The optimum parameter for the duration of performing the reinforcing and reducing method by twirling and rotating the needle: one to three minutes for each point. This parameter was put forward after investigation and comparison one after another on 365 points from the regular meridians and fifty points from the extraordinary meridians. d. The optimum parameter for the interval between two needlings is three to six hours. The effect-sustained time after the needling varies with the diseases. In order to find out the effectively sustained time after the needling, Dr. Shi, after a thorough study on more than fifty diseases, put forward the optimum effect-sustained time for each point in the treatment of various diseases. For example, when Renying (S 9) is needled to treat the cerebrovascular diseases, the most obvious change in the rheoencephalogram can be found at the time three minutes after the needling. The cerebral blood supply becomes lessened six hours after the needling. Therefore, the treatment of this disease should be given every six hours. Another example is the acupuncture treatment of asthma. Three minutes after the reinforcing method is performed by twirling and rotating the needle,

the wheezing sound becomes weaker and the symptoms are alleviated. The optimum effectiveness of the treatment can last three to four hours, suggesting that another treatment should be given four hours later. The advancement of the four major factors is an encouraging attempt to the standardization and unification of the acupuncture quantitation.

2) *The clinical experiment* Dr. Shi's studying method—selecting the research subject from the difficult and severe cases and testing it in the clinical practice—runs through the whole process of the study on the acupuncture quantitation. The summary is as follows:

a. The clinical experiment on the improvement of the insufficient blood supply of the vertebrobasilar artery:

For fifty-four cases who were diagnosed as cerebral arteriosclerosis with the syndrome reflecting in the vertebrobasilar artery or insufficient blood supply caused by compression due to cerevical proliferation tested by EEG, rheoencephlogram and microcirculation, Dr. Shi selected the coupled Fengchi (G 20) and Wangu (G 12) of the Gallbladder Meridian of Foot-Shaoyang and Tianzhu (B 10) of the Bladder Meridian of Foot-Taiyang. On each point, the reinforcing method by twirling and rotating the needle at low amplitude and high frequency was performed for three minutes, twice daily. The symptoms, such as dizziness, vertigo, irritability and insomnia, were relevantly relieved. At the same time when the manipulation was performed, the occipitalmastoid leading figures at the time immediately after the needling, two hours later, four hours later and six hours later were recorded, showing that the wave amplitude was higher than that recorded before the needling and there appeared heavy pumping waves. All this revealed that the cerebral blood supply improved and the elasticity of the blood vessels had increased. This change was in accordance with the improvement of the clinical symptoms.

b. The clinical experiment on the treatment of cholelithiasis:

For 102 cases who were diagnosed as cholecystolithiasis by cholecystography and B-ultrasonic examination, Dr. Shi needled the bilateral Taichong (Liv 3) of the Liver Meridian of Foot-Jueyin and Yanglingquan (G 34) of the Gallbladder Meridian of Foot-Shaoyang and the right Riyue (G 24) with the reducing method by twirling and rotating the needle for one minute on each point. With the performance of this manipulation, the patient could feel a jerking sensation on the upper abdomen. Stones, especially the sand-like stones, could be discharged after three to seven treatments. An observation on the cholecystography films taken before and after the needling have been made in thirty cases. The films were taken immediately after the reducing method by twirling and rotating the needle at large amplitude and low frequency for one minute and with the position of the patient unchanged. The blurring of the films suggested the contraction of the gallbladder. The film taken three minutes after the manipulation was performed, showing a round stone in the gallbladder being moved to the neck of the gallbladder. Both the clinical experiments and physical observation have confirmed strongly that the application of the standardized quantitation in the reducing method by twirling and rotating the needle is conducive to bile excretion, to promote the expansion of the Oddi's sphincter and accelerate the discharge of the stones.

c. The clinical experiment on the treatment of the coronary heart disease:

For 380 cases who were diagnosed as having coronary heart disease by EEG, cardiac ultrasound and heart monitor, Dr. Shi needled Neiguan (P 6) of the Pericardium Meridian of Hand-Jueyin, Shenmen (H 7) of the Heart Meridian of Hand-Shaoyin, Xinshu (B 15) and Geshu (B 17) of the Bladder Meridian of Foot-Taiyang and Tanzhong (Ren 17) of the Ren Meridian with the reinforcing method by twirling and rotating the needle for three minutes. The oppressed feeling of the chest and stabbing pain of the left shoulder and arm lessened. An electrocardiogram showed that the S-T section was restored from the original basis and the amplitude of the T wave was raised, suggesting that the blood supply of the coronary artery and the oxygen consumption of the myocardium improved.

3) *The basic research* In order to find out whether there is any difference on each point treated by different quantitative manipulation, Dr. Shi has made an experimental comparison on the blood rheology and blood-lipid with the double blind method. The objects for observation were the in-patients who had suffered from windstroke for less than ten days. Most of them were ischemic cerebrovascular diseases at the acute stage with cerebral embolism. There were thirty cases in the first group, in which the standardized needling method to refresh the mind for resuscitation was applied. In the second group consisting of thirty cases, the needling method of refreshing the mind for resuscitation was still used, but the manipulation used was the traditional one. Then the following seven indexes, i.e. whole blood viscocity, packed cell volume, erythrocytic electrophoresis, platelet electrophoresis, cholesterol and high density lipoprotein were determined. The experimental results proved that the difference is not significant before the treatment by applying the method of refreshing the mind for resuscitation in comparing the standard quantitation with the non-standard quantitation. However, the seven indexes after the treatment changed greatly. The difference is significant ($P < 0.01$). The experimental results showed that the therapeutic effect was not only related to the point selection and point combination, but also to the difference of the manipulations. This has confirmed that the raising of the standardization of the quantitation of the needling manipulation is very important, and also has proved the scientific and application value of this method.

3. The application of differentiation according to the meridians and muscle regions

1) *The lumbocrural pain (sciatica)* This disease, which falls within the range of Bi-syndrome, can be induced by the disorders of the spinal joints and caused by the wind, cold and dampness. According to the main symptoms, severe pain from the waist to the buttock to the popliteal and ankle, Dr. Shi thinks that this disease is due to the affection of Taiyang and Shaoyang meridians. The symptoms are the same as those recorded in *Miraculous Pivot*: "Lumbago with a sensation as the waist being broken up, and inability to bend the hip joint, stiffness of popliteal fossa as being tied up, and pricking pain in the gastrocnemius muscles, and pain of all the joints." So Dachangshu (B 25), Zhibian (B 54), Weizhong (B 40) and Yanglingquan (G 34) of the Taiyang and Shaoyang meridians are selected. For the pain with long duration, Renzhong (Du 26) is added. The main point of the manipulation: Dachangshu (B 25) is needled at the prone position and

the needle is inserted 2 to 2.5 cun deep perpendicularly. The reducing method is used by lifting and thrusting the needle. The needling sensation is directed downwards to the heel or to the toes. Zhibian (B 54) is needled at the prone position with the needle inserted 3 to 3.5 cun perpendicularly. The reducing method by lifting and thrusting the needle is used to direct the needling sensation downwards to the tips of toes. The lower limbs should convulse three times. Weizhong (B 40) is needled at a supine position with the leg lifted. The needling sensation is directed downwards to the tips of the toes. The reducing method is used by lifting and thrusting the needle and the lower limbs should convulse three times. Yanglingquan (G 34) is needled obliquely 2 cun deep with the needle pointing downwards. The reducing method is used by lifting and thrusting the needle. The needling sensation is directed downwards to the tips of the toes. Renzhong (Du 26) is needled with the sparrow-pecking method. The needling can be stopped when the eyes have tears.

Dr. Shi has treated 110 cases of sciatica, among which the shortest duration of the disease was one month and the longest was eighteen years. The disease is mostly the secondary diseases due to spinal joints disorders, such as hyperplastic spondylitis, occult cleft spine and regressive degeneration of the interventebral discs. Some of them are the injury of piriformis, sacro-iliilis, coxarthritis, and injury of the lumbar soft tissues. With the above-mentioned method, the clinical cure rate was 83.6 percent and the total effective rate was 99 percent.

2) *Rheumatism with the blood vessels involved (pulseless syndrome)* This disease is often caused by the invasion of cold and dampness in the meridians, leading to short nourishment of qi and blood in the areas where the meridians pass through. There may appear weak pulse at the cun region, Chongyang (S 42) and Qi Street, and pain, cold and weakness. In case of long-standing presence, the disease will affect the zang-fu organs from the meridians. Such symptoms as palpitation, short breath, dizziness and blurring of vision may appear. According to the differentiation, Dr. Shi thinks that this disease is "arm syncope" of the Lung Meridian of Hand-Taiyin and the Heart Meridian of Hand-Shaoyin and "leg syncope" of the Stomach Meridian of Foot-Yangming. Therefore, he sets up the principle of treatment of dredging the meridians and selects Taiyuan (L 9) of the Lung Meridian of Hand-Taiyin and Renying (S 9) of the Stomach Meridian of Foot-Yangming as the main points. For no pulse on the upper limbs, linear needling is added on the Heart and Lung Meridians; for pulseless on the lower limbs, the linear needling is added on the Spleen and Stomach Meridians. For headache and dizziness, Fengchi (G 20) is added; for hyposia, Jingming (B 1) and Zanzhu (B 2) are added. For precordial pain and chest distress, Xinshu (B 15) is added. Taiyuan (L 9) is the Yuan-Source point of the lung and the Influential Point of the pulse. Needling of this point can reinforce qi and dredge the meridians. Renying (S 9) is the point where the meridian qi of the Stomach Meridian of Foot-Yangming is originated and a crossing point of the Yangming and Taiyang. There is plenty of qi and blood on this point and needling it can regulate qi and blood and dredge the meridians. The linear needling on the Heart, Lung, Stomach and Spleen Meridians is performed in order to dredge the meridians and regulate the qi and blood, and to disperse the yang qi. Fengchi (G 20) can dispel the wind and eliminate the pathogenic factors to clear away the dizziness. Xinshu

(B 15) can relieve the depression of the chest and reinforce qi, reduce the heart fire and tranquilize the mind. Jingming (B 1) can dispel the wind and reduce the pathogenic fire nourish the yin and brighten the eyes. The main points for manipulation: Taiyuan (L 9) is needled 0.5 cun perpendicularly with the reinforcing method by twirling and rotating for three minutes. Renying (S 9) is needled 1 to 1.5 cun perpendicularly with the reinforcing method by twirling and rotating for three minutes. The needling sensation is directed upwards along the lower teeth to the head and backwards to the back of the body diffusing to the front chest or the electric shock sensation travels along the shoulder, arm to the tip of the fingers. Needling along the meridian: Needling is performed on every other cun and the depth is one cun. The reinforcing method is used by twirling and rotating the needle and the needling sensation travels along the meridian. Fengchi (G 20) is needled with the needle tip pointing to the eyeball on the opposite side. The needling depth is 1 to 2 cun and the reinforcing method is applied by twirling and rotating the needle for three minutes. The needling sensation is directed to the vertex of the head. Xinshu (B 15) is needled obliquely to the direction of the spinal process, 1 to 1.5 cun deep, with the reinforcing method by twirling and rotating the needle. The needling sensation is directed along the hypochodrum to the chest. Jingming (B 1) is needled perpendicularly 0.3 cun deep until the local soreness and distention appear.

Dr. Shi once treated eighty-three cases of pulseless patients, among which seventy-nine cases had no pulse on the upper limbs with disappearance of the pulsation of the radial artery and the blood pressure of the upper limbs 0, and four cases with the affection below the descending aorta, weakness of pulsation of the femoral artery and disappearance of the pulsation of the dorsal arteries of the foot. The patients' ages ranged from twenty-one to twenty-three. All of them had dizziness, headache, chest fullness, cold limbs and low fever. After being treated with the above mentioned method, the clinical curative rate was 38.46 percent, the effective rate, 61.53 percent.

3) *Facial paralysis* For the patient who had the disease for a short duration with facial muscle atrophy, Dr. Shi, according to the characteristics that most of the running courses of the Hand and Foot-Yangming, and Hand and Foot-Shaoyang Meridians on the face and head, and the Muscle Regions located on the superficial portion of the body, thinks that the disease belongs to "real windstroke." The mechanism of the disease is the deficiency of qi, instability of the defensive yang and wind invading the muscle regions, leading to twisting of the mouth and eyes. Long duration of the disease will cause the loss of the nourishment on the muscle regions and muscular atrophy. So he set up the principle of dispelling the wind and promoting the blood circulation and soothing the muscle regions. The shallow needling with multipoints and penetration towards multidirection are adopted. The points selected were Yangbai (G 14) penetrating Touwei (S 8), Shangxing (Du 23), Jingming (B 1) and Sizhukong (SJ 23) to soothe the muscle regions on the forehead angle; Taiyang (K 1) penetrating Dicang (S 4), and Dicang (S 4) penetrating Jiache (S 6) to correct the twisting of the mouth and eyes. Because of the muscle atrophy caused by the long-standing pathogenic factors and the blood stasis on the muscle regions, Taiyang (Extra 2), Quanliao (SI 18) and Jiache (S 6) are needled with the bloodletting method in combination with cupping to remove the blood stasis and activate the blood circulation. The main points for manipulation: All of the points are

needled with the reducing method by twirling, rotating, lifting and thrusting for one minute each. The amount of bleeding for each bloodletting puncture is 3 to 5 ml.

Fifty cases of facial paralysis were treated with the above-mentioned method. All of them had a duration of over one year accompanied with facial muscle atrophy of different degrees. Among them, forty-seven cases were cured within one month. The average number of days for the patient to be cured was forty-one and the total effective rate was 94 percent.

4) *Constipation* Dr. Shi thinks that the main pathogenesis of the disease is excessive heat in the Yangming Meridian, and failure of the intestines in transmitting the wastes. The Lower He-Sea point of the Large Intestine Meridian of Hand-Yangming—Shangjuxu (S 37) is selected as the main point and the left Shuidao (S 38), Guilai (S 29) and the two points 2 cun lateral to the left Shuidao (S 38) and Guilai (S 29) (temporarily named as Waishuidao and Waiguilai) as the auxiliary points. The main points for manipulation: Based on the four major factors, first needle the bilateral Shangjuxu (S 37) for 1 to 1.5 cun, then needle Shuidao (S 38), Guilai (S 29), Waishuidao and Waiguilai on the abdomen. The needle tip should be inserted obliquely downwards 2.5 to 3 cun deep. The reducing method is used by twirling and rotating the needle and retaining of the needle for twenty minutes.

With this method, 250 cases of constipation were treated, among which, 214 cases had primary cerebrovascular diseases, 15 cases of habitual constipation, 8 cases of gastroptosis, 7 cases of traumatic paraplegia, 3 cases of hyperplastic spondylitis of the lumbar vertebrae, 1 case of myelitis, 1 case of amyotrophic lateral sclerosis and 1 case of fracture of femoral shaft. One third of the patients could pass stools twenty minutes after the needling and most of them could pass stools around one hour after the needling. Fifteen cases of habitual constipation could pass stools normally after the treatment for one week. The total effective rate was 94.6 percent.

4. The application of the venous bleeding with cupping

Dr. Shi uses the method of venous bleeding with cupping in clinic to treat asthma, pain of the supra-orbital bone, trigeminal neuralgia, brachial plexus neuralgia and periarthritis of shoulders.

The venous bleeding method comes from the *Miraculous Pivot*. The function is to reduce the excessive yin and yang, but not to harm the body resistance. The main point is to control the amount of blood. Only when the diseased blood is removed can the pathogenic factors be eliminated. Howeve, with the traditional bloodletting method, the blood may flow out naturally. It is difficult to clear away all the diseased blood. Cupping is used immediately after the venous bleeding at the affected area. The operator can observe through the transparent cup the amount of blood. When the expected volume is reached, remove the cup. When the diseased blood is completely removed and the pathogenic factors are eliminated, the therapeutic effect can be achieved more quickly.

Dr. Shi treated an old woman, who could only sit in bed supported by her arms. She had a pale and flabby face with the mouth open, flaring nostrils, and stridor in the throat. The patient complained that she had had the disease for thirty-one years, which became worse in winter and spring. She had visited many doctors, but the disease could not be cured. Dr. Shi thought that for long-term asthma, there must be deficiency of the body resistance and excess of the symptoms. The treatment should reinforce the lung qi and remove the pathogenic factors by venous bleeding. The Back-Shu points from Dazhu (B 11) to Geshu (B 17) were needled with the reinforcing method by twirling and rotating the needle for one minute. Then the bilateral Feishu (B 13) and Geshu (B 17) were needled with a three-edged needle. When the blood was seen, the points were cupped with glass cups. The cups were removed when the blood reached 10 ml in each cup. Immediately after the cupping, the patient had smooth breathing. Twenty minutes later, she began to feel comfortable in the chest. On auscultation, it was found that the dry and wet rales became more alleviated than before. After only ten treatments, the patient was cured and no relapse was found until the present time. In twenty years, Dr. Shi has treated altogether 160 cases of asthma, among which 78 had had the disease more than 15 years; 34 cases were complicated with pulmonary emphysema, 17 cases with pulmonary infection and 11 cases had erythrophage higher than normal. After being treated with the needling combined with the venous bleeding, two thirds of the cases had their symptoms removed after one treatment and one third of the cases had their symptoms removed after twenty to thirty treatments. The total effective rate was 95.6 percent.

In winter, Dr. Shi treated a patient with trigeminal neuralgia who had the disease for twenty-five years. He had received nerve blocking three times, but relapses were always found two years after the operation. The patient then had severe paroxysmal pain in the left forehead, zygomatic and mandibular regions and he could not wash, drink and take food. He had lassitude and was thin. Dr. Shi thought that this disease was due to excess-heat of the spleen and stomach, long-standing depression transforming into fire, which goes upward to disturb the head along the meridian and blocks the meridian qi and blood. The principle of treatment should promote the blood circulation to remove the blood stasis and dredge the meridians to kill the pain. First Taiyang (Extra 2) was penetrated towards Dicang (S 4) and Zanzhu (B 2) with the reducing method by twirling and rotating the needle for one minute. Then Taiyang (Extra 2), Quanliao (SI 18) and Jiache (S 6) were selected with the method of venous bleeding followed by cupping. The amount of blood in each cup was 5 ml. When the manipulation was over, the patient began to feel alleviation of the pain. After another seven treatments, the case was cured. In recent years, Dr. Shi has treated altogether 83 cases of trigeminal neuralgia, among which, 13 cases of which had a duration of one year, 15 cases of 1 to 3 years, 24 cases, 3 to 5 years and 21 cases, over 5 years. About 90 percent of the cases were cured within one week of treatment using the method of venous bleeding in combination with cupping.

In summer, a patient came to Dr. Shi for help. The patient had frequent spasms of the right facial muscle, especially during mental stress. The disease was caused by the wind seventeen years ago. Treatments of thread burial therapy and drug injections were unsatisfactory. Dr. Shi held that this disease was due to the blockage of meridians by the six exogeneous pathogenic factors, which were turned into dryness and wind because of the long-standing depression. The treatment should promote the blood circulation to eliminate the wind and dredge the meridians to stop the pain. Dr. Shi first penetrated Taiyang (Extra 2) towards Dicang (S 4) with the reducing method by twirling the needle for one minute. Then the method of venous bleeding combined with cupping was performed at Taiyang (Extra 2), Xiaguan (S 7) and Quanliao (SI 8). The amount of blood in each cup was 5 ml. After the manipulation, the spasm was stopped. Though the relapse appeared again three hours later, the degree was greatly reduced. After twenty treatments, the disease was cured completely. In recent years, fifty-five cases of facial spasm have been treated by Dr. Shi, all satisfactorily using the above method.

II. Case Analysis

Case 1: Windstroke (hemorrhage in basal ganglion)

Name, Sun x x; sex, male; age, 46; date of the first visit, March 11, 1986.

Complaints He suffered from hypertension for ten years, and he suddenly had difficulty in moving his right limbs, slurred speech and left migraine twenty days before. Five minutes later, he had paraplegia on the right limbs. The lumbar puncture performed in a Western hospital revealed hemic cerebrospinal fluid and the CT scan showed hemorrhage of left basal ganglion and bleeding into the cerebral chamber. The patient was in a dispirited state. He could respond to questions but with slurred speech. The patient had central facial paralysis on the right side and the myodynamia was degree zero. His tongue proper was red with a thin white coating and the pulse was irregularly intermittent. The rheoencephalogram showed that the occipitalmastoid wave amplitude was low and flat. The X-ray film of the chest showed aortic type of heart and ECG showed chronic coronary insufficiency of blood supply and ventricular premature beat. The nervous system: Right Hoffmann's sign (+), bilateral Bard's sign (+).

Differentiation Excess yang qi invading upwards to disturb the brain and the mind. The treatment should refresh the mind for resuscitation and dredge the meridians.

Prescription Neiguan (P 6), Renzhong (Du 26), Sanyinjiao (Sp 6), Jiquan (H 1), Chize (L 5), Weizhong (B 40) and Hegu (LI 4).

Treatment procedure After two months' treatment with the method of refreshing the mind for resuscitation, the patient's speech and motor abilities were totally recovered. The CT reported the hematoma absorbed.

Case 2: Clonic convulsion (major chorea)

Name, Wang x x; sex, male; age, 59; date of the first visit, April 15, 1986.

Complaints The patient used to get angry easily. One week before he was attacked by wind after physical labour. He began to suffer from aching and weakness all over the body and then involuntary movement appeared. The symptoms would become aggravated by mental distress and external irritation. The tongue proper was red with thin yellow coating and the pulse was deep and slippery. No abnormal findings in the examination of various kinds.

Differentiation Stirring of the liver wind. The treatment must be directed to refresh the mind for resuscitation and suppress the liver-yang and eliminate the wind.

Prescription Neiguan (P 6), Renzhong (Du 26), Hegu (LI 4), Taichong (Liv 3),

Sanyinjiao (Sp 6) and Taixi (K 3).

Treatment procedure After the treatment with the above method for half a month, the amplitude of the limbs' movement was lessened and the involuntary movement disappeared one month later.

Explanation Usually this disease is treated with the method of nourishing the liver and stopping the wind. However, Dr. Shi, according to the theory "the wind controls the movement of the four extremities," set up the method of refreshing the mind for resuscitation. He treated the disease with Neiguan (P 6) and Renzhong (Du 26) (the main points for major regulation of the mind) and Taichong (Liv 3) and Hegu (LI 4) (the main points for minor regulation of the mind). Because the patient was over sixty years old and he had deficiency of the liver and kidney, Sanyinjiao (Sp 6) of the Spleen Meridian of Foot-Taiyin and Taixi (K 3) of the Kidney Meridian of Foot-Shaoyin were selected to stop the wind and recover the mind. The patient was then cured with satisfactory effect.

Case 3: Inflammation of the throat (pseudobulbar paralysis)

Name, Xu x x; sex, female; age, 70; date of the first visit, April 24, 1986.

Complaints On April 4, 1986, the patient suddenly had weakness of the right side of the body. She was diagnosed by CT in the First Affiliated Hospital of Tianjin Medical College as having an embolism of the left thalamus. Two days later, there appeared aphasia and choking of the water and food. The patient had to take food by nasal feeding. Examination: Dysphagia, aphasia and weakness of the right side, normal uvulae, unable to lift the soft palate, sluggish pharyngeal reflex, normal tongue, sluggish left physiological reflex and the left Bard's sign (+). No other abnormalities were found.

Differentiation Dysfunction of the house of the mind, leading to inflammation of the throat. The treatment was to refresh the mind for resuscitation and relieve the sore throat and remove the stagnation of qi.

Prescription Neiguan (P 6), Renzhong (Du 26), Fengchi (G 20), Wangu (G 12), Tianzhu (B 10) and Shanglianquan (Extra 3).

Treatment procedure With the above-mentioned method, the patient was treated for three weeks. Then she was discharged from the hospital with recovered swallowing function.

Explanation The main symptom of the inflammation of the throat is disturbance of the swallowing function. Generally nasal feeding is given. Most of the patients are thin and weak. Dr. Shi thinks that this disease is due to disturbance of the mind caused by dampness and heat, phlegm turbidity, yin deficiency and yang hyperactivity. The mechanism of the disease is also the disturbed mind, leading to the dysfunction of the throat and tongue. Therefore, Neiguan (P 6) and Renzhong (Du 26) were selected to refresh the mind for resuscitation. Fengchi (G 20), Wangu (G 12), Tianzhu (B 10) and Shanglianquan (Extra 3) were selected to relieve the sore throat and remove the stagnated qi. Needles of No. 32 were used and the needle tip was directed to the laryngeal protuberance. The needling depth was 2.5 to 3 cun and the reducing method was used by twirling and rotating the needle. When Shanglianquan (Extra 3) was needled, the tip of the needle should be pointed towards the hyoid bone and the depth was 2 to 2.5 cun. The reinforcing method was used by twirling and rotating the needle. Each point was needled for three minutes. According to the clinical observation on 130 cases, this prescription and manipulation were found to have very good therapeutic effect on the throat inflammation (pseudobulbar paralysis). The total effective rate was 97 percent.

Case 4: Hypochondriac pain (cholelithiasis)

Name, Xu x x; sex, female; age, 51; date of the first visit, March 9, 1974.

Complaints The patient suffered from colicky pain of the right upper abdomen which was induced by the emotional stress for four months. The pain was relieved by antispasmodics, but became clonic. Usually the attack was accompanied by vomiting, high fever and heavy sensation on the back. The patient was found to be in an exhausted state with a sallow and lustreless complexion. The tongue was red with dark purple margins. The pulse was string-taut and thready. Examination: Temperature, 39.6℃; Murphy's sign, (+); WBC, 22000/mm^3; neutrality, 89 percent. Blood amylase, 32 units. Eight pieces of round stones could be seen by a cholecystography.

Differentiation Retention of dampness and heat in the liver and gallbladder. The stones were formed by long stagnation. The treatment should soothe the liver and nourish the gallbladder.

Prescription Right Riyue (G 24), Yanglingquan (G 34), Fenglong (S 40), right Ganshu (B 18) and Danshu (B 19).

Treatment procedure After being treated with the above-mentioned prescription, the patient felt that the symptoms were apparently relieved one week later. The appetite and body temperature became normal. Debris of the stones were discharged intermittently. After one month treatment, no stone was found in the cholecyotography and the patient was cured.

Explanation Most of the cholelithiasis are due to the stagnation of qi and damp heat in the gallbladder so that the heat will burn the bile and long stagnation will form stones. Dr. Shi adopted the method of combining the Back-Shu points with the Front-Mu points and he selected the points Ganshu (B 18), Danshu (B 19), and the Front-Mu point Riyue (G 24) as the main points and the He-Sea point of the Gallbladder Meridian Yanglingquan (G 34) as the auxiliary point to treat the internal organs. Fenglong (S 40) of the Stomach Meridian of Foot-Yangming was added to promote the function of the intestines and remove the stagnation to discharge the stones.

Case 5: Headache (vascular headache)

Name, Zhang x x; sex, male; age, 29; date of the first visit, April 18, 1986.

Complaints The patient was so addicted to the wine that his daily intake was one fourth of a kilogram. After a heavy drink one week before, he began to suffer from severe headache the following day. The findings of the lumbar puncture and cerebrospinal fluid examinations were normal. No response was found to sedative drugs. When the patient was transferred to our hospital, he was conscious and the headache was paroxysmal. During the attacks, the pain in the bilateral Taiyang regions, Wangu (G 12) point behind the ear and the posterior occipital regions was especially severe. The tongue proper was dark red with yellow and greasy coating. The pulse was string-taut and tense. Examination: Eyeground (-), rheoencephalogram, extremely low frontalmastoid leading wave and extremely irregular occipitalmastoid leading wave, suggesting poor blood-supply of the cerebral artery.

Differentiation Dampness and heat going upwards to disturb the mind. The treatment was to clear away the heat and eliminate the dampness, and dredge the meridians and stop pain.

Prescription Fengchi (G 20), Wangu (G 12), Tianzhu (B 10), Taiyang (Extra 2), Yintang (Extra 1), Sanyinjiao (Sp 6) and Renzhong (Du 26).

Treatment procedure After two treatments with the above-mentioned points, the disease was basically relieved. One week later, the patient began to have a clear mind. The rheoencephalogram showed higher frontalmastoid and occipitalmastoid wave amplitudes. After another week consolidating treatment, the patient was discharged from the hospital.

Explanation According to the theory of the meridians and collaterals, Dr. Shi thought that the pain was located on the places where Hand and Food-Shaoyang and Foot-Taiyang Meridians pass through. Therefore, he selected the Shu points Fengchi (G 20), Wangu (G 12) and Tianzhu (B 10) of the affected meridian as the main points combined with Renzhong (Du 26) and Yintang (Extra 1) in order to regulate the mind, with Sanyinjiao (Sp 6) and Taiyang (Extra 2) to reduce the dampness and heat of the head and eyes. Because the treatment was proper, the pain was stopped.

Case 6: Pain of the shoulder and arm

Name, Su x x; sex, female; age, 49; date of the first visit, July 31, 1985.

Complaints The patient began to have pain of the right shoulder and arm which was induced by strain three years before. The pain would become more severe on exertion. The patient had difficulty in rotation and lifting the upper arm, inability to comb her hair and take off her clothes. The tongue proper was dark red with thin and white coating. The pulse was deep and string-taut. Examinations: Limitation in abduction, forward and backward rotation of 45°. The pulling test of the brachial plexus (+). There were no other abnormal findings.

Differentiation Deficiency of qi and blood stasis. The treatment was to remove the blood stasis and promote the blood circulation and dredge the meridians to stop the pain.

Prescription Venous bleeding combined with cupping at Jianyu (LI 15) and Naoshu (SJ 10).

The amount of blood for each point is 5 to 10 ml/time. The reducing method is used by lifting and thrusting the needle at Jianyu (LI 15), Jianzhen (SI 9) and Wangu (SI 4).

Treatment procedure After three treatments with the above method, the pain disappeared. No relapse was found up to now.

Explanation The patient used to have a weak constitution. The root cause of the affection of the right arm is the deficiency. In case qi fails to command the blood, the blood stagnation occurs in the shoulder and arm and causes pain. She in fact had deficiency in root cause and excess in symptoms. According to the theory of "treating the acute symptoms in case of emergent cases," Dr. Shi combined the venous bleeding with cupping. The case was cured after three treatments.

Case 7: Chronic colitis

Name, Zhang x x; sex, male; age, 31; date of the first visit, June 25, 1981.

Complaints The patient suffered from disease of the intestines due to an attack by cold five years before. The disease attacked intermittently. The pain in the left abdomen became more and more severe and the patient had to move the bowels four to seven times a day. The patient had lassitude, sallow complexion, emaciation, loss of appetite, indigested food, mucus stool, pale red tongue, thin white and greasy coating, and slow and weak pulse. Examinations: Stool routine, "mucous stool." The results of the other tests were all normal.

Differentiation Stagnation of cold in the intestines and failure in digestion and transportation of the spleen and stomach. The treatment was to strengthen the function of the spleen and stomach.

Prescription Zhangmen (Liv 13), Tianshu (S 25), Guanyuan (Ren 4), Shuidao (S 28), Pishu (B 20) and Zusanli (S 36).

Treatment procedure All of the symptoms were relieved after two weeks' treatment with the above-mentioned points. The patient began to move bowels once daily and the routine examination of the stool was normal. No relapse was reported in the follow-up visit until the present time.

Explanation Dr. Shi thought that this disease was caused by the cold. When the disease lasted a long time, the primary qi became weak and the intestines lost their astringency. This is why the patient had diarrhoea for five years. As it said in *Miraculous Pivot* that "the large intestine dominates the essence and the small intestine dominates the fluids." Tianshu (S 25), the Front-Mu point of the Large Intestine Meridian of Hand-Yangming and Guanyuan (Ren 4), the Front-Mu point of the Small Intestine Meridian of Hand-Taiyang were selected as the principal points to regulate the intestines. Pishu (B 20), Zhangmen (Liv 13) and Zusanli (S 36) points were taken as the auxiliary points to reinforce the primary qi. Shuidao (S 28) was used to treat diarrhoea by means of diuresis. Then the disease was cured.

Case 8: Herpes zostor

Name, Lin x x; sex, female; age, 66; date of the first visit, March 18, 1986.

Complaints The patient was admitted to the hospital for windstroke. One day before she visited the hospital, she ate fish and shrimps. Then rashes were found around her waist the following day. The rashes were the size of rice grains, red in colour, with a small amount of purulent secretion, mild burning felt by palpation with burning and stabbing pain. The tongue proper was red with yellow coating, and the pulse was string-taut. No abnormalities were found on examinations.

Differentiation Heat resulted from the greasy food overflowing the skin. The treatment was to reduce the heat, remove the dampness and stagnation and dredge the meridians.

Prescription Prick the place where the rashes located with a three-edged needle. When bleeding appears, the cupping should be used. The amount of blood for each cup was 5 ml.

Treatment procedure Only after two treatments with twelve cups, the rashes were subsided and the case was cured.

Explanation Because the patient ate a lot of fish, the heat was stagnated in the spleen and stomach. The heat overflows the skin and herpes developed. When the cupping method was adopted, the pathogenic blood was expelled and the disease was cured.

PROFICIENCY IN PENETRATING POINTS WITH THE GOLD NEEDLE

—Ye Xinqing's Clinical Experience

Ye Xinqing (1908-1969), a native of Dayi County, Sichuan Province, learned medicine from a famous doctor Wei Tingnan in Hankou in 1921, and finished his studies in 1933. After graduation, he returned to Sichuan, and ran a clinic with his colleagues Gong Zhixian, Zhang Letian, Tang Yangchun in Chongqing. He practised medicine first and then started to train students. He helped establish the Academy of Traditional Chinese Medicine in 1955. Dr. Ye was busy in his clinic, and so he left no works for the public.

I. Academic Characteristics and Medical Specialities

1. Treating aplastic anemia by nourishing the liver

Dr. Ye held that the liver was the first one to be affected by emotional factors. Instead of maintaining the patency for the flow of qi, the disfunctioned liver qi will transversely attack the spleen, which leads to failure of the spleen in transportation and transformation, thus resulting in deficiency of kidney water and retention of deficiency-heat. For the treatment, the stress should be put on the liver and spleen. To nourish yin should be done first. The liver should be regulated, the spleen strengthened, and the kidney nourished. Points Zusanli (S 36) and Sanyinjiao (Sp 6) were bilaterally needled with retaining the needle and Qimen (Liv 14) and Zhongwan (Ren 12) were pricked for the purpose of bringing about the free flow of qi. In June of 1953, a 52-year-old female patient came to Ye's clinic, complaining of dizziness, vomiting, shortness of breath and weakness of the legs, and loss of appetite. She had pallor, red and slippery tongue without coating, thready and rapid pulse, the hematochrome 2.5g%, RBC 860.000/mm^3, and blood platelet 40.000/mm^3. Aplastic anemia was diagnosed by the osteostixis. She was sent to many hospitals and treated for eight months. She had fourteen blood transfusions totalling 3300 ml blood, but no response was found. Dr. Ye needled Zusanli (S 36) and Sanyinjiao (Sp 6) points once every other day, retaining the needles on both sides alternatively for thirty minutes. After withdrawing the needle, Qimen (Liv 14) was pricked in combination with Chinese herbs, such as dried Radix Rehmanniae, Rhizoma Dioscoreae, Fructus Corni, Radix Ophiopogonis, Radix Codonopsis Pilosulae, and Semen Coicis to nourish yin of liver and kidney, and Radix Stellariae, Mountain Radicis, Cynanchi Radix, Rhizoma Anemarrhenae, and Certex Phellodendri to regulate the liver and reduce the heat. After being treated for eighty days, the symptoms disappeared and the patient could do some light work.

2. The combination of dispersing with the gold needle and reinforcing and reducing with herbs

Dr. Ye preferred to use a self-made gold needle. Making the gold needle: 10 percent red copper is added to 90 percent gold, refine the mixture, remove the residues and draw it into needle 0.28 mm in diameter, which is similar to the No. 32 stainless steel needle used at present. The gold needle is divided into 3 cun (75 mm) and 5 cun (125 mm), and characterized by a thin and long body, short handle and soft quality.

When the needle is inserted, the lower portion of the needle is held by the thumb and index finger of the puncturing hand. The thumb is almost perpendicular to the needle body. An angle of 15° to 30° is formed between the needle body and the skin. The thumb of the pressing hand is against the needle tip and presses the skin while the puncturing hand inserts the needle forcefully into the point. This special inserting technique is not only suitable for the characteristics of the fine, long, and soft gold needle, but also practical for preventing pain during the insertion. The pressing hand could feel the arrival of qi and at the same time fix the point. Dr. Ye described the arrival of qi as "fish eating the bait," neither too strong nor too gentle. A warm sensation would be appreciated because it results in remarkable improvement. If the warm sensation travels along the running course of the meridian to the diseased area, the curative effect would be even better.

It is stated in *Plain Questions* that "the herbs are treating the diseases deeply located inside the body, while acupuncture is better for the treatment of those on the superficial portion of the body." Dr. Ye put forward the combination of these two, because the herbs function well in reinforcing or reducing, while acupuncture functions well in regulating qi circulation. For example, the bolus "Wumeiwan" (Mume pills) for Jueyin disease mentioned in *Treatise on Febrile Diseases* (written at the end of the Han Dynasty, 206 B.C.-220 A.D. by Zhang Zhongjing) is originally used for the acute abdominal pain with cold limbs brought on by ascarisis. Dr. Ye adapted it to a decoction based on the principle that the herbs of cold and hot natures used together reduce the pathogenic factors and reinforce the body resistance at the same time. It is effective when the decoction of "Wumeiwan " (Mume pills) prescribed for the complicated cases of those who failed to respond to the repeated treatments, such as deficiency-cold headache, dizziness, prolonged dysentery, ulcer, and functional gastrointestinal disorders. The key link in differentiation is that the tongue coating is white but not dry, the pulse is deep but not rapid. The administration depends on the practical application. The amount of Cortex Cinnamomi and Radix Aconiti Praeparata is reduced but that of Rhizoma Coptidis and Certex Phellodendri is added in case of excessive heat. On the contrary, the amount of Cortex Cinnamomi and Radix Aconiti Praeparata is added, but that of Rhizoma Coptidis and Certex Phellodendri is reduced if the cold is preponderant. A patient aged twenty-seven suffered from severe migraine on the right side for three years. She had pallor, nausea and vomiting during attack. No response was found after being treated by Chinese and Western medicine as well as acupuncture and moxibustion. Dr. Ye needled Taichong

(Liv 3), the Front-Mu and Yuan-Source point of the Liver Meridian, and Qimen (Liv 14) in combination with Fengchi (G 20), Touwei (S 8), and Taiyang (Extra 2) to eliminate the pathogenic wind-cold in the Liver Meridian. Shuaigu (B 8) was needled too to nourish the liver, activate the blood circulation and eliminate the wind. Treat once every other day with acupuncture and administering of "Wumeiwan" (Mume pills) every day. Nine g of the Radix Aconiti Praeparata slices were boiled for half an hour first, and then 3 g of Cortex Cinnamomi, 3 g of Herba Asari, 6 g of dry ginger slices, 1 g of Pericarpium Zenthoxyli, 6 g of Rhizoma Coptidis, 6 g of Certex Phellodendri, 12 g of Radix Condonopsis Pilosulae, 12 g of Radix Angelicae Sinensis and 9 g of Mume are added. The migraine stopped after ten acupuncture treatments and no recurrence was found since then.

3. Penetrating along meridians, retaining to wait for qi

Dr. Ye laid stress on penetrating. His techniques are as follows: 1) A 15° to 30° angle is formed between the needle body and the skin. After insertion, the needle is lifted and thrust in accordance with the direction of meridian. 2) Obliquely insert the needle to penetrate several points without diverging from the meridian.

The following are the combination of points:

1) *Penetrating the points of the same meridian* For instance, Waiguan (SJ 5) to Zhigou (SJ 6)—febrile diseases, headache, tinnitus, hypochondriac pain, shoulder and arm soreness and numbness of the fingers; Jianshi (P 5) to Neiguan (P 6) and Daling (P 7)—heart pain, palpitation, epilepsy, vomiting, spasm of elbow, and swelling of axilla; Zusanli (S 36) to Shangjuxu (S 37)—dyspepsia, borborygmus, diarrhoea, abdominal distention, poor appetite, abdominal pain due to appendicitis; Zusanli (S 36) to Xiajuxu (S 39)—Wei and Bi-syndrome of the lower extremities, and mastitis; Qihai (Ren 6) to Guanyuan (Ren 4)—lumbago, prolonged dysentery, dysmenorrhea, enuresis, impotence and ejaculation praecox; Zhongwan (Ren 12) to Xiawan (Ren 10)—sinking of qi of the middle jiao, weakness of the spleen and stomach.

2) *Penetrating the points of different meridians* For example, penetrating five points with one needle. Insert the needle into Quchi (LI 11), penetrated to Chize (L 5), Quze (P 3), Shaohai (H 3), and Xiaohai (SI 8) for diarrhoea, elbow and joint pain. Penetrating three points with one needle: Penetrate Taiyang (Extra 2) to Xiaguan (S 7), Yifeng (SJ 17) to Tongziliao (G 1), Dicang (S 4) to Jiache (S 6) for facial pain (trigeminal neuralgia), and facial paralysis, aphasia, salivation and clenching of teeth due to windstroke; Waiguan (SJ 5) to Sanyangluo (SJ 8) for motor impairment of the upper extremities due to windstroke; Yanglingquan (G 34) to Yinlingquan (Sp 9) for paralysis of the lower extremities due to windstroke; Neixiyan (Extra) to Waixiyan (S 35) for all the diseases of knee joints; Ligou (Liv 5) to Guangming (G 37) for eye disorders; Zhongwan (Ren 12) to Tianshu (S 25) for stomach and intestinal diseases.

Miraculous Pivot says that "the crux of acupuncture is to get the arrival of qi. Only when the arrival of qi is obtained can the therapeutic effect be achieved." Dr. Ye manipulated the needle to promote the arrival of qi and direct the qi to the diseased area. In addition, he maintained in the spirit of *Compendium of Acupuncture and Moxibustion* that the needles should be retained for half an hour in the main points to wait for the arrival of qi. By doing this, better results can be achieved, as the body resistance is increased in case of the arrival of qi.

II. Case Analysis

Case 1: Insomnia

Name, Xi x x; sex, male; age, 62; date of the first visit, December 6, 1960.

Complaints The patient began to have difficulty in falling asleep when he was twenty years old because of mental tension and overstrain. The symptom was aggravated gradually, and he could sleep two or three hours only every night and always disturbed by bad dreams, accompanied with irritability, hot temper, paroxysmal burning pain lasting for half an hour each time on the left cheek, flushed face, red eyes, general dryness and heat. Sometimes all the symptoms disappeared after a few days. He was attacked twice that year before he came to China. He had been to many countries for treatment, but in vain. He asked for treatment by traditional Chinese medicine. Neurosis was diagnosed because nothing abnormal was found in the examination. The tongue coating was yellow and thin, the pulse was deep, thready and rapid.

Differentiation Flaring up of deficiency-fire due to deficiency of the liver and kidney. The principle of treatment was to nourish yin and calm the mind. This is what is known as replenishing the water, especially that of kidney and liver, to check the fire.

Prescription Sanyinjiao (Sp 6), Taixi (K 3), Ligou (Liv 5), Qimen (Liv 14), Zhongwan (Ren 12), and Shenmen (H 7).

Treatment procedure Puncture bilaterally Sanyinjiao (Sp 6), Taixi (K 3), and Ligou (Liv 5) with slow insertion and withdrawal of the needle and retaining the needles to wait for the arrival of qi. Prick the right Qimen (Liv 14), with rapid insertion and withdraw the needle for reducing, and prick Zhongwan (Ren 12) and Shenmen (H 7) bilaterally with an even movement. Treat once a day. After ten days treatment, the patient could sleep eight or nine hours at night, the irritability disappeared.

Explanation The patient was overtired in mental work which consumed yin and essence. Dr. Ye selected Sanyinjiao (Sp 6), the meeting point of the three yin meridians, as the main point, combined cleverly Taixi (K 3) to nourish water, Ligou (Liv 5) and Qimen (Liv 14) to moisten the wood, Shenmen (H 7) to ease the mind, and Zhongwan (Ren 12) to protect the stomach. The points selected were so exactly to the pathogenesis that the effect was remarkable.

Case 2: Disharmony between the liver and stomach

Name, a foreign visitor; sex, female; age, 43; date of the first visit, February 15, 1959.

Complaints The patient had had a dull pain in the epigastrium since 1955. The gastric analysis showed the gastric acidity was low. She was once treated for chronic gastritis. She went to the Soviet Union for treatment as she felt it becoming worse in

1958. She vomited after eating. She left the Soviet Union for home until the symptoms were relieved forty-five days later. But she suffered again after several months and the condition was even worse. A mild duodenal stagnation was spotted by the barium meal examination. An abortion was done on February 3, 1959. After operation, the epigastric distention was relieved, but the vomiting was as serious as before. She suffered from over excitement, unreasonable crying and laughing, and constipation. She turned pale when talking about the meal owing to the terrible vomiting. Admitted to the Friendship Hospital, she was diagnosed as having nervous vomiting. No relief was found after the treatment with sedatives and antispasmodics. The amount of vomit was at first about 600 ml. The vomiting happened one or two hours after eating, but later nearly half an hour once. There was no coating on the tongue. The pulse at "guan" region was deep and string-taut. Differentiation: Disharmony between the liver and stomach, leading to transformation of qi into fire. The principle of treatment was to clear the liver, harmonize the stomach, descend the perverted qi and stop vomiting.

Prescription Taichong (Liv 3) and Yanglingquan (G 34) with reducing method; Zusanli (S 36), Zhongwan (Ren 12), Neiguan (P 6), and Tanzhong (Ren 17) with even movement; retain the needle for thirty minutes. Treat once a day. The decoction was administered too. The prescription includes 6 g of Radix Ginseng, 3 g of Fructus Euodiae, 12 g of Radix Ophiopogonis, 12 g of Poriae Cocos, 6 g of fried Hordei Vulgaris Germinantus, 3 g of Retinervus Citri Reticulatae Fructus, 2 g of Rhizoma Coptidis, 6 g of Endothelium Corneum Gigeriae Galli, 12 g of Radix Paeoniae Alba, 2 g of Radix Aucklandiae, 12 g of Herba taraxaci and 2 g of Radix Glycyrrhizae.

Treatment procedure Two days later after treatment, vomiting was relieved and eight days later vomiting stopped. The patient felt a little headache and sore arms, which were controlled by puncturing Yintang (Extra 1), Jianyu (LI 15), and Quchi (LI 11) five times. After half a year of recuperation, there was no recurrence.

Explanation This is a case of wood stagnation , fire overacting on the stomach, disharmony between the liver and stomach, which causes vomiting and constant regurgitation. Dr. Ye knew that regulating the qi mechanism should be the key to the treatment. So he selected Taichong (Liv 3), the Yuan-Source point of the Liver Meridian, Yanglingquan (G 34), the He-Sea point of the Gallbladder Meridian, in combination with Tanzhong (Ren 17), the point of qi, Zusanli (S 36), the He-Sea point of the Stomach Meridian, Zhongwan (Ren 12), and Neiguan (P 6). Only when the qi mechanism is regulated could the liver and stomach be harmonized and the vomiting be stopped automatically.

Case 3: Hypochondriac pain due to cold-damp

Name, Liang x x; sex, male; age, 55; date of the first visit, October 24, 1963.

Complaints The patient suffered from the right hypochondriac pain radiated to the right shoulder for five years, accompanied with fever, jaundice, and vomiting. The frequency of attacks increased during that year. He was admitted to a hospital, where the acute attack of chronic cholecystitis and cholelithiasis were diagnosed by cholecystography. No improvement was achieved after the treatment of both Western and Chinese medicine.

Examination Pain of the right hypochondrium, abdominal distention, poor appetite, loose stools, white and sticky tongue coating but yellow at the root, deep and string-taut pulse. Differentiation: Retention of cold-damp and disharmony between the liver and spleen. The principle of treatment was to warm yang, dispel cold and harmonize the functions of the liver and spleen.

Prescription Gongsun (Sp 4), Neiguan (P 6), Zusanli (S 36), half an hour retaining. Pricking Zhongwan (Ren 12), Qimen (Liv 14), and Ganshu (B 18).

Treatment procedure Treat once every other day. The extract of "Wumei" (Mume) was administered one dosage every other day. The pain stopped and appetite increased after ten days of treatment. No relapse was found after half a year.

Explanation It is stated in *Miraculous Pivot* that "if the liver is ill, there must be hypochondriac pain." The case mentioned above is that the cold-damp causes the pain in hypochondrium. Reinforcing the spleen in transportation and transformation, and regulating the liver in keeping the free flow of qi are the important methods. Gongsun (Sp 4) and Neiguan (P 6)—one pair or the Eight Confluent Points, Zhongwan (Ren 12)—the Front-Mu point of the stomach, and Zusanli (S 36)—the Lower He-Sea point of the stomach are combined with Qimen (Liv 14) and Ganshu (B 18) to eliminate the cold-damp. When qi of the liver is regulated, the hypochondriac pain is removed.

POINT APPLICATION AND HERBAL MOXIBUSTION

—Tian Conghuo's Clinical Experience

Tian Conghuo, a native of Jinzhou, Liaoning Province, was born in 1927. After he graduated from the Chinese Medical College in 1951, he acknowledged Zhu Lian and Gao Fengtong as his masters in the Acupuncture Experimental Institute of the Ministry of Public Health in 1952. He became a teacher of the South-China Training Course for Teachers of Acupuncture and Moxibustion in Wuhan in 1953. He has been engaged in acupuncture clinical practice, teaching and research for more than thirty years, emphasizing the combination of acupuncture, moxibustion, herbs and massage in his clinical practice. The adhesive plaster for relieving asthma made by Tian and his colleagues achieved the research prize of the Ministry of Public Health. He has published more than thirty treatises, among which some of them were published in foreign countries. His works include *Experiences in Acupuncture and Moxibustion* and *Essentials of Chinese Moxibustion*. Now he is a research fellow in the Second Clinical Institute of China Academy of Traditional Chinese Medicine, a member and vice-secretary-general of the Standing Committee of China Society of Acupuncture. He was invited to be an honorary member of the Spanish Acupuncture Society and the Polish Acupuncture Society.

I. Academic Characteristics and Medical Specialities

1. Advocating the point application

Point application, guided by the theory of meridians and collaterals, is a method in which external medicine is used to stimulate the points. Dr. Tian has found out the laws through his thirty years of clinical practice and research.

1) *The characteristics of Chinese medicine applied to points*

a. Pungent, penetrating, restoring consciousness clearing and activating the meridians: e.g. borneol, musk, cloves, herba menthae, herba asari, pericarpium zanthoxyli, semen sinapis albae, spina gleditsiae, ginger, onion, semen allii tuberosi and garlic, etc.

b. Strong taste and vigorousness, poisoning and used freshly e.g. fresh arisaema cum bile, fresh rhizoma pinelliae, radix aconiti, radix euphorbiae kansui, fructus crotonis, mylabris, and calomel, etc.

c. Animals or organs of animals, e.g. sheep liver, pig kidney and crucian, etc.

According to Dr. Tian's experience, the herbs with hot nature function effectively while those with cool nature next; the herbs with eliminating nature function quickly, while those with reinforcing nature next.

2) *The principles of selecting points and commonly used points* The principles of selecting points are almost the same with those of acupuncture. The use of sneezing for

upper disease, that of filling in for middle disease and that of sitting for lower disease are the principles for external medicine in ancient China. Based on this principle, Dr. Tian proposes that:

a. For the diseases of the upper jiao, Tanzhong (Ren 17), Xinshu (B 15) and Laogong (P 8) points are mostly selected; for the diseases of the middle jiao, Shenque (Ren 8), Zhongwan (Ren 12), Zhangmen (Liv 13) and Qimen (Liv 14) points mainly used; and for the diseases of the lower jiao, Guanyuan (Ren 4), Mingmen (Du 4), Shenshu (B 23) and Yongquan (K 1) points often chosen.

b. The corresponding Back-Shu and Front-Mu points are commonly used for diseases of zang-fu organs.

c. Mental disorders and the ptosis of visceral organs due to qi deficiency are mostly treated by Baihui (Du 20), Dazhui (Du 14), Tanzhong (Ren 17) and Qihai (Ren 6) points.

d. For local inflammation, sprain, wind-damp Bi-syndrome and masses in abdomen, local or adjacent Ashi points are appropriate.

In a word, the number of points to be selected is comparatively less, one or two points for each treatment. The commonly used points are more than forty, especially the points located in the chest, abdomen, low back and back.

3) *The forms of processed drugs* Mashed, exudate, extract, powder, paste, pill, medicinal cake and lozenge, which are selected according to the pathological conditions, locations of diseases, and individual and seasonal conditions. For instance, mashed garlic is applied to Yongquan (K 1) to treat hemoptysis and epistaxis, mylabris exudate applied to Pishu (B 13) and Tanzhong (Ren 17) to treat asthma. In addition, there are adhesive plasters for asthma, powder for lumbago, paste for irregular menstruation, cakes for malaria, lozenge for phlegm-humour and so on.

4) *Indications* Point application can be used for more than eighty kinds of diseases of all departments. Among which thirty kinds are common indications, such as arthritis, ganglion, mastitis, allergic rhinitis, malaria, bronchitis, asthma, hemoptysis, ulcer, chronic enteritis, chronic dysentery, hypertension, coronary heart disease, dysmenorrhea and enuresis, etc.

5) *Precautions*

a. The duration of application should be strictly controlled. The medicines with strong stimulation and great toxicity should be applied to small areas for not more than four to six hours to prevent blisters from occurring in large areas or medicine poisoning. Careful attention should be paid when it is used for children.

b. If the patient is allergic to the medicine, the application should be stopped immediately and desensitization should be employed if necessary.

c. For pregnant women, strong stimulation and toxic medicines must be especially carefully used.

d. The medicines should be applied within the period of validity and should be used as quickly as possible if mixed.

e. The medicines which cause blisters are generally avoided for facial application to prevent pigmentation.

Dr. Tian used point application to treat many kinds of diseases, especially to treat asthma successfully. Asthma and bronchitis, frequently encountered diseases, have been short of effective methods in prevention and treatment for many years. Dr. Tian has observed thousands of patients with the point application, and has created the adhesive plaster for relieving asthma with winter disease treated in summer, based on the ancient prescription after changing some herbs and points. It prevents reoccurrence.

The preparation of herbs and application of the adhesive plaster for relieving asthma:

Grind 21 g of the baked semen sinapis albae and rhizoma corydalis, and 12 g of radix euphorbiae kansui and herba asari into fine powder. The quantity should be enough for one patient for one year's use. On hot summer days, one third of the powder is mixed with raw ginger juice. A hundred g fresh raw ginger after cleaning is immersed in the water and then ground into pieces to squeeze the juice out, then placed on six pieces of paper or plastic cloth 5 cm in diameter each. Stick them with adhesive to Feishu (B 13), Xinshu (B 15) and Geshu (B 17) bilaterally for four to six hours in general. If a burning sensation or pain exists in the local region, remove them in advance. Keep them on the back longer if there is itching, hot and a comfortable feeling. Apply once every ten days. No matter whether the patient is in remission or during the attack, the asthma plaster can be applied, generally for three years continuously. This method is effective for patients who have yang deficiency and cold excess such as cold feeling in the body and on the back and spitting white thin sputum, but not so good for those who have heat signs such as aversion to heat and spitting yellow thick sputum. It is not advisable for patients who have a fever due to the lung infection complicated with brochiectasis resulting in hemoptysis. The best time to apply the plaster is at noon on a sunny day. The therapeutic result is not very effective if it is applied on a cloudy day. Before the plaster is removed from the back, the patient is asked not to move quite often to prevent the herb paste from falling down. In 1976 and 1977, Dr. Tian followed up 1,074 patients who had been treated by the plaster. Among these, 785 were asthmatic bronchitis patients, the effective rate was 79 percent; 289 were bronchial asthma patients, the effective rate was 83.7 percent; 59 patients of which had no reoccurrence within three to six years. The curative rate was 23.1 percent. Through the tests of the ability of phagocytose of macrophagocyte in the blisters' fluid, the immunoglobin A and G content of the blisters' fluid and the rate of lymphocyte blastogenesis, we have found that after the point application, the nonspecific immunity of the body was increased; the oxyphil cells in blood obviously decreased, suggesting that the application could reduce the hypersensitivity of the body. The great increase of cortisol in blood plasma indicates the improvement of the functions of the thalamus-pituitary body-adrenal cortex system. Thus the functions of the plaster in preventive treatment were ensured. In addition, the stimulation to the points by point application and the absorption and metabolism of herbs, the influences to the physical-chemoreceptors concerned to the lungs directly or reflexly regulate the functions of the cerebral cortex and vegetative nervous system in improving the reaction of the body and in increasing the antipathogenic qi. Thus, the prophylactico-therapeutic purpose is achieved.

2. Magical moxibustion

1) *Taiyi moxa-stick for treatment of retention of urine* In October, 1984, Dr. Tian was invited to see a 63-year-old female patient who suffered from retention of urine. Enuresis occurred after the operation of retinopathy. A catheter was kept in her urethra for twelve days leading to infection. Treatment of both Western and Chinese medicine, as well as acupuncture was tried but with no improvement. Dr. Tian thought it was due to obstruction of qi and blood in the lower jiao, which resulted in a disturbance of the free flow of qi in Sanjiao and the blockage of the water passage. Therefore, he treated her with Taiyi moxa-stick to remove the obstruction and to disperse stagnation. In the first treatment, Qihai (Ren 6), Shuifen (Ren 9), Shenque (Ren 8) and Tianshu (S 25) points were bilaterally selected, and Taiyi moxa-stick wrapped with six layers of white cloth was used to pack the points respectively. After three treatments of moxibustion in this way, the patient had a desire to urinate. The treatment was continued when the patient was sitting on a bedpan. She felt the abdominal distention was much relieved while the urine dripped. On the following day, the same moxibustion method was applied to points Guanyuan (Ren 4), Shuidao (S 28) and Shenque (Ren 8). After being treated three times on the same day, the urine could be discharged, but the patient felt difficulty urinating and had a feeling that she could not discharge her urine completely. After the treatment on the third day, she discharged urine smoothly. There was no longer any disturbance of urination when the treatment was carried on for five days. Taiyi moxa-stick was developed by changing the prescription of herbs based on the thunder-fire moxa-stick. Taiyi Moxa-Stick Technique was the earliest special work dealing with the Taiyi moxa-stick, which is made by rolling the moxa wool and the herbs with pungent and fragrant, dispersing cold, distributing and promoting resuscitation in nature. Its functions are to warm and remove obstructions from the meridians, disperse cold, induce resuscitation and stop pain. Dr. Tian used such a method quite often for the intractable wind-cold-damp Bi-syndromes, Wei-syndromes, abdominal pain and retention of urine. The manipulation is special. One method is to cover the point with ten layers of cotton paper or five to seven layers of cotton cloth, then press the ignited moxa roll on the point for one or two seconds. If the fire is put out by pressing, ignite the roll again. Repeatedly press each point about ten times. Another method is to wrap the ignited end of the roll with seven layers of cotton cloth, and press it tightly on the point. If the patient feels too hot, the needle can be lifted a little, when the heat is reduced, press it on the point again. Repeat the procedure on each point five to seven times.

2) *Indirect moxibustion with medicinal cake to Baihui (Du 20) to treat ptosis of visceral organs* Dr. Tian used to treat prolapse of the uterus or gastroptosis with herbal cake moxibustion in the following way: Galla Chinesis is first ground into fine powder and mixed with Castor-bean of the same quantity, and then pounded again, made into cake 2 cm in diameter and 0.3 cm to 0.5 cm in thickness, and 10 g in weight each. Put the cake on the Baihui (Du 20) point with the medium sized moxa cone on the cake to do moxibustion, ten to twenty cones in each treatment. Treat once daily. Five to six treatments constitute one course. Dr. Tian has treated thirty cases of

prolapse of the uterus and ten cases of gastroptosis with this method and achieved good results. Both Galla Chinesis and Castor-bean have the function of contraction and checking the sinking. Thus they are frequently used for ptosis of internal organs. Baihui (Du 20), a point of the Du Meridian, functions well in lifting yang qi and checking sinking. Cake moxibustion is effective for prolapse, because it can reinforce the Du Meridian with its warmth and increase the function of herbal cake in checking the sinking. When this technique is applied, a sitting position is mostly selected with the head bent forward a little. During the treatment, the patient generally has a feeling just like mild dizziness, warm in the brain, warm in the trunk even in the whole body and a lifting sensation in the lower jiao. The moxibustion cannot be stopped until the patient feels warm in his body, no matter how many cones are used.

3) *Incense moxibustion to treat bronchitis, throat itching and cough* The patients who have acute bronchitis, throat itching and cough are treated by incense moxibustion to Tiantu (Ren 22), Fengmen (B 12) and Feishu (B 13) points. After one or two treatments, the symptoms can be relieved. The method is to ignite the incense, quickly put it on the point and swiftly withdraw it from the point when there is a sound on the skin heard. One treatment for each point. The manipulation should be done on the exact location of point with rapid pressing and removing. Heavy force shall in no case be applied. For instance, a female patient, aged fifty-one had itching throat followed by continuous coughing after catching cold. She coughed when she smelled strong odours. She was treated by medication without any improvement. Dr. Tian treated her every other day with incense moxibustion to Tiantu (Ren 22) and Fengmen (B 12) in the first time, and Dazhui (Du 14) and Feishu (B 13) in the second time. The patient was recovered and no relapse was found in the follow-up visit. Dr. Tian also applies this method to treat asthma and epigastric pain. It is especially good for the patients with a weak constitution and the elderly.

3. Deep insertion of Dazhui (Du 14) to treat tetanus

During the war in Korea in 1951, Dr. Tian treated eleven tetanus cases with acupuncture, of which nine were cured.

Method: No. 26 needle is used for deep insertion of Dazhui (Du 14). After the needle is inserted into the skin, the needle tip is directed obliquely upward at an angle of 40° along the upper border of the spinous process of the first thoracic vertebra and slowly inserted 2 to 2.5 cun to the dura mater spinalis without penetrating it through. Stop insertion when a feeling of resistance appears. Rotate the needle at the small amplitude of 200 to 500 times/min. (less than 90°). Retain the needle for one hour or even longer until the convulsion and opisthotonos are relieved. During retention, manipulate the needle once every five minutes. This method can be repeatedly used when each attack occurs. Generally, two or three treatments may achieve the effects. Some cases had good results with only one treatment and at most with five treatments.

4. Selecting the points in imitation of Monarch, Minister, Assistant and Guide in prescription of herbs

Dr. Tian has experienced that the five links such as the theory, the principle, the prescription, the points and the techniques should be mastered very well in the acupuncture treatment which guided the theory of TCM. Among them, prescription of points is the most important. The points should be selected and combined flexibly according to the relationship between meridians, collaterals and zang-fu organs, the properties and functions of the points, and the differentiation. Points for each prescription are fewer but better. One point can be selected with several usages and the combination of points must be rigorous and suitable. The principle of monarch, minister, assistant and guide should be reflected between the points of a group. For example, irregular menstruation was treated by selecting Guanyuan (Ren 4) as a monarch to regulate the Chong and Ren Meridians and soothe the chamber of blood—uterus, Sanyinjiao (Sp 6) as a minister to reinforce the spleen and stomach—the production of blood, Xuehai (Sp 10) as an assistant to be reduced in order to activate the blood circulation and regulate the menstruation in case of heat in blood, in combination with Zhigou (SJ 6) as a guide with reducing method to clear the middle jiao. The points combined are Yanglingquan (G 34), acting as an assistant, for strengthening the spleen and stomach and reinforcing qi and blood, and Quchi (LI 11), acting as a guide to readjust qi and blood.

In addition, there are some other prescriptions with fewer but better points. The points supplement each other and thus bring good effect. For example, the combination of Jianyu (LI 15) and Quchi (LI 11) can be used for all the symptoms caused by stagnated heat, qi stagnation, fullness of the chest, irritability, hiccup and poor appetite. The combination of Tongli (H 5) and Zusanli (S 36) are used for insomnia. And Yinbai (Sp 1) together with Sanyinjiao (Sp 6) for uterus bleeding.

As to the monarch, minister, assistant and guide, first of all, the differentiation and functions of points, especially the minute difference among the points with same functions must be learned very well. For example, the points of promoting resuscitation, Shixuan (Extra) is to promote resuscitation by clearing heat; Renzhong (Du 26) is by clearing heat and restoring yang; Baihui (Du 20) by regulating the Du Meridian and reinforcing qi; Chengjiang (Ren 24) by leading yang from yin and opening the mind; Laogong (P 8) by clearing heart and restoring consciousness; Xinjian (Liv 2) by removing fire from liver; Shenmen (H 7) by clearing heart and opening the mind; Hegu (LI 4) by clearing heart and improving brain and opening the mind; Neiguan (P 6) and Sanyinjiao (Sp 6) by clearing yin fire and calming the mind in heart. Only if the properties of the points are studied well, can the prescriptions be made correctly. Just like prescribing herbs, the primary and secondary should be noted.

5. Moxibustion to Shenzhu (Du 12) to treat cold back and limbs due to yang deficiency

Shenzhu (Du 12) indicates in pain diseases. It is recorded in literature of generations as for treating the stiff pain in the spine and lumbar region, consumptive diseases, asthmatic cough, clonic convulsion, manic-depressive disorders and infantile convulsion and so on. There are the records in which Shenzhu (Du 12) is said to treat fever too. But no records say it is used for cold back and limbs due to yang deficiency. From 1982, Dr. Tian had five patients who suffered obviously from cold back penetrating to the heart and abdomen and cold extremities. Dr. Tian treated them with ginger moxibustion to Shenzhu (Du 12), ten to twelve cones for each treatment, once or twice daily. After one or two weeks of treatment in average, they were cured. For example, a female patient aged fifty had a cold feeling on her back as if an ice compress were on it, chills, cold extremities, complicated with insomnia, spontaneous sweating and poor appetite for four years. She was treated by many methods, but without results. She came from Yunnan to Beijing and was admitted to the hospital in November, 1983. The treatment for her was the simple moxibustion to Shenzhu (Du 12) as mentioned above, the cold feeling on her back was reduced, chills stopped after the first moxibustion, and disappeared after five treatments. Ten treatments were given in all and the symptoms were gradually relieved. Two weeks later, she was discharged from the hospital.

Shenzhu (Du 12), a point of the Du Meridian, is located below the spinous process of the third thoracic vertebra between the two Feishu (B 13) points. The Du Meridian is the sea of yang meridians and governs all yang in the whole body; Feishu (B 13) is the place where the lung qi is infused. The lung regulates the mechanism of qi, which is the commander of blood. Shenzhu (Du 12) is the door from which the Du Yang comes in and goes out. The Du Yang helps the lung qi to inspire the heart yang. "Yang deficiency will lead to the interior cold." Therefore, the moxibustion to Shenzhu (Du 12) can inspire the Du Yang, improve the lung qi, promote blood circulation. The cold limbs can be warmed because the qi and blood are abundant. In case the qi of the Du Meridian is reinforced, the qi of all other meridians is replenished. The cold feeling on the back and on the extremities disappeared owing to the accumulation of yang resulting in the consumption of yin.

II. Case Analysis

Case 1: Cough and asthma (asthmatic bronchitis, emphysema)

Name, Ma x x; sex, female; age, 65; date of the first visit, July 14, 1978.

Complaints The patient had a cough and asthma especially during the winter for thirty years. The condition was worse in the last ten years. Although she had treatment with both Western drugs and Chinese herbs, her disease was not cured. The patient was emaciated, tired, had a low voice, mild cough with white frothy thin sputum of medium quantity, asthmatic breathing on exertion with exhaling more but inhaling less, aversion to cold, cold limbs, palpitation, spontaneous sweating, poor appetite, weak, and easily got a common cold. But now the disease was stable. Her tongue was pale with a thin white coating. The pulse was deep and thready. It was the deficiency of both lung and kidney. The treatment was to reinforce the lung and kidney for receiving qi in order to stop asthma.

Prescription Asthma plaster applied to acupoints.

Treatment procedure She was treated with the asthma plaster (the method as mentioned above). The follow-up visit in July of the following year showed that cough and asthma were both relieved, appetite increased, the frequency of colds reduced, the attacks during winter minimized more than two thirds. The plaster was used continuously, and another follow-up visit in the third year showed that cough and expectoration stopped. Asthma was remarkably relieved, her physical strength was increased and she could undertake general physical work. The treatment was continued with the same method, and the follow-up visit in 1984, the sixth year since she began the treatment, revealed no attack of cough and asthma except shortness of breath on exertion. She has stopped medication and herbs since then.

Explanation The asthma was due to deficiency of both lung and kidney. The key point of treatment is to reinforce qi of lung and kidney and to strengthen resistance against the pathogenic factors. The application of asthma plaster on hot summer days is to reinforce qi of lung and kidney and to clear the summer heat. Yang qi is easily lost in summer. Reinforcement of yang qi will not lead to weakness when it is deficient in winter. This is the reason that the body resistance increased, the colds decreased and the cough and asthma were controlled.

Case 2: Chronic diarrhoea

Name, Li x x; sex, male; age, 47; date of the first visit, May 10, 1982.

Complaints The patient generally had an improper diet with a preference for cold and raw food. He started to have abdominal pain and diarrhoea very often since 1974. The condition was intermittent with dull pain on the abdomen, which was relieved by pressure, but aggravated by eating cold food. He had loose stools, three to six times a day, sometimes with a white frothy pus-like discharge and a bearing-down feeling and a sallow complexion without lustre. In the last three years, the symptoms were getting worse. He couldn't take any cold food. He had a bowel movement four to seven times a day, diarrhoea at dawn, abdominal pain after eating, especially around the umbilicus, sometimes serious pain, a desire to defecate whenever the pain appeared, abdominal distention, spontaneous sweating, weakness of the four limbs and emaciation, pale tongue proper, flabby tongue with toothmarks on the tongue, white and slightly thick tongue coating, and deep thready pulse. The routine examination of stools was made and nothing abnormal was found. He was treated with various antibiotics, but there was no marked improvement. Dr. Tian thought it was yang deficiency of spleen and stomach. The treatment was directed to warm the middle jiao, reinforce the spleen, and lift yang to check diarrhoea.

Prescription of points

1) Tianshu (S 25), Shenque (Ren 8), Guanyuan (Ren 4) and Zusanli (S 36).

2) Pishu (B 20), Shenshu (B 23), Dachangshu (B 25) and Mingmen (Du 4).

Treatment procedure Except a warming needle to Zusanli (S 36) point, indirect moxibustion with ginger was used for all other points, five cones each in every treatment. Treat once a day. Ten treatments constitute one course. Rest for five days between the courses. Two groups of points are used alternately.

After the two courses of treatment, all the symptoms were cured. The follow-up visit for one year showed no relapse.

Explanation Abdominal pain and diarrhoea for eight years led to deficiency of spleen and kidney, consumption of primary yang, failure of fire in warming the earth, dysfunction of the spleen in transportation and transformation. It was a difficult case. Moxibustion with ginger to Guanyuan (Ren 4) and Mingmen (Du 4) is to warm and reinforce the root of primary yang, thus the kidney yang is abundant; Zusanli (S 36) and Tianshu (S 25) are reinforced to activate the spleen yang. The dampness is eliminated, cold is dispersed and transportation of dampness is improved in case yang is activated. Therefore, abdominal distension and diarrhoea stopped. Eliminating the stubborn cold by warming yang is a function of moxibustion.

EXPOSITION OF PENETRATING ACUPUNCTURE WITH LONG NEEDLES

—Feng Runshen's Clinical Experience

Feng Runshen, a native of Ningjin County, Hebei Province, was born in April of 1929. He went to an old-style private school when he was young. But he was obliged to discontinue his studies because of his poverty. Influenced by his uncle, a doctor of traditional Chinese medicine, he became an apprentice in the Huazhou Pharmacy in Taiyuan. In the winter of 1945, he was admitted to the training course for medical workers of Taiyuan. After he passed the examination for doctors in Baotou municipality in 1949, he practised medicine in Baotou. He was appointed by the Public Health Bureau of the Suiyuan Region as the principal of Suidong Central Banner Hospital. In 1960, Feng did a special course of *Internal Classic* in Beijing College of Traditional Chinese Medicine. He was transferred to the Chinese-Mongolian Medical Institute of the Inner Mongolia Autonomous Region in 1962. In his clinical acupuncture practice, he put forward a proposal of acupuncture standardization and the importance of peculiarity of meridians and points. He maintained the comprehensive treatment of the combination of acupuncture and medicine. Feng has been engaged in research work of the theory of "Ziwuliuzhu" and has sound judgement about it. At present, he is a committee member of the All-China Commission for the Systematization and Research of the Theory of Traditional Chinese Medicine, a member of the Chinese Acupuncture Society, a member of the Standing Committee of the Society of Traditional Chinese Medicine in Inner Mongolia Autonomous Region, director of the Society of Acupuncture of Inner Mongolia Autonomous Region, and the vice-chief physician of the Institute of Chinese-Mongolia Medicine.

I. Academic Characteristics and Medical Specialities

Penetrating technique, which is also named as passing sea, crossing beam, going through the thorax and rough method, is a special needling method which works by inserting a long filiform needle in the direction from one point towards the other point passing some tissue in order to strengthen the regulation of qi circulation of the meridians. It is more effective than puncturing one point with one needle. The effect of one needle for each point is not satisfactory for treating scrofula, chest pain, facial paralysis and so on. The point which is inserted is called penetrating point, the point which is penetrated to is named arriving point and the point which is passed through is known as the central point. The classification of the penetrating technique according to the different directions, angles and meridians is as follows:

1. Classification according to penetrating direction

1) *Unidirection* Because of the location and purpose of treatment, the penetrating direction is set only from A to B. For example, penetrating Hegu (LI 4) towards Laogong (P 8), Yanglao (SI 6) towards Tongli (H 5).

2) *Multidirection* The needle is inserted from a certain penetrating point and reaches the arriving point. After arrival of qi, the needle is lifted to the penetrating point and inserted towards another arriving point. For instance, Yintang (Extra) towards Yuyao (Extra) bilaterally, Baihui (Du 20) towards Sishenchong (Extra) multidirectionally.

3) *Mutualdirection* The needle can be inserted from A to B and vice versa. Both the A and B points can be penetrating point and arriving point. For example, Dicang (S 4) towards Jiache (S 6), Jiache (S 6) towards Dicang (S 4), Fengchi (G 20) towards Fengchi (G 20).

4) *Surrounding penetration* It is mostly used for tendon knots formed on the body surface and local numbness of the skin. The procedure is just as in the description in *Miraculous Pivot*. "Quintupe puncture is a method in which the needles are inserted at five spots with one perpendicularly in the centre and the four scattered obliquely or horizontally around it and towards its tip." If the disease is located deep in the muscle, the needles scattered around can be inserted a small distance from the diseased area. A suitable angle should be made with the long axis of scattering needles towards the penetrating points. The tips of the needle in the centre and the needles around it should be all concentrated to the base of the disease, just as what is required in *Miraculous Pivot* that all tips of the needles surrounding are towards the diseased base.

2. Classification according to the angle formed by the needle and the skin surface

1) *Horizontally* After insertion, the body of the needle is between the skin and muscle. Both the penetrating and arriving points are superficial. For example, Taiyang (Extra) towards Shuaigu (B 8), Yangbai (G 14) towards Yuyao (Extra).

2) *Perpendicularly* The right angle is formed by the long axis of the needle and the skin of the penetrating point. The needle is inserted perpendicularly to the arriving point. This method is commonly used in the areas, e.g. forearms and legs where the two points locate oppositely: Neiguan (P 6) towards Waiguan (SJ 5), Juegu (G 39) towards Sanyinjiao (Sp 6).

3) *Obliquely* The needle is inserted with a suitable angle (not a right angle) formed by the long axis of the needle and the skin of the penetrating point. After insertion, the angle is readjusted in order to thrust the needle to the arriving point. The oblique penetration is applied in the area around the joints of the four extremities, e.g. Yanglao (SI 6) towards Tongli (H 5), Qiuxu (G 40) towards Zhaohai (K 6).

3. Classification according to the meridians

1) *The same meridian* The two points on the same meridian are penetrated to excite

and regulate qi of that meridian. Horizontal method is generally a part of this category, e.g. Baihui (Du 20) towards Houding (Du 19), Yemen (SJ 2) towards Zhongzhu (SJ 3), Yangchi (SJ 4).

2) *The different meridians*

a. The exterior-interior yin-yang meridians: The penetrating point and the arriving point located on different meridians which are exteriorly-interiorly related to each other, e.g. on the extremities, Jianshi (P 5) towards Zhigou (SJ 6), Fuliu (K 7) towards Fuyang (B 59).

b. Non-exterior-interior yin-yang meridians: Although among the meridians of the penetrating point and arriving point, one is yin, while the other is yang, there is no exterior-interior relationship between them, e.g. Xiangu (S 43) towards Yongquan (K 1), Zhongzhu (SJ 3) towards Shaofu (H 8).

c. The adjacent meridians with the same nature of yin or yang: The two meridians penetrated are both yin and yang and adjacent to each other, e.g. Tiaokou (S 38) towards Chengshan (B 57), Taichong (Liv 3) towards Yongquan (K 1).

4. Precautions for penetrating acupuncture

1) *Needles* Stainless steel filiform needles, 6 to 7 cun, at least two cun in length, Nos. 26 to 28 in diameter, are used for penetrating. Prior to treatment, they should be inspected carefully to prevent accidents from loose handles and bent needles.

2) *Training of finger strength* Because the needles for penetration are comparatively longer, if the finger strength is not forceful enough, the insertion will be difficult, the needles easily bent and the tips cannot reach the arriving point smoothly. Thus the therapeutic effect will be decreased. Therefore, the finger strength with long needles should be trained as the following two steps: First, practise increasing the finger strength. Smooth insertion and withdrawal are respected to increase the finger strength of the puncturing hand. Second, practise willpower. Based on practice of finger strength, concentration is drawn greatly to the tip of the needle and insert and thrust the needle forward with willpower. Determine where the tip of the needle reaches at all times and change the direction and depth if necessary according to the finger sensation from the tip and body of the needle.

3) *Posture of the patient* The principle is that the patient should be in a comfortable position which can be kept for retention of the needle, and is convenient for the doctor to do acupuncture. Prone position and sitting in a chair are appropriate in clinic.

4) *Sterilization* Sterilization in penetrating acupuncture is stricter than that of simple acupuncture, because the tip of the needle is inserted passing through tissues deep in the body.

a. Sterilization of the needles: Boil the needles wrapped in gauze for thirty minutes or sterilize in an autoclave. The water scale on the needle should be cleaned with a 75 percent alcohol cotton ball. The needles should be soaked in 75 percent alcohol for fifteen minutes in case of urgent need.

b. Sterilization of the points: The areas of the penetrating point and the arriving point must be sterilized. First, clean the skin with soap, second with iodine and then with alcohol. Don't let the needle tip puncture the skin of the arriving point, so as not to bring pathogenic bacteria into the body which can cause infection. Sterilize only the penetrating point if the doctor is skillful enough.

c. Sterilization of the practitioner's fingers: Both the left and right hands of the practitioner should be washed clean and sterilized by iodine and 75 percent alcohol for the needle is inserted not only by the puncturing hand but also with the help of the pressing hand.

5) *Holding the needles* The method of holding needles is important in penetrating acupuncture. Because the needles for penetrating are longer, they are comparatively thin, soft and bend easily. On the other hand, the patient may have a tendency to faint if he is afraid of long needles. What is preferred is Feng's technique: Avoiding fear by hiding the needle.

Hiding the needle completely: The index finger of the right hand is in flexion and the handle of needle is held in the flex crease of the middle section of the index finger. The other four fingers are naturally flexed-stretched and help the left hand press the point. The patient does not know the needles are hidden in the practitioner's hand. To avoid that the patient sees them, the needle is pushed out by the right thumb during insertion. Hold the needle with the thumb, index and middle finger.

Hiding the needle incompletely: The right thumb and the index finger hold the body of the needle with 1 cun more or less of the tip exposed. The rest of the needle body and handle is hidden in the palm to show the patient that it is not long. The needle is inserted section by section directly to the arriving point.

6) *The pressing hand and insertion* The left hand is the pressing hand, which plays an important role in inserting and helping push the needle tip to the definite spot. It can not only fix the skin of the penetrating point and limit the direction of insertion, but it also feels and conducts where the needle tip reaches. "An experienced acupuncturist believes in the important function of the left hand, while an inexperienced believes in the important function of the right hand," showing the significance of the pressing hand described in *Classic on Medical Problems*. The needles must be sterilized prior to insertion. The practitioner should be calm, regulate his respiration and concentrate on the needle tip during insertion. Just as stated in *Internal Classic*, "The key in acupuncture is that the practitioner should concentrate his mind. No matter the insertion is deep or shallow, the point close or distant, the practitioner must be wholly absorbed into his manipulation, as facing an abyss and a tiger." The patient will be reassured if the doctor is calm and fainting can be avoided and the therapeutic effect increased. What's more, the doctor is aware of his needle with his concentrated attention. The commonly used methods of insertion with the pressing hand are given in the following:

a. The method with the thumb pressing the needle and the middle finger feeling the sensation:

Flex the thumb and put it on the penetrating point with a right angle formed by the palm and the skin. Press the penetrating point with the thumb, and put the left middle finger abdomen on the arriving point. The needle is inserted to the arriving point with a right angle formed by the needle body and the palm. Stop the insertion when the left middle finger feels the sensation which the needle tip is coming. This method is mostly used on the extremities for the perpendicular penetrating, e.g. Quchi (LI 11) towards Shaohai (H 3), Xiyangguan (G 33) towards Ququan (Liv 8).

b. The method with the thumbs pushing the needle and the middle finger feeling the sensation:

Press the left thumb abdomen on one side of the penetrating point and hold the needle with the right thumb, index and middle fingers keeping the needle tip towards the arriving point. Push the needle swiftly into the skin with the both thumbs, and still keep the left thumb on the penetrating point. After insertion, put the four fingers on the skin to feel where the tip reaches and help guide its direction and stop it when it reaches the arriving point. The method is appropriate where the skin is loose, e.g. Tianjing (SJ 10) towards Binao (LI 14), Taiyang (Extra) towards Shuaigu (B 8).

7) *Arrival of qi and promoting qi* When qi arrives, the operator feels tenseness around the needle. Meanwhile, the patient feels soreness, numbness, distension, hot, cold and heaviness. Sometimes the feeling is like something pouring into his body or like an insect walking. If qi fails to arrive, measures have to be taken, such as lifting, thrusting, rotating and pressing. After two or three times promoting qi, arrival of qi should be obtained. If not, the direction of the needle needs to be changed.

8) *The manipulations and reinforcing and reducing* After arrival of qi, manipulate the needle every ten minutes. Manipulation means the corresponding methods applied for purpose of reinforcing and reducing.

9) *Withdrawing the needle* Withdrawing the needle quickly or slowly depends upon the condition of reinforcing or reducing. On withdrawing the needle, besides keeping the hole open or close, the cooperations of the pressing hand is important too. The right hand holds the handle, and the left thumb presses tightly the sterilized cotton ball on the penetrating point. The rest four fingers of the left hand put on the skin between the penetrating and arriving points and fix the skin of arriving point. The right hand rotates the needle slightly and withdraw it gently if not stuck. Press gently between the penetrating and arriving points with the left hand to prevent qi stagnation and hematoma that may occur.

5. Examples for penetrating technique

1) *Dicang (S 4) towards Jiache (S 6)* The patient is asked to sit erect. Puncture the right side in case of the deviation to the left side and vice versa. The left thumb presses Dicang (S 4), the index, middle and ring fingers put between Dicang (S 4) and Jiache (S 6). The right hand holds the needle on Dicang (S 4), while the left thumb pushes the needle tip. With the help of the left index, middle and ring finger, the needle is pushed directly to Jiache (S 6) after the arrival of qi. The needle should be kept going inside the muscle, not penetrating through it to the mouth cavity.

In case of the deviation of the mouth caused by wind attacking the facial collaterals of Yangming Meridian, Dicang (S 4) towards Jiache (S 6) is used with the reducing method, in regulating qi and blood circulation of Yangming Meridian and dispersing pathogenic wind.

2) *Tanzhong (Ren 17) towards Juque (Ren 14)* The patient is sitting erect or in a

supine position. The doctor puts the left thumb inferior to Tanzhong (Ren 17) and holds a needle of 3 to 4 cun long with the right hand on the point. Insert the needle obliquely a little into the point. After arrival of qi, horizontally penetrate along the sternum through Zhongting (Ren 16) and Jiuwei (Ren 15) to Juque (Ren 14).

The indications of penetrating Tanzhong (Ren 17) towards Juque (Ren 14) are the symptoms due to ascending of the perverse qi, asthma, cough, chest pain and fullness. "Mu" is the place where qi of zang-fu assembles. Tanzhong (Ren 17) is the Front-Mu point of the pericardium; and Jiuwei, the Frout-Mu point of heart. Penetrating these two points can not only regulate qi circulation of Sanjiao, relax chest, remove stagnation, promote transportation of middle jiao and resolve dampness, but also strengthen the functions of the heart and pericardium and regulate yang qi of the chest.

3) *Tianshu (S 25) towards Huangshu (K 16)* Press the thumb of the left hand on Tianshu (S 25) and the middle finger on Huangshu (K 16). Hold the needle with the right hand and insert it into Tianshu (S 25) point, 0.8 cun deep. After arrival of qi, lift the needle tip with 0.5 cun left in the point and penetrate horizontally to Huangshu (K 16) with slight rotation. Retain the needle when qi arrives, or penetrate Huangshu (K 16) towards Tianshu (S 25).

The penetration of these two points is very effective for headache due to phlegm and diarrhoea. The headache due to phlegm mostly occurs in patients who have a yang deficient constitution and excessive cold-damp in middle and lower jiao. When it attacks, the perverse qi ascends from both sides of abdomen, shortness of breath and dizziness occur. Subsequently, drilling pain of the forehead, cold salivation, pallor, deep thready and string-taut pulse, which may relieve after a while. Penetrating Tianshu (S 25) towards Huangshu (K 16) functions in promoting spleen, resolving dampness, ascending clarity and descending turbidity, regulating Chong Meridian and sending the perverse qi downward. Diarrhoea is usually caused by cold or damp, or by stagnation of damp-heat, but also due to dysfunction of spleen and stomach, or due to dysfunction of the intestines. Penetrating Tianshu (S 25) towards Huangshu (K 16) helps greatly in regulating spleen and kidney, harmonizing the stomach and restoring the intestinal function.

4) *Tianjing (SJ 10) towards Binao (LI 14)* The patient is asked to sit erect with the affected side elbow bent, keeping the flexed arm as forward as possible. After sterilization, the doctor puts the tip of his left thumb superior to Tianjing (SJ 10) and the four fingers between Tianjing (SJ 10) and Binao (LI 4). Hold the needle tip with the thumb and the index finger of the right hand, keeping 1 cun exposed above Tianjing (SJ 10). Insert the needle when the patient inhales, with the left thumb pushing the needle tip. Generally, qi arrives when the needle is inserted 0.5 cun deep. Lift the needle slightly and penetrate towards Binao (LI 14). Press Tianjing (SJ 10) tightly with the left thumb and try to feel where the needle tip reaches with the four fingers until the needle reaches Binao (LI 14). When the patient feels hot in the humerus region or pain radiating to the shoulder, it means the arrival of qi, and reducing is performed. During penetrating, if the needle tip deviates from the direction or is too shallow in the skin, lift the needle slowly, correct the direction and insert it again. When withdrawing the needle, press Tianjing (SJ 10) with the left thumb and fix the skin between Tianjing (SJ 10) and Binao (LI 14), with the four fingers holding the needle handle with the right hand and rotating

it slightly, withdraw the needle slowly and rub the skin for a while after withdrawal. Treat once every other day on both sides alternatively.

This method is good for facial swelling and pain caused by fire due to qi stagnation of Sanjiao, sore throat and inflammation of the throat, scrofula and mumps, especially effective for the early stage of scrofula when the pus is not yet formed. The occurrence of scrofula is from the combination of fire due to Shaoyang stagnation and phlegm-damp in the meridian. Tianjing (SJ 10) is a He-sea point of Hand Shaoyang. Needling it can reduce fire of the gallbladder and Sanjiao and remove obstruction of Shaoyang Meridian. Binao (LI 14) is a meeting point of Yangming Meridian of Hand, and is an important point for scrofula. Penetrating Tianjing (SJ 10) towards Binao (LI 14) functions not only in reducing the pathogenic fire due to stagnation of Sanjiao and pathogenic heat and resolving the phlegm in the meridians but also in dispersing qi and blood of Yangming Meridian and resolving stagnation and masses of all the meridians in the neck. This is why it is especially effective for scrofula. (Note: Prick Tianjing with a three edged needle in a line, squeeze out five or six grain-like things, cover with adhesive plaster. The wound will be healed after seven days.) If the primitive scrofula is not healed, apply penetrating acupuncture to the opposite side as the above mentioned.

5) *Yanglao (SI 6) towards Tongli (H 5)* The patient is asked to sit erect with palm facing downward. Press the head of the ulna of the patient with the operator's left thumb, and direct the index finger to Tongli (H 5) point. Hold the needle with the right hand and insert it 0.5 cun deep into Yanglao (SI 6), push the needle to Tongli (H 5) after arrival of qi, and keep the needling sensation radiating to the posterior aspect of the wrist and retain the needle there.

Irregular menstruation, hysteria and palpitation respond to penetrating Yanglao (SI 6) towards Tongli (H 5). Over-exertion, emotional disorders and exhaustion of blood may lead to disturbance of heart and spleen, irregular menstruation, even amenorrhea, afternoon fever, emaciation, sallow and dim complexion. Exactly as described in *Internal Classic*, "Both heart and spleen yang deficiency will give rise to irregular menstruation." Hysteria is usually caused by yin exhaustion due to stagnated fire, excessive heat in the blood system due to liver disturbance. As we can see, both of them result from yin deficiency, heat in blood, depression of liver and qi stagnation. But the function of penetrating Yanglao (SI 6) towards Tongli (H 5) is good to activate blood circulation, remove obstruction from the meridians, reinforce the liver and kidney, clear deficiency-heat and calm the mind.

SIMPLE TABLE OF PENETRATION ACUPUNCTURE

	Penetrating point	*Arriving point*	*Indications*
1	Fengchi	Fengfu	Hemiplegia, stiffness and pain of neck
2	Taiyang	Jiaosun	Eye diseases, headache
3	Sizhukong	Shuaigu	Migraine, deviation of mouth and eyes
4	Zanzhu	Yuyao	Pain in supraorbital region
5	Yingxiang	Sibai	Epistaxis, obstruction of nose, facial paralysis

6	Qianding	Baihui	Vertical headache, prolonged diarrhoea
7	Yintang	Yuyao	Infantile convulsion, redness, swelling and pain of eyes (epidemic hemorrhagic conjunctivitis)
8	Quchai	Linqi	Wind-syndrome of head, epistaxis, eye diseases
9	Tongziliao	Yuyao	Pain in supraorbital region, eye diseases
10	Touwei	Tongtian	Hemiplegia, vertical headache
11	Renzhong	Dicang	Facial paralysis
12	Yangbai	Yuyao	Inability of closing eyes
13	Yuyao	Yuwei	Eye diseases, ptosis of eyelids
14	Yingxiang	Jingming	Deviation of mouth, nose diseases
15	Shengting	Linqi	Frontal headache, redness of eyes
16	Zhangmen	Jingmen	Liver depression, hypochondriac distension and pain
17	Jianzhongshu	Dazhui	Back and spinal pain, torticollis
18	Guanyuan	Qugu	Diseases of lower jiao
19	Tanzhong	Huagai	Cough, asthma, fullness in chest
20	Ganshu	Zhiyang	Stagnation and heat of liver and gallbladder, jaundice
21	Dingchuan	Dingchuan	Asthma
22	Jianwaishu	Shenzhu	Atrophy of lower extremities
23	Zhishi	Mingmen	Diarrhoea at dawn, impotence
24	Zhongzhu	Shaofu	Sudden precordial pain
25	Jianshi	Zhigou	Profuse sputum, precordial pain, fullness and discomfort in chest and hypochondrium
26	Hegu	Laogong	Sudden precordial pain, sores in palm
27	Yangchi	Daling	Diabetes, wrist pain, irritability
28	Yanggu	Wangu	Mental disorders, febrile diseases, tinnitus, toothache
29	Lieque	Taiyuan	Cough due to wind-cold
30	Yinxi	Yanggu	Epistaxis, distension and fullness in chest and hypochondrium
31	Naohui	Binao	Sore throat, pustule of finger tip
32	Jianyu	Binao	Shoulder and back pain
33	Xiangu	Yongquan	Syncope, epidemic hemorrhagia conjunctivitis, vertical headache
34	Fenglong	Lougu	Asthma due to phlegm obstruction and perverse qi
35	Kunlun	Taixi	Precordial pain with cold limbs, diarrhoea at dawn, frequent urination
36	Yanglingquan	Yinlingquan	Abdominal distension, difficult urination, diseases of lower jiao
37	Qiuxu	Zhaohai	Hypochondriac pain, globus hystericus

38	Gongsun	Yongquan	Diarrhoea with undigested food in stool
39	Taixi	Zhaohai	Atrophy, Bi-syndrome
40	Shangqiu	Jiexi	Abdominal pain, ankle pain
41	Liangqiu	Yinshi	Epigastric pain, knee pain
42	Taiyang	Shuaigu	Migraine, deviation of mouth and eyes
43	Fengchi	Fengchi	Windstroke, hemiplegia, headache, eye diseases, anhidrosis of exogenous febrile disease
44	Yintang	Zanzhu	Dizziness, vertigo, eye diseases, headache, convulsion
45	Zanzhu	Jingming	Eye diseases
46	Shenting	Shangxing	Headache, dizziness, vertigo
47	Daying	Jiache	Swelling and pain of cheek
48	Baihui	Sishengchong	Dizziness, vertigo
49	Wuchu	Shuaigu	Headache of wind-syndrome, hyperphoria with fixed eyeballs, epilepsy
50	Qubin	Tinghui	Deviation of mouth and eyes, swelling cheek, appetite-prohibiting dysentery
51	Chengjiang	Dicang	Intractable deviation of mouth
52	Tianzhu	Yamen	Vertical headache, spinal pain
53	Taiyang	Jiache	Facial paralysis, facial spasm and pain
54	Chengqi	Jingming	Eye diseases
55	Ermen	Tinggong	Tinnitus, deafness
56	Renying	Tiantu	Goiter
57	Shangwan	Zhongwan	Epigastric pain, indigestion
58	Fengmen	Dashu	Cough, chest pain
59	Qihai	Guanyuan	Diseases of lower jiao
60	Feishu	Dingchuan	Asthma, cough
61	Danshu	Zhiyang	Stagnation and heat of liver and gallbladder, jaundice
62	Dazhui	Dashu	Back and spinal pain, torticollis
63	Yaoshu	Yaoyangguan	Epilepsy (due to perverse phlegm), irregular menstruation
64	Ximen	Sanyangluo	Precordial pain, sudden loss of voice, insomnia
65	Quchi	Shaohai	Hemiplegia, elbow pain
66	Neiguan	Waiguan	Discord between spleen and stomach, precordial pain, mental disorders, pain syndromes
67	Houxi	Laogong	Alternate spells of fever and chill, sudden sprain in lumbar region
68	Jianqianshu	Jianzhen	Shoulder swelling and pain, motor impairment of upper extremities
69	Sanjian	Houxi	Sore throat, toothache
70	Lingdao	Shenmen	Precordial pain, sudden loss of voice,

			redness and pain of eyes
71	Jianyu	Jiquan	Omalgia
72	Shousanli	Wenliu	Soreness and weakness of upper extremities
73	Jianyu	Naohui	Shoulder and back pain
74	Fuliu	Fuyang	Edema due to Yang deficiency of spleen and kidney, lumbago, backache
75	Xiyangguan	Ququan	Arthroncus of knee, atrophy of lower extremities
76	Dubi	Xiyan	Arthroncus of knee
77	Juegu	Sanyinjiao	Gynopathy, spermatorrhea
78	Taichong	Yongquan	Syncope, lower abdominal pain
79	Jiexi	Zhongfeng	Atrophy of lower extremities, cold limbs, external genitalia pain
80	Qiuxu	Shenmai	Paralysis, fullness, hardness and pain in abdomen
81	Tiaokou	Chengshan	Cholera, vomiting and diarrhoea, atrophy of lower extremities
82	Shuiquan	Zhaohai	Irregular menstruation

II. Case Analysis

Case 1: Scrofula

Name, Su x x; sex, female; age, 28.

Complaints Two months ago, the patient began to have a pain in her chest and hypochondrium, emotional depression and loss of appetite after she had a quarrel with somebody. Several days later, she was gradually better. But she happened to discover that she felt a mass and pain below her right ear about twenty days ago when she washed her face. She came to see a doctor because she was diagnosed as having tuberculosis of cervical lymph nodes in a hospital. She used to suffer from scrofula nine years ago. It was broken and was not healed. Two years later after many methods of treatment were tried, a scar was formed. Examination: Medium physique, sallow complexion, dark eyesockets, below the right ear a walnut-size mass of tissue which was redish, tender, fixed and hard; there was a scar of scrofula about one finger-breadth below the mass; on the left side of the mass there was a scar too; afternoon fever, absence of night sweating, fatigue, general weakness, thirst, restlessness due to deficiency, loss of appetite, urine and stools normal, the pain radiating to shoulder when she turned her head with a large amplitude; a thin yellow tongue coating, string-taut, thready and rapid pulse. ESR: the first hour 25 mm. Hemogram: Leukocyte 7000, neutrophil 60 percent, lymphocyte 24 percent. Diagnosis: Scrofula (tuberculosis of cervical lymph nodes). Treating principle: Reduce fire of Shaoyang, clear phlegm and resolve mass.

Prescription Tianjing (SJ 10) towards Binao (LI 14)

Treatment procedure Needle Tianjing (SJ 10), as soon as qi arrives, penetrate towards Binao (LI 14) with reducing method. The needling sensation should go upward to the shoulder. Treat once daily with the points penetrated from either side alternatively. The mass was gradually reduced after ten treatments. With another treatment, it was reduced to the size of a date-pit. The pain was also much relieved. ESR of the first hour was improved to 15 mm from 25 mm. All the symptoms were almost completely finished with the third ten treatments.

Explanation The disease starts with the emotional depression, which injures the liver by anger, resulting in fire due to prolonged stagnation. The phlegm-damp is combined with fire at the cervical region obstructing Shaoyang Meridian, leading to fire, which makes the tissue bad and produces the scrofula. Tianjing (SJ 10) is a He-sea point of Hand Shaoyang Meridian. Reducing method is applied to clear fire and to remove obstruction from Shaoyang Meridian. Penetrate Binao (LI 14) is to regulate Yangming Meridian and resolve phlegm and scrofula. Tianjing (SJ 10) penetrated with Binao (LI 14) to clear fire from Shaoyang Meridian and to dissolve scrofula. Therefore, the therapeutic effect is successful.

Case 2: Ulcer of cronea

Name, Li x x; sex, female; age, 2.

Complaints Two months ago, the patient had redness, swelling and pain in the eyes. She was treated by anti-inflammatory agent and eye douche as well as eye drops. She was much better one week later, but she still had photophobia, pain of the eyes and blurring of vision. With ten days of treatment, although the inflammation was almost completely reduced, a white patch and erosion appeared in her left eye on the cornea. Except the original treatment, cod liver oil pills were prescribed and some white medical powder was spread on the cornea. But the ulcer of cornea was worse. The patient came to see doctor in our hospital. Examination: Eyelids dark and swelling, inner canthus dark red as inflammation, full of pus and discharges, aversion to light, lacrimation, blurring of vision, turbid cornea of the right eye like the clouds covered it. The left cornea was more turbid with a big white patch of a broomcorn millet size in the lateral superior region. Below the white patch, there was an erosion of a green bean size with a depression in the middle. She had dry and red lips, but did not want to drink. The patient felt hot in the afternoon but without high temperature. Distended pain in the forehead and temples, loss of appetite, dry stools, scanty and yellow urine, red tongue and white coating, bigger, string-taut and forceful pulse. Differentiation: Erosion of the black eye (ulcer of cornea), heat stagnated in the liver and gallbladder, toxin and blood stagnation. The treating principle is to reduce heat from the liver and gallbladder, to activate blood circulation and dissolve stagnation.

Prescription Ganshu (B 18), Danshu (B 19), Qimai (SJ 18), Taichong (Liv 3), Qiuxu (G 40), Zhongzhu (SJ 3).

Treatment procedure All the points were punctured with reducing method, and the needles retained for thirty minutes. After withdrawal of the needle, a drop of blood was squeezed out. Cupping with pottery cups was used on the Back-Shu points to abstract drops of blood. Treat once every other day. The inflammation was cured after three treatments and the pain and aversion to light were greatly reduced too. Another five treatments followed and the nebula, white patch and erosion disappeared. The patient was asked to take the Chinese medicine "Huang Lian Yang Gan Wan" for one month in order to reinforce the good results. Follow-up for eighteen years, nothing wrong discovered in the cornea of the eyes.

Explanation The patient was treated at the beginning, although the inflammation caused by wind-heat was reduced, the stagnated heat in the liver and gallbladder was not eliminated. The stagnated heat prolonged and transformed into toxins which eroded the black part of eye (the cornea). The treatment should reduce the stagnated heat of liver and gallbladder as the principle for the purpose of eliminating the toxins in the meridian. Points Ganshu (B 18) and Danshu (B 19) are used to reduce heat from the liver and gallbladder. Taichong (Liv 3) and Qiuxu (G 40), the Yuan-source points, in combination with Zhongzhu (SJ 3), are needled for clearing the pathogenic factors of Shaoyang Meridian. Geshu (B 17) is able to dominate the blood, to activate blood circulation and dissolve stagnation. Qimai (SJ 18) is an effective point for all kinds of eye diseases. These points are punctured and bled to function well in reducing heat of liver and gallbladder, in activating blood circulation and in dissolving stagnation.

FIVE NECESSITIES IN ACUPUNCTURE AND RESEARCH ON THEIR MECHANISM

—Kuang Peigen's Clinical Experience

Dr. Kuang Peigen, a native of Wuxi, Jiangsu Province, was born in 1924 in an aristocratic family of traditional Chinese medicine. In 1949, she graduated from the state-run Shanghai Medical College and she has been practising in an acupuncture clinic since the 1950s. She summarized "Five Necessities in Acupuncture Stimulation" and published more than twenty articles on acupuncture research. She has won nineteen achievement awards in scientific research. At present she is the director and professor of the brain department of the Military Doctors' Refresher College of the People's Liberation Army of China, a councillor of the Society of Neurology and Psychiatry, CMA, and vice-chairman of the Beijing Branch of the Chinese Medical Association.

I. Academic Characteristics and Clinical Specialities

1. "Five necessities of acupuncture stimulations"

Dr. Kuang thinks that in the selection of acupoints along the corresponding meridian and according to clinical syndromes in coordination with neurological anatomy, neurological physiology and neurological pathology, and in the application of acupuncture techniques, one must pay attention to the five necessities, i.e., correct acupoints, right direction and depth of insertion, proper intensity of stimulation, appropriate stimulating duration, and proper body position in treatment.

1) *Correct selection of acupoints* Acupoints should be selected according to nerve point and motor point in the viewpoint that "the therapeutical effect reaches where the meridian goes." For example, a. Sequela of poliomyelitis: Acupoints should be selected in accordance with major affected muscle or muscles (See tables 1 and 2). b. Cerebellar ataxia: Huatuojiaji points (Extra) are advisable. These acupoints are selected 0.5 cun at the lateral borders of each process from the first thoracic vertabra to the fifth lumbar vertabra alternatively on both sides, one acupoint from every two processes, in total six to eight points are used in combination with Quchi (LI 11), Huantiao (G 30) and Chengshan (B 57). c. Peripheral facial paralysis: Every time three to four acupoints are selected from the motor points of trigeminal and facial nerves as well as mimetic muscle (Orbicularis Oris, Orbicularis Oculi and Musculus Quadratus Labialis, Frontalis in prominence). At the beginning nerve points are used as major ones and supplemented by corresponding motor points. After obvious improvement, motor points are taken as major acupoints. d. Hemiplegia: On upper limbs the major acupoints are Jianyu (LI 15), Quchi

(LI 11) and Hegu (LI 4); and on lower limbs the major acupoints are Huantiao (G 30), Yanglingquan (G 34) and motor points of nervus femoris, the motor points of musculus peroneus longus and brevis in the case accompanied by talipes calcaneovarus.

2) *Direction and depth of insertion* Generally, the needles are inserted at least 1 to 3 cm in the muscle, in order to have enough connection with the needle body in electric stimulation. In puncturing nerve points, needles should be inserted perpendicularly and along the nerve-trunk. In puncturing motor points, the needles can be inserted along the muscle, or to penetrate two or more muscles if required. In puncturing acupoints, oblique insertion is demanded on head and face; perpendicular, deep and penetrating insertions are needed on four extremities; inward insertion with an angle of 30° (towards spinal column) is demanded on the body trunk, such as on Huatuojiaji points (Extra). The needle must be lifted 1 to 2 mm if it hits bone.

3) *Intensity of stimulation* After qi arrival, electric stimulation can be applied in different diseases by different current frequency (0.3, 1, 15, 25, 75 times/sec.). Generally speaking, 0.3 to 1 time/sec. is required in hemiplegia and cerebellar ataxia, 25 to 75 times/sec. is the best for sequela of poliomyelitis and facial paralysis. The requirements of current intensity: a. The patient can tolerate and feel comfortable. b. Muscles and joints can have rhythmical contraction (for example, in the treatment of hemiplegia and cerebellar ataxia), but in the treatment of facial paralysis and various deformities, it is better for the muscle to have tetanic contraction.

4) *Duration of stimulation* Generally, it is thirty to sixty minutes. But at the beginning, the treatments can be given twice a day, with a two-to-four-hour intervals between two treatments. Physical exercises are demanded between two electric stimulations.

5) *Body position in stimulation* For the convenience in the treatment, the patient must be told to have a comfortable position and to put the paralyzed limbs in a place free for physical exercises. In correction of limb deformities, it is necessary for the patient with an inward-rotated foot to lie down and to put the diseased foot outwards, and vice versa. For example, in the correction of flat foot or pes varus, it is necessary to have a sitting position and to step flat on ground (See tables 1 and 2).

On the basis of five necessities in stimulation, the treatment of motor impairment must be coordinated with physical exercises. And in physical exercises, the active exercises must be coordinated with passive exercises (three or four times a day, fifteen to sixty minutes per time). The volume and programme in exercises must differ from individual patient. The exercises must be done appropriately and progressively. But in the patient with hemiplegia, attention must be paid to cardiovascular situation and physical exercises can only be done under the permission of cardiovascular abilities.

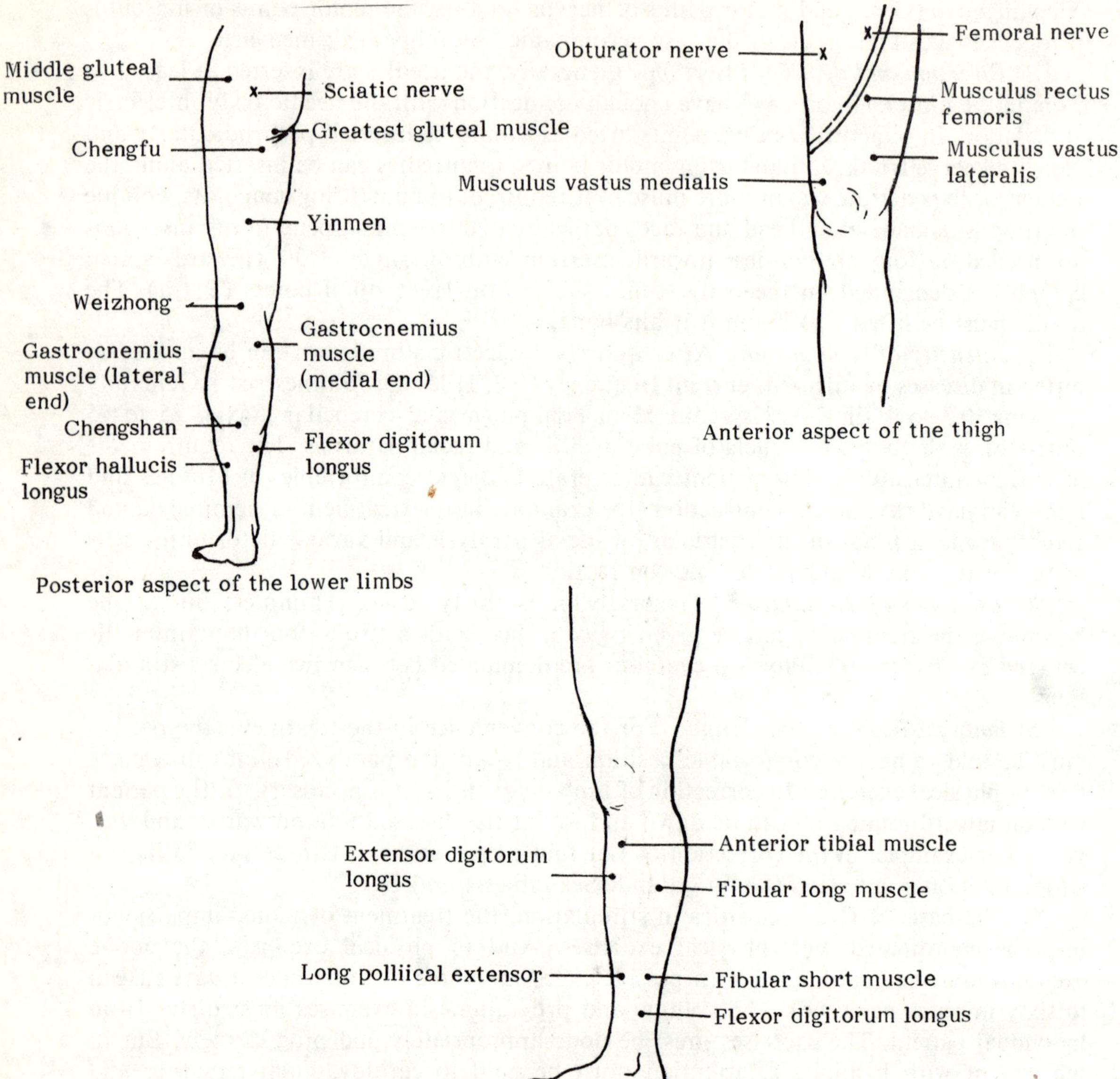

Fig. 1 Location of Points from the Muscle Group of the Lower Limbs

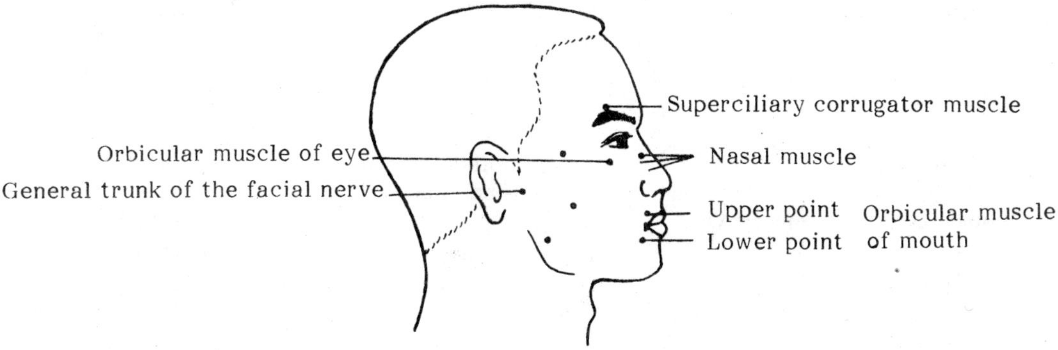

Fig. 2 Location of Points from the Face

TABLE 1. THE STIMULATING POINTS FOR THE TREATMENT OF SEQUELA OF POLIOMYELITIS

Motor impairment		Main affected muscles	Corresponding stimulating point (motor point)	Additional point (nerve point)	Body position
Hip	Disability of hip joint in extension	Musculus glutaeus maximus, hamstring muscles, femoris posterior	Motor point of muscular glutaeus maximus, Yinmen (B 37), Chengfu (B 36)	Sciatic nerve	Prone position
joint	Disability of hip joint in flexion	Musculus iliopsoas	Shenshu (B 23)	Nervus femoralis	Sitting position
	Disability of hip joint in abduction	Musculus glutaeus medius and minimus	Motor point of musculus glutaeus medius	Sciatic nerve	Prone position
	Disability of hip joint in adduction	Adductors	Wuli (Liv 10)	Shenshu (B 23), Qihaishu (B 24), Dachangshu (B 25)	Sitting position
	Disability of thigh in extorsion (intorsion of foot in walking)	Musculus piriformis, musculus obturator externus and internus, musculus glutaeus maximus, mimimus and medius, musculus iliopsoas	Sciatic nerve (perpendicular and deep insertion to bone)	Motor point of musculus glutaeus medius (deep insertion towards sciatic nerve)	Prone position with extension of lower leg
	Disability of thigh in intorsion (extorsion of foot in walking)	Musculus glutaeus medius and mimimus	Motor point of musculus glutaeus medius	One cun below motor point of musculus glutaeus medius	Prone position with intorsion of lower leg

Knee	Disability of knee in extension	Musculus quadriceps femoris	Motor point of musculus quadriceps femoris	Nervus femoralis	Sitting position with knees extended
joint	Disability of knee in flexion	Hamstring muscles	Yinmen (B 37)	Sciatic nerve, or corresponding point	Recumbent position with knees flexed
	Inversion (weakness of extroversing muscle)	Musculus peroneus longus and brevis	Motor point of musculus peroneus longus	Guangming (G 37)	Sitting position with knees flexed and feet flat on ground
Ankle	Extroversion (weakness of inversing muscle)	Musculus tibialis posterior and anterior	Zusanli (S 36) or motor point of musculus tibialis anterior	One cun below motor point of musculus tibialis anterior	Sitting position with knees flexed and feet flat on ground
joint	Drop foot (weakness of foot dorsum in flexion)	Musculus tibialis anterior	Zusanli (S 36) or motor point of musculus tibialis anterior	One cun below motor point of musculus tibialis anterior	Sitting position with knees flexed and feet flat on ground
	Tiptoed foot (weakness of musculus tibialis anterior, spasm of tends calcaneus)	Musculus tibialis anterior	Zusanli (S 36) or motor point of musculus tibialis anterior	One cun below Zusanli (S 36) or one cun below motor point of musculus tibialis anterior	Sitting position with knees flexed and feet flat on ground
	Weakness of metatarsal in flexion (usually accompanied by deformed heel)	Musculus triceps cruris	Motor point of musculus gastrocnemius	Sanyinjiao (Sp 6) connecting with Xuanzhong (G 39)	Sitting position or supine position
Toes	Weakness of toes in flexion	Musculus flexor digitorum longus pedis	Sanyinjiao (Sp 6)	Weizhong (B 40) or Chengshan (B 57)	Sitting position or supine position
	Weakness of hallux in flexion	Musculus flexor hallucis longus	Xuanzhong (G 39)	Weizhong (B 40) or Chengshan (B 57)	Sitting position or supine position
	Weakness of toes in extension	Musculus extensor digitorum longus pedis	Motor point of musculus extensor digitorum longus pedis	Motor point of musculus extensor hallucis longus	Sitting position or supine position
	Weakness of hallux in extension	Musculus extensor hallucis longus	Motor point of musculus extensor hallucis longus	Motor point of musculus extensor digitorum longus pedis	Sitting position or supine position

Notes: If two groups of muscles are stimulated simultaneously, one point can be selected for each group. But in the correction of deformed foot, two electrodes must be connected with one group of stimulating points similar in properties. For example, if three groups of muscles in anterior, lateral and posterior leg are injured seriously, tibial nerve point, Yinmen (B 37), Weizhong (B 40) and Yanglingquan (G 34) can be used. If there is serious injury in the whole leg, nerve points on femoral nerve and sciatic nerve can be used in alternation with the Back-Shu points in the lumbar region. Generally speaking, point selection and combination should be fewer and precise. In the electric stimulation, additional points also should be used accordingly.

TABLE 2. POINT SELECTION AND COMBINATION FOR THE TREATMENT OF DEFORMED FOOT

Commonly encountered deformed foot	Affected muscles in motor impairment	Point selection and combination	Body position
Drop foot with inversion (with or without tiptoed walking)	Musculus peroneus longus and brevis	Motor point of musculus peroneus longus and Guangming (G 37)	Knees flexed and feet flat on the ground
Drop foot with extroversion (with or without tiptoed walking)	Musculus tibialis anterior	Zusanli (S 36) or motor point of musculus tibialis anterior and one cun below it	Knees flexed and feet flat on the ground
Tiptoed walking	Weakness of myodynamia in musculus tibialis anterior, spasm of tends calcaneus	Zusanli (S 36) or motor points of musculus tibialis anterior and musculus extensor hallucis longus	Knees flexed and feet flat on the ground
Drop foot	Anterior muscles of legs	Zusanli (S 36) or motor points of musculus tibialis anterior and musculus extensor hallucis longus	Knees flexed and feet flat on the ground
Deformed heel	Musculus triceps	Motor point of musculus gastrocnemius and Sanyinjiao (Sp 6) toward Xuanzhong (G 39)	Sitting position

Generally, 1 to 4 courses of treatments are needed in the above-mentioned therapy. Each course of treatment is composed of 10 to 12 treatments (one treatment a day). Treatment can be repeated after a 3-to-5-day interval. The statistics show satisfactory effects in the treatment of above-mentioned four diseases. For instance, in 551 cases of sequela of poliomyelitis (disease duration ranges from 3 months to 58 years, mostly from 10 to 14 years), the obvious effect is 44.1 percent and improvement is 39.9 percent, the effective rate reaches 84 percent. In fifty-five cases treated with body acupuncture, obvious effect shows 29 percent and improvement is 41.8 percent, the effective rate reaches 70.8 percent. In 25 cases treated by determination of heat sensitivity, only 28.5 percent are improved. In 20 cases of cerebellar ataxia (disease duration ranges from 2 months to 14 years), the obvious effect is 50 percent, improvement is 15 percent, and the effective rate reaches 65 percent. In 100 cases of peripheral facial paralysis (disease duration in all cases is within 3 months, averaging 21 days), the basic cure is 80 percent, the obvious effect is 5 percent, improvement is 8 percent, and the effective rate reaches

93 percent. In 40 cases treated with body acupuncture, the basic cure is 70 percent, the obvious effect is 5 percent, improvement is 10 percent, and the effective rate reaches 85 percent. In 25 cases of hemiplegia (disease duration in all cases is within 3 months, averaging 22.6 days, with clear consciousness, but disability in independent walking), 36 percent of the patients are able to walk independently only after one treatment. And 76 percent of the patients are able to walk independently after seven treatments. By comparison, after the first treatment and seventh treatment with routine acupuncture techniques, only 4 percent and 39 percent of the patients respectively are able to walk independently.

Addition: Criterions of Therapeutic Effect
(After one to four courses of treatments)

1) *Poliomyelitis*

Basic cure: a. The patient with a limp walk and who falls easily is able to walk a long distance with no falls, even able to run and jump after treatments. b. The patient walking with support on a stick is able to walk without support with a stick a long distance.

Obvious improvement: a. The patient with a limp walk and who falls easily is able to walk a long distance with less falls after treatment. b. The patient walking with support is able to walk without support, but unable to walk a long distance.

Improvement: a. The patient with a limp walk and who falls easily has an increase in muscular power after treatment. b. The patient walking with support still walks with support, but walks longer after treatment.

Failure: The patient fails to meet the above-mentioned criteria, including those who stopped treatment before four courses.

2) *Facial paralysis*

Basic cure and full recovery: a. The functions recovered completely. b. No abnormal conditions on face can be noticed in still, smiling and laughing (full recovery). c. Completely normal in a resting pose, but a slight flat nasolabial groove still can be noticed in smiling and laughing (basic cure).

Obvious improvement: a. Most functions recovered, there is no influence to daily life. b. Facial expression seems normal in a resting state, but the mouth twists to the side in a smile.

Improvement: a. Partial functions recovered. b. Facial expression seems abnormal in a resting state, but there is obvious relief compared to before treatments.

Failure: No situations in above criteria appear.

3) *Cerebellar ataxia*

Cure: Completely normal and without any negative signs in the cerebellar system.

Obvious improvement: a. The patient who was unable to sit or to sit stably is able to walk a short distance after treatment. b. The patient who was unable to eat with a spoon is able to eat with a spoon or chopsticks after treatment. c. The patient who was unable to walk stably is able to walk more stably and longer. The patient in one of the above three situations is taken as an obvious improvement.

Improvement: a. The patient who was unable to sit or to sit stably is able to sit stably and walk a short distance under support. b. The patient who was unable to eat with a spoon is able to eat with a spoon if helped a little bit. c. The patient who was unable to walk stably is able to walk a longer distance indoors.

Failure: No above situations.

2. Clinical research on acupuncture mechanism

1) *Relationship between electric conductivity of auricular needle and auricular points, between headache and electric conductivity of auricular points, and between therapeutical effect in auricular treatment of headache and electric conductivity of auricular points* Is the electric conductivity of auricle able to reflect its change, and on which auricular acupoints is it able to reflect in headache? In order to provide reference data for auricular therapy, and to estimate the degree of headache by change in auricular electric conductivity for obtaining better therapeutic effect, Dr. Kuang observed forty-two cases of headache due to neurasthenia by meridian detector. It was found that auricular Occiput, Forehead and Chin reflected painful sensation (more obvious in auricular Occiput and Forehead) when headache attacked, accompanied by change in electric conductivity. The more serious the headache was, the higher the electric conductivity was. There is significant difference by comparison between average value and that in the control group. Therefore in the auricular treatment of these patients, the above points can be used accordingly. The change in electric conductivity can provide data for assessing the degree of a headache (particularly in severe headache). With 100 mA as the normal value, the results showed that accuracy in severe headache reached 95 percent.

On this basis, Dr. Kuang did further observations on the relationship between the therapeutical effect in the treatment of headache by auricular painful points and the change in electric conductivity. The method and result are the following: a. To puncture painful points detected by the meridian detector, the needling sensation is soreness, heat, distension, and numbness, etc. b. To puncture with a thumbtack-type auricular needle, which is stuck with plaster on points and retained for two to four days. During needle embedding, the patient is asked to press on embedded needle by himself when headache attacks. There is a one-to-two-day interval between two treatments. c. To puncture with filiform needle on auricular point 1 to 2 mm in depth, and retain the needle for thirty minutes, and manipulate the needle once every five to ten minutes. The treatment is given once a day. Therapeutical effect is evaluated on the next day of the last treatment. Clinically, effect is classified into three levels: Disappearance, relief, no change. The results showed that in forty-two cases, headache in severe and median degree disappeared in a respective 47.1 percent and 68 percent, headache was relieved in a respective 68.4 percent and 31.6 percent, and headache disappeared to a mild degree in 100 percent. The total disappearing rate was 64.3 percent, the relieving rate 35.7 percent. If the electric conductivity of auricular points is used as an index for calculation before auricular therapy, the average electric conductivity in the subjects with different therapeutical effect becomes lower than that before the treatment, and pre-treatment electric conductivity in a group where headache disappeared is lower than that in a group where headache was relieved. This indicates that there is a certain relationship between therapeutic effect and the value of the pre-treatment electric conductivity. Consequently, the electric conductivity of auricular points is able not only to display the degree of headache and therapeutical effect, but also to provide an index for pregnosticating therapeutical effect in auricular therapy, which is beneficial to the research in both Chinese and Western medical treatment of headache. The determination of electric conductivity in auricular points is a research method on individual specialities.

2) *Relationship between neurathenia and dermal resistance of the Yuan-Source point* The external manifestations of internal diseases appear on the Yuan-source point of the corresponding meridian. Dr. Kuang determined the dermal resistance of the Yuan-Source points before, during and after treatments on eighty-three patients with neurasthenia, in order to observe the relationship between neurasthenia and meridians. The results showed that among 83 cases of neurasthenia, there were 236 diseased meridians on which the Yuan-Source points changed, on average 2.84 meridians on each person; during treatment there were 59 meridians, on average 0.71 meridian on each person; after treatment there were only 43 meridians which failed to recover, on average 0.51 meridian on each person. After 24-day treatments, 193 meridians recovered, the rate was 81.7 percent. Among 236 diseased meridians, most external manifestations appeared on the Kidney Meridian of Foot-Shaoyin, the Sanjiao Meridian of Hand-Shaoyang, the Liver Meridian of Foot-Jueyin and the Gallbladder Meridian of Foot-Shaoyang. The symptoms and signs of kidney disease can be low-spirits, poor memory, dizziness, tinnitus, blurring of vision, lumbar soreness, weak legs, lassitude, and poor appetite, etc. Hyperactivity of liver yang causes irritability, bad temper, dizziness, blurring of vision, headache and insomnia; deficiency of liver yin gives rise to headache, dizziness, tinnitus, and blurring of vision. Deficiency of gallbladder can produce headache, vomiting, fearful and poor sleep; and excessive gallbladder will have blurring of vision, tinnitus, dizziness, chest fullness, hypochondriac pain, bitter taste in the mouth, vomiting of bitter fluid, bad temper, insomnia, dream-disturbed sleep. Sanjiao governs five zang and six fu organs, nourishes meridians and connects with qi everywhere. Therefore, the functions of Sanjiao related to all the organs in functions. As a result, the symptoms of the above four meridians are in agreement with those in neurasthenia basically. Dr. Kuang thinks that the changes of dermal resistance on the Yuan-Source points of the Kidney Meridian of Foot-Shaoyin, the Sanjiao Meridian of Hand-Shaoyang, the Liver Meridian of Foot-Jueyin and the Gallbladder Meridian of Foot-Shaoyang are the external manifestations of neurasthenia.

With the treatment and improvement of disease, the resistance of the Yuan-Source points on corresponding diseased meridians gradually displays changes of full recovery and basic cure (71 cases in total, accounting for 88.5 percent), the recovery rate is high in a respective 94.9 percent and 85.3 percent; the rate is lower (56.1 percent) in patients with obvious improvement. The difference is significant. The above explanation indicates the close relationship between therapeutical effect and recovery of diseased meridians. Dr. Kuang thinks that the changes of resistance on the Yuan-Source points, to an extent, can manifest the condition of diseased meridians pre- and post-treatment of neurasthenia, as well as recovery degree of neurasthenia. At present, under the lack of objective indexes for dealing with neurological patients, the determination of resistance on the Yuan-

Source points needs further research in future.

3) *Relationship between acupuncture and Plasma DBH* Dr. Kuang observed sixty-four cases of functional and vascular headache (all the patients were diagnosed by specialists in the neurological department with a careful inquiry of disease history, physical and neurological examinations, also with EEG and CBFG, and examination of lumbar puncture if required, excluding organic diseases and intake of any kinds of medicine before acupuncture therapy). Acupoints: Bilateral Hegu (LI 4) or Neiguan (P 6), Taiyang (Extra) or Fengchi (G 20). The needles were manipulated for about one minute with rotation, by stimulation within the patient's tolerance. The needles were retained for 15 minutes and remanipulated for 1 minute before taking them out. Among 64 cases, 55 cases of headache displayed slight relief, and 9 cases, medial relief during acupuncture. Blood was taken from veins 15 minutes before and after acupuncture respectively for the determination of Plasma DBH. The results showed that among 64 cases, headaches decreased in 49 cases (76.5 percent) of differing extents after treatment. Among 49 effective cases, the content of Plasma DBH tended to decrease. Among failed cases, the content tended to increase. There is no statistical significance, perhaps related to the lack of enough cases.

Besides, Dr. Kuang also observed Plasma DBH in another group of patients with headache (functional and vascular) treated by acupoint injection of Injectio Angelicae Sinensis. The therapeutical method: To inject 20 percent Injectio Angelicae Sinensis into the Back-Shu acupoints. The acupoints were selected according to the area of headache: Bashu (Extra) (1.5 cun lateral to the eighth thoracic vertebrae) and Weishu (B 21) for frontal headache; Bashu (Extra) and Danshu (B 19) for temporal headache; Bashu (Extra), Ganshu (B 18) and Pangguangshu (B 28) for occipital headache; and Dazhui (Du 14), Bashu (Extra) and Ganshu (B 18) for vertex headache. The method was to insert a syringe needle (No. 22) perpendicularly into acupoint about 1 cm and then inject 20 percent Injectio Angelicae Sinensis into acupoint after the arrival of the needling sensation. Each acupoint was injected with 1.5 ml and four acupoints were used in each treatment. Blood was taken thirty minutes respectively before and during treatment for determination of Plasma DBH. The immediate effect in the first treatment was: Among 36 cases presenting headache in treatment, headache decreased in 22 cases (61.9 percent) in different extent 30 minutes later. Simultaneously, it was found that the content of Plasma DBH dropped obviously after the treatment in the patients who had headaches and obtained effect, while the content of Plasma DBH did not change prominently in the patients who had no headache during treatment and those who had headaches failed to obtain effect after treatment.

Dr. Kuang also treated thirty cases of headache due to internal injury according to syndrome-differentiation by meridian theory, and observed the relationship between therapeutical effect and activity of Plasma DBH. Among 30 cases, 12 cases were headache of yin deficiency, 8 cases were headache of liver yang, and 10 cases were headache of turbid phlegm. The method was as same as the above one. Each acupoint was injected 1.5 ml of 20 percent Injectio Angelicae Sinensis, and Bashu (Extra) was taken as the main pain-killing acupoint in each treatment. Afterwards other acupoints were added according to syndrome-differentiation. Plasma DBH was determined fifteen minutes before and after treatment respectively. The immediate effect was prominent in yin-deficiency headache than in liver-yang headache and in turbid-phlegm headache, while there was no significant difference between liver-yang headache and turbid-phlegm headache. This indicated that the therapy by syndrome-differentiation of meridian theory was best in effectiveness for yin-deficiency headache, good for liver-yang headache and worse for turbid-phlegm headache. Before treatment, there was no significant difference in activity of DBH between groups except that the activity of DBH was obvious higher in the group of turbid-phlegm headache than in liver-yang headache. After treatment, the activity of plasma DBH didn't decrease obviously in other groups except the group of yin-deficiency headache.

DBH is the last synthetase in the synthetic process of noradrenaline. It is believed that the determination of activity in DBH can be taken as an index for checking functions of the sympathetic system. Judging from the experiments in the above three groups, DBH tended to decrease and decreased prominently in all effective cases, regardless of acupuncture therapy, or injecting therapy with Injectio Angelicae Sinensis. The result showed that the above two therapies can perform the regulating abilities by sympathetic system.

4) *Relationship between acupuncture, RBCACHE and nail microcirculation* Is the pain-relieving effect in the acupuncture treatment of headache also related to the influence of the peripheral cholinergic system? Hydrolysis of acetylcholine deactivates under the functions of cholinesterase. Therefore, it is believed that the determination of RBCACHE can be an index for reflecting the activities of the peripheral cholinergic system. Dr. Kuang determined the activities of RBCACHE in fifty-three cases of headache (functional and vascular) treated by acupuncture therapy. Electric acupuncture was applied on bilateral Hegu (LI 4), Taiyang (Extra), Yangbai (G 14) or Fengchi (G 20) with an Electric Stimulator (Model BH-6, Wave Type-I, Interval Frequency 14 times/min, Fixed Frequency F1=0, Frequency Conversion F2=20 times/min). The points were stimulated for fifteen minutes with the intensity of stimulation under the patients' tolerance, and all the needles were twisted for one minute (200 times/min) before, during and after electric stimulation. RBCACHE was determined and nail microcirculation was observed before acupuncture and after stimulation in order to find the regulating ability of acupuncture toward peripheral blood vessels. It was found out that among 53 cases, 45 cases (84.9 percent) got immediate effect after electric acupuncture, and 8 cases (15.1 percent) failed. Among effective cases, the activities of RBCACHE decreased in 34 cases with treatment. There was no change in 1 case and there was an increase in 10 cases. Among 8 failed cases, RBCACHE decreased in 3 cases, and increased in 5 cases. By comparison between two groups, the decrease of RBCACHE was in the majority in effective cases, and the increase, in the majority in failed cases. There was significant difference between two groups. At same time it was detected that the average value in the content of RBCACHE decreased prominently after treatment than that before electric stimulation, and increased obviously in failed cases. Also it was found out that in effective cases the speed of nail microcirculation quickened after treatment. These results indicated that peripheral cholinergic mediator participates in acupuncture analgesia.

Besides, Dr. Kuang also observed the relationship between therapeutical effect and activities of RBCACHE in another group of sixty-five cases of functional and vascular headache treated by auricular acupuncture. Of them, fifty-five cases were under the attack of headache, and ten cases were in the interval of headache. Auricular therapy: During attack of headache, the corresponding points were selected bilaterally according to painful area (for example, Point Forehead for frontal headache, Point Taiyang for temporal headache and Point Occiput for occipital headache), at same time plus Point Nervus Occipitalis Minor, Point Subcortex and Point Ear-Shenmen. The points were punctured perpendicularly 1 to 2 mm in depth, the needles were twisted once and retained for fifteen minutes. For the interval of headache, the corresponding points also were selected in accordance with painful area where the headache attacked. The result showed that after auricular therapy, headache decreased and disappeared immediately in forty-two cases (76.4 percent), and failed to improve in thirteen cases (23.6 percent). In the determination of RBCACHE before and after treatment, it was found out that RBCACHE decreased obviously in the effective cases and had an increasing tendency in failed cases among fifty-five cases with attack of headache, but there was no significant difference. In the group of headache intermittence, there was no obvious change in RBCACHE after auricular therapy.

Clinical experiment and research demonstrate that in the effective cases, there are changes in the cholinergic system and noradrenaline system, as well as change in microcirculation, indicating that various acupuncture therapies can regulate functions of meridians via the above two systems.

II. Case Analysis

Case 1: Sequela of cerebral trauma

Name, Kang x x; sex, female; age, 18.

Complaints The patient had an accident during farmwork and lost conciousness for forty-five days. After regaining consciousness, the patient walked unstably and had trouble speaking. The patient was transferred to be treated in the acupuncture department on February 12, 1971. Neurological examination showed: Ambiguous and vague speaking, myodystony in the four limbs, decreased tendon reflex, all prominent on the right side of the body. Finger-nose test and heel-knee test confirmed prominent symptoms on the right side of the body, accompanied by unstable walking, and unrestrained cry and laugh. Diagnosis: Sequela of craniocerebral trauma. The patient's accident was very extensive. Among the symptoms, cerebellar ataxia was the major one seriously affecting patient's ability in daily life. Therefore the therapy with five-necessities stimulation was applied.

Prescription Huatuojiaji (Extra), bilateral Huantiao (G 30) and Quchi (LI 11).

Treatment procedure Huatuojiaji points (Extra) are located 0.5 cun lateral to lower border of each spinous process from the first thoracic vertebra to the fifth lumbar vertebra. The points, one from every other process and selected alternatively on both sides, were six to eight in number. The needles were punctured obliquely with an angle of 30° and lifted about 1 to 2 mm, if bone was hit. After insertion, the needles were twisted one or two times with large amplitude and then retained. The needling sensation should radiate to head upwards and to lumbosacral region downwards. Huantiao (G 30) was punctured perpendicularly and the needle was twisted one or two times with large amplitude, with needling sensation radiating to the foot and afterwards the needle was retained. Electric frequency: 0.5-1 time/sec.; electrode pole: alternatively applied. One electrode was applied to the left side of body and then the other one, applied on the opposite Huatuojiaji point (Extra). Electrodes on Huatuojiaji points (Extra) were exchanged once every ten minutes from bottom to top. The electrodes on Huantiao (G 30) and Quchi (LI 11) were alternated once every fifteen minutes. Stimulating time: sixty minutes.

Treatment course One treatment every day or every other day, twelve treatments as one course, three to five days' rest between two courses of treatments. Three treatments later with the above therapy, the patient was able to stand stably for one minute. One course of treatments later, the patient was able to stand longer, walk more stably and faster, and to speak understandably.

Precautions 1) Electric stimulation must be adjusted to a certain degree able to have obvious muscular contraction on limbs. If symptoms are not similar on both sides, electric stimulation can last longer on the side with serious symptoms. Attention must be paid to avoid needle dropping (the needles come out easily because of muscular contraction), theefore the needles must be reinserted to former depth and retwisted once to twice with large amplitude when electrodes are exchanged. 2) Physical exercises cannot be neglected and must be done for one to two hours. The programmes in physical exercises are learning to stand, walk and squat, and to learn finger-nose actions as well as to repeat actions alternatively and faster. Physical exercises should proceed from the easy to the difficult.

Explanation Dr. Kuang realizes that in the treatment of cerebellar ataxia, electric stimulation on acupoints with low frequency by the method of five-necessity stimulation, plus physical exercises obtains a better effect.

Case 2: Vertigo (primary hypertension)

Name, Gao x x; sex, female; age, 43.

Complaints For half a year because of frequent headache, dizziness and palpitation, the patient sought medical service and was diagnosed as primary hypertension by internal medical and neurological departments. Her blood pressure did not decrease obviously with the use of both Chinese and Western medicine. Her blood pressure fluctuated between 170/140 and 140/100 mmHg.

Prescription Blood-Pressure-Regulating Point (Line) (Extra).

Treatment procedure The patient took a sitting position and looked straight ahead. The Blood-Pressure-Regulating Point (Line) is located on the horizontal line behind auricular lobe, at the conjunction of anterior one-third and middle one-third of musculus sternocleidonmastoideus, from where the place within 0.5 to 3 cm below the conjunction of the anterior and middle one-third of this muscle is the Blood-Pressure-Regulating

Point (Line). The needles were punctured perpendicularly and lifted a little bit when hitting bone. Needling depth: Generally 2 to 3 cm in adults. Needling technique: The needles were slightly twisted 2 or 3 times with a small amplitude, and afterwards the needles were retwisted slightly 2 or 3 times with a small amplitude every 5 to 15 minutes in accordance with the condition of blood pressure, the needles were retained for 1 to 2 hours and retwisted slightly before taking them out. Needling sensation: It must be made to radiate to the head of the same side, accompanied by a cool sensation. After treatment: Blood pressure was 124/96 mmHg 20 minutes later; 130/92 mmHg 30 minutes later; 128/88 mmHg 45 minutes later; and 112/84 mmHg 2 hours later. Simultaneously the patient felt clear and comfortable in brain. Follow-up check: The patient was treated four times, and the symptoms were obviously relieved after first treatment. The next day the patient was able to work and to stop taking any hypertensive medicine. Although her work was stressful, the symptoms decreased gradually, and blood pressure was kept to a normal level. In a visit to the clinic one month later, blood pressure was 130/90 mmHg. In the follow-up half a year later, blood pressure was still kept to a normal level, with better subjective sensation.

Explanation Thirty cases of hypertension had been treated with the above-mentioned method. In accordance with the disease duration, cases were classified as 1 case of Ia degree, 4 cases of Ib degree, 9 cases of IIa degree, 15 cases of IIb degree and 1 case of IIIb degree. Cases of II degree were in the majority, accounting for 24 cases (80 percent). By the comparison before and after acupuncture treatment, blood pressure dropped to a normal level in 14 cases (46.7 percent), decreased to obvious effect level in 3 cases, decreased to effect level in 7 cases. There were 24 cases (80 percent) obtaining result above effect level. Judging from fourteen cases whose blood pressure was restored to a normal level, they were mainly cases of Ia and IIa degree. It must be noticed attentively that in fifteen cases of Ia and IIa degree, there were eleven cases whose blood pressure dropped to a normal level. It was observed that the decrease of blood pressure could appear very soon after acupuncture. Apart from Blood-Pressure-Regulating Point as the major point, Neiguan (P 6) also can be selected in accordance with the dropping range of blood pressure.

RESEARCH AND APPLICATION OF THE NEW NINE NEEDLES

—Shi Huaitang's Clinical Experience

Dr. Shi Huaitang, born in Changzi County, Shanxi Province, in 1922, began from his childhood to learn acupuncture in his family. He completed a one-year course in the Central Experimental Institute of Acupuncture and Moxibustion of the Ministry of Public Health in 1953. Then he became the chief of the Acupuncture Department, Internal Medicine Department and Massage Department of Shanxi Provincial Hospital. He wrote more than twenty major papers, including *The Inheritance, Development and Clinical Application of the Nine Needles,* and *The Clinical Application of the Plum-blossom Needle and the Scalp Therapy.* He is also the author of *The Practical Acupuncture and Moxibustion.* One of his papers *The Reformation and Clinical Application of the Nine Needles* received the scientific and technological achievement award of Shanxi Province. These nine needles of a new type have filled in gaps in the field of acupuncture therapy. For instance, the round magnetic needle treats phlebeurysma; the fire needle treats leukoplakia vulvae; and the fire blunt needle treats angioma. Now he is the director of the Shanxi Institute of Acupuncture and associate chief-physician.

I. Academic Characteristics and Medical Specialities

1. Creating the new nine needles

During his forty years of clinical acupuncture practice, Dr. Shi has researched the clinical application of the ancient nine needles. After five modifications he created the new nine needles, in which except for the filiform needle (including the long needle) and the three-edged needle, the other six needles were improved, i.e. the sagital needle, the magnetic round needle, the blunt needle, the sharp-hooked three-edged needle, the sword-like needle and the fire needle. He has also improved the plum-blossom needle. Dr. Shi has applied these new needles in his clinical practice in accordance with their indications and affects, which, comparatively speaking, widened the indications by simply using the filiform needles, and shortened the course of treatment and raised the therapeutic effect. The application of the new nine needles has also achieved satisfactory results in treating some difficult cases. The following is a brief introduction to the new nine needles:

1) *The sagital needle* It is one of the nine ancient needles. As said in the *Miraculous Pivot*, "it is 1.6 cun long, and has a large head and a sharp tip, and it may be used to reduce yang qi to treat general heat and heat of the head." Unfortunately, the acupuncturists of the later generations seldom used this needle and it almost vanished.

Dr Shi has found that this needle has special effects in the treatment of many diseases, especially effective for gastrointestinal diseases, skin problems and facial paralysis.

a. Making the needle: The needle consists of two parts, the body and the handle. The body is made of molybdenum 10 cm long, while the later is made of wood, 4 cm in length. A part of the needle body is in the wood handle, leaving the tip 0.5 cm. Extended with a sharp arrow head (See Fig. 1). Molybdenum is a heat-resisting material, which could be hardly out of shape, neither annealed in high temperature for sterilization. The edge of the needle is easily sharpened.

b. Manipulating the needle: Hold the needle handle with the thumb, index and middle fingers of the right hand and cut the selected area to cause slight bleeding. This needle is mainly used to cut perpendicularly the white or purplish cord on the buccal mucosa, with a distance 1 cm long. The numbers of the cuts are based on the length of the cord. This method is used for treating many gastrointestinal disorders and facial paralysis. In treating skin diseases, this needle is applied to cut gently the medial and posterior aspects of the ear, or the corresponding area according to the ear-points. Only three to five points or places are selected in each treatment. In treating the disorders caused by exogenous pathogenic wind, points from the Bladder Meridian may be cut up and down along the course of the meridian.

c. Indication: Diseases attacked by the exogenous pathogenic wind, deviation of the mouth due to windstroke, gastrointestinal disorders with white or purplish cord on the buccal mucosa, eczema, abscess, and chloasma. For example, a male patient aged sixty-four suffered from chronic gastroenteritis for many years.

In 1973, he noticed some white spots appeared on his buccal mucosa of both sides inside the mouth, which was diagnosed as cancer at an early stage by Beijing Hospital and Ritan Hospital. The treatment in the hospitals failed and in January of 1976, he came to see Dr. Shi for treatment, in which a sagital needle was applied to cut the white cord spots on the buccal mucosa. After three treatments, the white spots disappeared and he recovered from gastroenteritis.

2) *Magnetic round plum-blossom needle* This needle is a new creation of the ancient round needle in combination with the magnetic therapy of modern times. The round needle is one of the nine needles of ancient times, 1.6 cun long with a cylindrical body

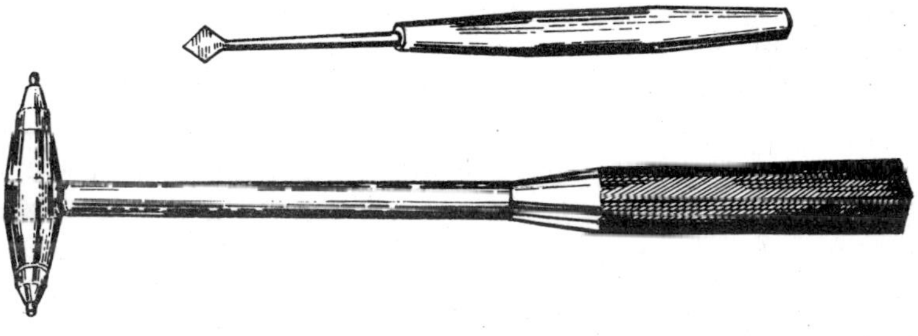

Fig. 1 Sagital Needle (Upper)
Fig. 2 Magnetic Round Plum-Blossom Needle

and an oval tip. It is often used to treat the skin and vessel disorders by pressing the points or meridians. In his clinical practice, Dr. Shi noticed the effect of either the plum-blossom needle or magnetic therapy in treating some chronic and intractable skin disorders. So the magnetic round plum-blossom needle was created. Since the shape of the both ends of the head is different, the functions of the needle vary (See Fig. 2).

a. Making the needle: The magnetic round plum-blossom needle is divided into two parts, the head and the handle. The handle consists of two parts connected by screws. The front part is thin and 12 cm long, while the back part is thick and 10 cm long. The handle is made of nylon 101. The head looks like a hammer, on which the high magnets are laid on both ends. One end is as round as a mung bean, called magnetic round needle, and the other end as the plum-blossom needle, known as the magnetic plum-blossom needle. The two heads and the handle are connected by screws.

b. Indication: This new type needle has the combined effects of the magnetic therapy, round needle and the plum-blossom needle. It is indicated in soft tissue injury, scapulohumeral periarthritis, varicose veins, gastroptosis, arteritis, phlebitis, bedwetting, arteriosclerosis, insect bites, hemotoma or swelling due to injury, tinea unguium, neurodermatitis (with the head of the magnetic plum-blossom needle); infantile diarrhoea, acute or chronic gastroenteritis, chronic enteritis, dysentery, rheumatic or rheumatoid arthritis, external and internal humeral epicondylitis, consumption disease, neurasthenia, prolapse of the rectum, prolapse of the uterus and infertility in women.

c. Manipulating the needle: Hold the handle tightly with the right hand, keeping the elbow flexed at an angle of 90°, tap the meridians, especially the points with the movement of the wrist five to ten times each. The principle for selecting the points is the same as that for acupuncture, and the procedure for the magnetic plum-blossom needle same as that for plum-blossom needle. The reinforcing, reducing and even movement are performed by tapping along or against the meridians and according to the intensity of stimulation. Mild tapping along the course of the meridian is considered reinforcing, heavy stimulation against the course of the meridian is reducing; medial tapping on the meridian back and forth is considered even movement, which is still under research. For example, a female patient aged forty-eight suffered from popliteal neurodermatitis for eight years, accompanied with severe itching which worsened at night. She was treated in many hospitals by both herbal medicine and Western drugs, but with little result. The patient also had varicosis on her lower limbs but she refused to have surgery. She came to see Dr. Shi in February, 1982. Examination: Lichenoid change 8 x 4 cm in size, skin thickened, desquamation, keratoses, and a little bleeding by scratching, limbricoid varicosis along the two legs with slight swelling.

Treatment: Tap the affected area heavily with the head of the magnetic plum-blossom needle until it reaches congestion, and also tap heavily the three yin meridians against their running courses. After three treatments the itching was much alleviated and the skin was smoother. After ten treatments she recovered from the neurodermatitis. A following visit was made three months later and there was no relapse. Tap the varicosis heavily from below to up until prominence appears. One treatment cured the case.

3) *Blunt needle* It is one of the nine needles of the ancient times. As said in *Miraculous Pivot*, it is 3.5 cun long and its tip looks like a piece of broomcorn millet.

The needle is mainly used to massage the diseased area to dispel the pathogenic factors, but not too deep. However, it was seldom used by the later generations. Dr Shi made a copy of the needle and applied in the clinic. This needle has particular effect on some diseases, especially on pediatric disorders, infantile indigestion, diarrhoea and sprain. When it is burnt for cauterization (a detailed discussion of the method will be given in "Fire Needle"), it can treat small angioma, verrucous vegetation, superficial pigmented nevus, senile plaque, chronic ulceration, anal fistula and fissure.

a. Making the needle: The blunt needle is 12 cm long, of which the wood handle is 9 cm long, and the molybdenum body is 3 cm long. The tip looks like a piece of broom-corn millet (See Fig. 3).

b. Manipulating the needle: Hold the handle with the thumb, index and middle

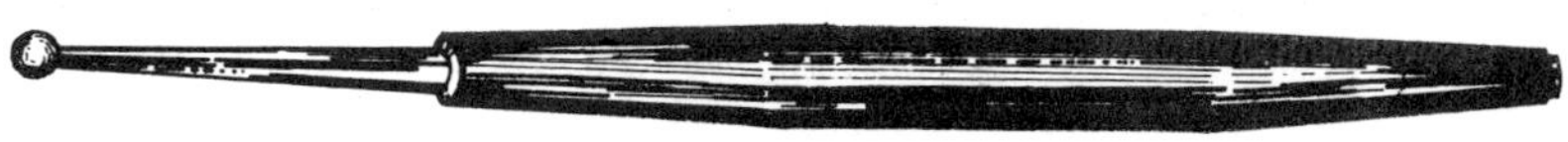

Fig. 3 Blunt Needle

fingers as though holding a pen, then press the selected points for a while to cause a clear depression until the needling reaction appears.

c. Indications: It is mainly used for children for malnutrition, infantile vomiting or diarrhoea, indigestion, or for finding the tenderness, reaction point, Ashi point or for causing a depression as a marking in cauterization. For example, a female patient aged sixty came to see Dr. Shi on January 11, 1980, complaining of sprained right ankle joint, accompanied with red swelling, pain and difficulty walking. The next day the redness and swelling turned blue, and the pain worsened. She was then treated with a blunt needle pressed hard at the corresponding area of the left wrist. Ten minutes later she could move the right ankle, but she still could hardly walk. As there was bruise and swelling from the stagnation of blood in the collaterals, the plum blossom needle was applied to tap the local area for half an hour, then the patient could move on the ground and she recovered the next day.

4) *Sharp-hooked three-edged needle* One of the nine needles, 1.6 cun long with a prismatic sharp tip used to treat intractable diseases. The three-edged needle used today is derived from it. The hooked needle is very popular among the ordinary people for it is often used to treat boils. During his clinical practice, Dr. Shi combined the two needles into one unit to make a sharp-hooked three-edged needle. (See Fig. 4)

a. Making the needle: It is made of stainless steel, 4 cm in length, with the thick middle part and thinner ends. The head is hooked with three sharp edges; but the sizes of the two tips are different, as they may be selected correspondingly according to the different locations or the nature of the diseases. So the needle in one hand can be used to puncture the vessels by causing bleeding to alleviate blood stagnation; or on the other hand, by lifting-thrusting the needle, to cut down the fatty tissue or muscle fibre in order to remove the obstructions. As the tip of the needle is only 3 mm, it causes less pain with

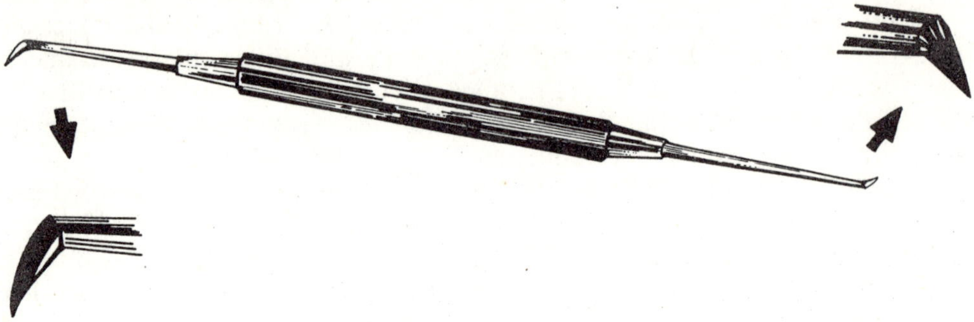

Fig. 4 Sharp-hooked Needle

a very small cut, when it is used for cutting purpose, but gives high effect and offers large indications.

b. Manipulating the needle: First, a routine sterilization is given to the selected needling area, and the needle is dipped into 75 percent alcohol for a while before puncturing. The right hand holds the needle while the index and middle fingers of the left hand stretch the skin of the needling area, then the right hand punctures the needle quickly into the skin. For cutting purpose, the needle is first punctured under the skin, then turned perpendicularly to the skin, and lifted and thrust slightly, a crack sound can be heard when the needle cuts the muscle fibre. The needle should be turned back to the original puncturing angle before withdrawing it, in order to avoid any further skin injury. Afterwards, a piece of cotton ball is used to press the needling spot.

c. Indications: Local functional disturbance due to some chronic diseases, intractable pain problems (scapulohumeral periarthritis, nervous headache, lumbar muscle strain, tenosynovitis, sequela of cerebral thrombosis, bronchitis, asthma and gastro-spasm), some acute infectious disorders (such as acute conjunctivitis, tonsillitis, acute or chronic pharyngitis, shock, and aphonia). For example, a male patient aged forty-six came to see the doctor on May 14, 1980, complaining of intermittent migraine on the left side for two months, attacks occurring at lunch time. Drugs such as analgesics and rotundin did help him, but could not cure the disease. The patient was subsequently diagnosed in a hospital as having nervous headache. He was treated with Western medicine, but with little result before he came to see Dr. Shi. Examination: Good development, listlessness, normal heart and the lung; normal liver and spleen, ECG. normal, BP: 140/90 mmHg, throbbing sensation at the left temple area on pressure, deep and forceful pulse, dark red tongue with some small purplish spots. He was treated with sharp-hooked three-edged needle by puncturing Dazhui (Du 14), Tianzhu (B 10), Fengchi (G 20) and Taiyang (Extra) to cause bleeding, and the pain stopped immediately. On May 16, 1980, he came back to tell the doctor that the pain had completely gone, and there was no relapse.

5) *Sword-like needle* It is also one of the nine needles. As it says in *Miraculous Pivot*, "The sword-like needle is 4 cun long and 0.2 cun wide. Its tip looks like a sword, which is used to treat abscess." However later generations did not use this needle in

acupuncture treatment. Dr. Shi tried to apply it in the treatment of some diseases which had never been treated by acupuncture before and he noticed a good result. But the method now he uses is entirely different from the one in ancient times. Actually, he uses this needle in combination with the fire technique, with which he called cauterization and cutting method, such as the treatment of neoplasm, anorectal polynus or big wart. This method is easy and effective and causes neither infection nor bleeding.

a. Making the needle: The method and material are generally the same as those for the arrow head needle, only the tip of the needle is in the shape of a sword head, 2 cm long and 0.5 cm wide. The tip and both sides are sharp. As with the arrow head needle, this needle is also heat-resistant, hardly annealed in high temperature, and difficult to break, but may be sharpened again. (See Fig. 5)

b. Manipulating the needle: Burn the tip of the needle on the flame of a spirit lamp until it gets red, then hold the needle horizontally with the thumb, index and the middle fingers of the right hand, keeping the sword tip towards the medial aspect of the operator and the handle of the needle to the lateral aspect, and with the forceps in the left hand, lift the diseased tissue (such as neoplasm, polynus or dermatoma) and then cut it off from the end of the tissue quickly. One treatment is usually enough. Observe the cut for five minutes. If there is any blood oozing, a blunt needle is applicable to cauterize the cut, and then press there for a while before binding the cut.

c. Indications: It is mainly used to treat skin disorders, such as big verrucous vegetation, anoretal polynus, or polynus exposed clearly on some other parts, benign dermatoma, old anal fissure and external hemorrhoids. For example, in March, 1981, a woman came to see Dr. Shi, complaining of a small tumour superior on the right breast which had been there for years, pain due to friction of her clothes. She was asked to have surgery in another hospital before she came, but she was afraid. Examination: Good health, tumour 2.8 x 2 cm in size directly above the right breast, thin, soft and long, the top red. Treatment: The cauterizing and cutting method with a sword-like needle was used to cut off the tumour from its end and there was no oozing of blood. The pain was gone after binding. Half a year later, the patient was still healthy.

6) *Fire needle* Fire needle therapy is noted in *Miraculous Pivot* as burning needle of fire acupuncture, and called in *The Treatise on Febrile Diseases* heating needle, and in *A Classic of Acupuncture and Moxibustion Therapy*, white needle. It has been called fire needle in the books of *High Light of Acupuncture*, *Compendium of Acupuncture* and *Complete Works of Acupuncture* since the Ming and Qing dynasties. The clinical application of the fire needle is much more progressive today than in ancient times.

a. Making the needle: The fire needle made of wolfram is classified into six kinds

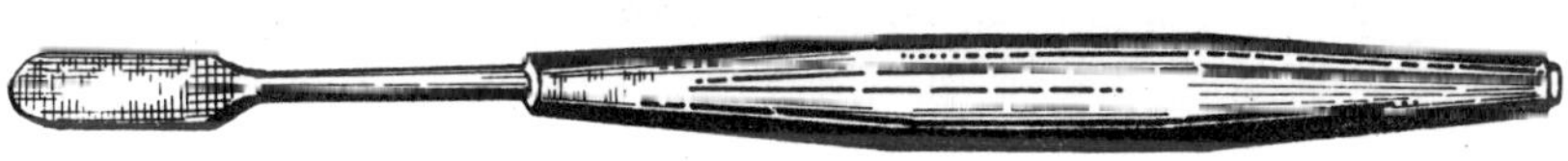

Fig. 5 Sword-shaped Needle

according to the different requirements of diseases. This needle is heat-resistant, free of change in its shape, neither annealed nor broken, but harder in high temperature. The six kinds of fire needle are thin fire needle, 0.5 mm in diameter; medium-sized fire needle, 0.75 mm in diameter; thick fire needle, 1.2 mm in diameter; three-headed fire needle, three needles bound together 0.75 mm in diameter each; blunt fire needle, similar as an ordinary blunt needle; and sword-like fire needle, like the common sword-like needle as mentioned above. The handles of the fire needles 5 cm long are all made of wood except the fire three-headed needle, 9 cm long, which is made of stainless steel. The length of the needle body is 5 cm, but that of the three-headed needle is 1 cm. (See Fig. 6)

b. Manipulating the needle and indications: An alcohol burner and several different fire needles are prepared. A routine sterilization is applied to the selected points prior to the treatment. A blunt needle is then used to press a dent on the skin in order to make a marking for the treatment (it is not advisable to use any staining material to mark the dent to prevent black staining). Take a prone position when the treatment is given. According to the different cases, either the prone position, or supine position or lateral recumbent position, may be selected. Hold the fire needle with the operator's thumb, index and middle fingers of the right hand as though holding a pen, and hold up an alcohol burner with the left hand, put the burner close to the treatment area, and burn the needle on the flame with an angle of 45° until it gets white, red or pink. Rapid insertion, quick shallow pricking, or slow cauterization may be used respectively according to the purpose of the treatment. No matter which method is applied, the needling spots should be pressed hard immediately after the manipulation to prevent bleeding. Rubbing or rotating shall in no case be used.

As said by an ancient physician, "The fire needle might be applied to any part of the body but the face." Dr. Shi thinks the face is not really forbidden for fire needle treatment, but great care should be taken when the points around the sense organs are selected. In that case quick shallow pricking or slow cauterizing is mostly used.

Selection of the points: Either the regular points, Ashi points or the diseased area

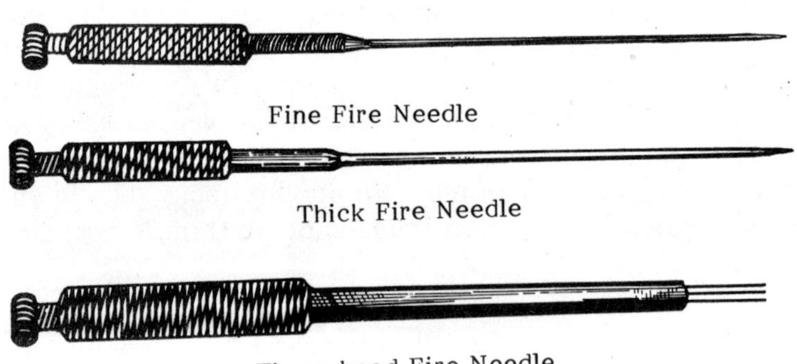

Fig. 6 Fire Needle

may be selected according to the nature or location of a disease. The course of the treatment also varies. Generally speaking, the method for selecting the points according to differentiation is mostly used in clinical treatment today.

Deep rapid insertion: The needle is inserted to the deep area of a point as though to insert with an ordinary filiform needle. The needle is first burnt to white and bright, then quickly punctured into the point, and immediately taken out. This method is mainly used to treat chronic gastroenteritis, chronic colitis, rheumatic and rheumatoid arthritis, or regressive and traumatic arthritis, scapulohumeral periarthritis, tennis elbow, lumbar muscle strain, sciatica, chronic dysentery, leukoplakia vulvae, trigeminal neuralgia, sequela of windstroke, tuberculosis of spine, osteoraticular tuberculosis, intractable insomnia, impotence, chronic pelvic infections, dydrarthrosis, muscular rheumatism, subdermal cyst, bursitis, thyroid enlargement, hydrarthrosis, abscess or boils, and purulent mastitis. The needle is inserted to get through both the upper and lower walls of the cyst for treating lipoma; the needle should be inserted towards the centre of the tubercle for treating scrofula; and the needle is inserted down to the end of the hard tissue for treating clavus. Though a deep insertion is needed for the treatment of above-mentioned diseases, the depth of the needle should still be varied according to the patient's constitution, the nature of the disease and the location of the point. However, the depth of a normal filiform needle insertion may be taken for reference when the deep rapid insertion of the fire needle is applied.

Shallow pricking method: Burn the needle to red, then rapidly prick and remove the needle. This method is mainly indicated for various kinds of pigmented nevus, small verruca vulgaris, flat wart, soft wart, angioma in small size, arthritis of phalangeal joints, intractable facial paralysis, trigeminal neuralgia, auditory vertigo, supraorbital neuralgia, intractable ulceration, mucosal ulcer, tinea unguium, tuberculoderm, vulva lichen, and peripheral neuritis.

Slow cauterizing method: Burn the needle to a little red, and then cauterize the superficial skin of the diseased area gently and slowly. This method is mainly used to treat pigmented nevus more than 5 mm in diameter, various kinds of warts, intractable ulcer, ulcer due to varicosis of lower extremities, senile plaque, ephelis, superficial angioma, internal and external hemorrhoids, fissure in ano and leukoderma of small size.

Methods for selecting the six kinds of fire needles: Generally, the medium-sized fire needle and the thick fire needle are mainly used to treat hydrarthrosis, cystis, mucous ulcer in small area, mastitis, inducing pus in abscess or boils, lipoma, pigmented nevus of small size, angioma, and various kinds of warts. The sword-like fire needle and blunt fire needle may be used in combination. The sword-like fire needle is used first to cut or cauterize the diseased part and then the blunt fire needle follows to iron and mend the cut or the cauterized part to stop bleeding, treating external hemorrhoid, skin vegetation, or prominent warts, verruca and small tumour, all of which could be cut down to the level of the skin, and then covered with some sterilized dressing over the treated area. The blunt fire needle may also be used to treat a superficial ulcer, fissure in ano, superficial angioma, superficial pigmented nevus of large area, senile plaque, internal hemorrhoid and leukoderma. The three-headed fire needle is mainly applied to cauterize diseases like medium-sized nevus, vegetation 0.5 mm higher than the skin, ephelis, senile plaque and mucosal ulcer.

Precautions:

1) When deep rapid insertion method is applied, the needle should be burnt until white and bright, otherwise, the needle would be inserted or removed with severe pain. Withdrawal of the needle should be rapid and forceful to avoid entangling the needle with the fibrous tissue.

2) Needle should be away from the areas close to the internal organs, the sense organs and the major arteries; and the depth of insertion around these areas should be shallow.

3) Strict sterilization is required before the treatment, and after the treatment the patient should be told to be careful with his needling spots or the cuts in order to avoid infection.

4) The needles, such as the medium-sized fire needle, the thick fire needle, the three-headed fire needle, the blunt fire needle or the sword-like fire needle should be selected according to the pathological conditions. A large needle is used if the diseased area is large; and vice versa. The cutting or cauterizing method is applied based on the nature of a disease. But in general, localized anesthesia is required before treatment.

Case examples:

1) Name, Luo x x; sex, male; age, 41.

The patient complained of a wart on the right side of the lower lip of the mouth in 1984. It was as big as a grain of rice without pain or itching, and broke when he ate one day in the summer of 1985. After that, it was infected with a swollen mouth and sharp pain. The infection improved five days later after he had been treated with antibiotics in a local clinic. Then the patient was referred to the Shanxi Second Hospital to treat the wart, but with no result after two treatments by crymotherapy. The wart grew bigger and troubled the patient in his daily life. Examination: Verruca vulgaris 1 x 0.8 cm in size on the mucous membrane of the right side of the lower lip, clear edge with oozing of blood on the top, pain on pinching. Treatment: Prick the affected area with a three-headed fire needle seven times after local sterilization, then apply the blunt to cauterize the scab area slightly and dress the treated area. The follow-up visit ten months later showed that there was no scab left on the original place.

2) Name, Zhang x x; sex, male; age, 37.

Chief complaints: Chronic colitis for twelve years, accompanied with intermittent abdominal pain, diarrhoea, loose stool with excess mucous and undigested food, loss of the weight to 13 kg, general lassitude, and poor appetite. After the colonofiberscope examination, he was diagnosed as having chronic colitis. He was then treated by medication, injections, and enemas of both TCM and Western medicine, but with little improvement. The patient had problems in the summer of 1982 after eating some muskmelon, and the disease soon developed. He was treated in Shanxi Provincial Academy of Traditional Chinese Medicine by more than sixty herbal remedies, and by herbal enema for two months, but with little help. In the spring of 1984, the patient was referred to Dr. Shi. Examination: Lassitude, emaciation, general aversion to cold, cold limbs, sallow complexion, weak voice, dent of the lower abdomen, touching of the spinal cord on slight palpitation, clear tenderness on the left side of the lower abdomen, deep slow and forceless pulse, especially at the right "Chi" region, pale slippery tongue with white sticky coating.

Differentiation: Dysfunction of the spleen in transportation and transformation due to deficiency of yang of both kidney and spleen.

Treatment principles and method: Invigorating yang, resolving damp, strengthening the spleen and stopping diarrhoea by applying the thin fire needle pricking at points of Shuifen (Ren 9), Zhongwan (Ren 12), Tianshu (S 25), Zhixie (Extra), Dachangshu (B 25), Xiaochangshu (B 27), Yinlingquan (Sp 9), and Mingmen (Du 4).

The second visit took place five days later and the patient was much improved, except for loose stools. His appetite increased, and the tongue coating was thinner. The same prescription was given again and there were no more symptoms after his third treatment. But the patient insisted to have one more treatment for consolidation.

Dr. Shi has been applying the fire needle method to treat nearly sixty kinds of symptoms and diseases. He has noticed that this method has a high and quick effect. Usually one treatment is enough for many symptoms or diseases, such as various kinds of warts, vegetation, pigmented nevus, external hemorrhoid, fissure in ano, etc. The selection of different kinds of needles varies in accordance with the nature of the disease, as *Miraculous Pivot* says, "Nine needles are designed for various purposes; as they are in different sizes and shapes, the diseases will not be eliminated if the needles are used in a wrong way." According to his clinical experience, Dr Shi reformed the fire needle in six sizes and had great success in the treatment. However, the nature of the disease of cold or heat, deficiency or excess may be neglected when the fire needle method is applied. Just as *Highlights of Acupuncture* says, "Fire needles invigorate qi circulation with heating. So there is neither reducing nor reinforcing nor any harm towards a deficiency or an excess case. But the other kinds of needles invigorate qi circulation through reinforcing or reducing, or deep or shallow insertion to bring about the antipathogenic qi, or to dispel the pathogenic factors. It will be harmful if the methods are wrongly used against the nature of a disease, as reducing for a case of deficiency, reinforcing for a case of excess." Acute rheumatic arthritis with red, swollen, hot and painful joints is an excess with heat condition. But the fire needle still can be used to treat it by warming and clearing the meridians and collaterals, so as to remove the stagnation of pathogenic heat. Pain then may be relieved and swelling alleviated. The fire needle method may also be applied to treat some facial problems, such as senile plaque, ephelis, pigmented nevus, angioma or vegetation.

7) *Plum-blossom needle* The plum-blossom needle is an instrument used to tap or prick the superficial skin. It is not included among the ancient nine needles, but it has been developed from the ancient needling techniques of shallow needling, extremely shallow puncture and centro square needling.

a. Making the needle: It is made of five to seven needles bound together with their tips at the same level and fixed at one end of a small stick. The one composed of five needles on its end is known as plum-blossom needle, while that with seven needles is known as the seven-star needle. Though the names are different, the therapeutic effect of the two needles is the same. According to his clinical experience, Dr. Shi also reformed the traditional plum-blossom needle. The handle of the needle consists of two parts, made of nylon, 4 cun long each, connected by a stainless steel junction. The sharp tips are

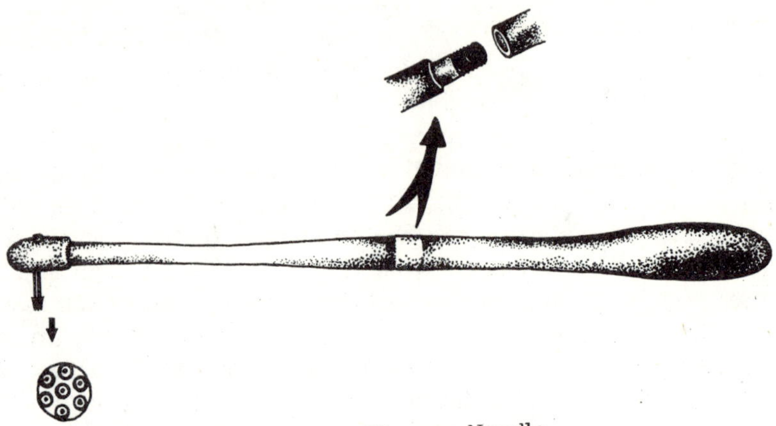

Fig. 7 Plum-Blossom Needle

replaced by the blunt tips, thus the patient's suffering is reduced.

b. Manipulating the needle: Burn the head of the needle on an alcohol burner, and sterilize the tapping area with a 75 percent alcohol cotton ball prior to treatment. Hold the handle with the four fingers of the right hand except the index finger which presses on the top of the handle, leaving the end of the handle on the transverse crease of the wrist. Tap the skin surface with a flexible movement of the wrist with an even movement. Tapping may be divided into light, medium and heavy stimulation according to the pathological condition.

c. The intensity of stimulations and course of treatment: The intensity of stimulation is divided into light, medium and heavy according to the location for tapping, the patient's constitution and the nature of the disease.

Generally, ten treatments constitute a course. The second course is usually started within a two or three day interval after the first course.

d. Tapping area: Tap along the running course of the meridians. Commonly used are: Head-Du Meridian, Taiyang and Shaoyang Meridians; Back-Du Meridian, Huatuo Jiaji, Taiyang Meridian; Abdomen-Ren Meridian; and Four Limbs-Points from the regular meridians below the elbow or knee. The tender points and the affected area are often tapped locally.

e. Indications: General disease, especially for headache, dizziness, nervous system disorders, skin disease, sequelae of cerebral accident, gas poisoning, insomnia, cerebral arteriosclerosis, sprain, infantile diarrhea and dysentery, etc. As the needle is used to prick the skin superficially, it is good for children, thus it is also called the child's needle.

THE STIMULATING METHOD AND LOCATION

Intensity of stimulation	Manipulation method	Requirements	Indications		
			Location	Constitution	Nature
Light	Gently flexible movement of the wrist, high frequency of tapping with a very short distance of the needle moving up and down	Slight redness at the local area	Head and face	Old people, weak constitution and children	Deficiency and chronic cases
Heavy	Heavy flexible movement of the wrist, low frequency of tapping with a high distance of the needle moving up and down, flexible movement of the wrist	Redness at the local area with a little bleeding	Back, buttock, the four limbs and the local diseased area	Young adults, people with strong body constitution	Excess and new disease
Medium	Redness at the local area between the heavy and light manipulation	General area without bleeding	General location	General	Mixture of deficiency and excess, cold and heat

2. Sticking needle method

This method is used to continue maintaining the strong needling sensation during acupuncture treatment. If the needle is accidentally stuck, a tension is felt under the needle which is difficult to lift or thrust, because the needle is entangled with the muscular tissue. However, this method differs from the needle that is accidentally stuck, as the sticking needle is only to touch the muscular tissue at its tip. The other part of the needle is not entangled with any muscular tissue or superficial skin tissue. The sticking of the needle may be withdrawn easily with several gentle backward rotations. The method has the effect of strengthening the needling sensation, spreading the propagated range, and bringing the qi to the diseased area. Good results have been obtained in the treatment of some painful disorders due to tissue accretion in some chronic infectious diseases, or disorders due to the functional disturbance.

Manipulation: When the needle is retained, place the index and middle fingers of the left hand separately in front and behind the point, while the thumb and index finger of the right hand hold the handle of the needle. The tip of the middle finger of the right hand touches a side of the point to make a triangle around the needle. The index and the middle fingers of the left hand stretch the skin. The needle is then inserted slowly to the expected depth by the thumb and index finger of the right hand lifting, thrusting and rotating until the needling sensation arrives. Afterwards, twirl the needle in one direction without any back and forth rotating; then lift the needle slightly and tension may be felt. Remove the left hand, the needle then is stuck. Now it is difficult to rotate, lift and thrust the needle with the right hand; the operator may feel tension and heaviness around the needle; and the patient at the same time will feel a strong needling sensation around the point.

Indications: Generally diseases except for deficiency cases, especially for numbness and painful disorders, tissue accretion in chronic infections (such as accretion due to periarthritis, which leads to difficulty in raising the arm), or adhesion of the intestine to the internal abdominal wall after surgical operation.

A case example:

Name, Wang x x; sex, female; age, 30; date of the first visit, March 5, 1974.

Chief complaints: Constant dull pain of the lower abdomen since hysterectomy six months before. The pain was aggravated when she straightened her back or coughed. She had to press the lower abdomen hard to walk, and working was impossible.

Examination: Heart and lungs were normal. The pain on the lower abdomen was aggravated by pressure, and there was tenderness below the cut. Dragging pain might be felt when the skin of the cut was gently lifted, but no any other abnormality.

Diagnosis: Postoperative intestinal adhesion.

Treatment: Sticking needle method on Ashi point was used. The tip of the needle went down to a depth where there was an adhesion of the intestine and the internal abdominal wall. The needle was then lifted slightly and there appeared a tenderness with a dragging sensation. Sticking the needle there by twirling the needle in one direction was performed and at the same time the index finger of the left hand pressed hard at the skin around the needle. The right hand lifted the needle vigorously while the left hand was removed. The patient let out a scream and the adhesion was separated. The skin around the cut was lifted after the withdrawal of the needle but there was no more dragging pain at all. She now could straighten her back without pain. Three days later she came again for another treatment in order to prevent further adhesion. The patient was advised to do certain exercises after the treatment. A follow-up visit 6 months later revealed no recurrence of the disease and she went back to work normally.

3. Method with multiple needles but shallow insertion

The method is manipulated by inserting three needles 0.1 cun deep at one point. The needles are inserted superficially, and the needle body is perpendicular, shaking along with the movement of the patient. This method is also called the suspending needling method. It is derived from "triple puncture," "perpendicular puncture" and "superficial puncture" noted in *Miraculous Pivot*. Triple puncture is to puncture the centre of the affected part with one needle and both sides with two needles respectively to treat the localized cold bi symptoms. Perpendicular puncture is to insert the needle subcutaneously by pinching the skin to treat the superficial bi syndrome. Superficial puncture is to needle shallowly lateral to the affected part to treat muscular spasm of cold nature. The method with multiple needles in shallow insertion is a comprehensive summary of the three needling techniques. Three needles are used together to puncture shallowly to treat superficial cold bi syndrome, i.e. the pathogenic factors only stay in the collaterals but not the meridians. Clinically, this method has a special effect in the treatment of facial spasm.

A case example:

Name, Fan x x; sex, male; age, 19; date of the first visit, June, 1980.

The patient had a spastic tic on the left lower eyelid and the left face in 1977. The disease progressively worsened from intermittent to continuous attack, accompanied with lacrimation and blurred vision. "Facial spasm" was diagnosed in some hospitals and was treated with various methods and medication before, but with little help. Treatment: Chengqi (S 1), Tongziliao (G 1), Zanzhu (B 2) and Sibai (S 2) were needled with multiple needles in shallow insertion. Good results were produced after each treatment. Seven treatments completely stopped his facial spasm.

4. The application of the Lower-Zhibian

The lower Zhibian is a point used by Dr. Shi for forty years. Since this point is located inferior to Zhibian (B 54), it was then named as lower Zhibian.

1) *Location* Take a lateral recumbent position with the knee flexed in an angle of 130°, and the body slightly tilted forward, then draw an equilateral triangle with one line joining the anterior superior iliac spine to the centre of the greater trochanter, while the other two lines meeting at the centre of the hip. The point is located at the junction of the later two lines in the centre of the hip.

2) *Indications*

a. Lower limbs disorders: Systremma, paralysis of the lower limbs, sciatica, injury of musculus piriformis, sequela of poliomyelitis, rheumatalgia of lumbar muscle, sequela of cerebral accident, paraplegia, polyneuritis, peripheral euritis, nerve injury of the lower limbs, and Buerger's disease.

b. Disorders of the urinary and reproductive systems: Cystitis, urethritis, urethralgia, enuresis, retention of urine, dysmenorrhea, leukorrhea, prolapse of uterus, vaginitis, leukoplakia vulvae, pruritus vulvae, uterine bleeding, irregular menstruation, enterospasm and impotence.

c. Disorders of the rectum and anus: Constipation, pruritus ani, prolapse of rectum, fecal incontinence, dyschesia and pain of the anus.

3) *Manipulation* Select a filiform needle gauge No. 28 3.5 to 5 inches long and insert perpendicularly to make the needling sensation radiate down to the leg and toes to treat the disorders of the lower limbs. Tilt the needle obliquely forward to the lateral abdomen with an angle of 10°, the needling sensation may reach the lower abdomen, external genitals or perineum to treat the disorders of the urinary and reproductive systems, while tilting the needle obliquely backward to the sacral region with an angle of 10°, the needling sensation may travel to the anus to cause a feeling of a bowel movement. Needling this point always causes a strong needling sensation with clear radiation and the patient may scream when qi arrives, or an abrupt movement of the lower limbs may appear. Lifting-thrusting and rotating techniques are sometimes given to obtain qi after insertion of the needle, and the sticking needle method is immediately used to radiate the qi to the diseased area. The needle should be retained for one or two minutes; otherwise, there may be a strong post-needling sensation.

5. A personal understanding about Huatuo Jiaji points

Huatuo Jiaji points (Extra), also called Jiaji, are located along the spinal column 0.5 cun lateral to the spinous process from the first thoracic vertebra to the first sacral vertebra, seventeen points on each side and thirty-four in all. Today, another fourteen points are added on both sides from the first cervical vertebra to the first thoracic vertebra, 0.5 cun lateral to the spinous process. Therefore, the total number of Huatuo Jiaji points (Extra) is forty-eight. They are named by Dr. Shi as Cervical Jiaji, Thoracic Jiaji or Lumbar-sacral Jiaji according to their locations respectively at the cervical, thoracic or lumbar-sacral vertebrae. The following is the generalization of the indications of Huatuo Jiaji Points (Extra) and the method of application:

Points	Indications	Needling method	Moxibustion method
C1-C77	Disorders of the head and neck	Perpendicular or slightly oblique inserting to the vertebra; 1 to 1.5 cun deep for the points of the cervical vertebrae and 2 to 2.5 cun deep for the points of the lumbar vertebrae	Three cones to each point, or 5 to 15 minutes with moxa sticks
C4-T1	Disorders of the upper limbs		
C3-T9	Disorders of the chest, heart and lung		
T5-T12	Disorders of internal organs in the upper abdomen		
L1-L5	Disorders of organs in the pelvic cavity		
L2-L5 Sacral Vertebra	Disorder of the lower extremities, the organs in the pelvic cavity		

1) *Huatuo Jiaji (Extra) may be used instead of Back-Shu Points* Huatuo Jiaji (Extra) points, corresponding to the Back-Shu points, have the similar indications and effects as the Back-Shu points. Since Huatuo Jiaji points (Extra) are convenient and safe in use, and provide a stronger needling sensation, they are much more effective in the treatment of the disorders of the four limbs. The needles may be inserted obliquely from the Back-Shu points towards the deep part of the corresponding Jiaji points (Extra) in case of treatment of zang or fu diseases. The Back-Shu points are all from the Bladder Meridian, and close to their corresponding zang or fu organs, they are indicated in the

disorders of the zang or fu organs or the related organs.

2) *The new use of Huatuo Jiaji Points (Extra)*

a. Eye disorders: Jiaji Points (Extra) from C 3-C 6 in combination with some positive reaction spots on the back may be pricked with a sharp-hooked three-edged needle to treat glaucoma and central vetinitis, to lower the intraocular pressure, and to treat chronic conjunctivitis or congestion, swelling of the eyes together with Taiyang (Extra) and Zanzhu (B 2) with pricking to cause bleeding.

b. Cervical vertebra disorders: A fire needle may be selected to puncture the Jiaji Points (Extra) on both sides of the diseased cervical vertebra with a deep rapid insertion. The therapeutic result is quite satisfactory.

c. Hyperplastic spondylitis: A thin fire needle is used with a deep rapid insertion to puncture Jiaji Points (Extra) on both sides of the diseased vertebra, which may warm and invigorate the circulation of qi and blood around the diseased part and then remove the obstructions from the local collaterals.

d. Rheumatic or rheumatoid arthritis: Jiaji Points (Extra) C 7-T 1 are selected for treating the diseases of the upper limbs; while Jiaji Points (Extra) from L 2-L 5 and Baliao points, i.e. Shangliao (B 31), Ciliao (B 32), Zhongliao (B 33) and Xialiao (B 34) are used for treating the diseases of the lower limbs. Jiaji Points (Extra) on both sides of the diseased vertebrae are punctured for treatment of rheumatoid spondylitis, which is effective not only for relieving pain and swelling, but also for dropping the E.S.R. in case the thin fire needles are used with a deep, rapid insertion.

e. Tuberculosis of spine: Jiaji Points (Extra) on both sides of the vertebra and Ashi points between the vertebrae may be punctured with thin fire needles by applying the method of a deep, rapid insertion. Ashi points in the center between the vertebrae are sometimes called Zhuijian Xue (between the vertebrae).

f. Sciatica and thromboangiitis obliterans (Buerger's disease): A thick filiform needle (about No. 26 in gauge) is used to puncture Jiaji Points (Extra) from L 3-L 5 3 to 4 cun deep. Only one point on the diseased side is needled for each treatment to keep the needling sensation going down to the toes.

II. Case Analysis

Case 1: Retention of urine (simple prostatomegaly)

Name, Wu x x; sex, male; age, 70.

Complaints The patient was admitted to the hospital on September 9, 1985 because of cough for half a month, fever for three days and retention of urine for one day. In the hospital he was treated with the method of anti-infection. His fever was gone, but the symptoms of distension and straining sensation in the abdomen and retention of urine still existed. The surgeons were invited for consultation. Rectal touch: Moderate hypertrophy of the prostate, the central groove turning flat and shallow. Impression: Simple prostatomegaly. Treatment: 1) Urinary anti-inflammatory agent. 2) Maintaining the urinary catheter. 3) 2 mg. b.i.d. with intra-muscular injection of 2 mg diethylstilbestroh twice a day. But there was little help for alleviating the retention of urine after the treatment, then orchiectomy was suggested, but refused by the patient because of his advanced age. Dr. Shi was then asked to give him acupuncture treatment. Differentiation: Downward disturbance of the lung heat to the urinary bladder. Principle of treatment: Remove the heat from the lower jiao.

Prescription Zhibian (B 54), Mingmen (Du 4), Yaoqi (Extra) and Baliao (B 31-B 34).

Treatment procedure Zhibian (B 54) on both sides were needled, retaining the needles twenty minutes for the first treatment. The needling sensation was required to reach the testis and urethra. The patient could have urination during the treatment. The second treatment took place on the next day and the patient felt the abdominal distension was much improved. In addition to the needling of Zhibian (B 54) with a filiform needle, Mingmen (Du 4), Yaoqi (Extra) and Baliao (B 31-B 34) were pricked by a sharp-hooked three-edged needle. The catheter was removed after this treatment. Five treatments stopped all the symptoms.

Explanation Chronic prostatitis is one of the common diseases of the urinary system and it is in the category of retention of urine in TCM. The onset of the disease in this case was due to the accumulation of lung heat which led to the dysfunction of the lung in regulating water passage and the heat then infused down to the urinary bladder to cause dysfunction of the bladder in evaporation. Retention of urine occurred. Reducing Zhibian (B 54) and Baliao (B 31-B 34) with the needling sensation going to the diseased area could eliminate the heat of the lower jiao, and regulate the qi of the urinary bladder. A sharp-hooked three-edged needle was used to prick Mingmen (Du 4) and Yaoqi (Extra) to invigorate yang qi (as these two points are from Du Meridian which dominates yang qi of the whole body) and then send yang qi down to the kidney to strengthen the evaporating function of the urinary bladder.

Case 2: Pruritus (hyperplasia of the collagen fibre of derma)

Name, Han x x; sex, male; age, 50.

Complaints The patient had pruritus for eleven years since 1970. It started with itching at the medial aspect of the right leg. At the beginning, the diseased area was as big as a finger nail, accompanied with dermostenosis, darkened skin, loss of the hair on the local part and sclerotic creases. It became larger in the size of 4 x 5 cm with every symptom worsening. The patient was treated with different methods including herbal medicine and Western medicine but without any help. He was then diagnosed as having "hyperplasia of the collagen fibre of derma."

Differentiation Stagnation of the pathogenic toxin which caused the obstruction of the circulation of qi and blood.

Prescription Tap the affected area with a magnetic plum-blossom needle.

Treatment procedure Four treatments with a magnetic plum-blossom needle cured the case.

Explanation Such kind of pruritus is not often seen in the clinic. But the disease seemed to be related to exogenous pathogenic wind and heat or some toxin of the insects. All these might be accumulated and then stagnated between the skin and muscles, leading to obstruction of the circulation of qi and blood which fails to nourish the skin, so the disease occurs. The application of the magnetic plum-blossom needle is actually a kind of combination of acupuncture and magnetic therapy. Local tapping with a plum-blossom needle eliminates the pathogenic factors, while the magnetic therapy dilates the local blood vessels to promote the blood circulation, thus helping regenerate the skin.

Case 3: Epistaxis

Name, Zhang x x; sex, male; age, 62.

Complaints The patient got a severe attack of epistaxis after exhaustion in August, 1979, and then he was admitted to a local hospital to have treatment for eight days with TCM and Western medicine but with little help. He was then transferred to the First Affiliated Hospital of Shanxi Medical College where he stayed for another fifteen days. Blood examination showed that the hemochrome was only 7 g. The patient then received a blood transfusion with renin gauze in the nose to stop bleeding by pressure and hemostat, but blood still oozed, and bleeding occurred after removing the gauze. Examination: General lassitude, sallow complexion, poor appetite, difficulty in breathing and deep thready pulse.

Differentiation Dysfunction of the spleen in controlling blood.

Prescription Yinbai (Sp 1), Zhiyin (B 67), Shaoshang (L 11), Shangyang (LI 1), Guanchong (SJ 1) and Shangxing (Du 23).

Treatment procedure Needle with the filiform needles with moderate stimulation. Retain the needles for twenty minutes. The next day the gauze was removed and bleeding stopped. The follow-up visit for three years found no relapse. The patient had another attack in 1982, and was cured only by one treatment. There is no recurrence of the disease so far.

Explanation The Jing-Well Points are either the terminal or starting points of the regular meridians, and are also the important connections of yin and yang meridians. Thus, they are considered as the fundamental points for regulating yin and yang of the body. For treating a hemorrhage case, no matter it is an excess or deficiency, the Jing-Well Points of the Heart, Lung, Liver, or Spleen Meridians or their related meridians may be selected according to the involved zang or fu organs. The reinforcing method is applied in case of deficiency and reducing in case of excess.

Case 4: Abdominal pain (acute intestinal obstruction)

Name, Li x x; sex, female; age, 60.

Complaints The patient noticed a sudden severe abdominal pain in the morning on November 17, 1982. The pain was intermittent, accompanied by nausea and vomiting. During the attack, a protuberance could be palpated in the abdomen, and there was also severe abdominal distension. She was then sent to a hospital and was subsequently diagnosed as having acute intestinal obstruction. The gastrointestinal decompression technique, infusion of fluid, and enema were given but with little help. The pain persisted and there was no bowel movements or passing gas. Then the patient was transferred to Dr. Shi's house at 11 that night for treatment. Examination: Grey and yellow complexion, extreme exhaustion, with eyes and mouth closed, cold sweating on the forehead.

Deep and thready pulse, tenderness or rebounding pain on the abdomen, and the muscular strain of the abdomen not clear.

Differentiation Stagnation of qi of the intestines.

Prescriptions

1) Dachangshu (B 28), Xiaochangshu (B 27), Ciliao (B 32) with even movement. 2) Changqiang (Du 1) with sticking needling method and retaining of the needle for several minutes.

Treatment procedure During the treatment the patient wanted to have a bowel movement. After withdrawal of the needles, she had some frothy stool in a moderate volume with gas. Her abdominal pain and distension were much alleviated after the bowel movement. Twenty minutes later, all the symptoms disappeared. The next day a relative came to say that the patient had recovered and went to work. She had another attack at about 7 o'clock in the evening on November 20, 1985 with the symptoms of abdominal pain, distension, nausea and vomiting, intestinal protuberance during pain, a little stool and gas, vomiting of food on pressure on the abdomen. Three hours later Dr. Shi was invited to give her a treatment. He considered the problem as incomplete intestinal obstruction. The same prescriptions were used and soon the patient had a bowel movement in a moderate volume with gas. The pain was much alleviated. The patient recovered the next day.

Explanation Intestinal obstruction is one of the common symptoms in acute abdominal diseases. TCM considers it as obstruction and rejection or intestinal stagnation. The disease will occur when there is stagnation of qi, calculation of blood, accumulation of heat, retention of cold, or retention of roundworm, all of which may lead to the derangement of the intestines in normal descending. Stagnation of qi and blood leads to the pain, qi stagnation causes distension; retention in the intestines leads to abnormal bowel movements. Nausea and vomiting result from the upward attack of stagnated cold. The principle of treatment is to remove the obstruction and stagnation. Changqiang (Du 1) is the Luo-Connecting Point of the Du Meridian communicating with Ren Meridian. Giving strong stimulation to this point may regulate the qi circulation of the Du Meridian and induce the qi downward. Needling Dachangshu (B 28), Xiaochangshu (B 27) and Ciliao (B 32) may remove the obstruction from the intestines and promote qi circulation in the intestines, and then bowel movement becomes easy.

Case 5: Infantile diarrhoea

Name, Wei x x; sex, male; age, 10 months; date of the first visit, September 9, 1985.

Complaints The patient had loose stool for over ten days. The stool was watery, green, sometimes with mucus. He had four or five bowel movements each day after meals, but no fever. The patient was sent to Taiyuan Children's Hospital where he was diagnosed as having infantile diarrhoea. He was treated with neomycin and pepsin orally for three days, but with little help. Then the patient was brought to Dr. Shi for acupuncture treatment. The child was also restless, his heart and lungs were normal, his abdominal wall was soft and there was no hepatosplenomegaly.

Differentiation Retention of excessive damp.

Prescription Dachangshu (B 28), Shenshu (B 23), Tianshu (S 25), bilaterally;

Shuifen (Ren 9), and Qihai (Ren 6).

Treatment procedure Fire needles were applied to all of the points. The patient recovered with only one treatment. A follow-up visit revealed no recurrence of the disease.

Explanation Children are considered to be major yang constitution, and both yin and yang are extremely tender. Prolonged diarrhoea must damage yin and further yang. Thus the principle of the treatment is to warm the yang and stop diarrhoea. Fire needles may warm up the yang. Tianshu (S 25), Shuifen (Ren 9) and Dachangshu (B 28) are needled to promote the function of the intestines in transportation and transformation, in order to clarify essence from the food and water, and keep the turbid downward. Shenshu (B 23) and Qihai (Ren 6) are needled again to warm the yang and stop diarrhoea.

PRIORITY FOR QI REGULATION AND MAGIC USE OF NEW POINTS

—Bi Fugao's Clinical Experience

Bi Fugao, a native of Shangshui County, Henan Province, was born in a medical family in September, 1923. He practised medicine at the age of sixteen, and opened his own clinic when he was twenty. In 1949, he worked in the United Traditional Chinese Medicine Clinic. He was sent to Henan College of Traditional Chinese Medicine for further training in 1958, and then was transferred to the Provincial Institute of Traditional Chinese Medicine. With a great interest in acupuncture, he has improved the use of Huatuojiaji points in his clinical practice therefore improving the curative effects for treatment of arachoid membrane paralysis, sequelae of windstroke, and Wei syndrome. He discovered the new point "Huanzhongshang Xue," which is very effective for prolapse of the uterus, ptosis of the anus, nocturnal enuresis and seminal emission. He was awarded the First Scientific and Technological Prize issued by Henan Province. He was director and deputy research fellow of the Research Office of Meridians and Collaterals of Henan Institute of Acupuncture and Moxibustion, vice president of Henan Association of Acupuncture and Moxibustion, vice president of Zhengzhou Society of Acupuncture and Moxibustion, and he is a member of the Henan Association of Traditional Chinese Medicine.

I. Academic Characteristics and Medical Specialities

1. Priority of qi regulation based on zang-fu organs

1) *Qi and blood* Dr. Bi holds that the mechanism for acupuncture and moxibustion lies in activating the flow of qi in the meridians, so priority should be given to qi regulation and then to promoting the blood circulation. Only by this way can the desired effect be achieved.

Procedure: a. Yangming, Shaoyang and Shaoyin Meridians which have abundant qi should be used to promote blood circulation. b. Reduce the meridian qi to promote the blood circulation, and reinforce the qi of zang-fu organs to activate the blood circulation. c. Reinforce the meridians and zang-fu organs which are abundant in blood.

2) *Number of the points* Dr. Bi holds that the number of points varies according to the patient's conditions. Generally, two or three points, but most of the time, only one point is selected for bi syndromes, while more than ten points, even twenty points are needled for facial paralysis. For bi syndromes, such as sciatica, the diseased areas are limited in Shaoyang or Taiyang Meridian, at most both meridians. The meridian route is straight for qi and blood circulation, so a few points will do. As for facial paralysis, three yang meridians are crossed on one side of the face, making the meridian routes

tortuous for qi and blood circulation, so more points are needed. For instance, a patient suffered from facial paralysis for several years. Having failed to get any positive results from various acupuncture treatments with few points, he came to Dr. Bi. Examination: Inability to raise the brow and to close the eyes, downward twisting of the mouth corner, all these indicating the involvement of three Yang Meridians, and also leaking of qi to whistle, failure in showing the teeth, emaciation and poor appetite. Prescription: The points from three Yang Meridians, based on reinforcing Zhongwan (Ren 12) and Zusanli (S 36). Beginning from the fifth treatment, some improvement occurred, and the patient was well in two weeks.

3) *Selection of the points from the left or right side* The points on the right side are selected for the disease located on the left side and vice versa. Based on this theory, Dr. Bi applies massage, thus rapid curative effects are achieved. In the autumn of 1985, he treated a female patient aged sixty suffering from sequelae of windstroke, complaining of severe pain on right Fengshi (G 31), which failed to respond to any posture. Examination: Normal skin colour, free from redness and nodules. It hurt slightly upon pressure. Dr. Bi punctured Fengshi (G 31) on the left side, with massage on the right side after the needling sensation was obtained. The patient first felt tightness and heaviness beyond her tolerance under the needle. After manipulation, she felt comfortable and could stretch, flex, lift and drop the leg at any position. In this case, the motor impairment is caused by obstruction of wind resulting in stagnation and pain. Since the twelve Regular Meridians, twelve Divergent Meridians, eight Extra Meridians and fifteen Collaterals are interrelated, forming the route for qi and blood circulation, puncturing one side can treat the other side. In cases of long-standing stagnation leading to deficiency of qi and blood, activating the meridian qi on the healthy side is not enough to dissolve the stagnation. Massage is added on the affected side to help eliminate the pathogenic factors.

4) *Zang-fu and meridians and collaterals* Though zang-fu organs and meridians and collaterals are different in their functions, there is still an inseparable relationship between them, because the meridians and collaterals are related to fu organ but pertain to zang, and related to zang organs but pertain to fu. In practice, detailed examination should be given to see whether the zang-fu organs or the meridians and collaterals are involved. Generally, the bi syndrome is a disease of the meridian because of a shallow and narrow diseased area, stress should be therefore laid on meridians and collaterals. The injury of the soft tissues may be treated by selecting the points along the meridian. As to zang-fu diseases such as spleen dampness, treatment should focus on regulating the qi activity of the zang-fu organs. Points are mainly selected from the Front-Mu, Back-Shu, Shu-Stream and He-Sea points, but seldom from the Xi-Cleft, Luo-Connecting, Jing-Well and Jing-River points. However, if the zang-fu disorders affect the meridians and collaterals, such as hypochondriac distension of the liver disease, stress should be laid on the zang-fu organ, while at the same time conduct qi to the affected area. Points are mainly selected from the Front-Mu and Back-Shu points in combination with Xi-Cleft and Luo-Connecting points. In 1980, Dr. Bi treated a female patient of forty-seven suffering from complete paralysis, aphasia and irritability. She was treated with the points from the four limbs and nape region, but failed to get any positive results. Dr.

Bi selected Qimen (Liv 14), Ganshu (B 18), Zhongwan (Ren 12), Pishu (B 20) and other related Shu points and local points. Five days later, the patient could walk and speak. She was completely cured after another five treatments.

5) *The root cause and the symptoms* Clinically, Dr. Bi regulates qi of zang-fu organs to treat the root cause, and differentiates the meridian qi to treat the symptoms. In the spring of 1981, he treated a girl, nineteen with wei syndrome, who suffered from complete paralysis for eight months, myodynamia on the left limb was 0, that on the right side II degree, incontinence of urine and stools, hypopsia of the right eye, weak constitution, superficial pulse, pale and flabby tongue and white coating. Diagnose: Arachnoid adhesion. Differentiation: Retention of lung heat and dampness in Middle Jiao. Principle of treatment: Clear away lung heat, and eliminate spleen dampness. He used the new Jiaji point on the thoracic and abdominal column to activate the lung qi and spleen qi. During the course of treatment, she often felt fever, pain of the limbs, loose stools, irritability and sore throat, which were more unbearable than the original complaints. Dr. Bi abided by the prescription and made alterations according to the change and finally cured the patient.

6) *Movement and quietness* Dr. Bi holds that the organic physiological function pertains to movement and is absolute, while the local focus caused by qi and blood stagnation pertains to quietness and is relative. Acupuncture is actually to promote qi and induce blood, that is to promote movement to eliminate stillness. Therefore, for the treatment of sequela of windstroke or bi syndrome, frequent manipulations are made in combination with the patient's active or passive massage movement. In case of deafness due to kidney qi deficiency or eye disorder due to hyperactivity of liver qi, manipulation is given to activate qi and induce blood. Generally, short retaining of the needles is for disease which the treatment can be combined with external movement, longer retaining is for the disease which the treatment cannot be combined with external movement, such as deafness and facial paralysis. The purpose for longer retaining of the needle is to transform the stillness into movement.

2. Discovery of new points based on the meridians

In his practice, Dr. Bi found some Ashi points effective for qi regulation and blood inducing. "Huanzhongshang Xue" is a point he found on Gallbladder Meridian during his treatment of sciatica. This point, 2.5 cun superior to Huantiao (G 30), can be inserted 4 to 6 cun deep. According to the different directions of needling, qi can be radiated to the toe, uterus, and anus. It is therefore able to treat many disorders. The new Jiaji points, thirty couples in all, including the pair points above the first vertebra and below the seventeenth vertebra, are located 0.5 cun lateral to the original Huatuojiaji points. The application of the new points raised the curative effects and widened the indications. Shangmiantanxue, 0.5 cun lateral to Taiyang (Extra), can be needled 2 cun deep with the needle tip penetrating Xiamiantanxue, which is below the midpoint between Dicang (S 4) and Jiache (S 6), and needled 2 cun deep with the needle tip directing Shangmiantanxue. Needles are retained for thirty minutes with synchronous manipulation and good results are achieved in the treatment of facial paralysis.

II. Case Analysis

Case 1: Windstroke (sequela of cerebral hemorrhage)

Name, Liu x x; sex, male; occupation, peasant.

Complaints The patient suffered from hypertension for more than ten years. He had a cerebral hemorrhage in January 1975. Two months treatment in a hospital restored his mental clearness, but failed to treat his hemiplegia. From then on he had deviated mouth and eyes, salivation, and an inability to blow the mouth. He came for treatment in November 1976. Examination: Clear mind, obese body, short breath, myodynamia on the right limbs III grade, myotony weakened. The right arm could be lifted to the chest, hand grasping force was 0. The lower limbs were weak, but he could lift his leg but he could not walk without help. Shallowed nasolabial groove, inability to blow the mouth, salivation, string-taut and rolling pulse, flabby tongue with tooth marks, yellow sticky coating. BP 118/80 mmHg. Diagnosis: Sequela of windstroke with the involvement of zang-fu organs. Differentiation: Phlegm-damp resulted from obese constitution, too much stress made yang hyperactive on the upper portion of the body and yin deficient on the lower portion. Liver wind in combination with phlegm attacked the mind. So symptoms of loss of consciousness, obstruction of the meridians, qi and blood blockage appeared, leading to deviation of mouth and eyes, and paralysis of the limbs.

Prescription Jiaji point on lumbar region, Jianyu (LI 15), Quchi (LI 11), Hegu (LI 4), Liangqiu (St 21), Yanglingquan (G 34), Xuanzhong (G 39), Bafeng (Extra), Shangmiantanxue, Xiamiantanxue.

Treatment procedure Treat once a day. Thirty treatments constitute a course. After being treated ten times, improvement could be seen on the right leg, the patient could walk three to five steps with a walking stick. On January 2, 1977, when the second course was completed, the patient could blow his mouth and lift his right arm over his shoulder. He could walk five meters without any help. On January 11, the facial paralysis was relieved and he could stretch or flex the right arm and walk stably on the right leg. The blood pressure remained 150/80 mmHg.

Explanation Jiaji points can activate the qi of zang-fu organs and Du Meridian, resolve phlegm and dampness. The combined use of two Miantan points can dredge the meridians and collaterals on the face. For facial paralysis, the points are mainly selected from Foot Yangming, Foot Shaoyin and three Hand Yang Meridians. Jianyu (LI 15), a crossing point of Yangming and Yangqiao Meridians, can treat contracture, obstruction and flaccidity of the upper limbs. Hegu (LI 4), a Yuan-Source point of Hand Yangming, is able to regulate the general functions and to activate the qi flow of the meridians. Quchi (LI 11), the He-Sea point of Hand Yangming Meridian, where the meridian qi infuses, can connect qi of the fu organs, and promote qi flow, and dredge the meridians. The combined use of Hegu (LI 4) and Quchi (LI 11) can treat facial paralysis, as well as paralysis of the upper limbs. Yanglingquan (G 34), the He-Sea point of Foot Shaoyang, is able to reduce the liver and subdue wind, activate tendons and collaterals. Xuanzhong (G 39), the Major Connecting point of the three foot yang meridians, and the influential point of marrow in combination with Bafeng (Extra) can treat difficulty in walking.

Case 2: Bi syndrome (sciatica)

Name, Hou x x; sex, male; age, 53; date of the first visit, February 24, 1976.

Complaints Lumbago for more than two years, which was aggravated on cloudy or rainy days, accompanied by pain of the legs, inability to walk, listlessness. The pain also got worse upon coughing. Examination: Tender points on both sides of Chize (L 5). The pain was radiated to the legs upon heavy pressure. Straight leg raising test (+) within 35°, motor limitation of the left leg, dark red tongue, white sticky coating. Differentiation: Pathogenic wind-cold and damp obstructing the meridians and collaterals and causing stagnation. Principle of treatment: Activate blood circulation to remove blood stagnation, eliminate wind to check pain.

Prescription Both sides of Shiqizhui, Huanzhongshangxue.

Treatment procedure Treat once a day. The pain disappeared after continuous treatment for seven days.

Case 3: Tinnitus

Name, Guo x x; sex, male; age, 56; date of the first visit, April 8, 1978.

Complaints Tinnitus for many years, which was like the sound of cicada and got worse upon exertion, accompanied with soreness and weakness of the lower back and legs, dizziness, blurred vision, irritability and insomnia. Medical examination showed nothing wrong with the ear. Examination: External ear, nose, throat, tonsil normal, BP 120/90 mmHg, thready and rapid pulse, red tongue, slight yellow coating. Differentiation: Kidney opens into the ear. Deficiency of the kidney meridian results in tinnitus. Kidney stores essence, brain is the sea of marrow. Kidney qi deficiency will result in dizziness and blurred vision. The kidney dominates the bones. The lumbar region is the place where the kidneys are located. Deficiency of the kidney will lead to soreness and weakness of the lower back and legs. Disharmony between the heart and kidney brings about insomnia and excessive dreams. Red tongue, thready rapid pulse are the signs of yin deficiency and hyperactivity of fire. Principle of treatment: Nourish kidney yin and calm the mind.

Prescription Shenshu (B 23), Sanyinjiao (Sp 6), Tinghui (G 2).

Treatment procedure Treat once a day with reinforcing method. After twenty treatments, tinnitus disappeared.

Explanation Shenshu (B 23), where the meridian qi is infused, is good for zang-fu disorders. Sanyinjiao, the crossing point of three Foot Yin Meridians, can nourish yin and blood. Tinghui (G 2), the crossing point of Shaoyang and Yangming Meridians, is good for ear disorders.

Case 4: Insomnia

Name, Kuang x x; sex, male; age, 46; date of the first visit, February 7, 1978.

Complaint Insomnia for three years, accompanied with dream-disturbed sleep, irritability, dry mouth, spontaneous sweating, dizziness, vertigo, tinnitus, palpitation, poor memory. Administering of sedatives and hypnetics failed to have any effect. Thready and rapid pulse, red dry tongue without coating. Differentiation: Overthinning injures the spleen, failing in producing the essence, short nourishment of the heart by blood. Principle of treatment: Calm the wind.

Prescription Pishu (B 20), Shenmen (H 7), Neiguan (P 6), Sanyinjiao (Sp 6).

Treatment procedure Treat once a day. Retain the needles for twenty minutes. After being treated for seven days, the patient could sleep for six to seven hours, and other symptoms disappeared.

Explanation Pishu (B 20) can nourish and strengthen the spleen and activate the spleen qi, Shenmen (H 7) is to regulate the qi of the Heart Meridian, and to calm the mind. Sanyinjiao (Sp 6), the crossing point of three yin meridians, is able to nourish yin and blood, benefit the kidney and regulate the spleen to strengthen the zang-fu organs.

Case 5: Nocturnal enuresis

Name, Yang x x; sex, female; age, 21; date of the first visit, May, 1977.

Complaints Nocturnal enuresis since childhood, sometimes twice a night, dizziness, soreness of the lower back. Examination: Normal development, heart, lung, liver and spleen normal, deep thready pulse, slight red tongue and white coating. Differentiation: Kidney qi deficiency. The kidney controls stools and urine. In case of dysfunction of the kidney, enuresis occurs. Dizziness and soreness of the lower back indicate kidney deficiency.

Prescription Huanzhongshangxue.

Treatment procedure Needle Huanzhongshangxue with the tip of the needle directing the anterior perineum, four cun in depth without rotating. Sparrow-pecking method was applied one or two times to conduct the needling sensation to the anterior perineum. Treat once a day. After five treatments, the patient was cured. No relapse was found during the follow-up visit two years later.

Explanation Huanzhongshangxue is effective for nocturnal enuresis.

Case 6: Impotence

Name, Li x x; sex, male; age, 36; date of the first visit, September 15, 1973.

Complaints For the past ten years, the patient suffered from dizziness, tinnitus, palpitation, shortness of breath, soreness and weakness of the lower back and legs, insomnia, excessive dreams and premature ejaculation. In 1966, he was impotent, and did not respond to any treatment. Examination: Dark complexion, tired appearance, dull eyesight, low voice, lung, liver and spleen normal, deep thready and weak pulse, pale tongue, thin white coating. Differentiation: Deficiency of kidney qi. Principle of treatment: Nourish the kidney.

Prescription Shenshu (B 23), Huanzhongshangxue.

Treatment procedure Reinforce Shenshu (B 23), needle Huanzhongshangxue with a 5-cun filiform needle 4 cun in depth without rotating, but the needle tip directed to the anterior perineum. The case was cured after one month treatment.

Explanation Huanzhongshangxue may have immediate effects on disorders of the genitals.

SYNCHRONOUS MANIPULATION AND COMBINATION OF PAIR POINTS

—Lu Jingshan's Clinical Experience

Dr. Lu Jingshan, a native of Luoyang, Henan Province, was born in November, 1934. When he was eighteen, he was enrolled in the Taiyuan Medical School in Shanxi Province. He studied in the Beijing College of Traditional Chinese Medicine at the age of twenty-one, and was assigned to work in the Shanxi Institute of Traditional Chinese Medicine after his graduation. From 1964 to 1965, he joined an acupuncture training course in aid of foreign countries sponsored by the Ministry of Public Health. From 1975 to 1977, he was a member of the medical team working in Cameroon. From 1978 to 1979, he studied further at the Beijing Union Medical College Hospital. His main works are *Practical Handbook of Acupuncture and Moxibustion* (in collaboration with Dr. Yang Zhanlin), *Dr. Shi Jinmo's Clinical Experience on Herbal Medicine*, which won the first prize for the National Excellent Scientific Books in 1982, and *The Clinical Experience on Selection of Pair Acupoints*. He has also written some articles, among which are *Application of Yanglingquan (G 34) in Clinical Practice* and *Application of Tanzhong (Ren 17), the Influential Point of Qi, in Clinical Practice*, won the third prize for the Excellent Articles of Shanxi Province. Now Dr. Lu is a vice chief physician and director of Acupuncture Department of Shanxi Institute of Traditional Chinese Medicine.

I. Academic Characteristics and Medical Specialities

1. Synchronous manipulation

This is to rotate the needle simultaneously with both hands at a frequency of 200 c/min, with the amplitude not more than 90°. Repeat the procedure two or three times after an interval for five to ten minutes between manipulations.

1) *Synchronous manipulation from the same meridian* Two or three points are selected from the same meridian for the manipulation. For instance: Huantiao (G 30) and Yanglingquan (G 34) are needled for bi syndrome due to cold, wind and damp, impairment of the lower limbs, flaccidity, clonic convulsion and sciatica to activate the meridians and promote the circulation of qi and blood. For another example, toothache and sore throat due to excessive heat of Yangming Meridian may be treated by selecting Quchi (LI 11) and Hegu (LI 4) to reduce Yangming heat, subdue swelling and relieve pain. For instance, in the winter of 1985, a middle aged male patient suffered from pain on the upper left tooth for three days, synchronous manipulation was applied on Quchi (LI 11) and Hegu (LI 4) (right side) for two minutes, which relieved the pain. Further manipulation for three minutes brought about a sensation of numbness, distension and

soreness on the painful area. The needles were retained for thirty minutes in all with three manipulations. After that, the pain disappeared.

2) *Synchronous manipulation on the points from the meridians of the same name* Synchronous manipulation is applied on the points of the meridians with the same name on the upper and lower extremities. For instance, synchronous manipulation on Zhigou (SJ 8), Yanglingquan (G 34) (left side) is applied to regulate the function of Shaoyang and qi, remove obstruction from collaterals and relieve pain, reduce heat to promote defecation in cases of hyperchondriac pain due to Shaoyang disorder, intercostal neuralgia, habitual constipation, pregnant constipation, premenstrual mastodynia and abnormal menstruation. For example, in early summer, 1978, a woman four months pregnant had been constipated for the last two months, with a bowel movement once every three to five days, accompanied by abdominal distension and fullness, a white sticky tongue coating, and a string-taut rolling pulse. Differentiation: Retention of heat leading to the unsmooth flow of qi in fu organs. She felt the fullness alleviated during the synchronous manipulation on Zhigou (SJ 8) and Yanglingquan (G 34). She had one bowel movement that night. This method is subsequently applied in case of appearance of constipation.

3) *Synchronous manipulation on the points on the left and right sides* In light of the theory of the Eight Confluent points, the points on the left and right sides of the upper and lower extremities are combined with rotation. For example, Houxi (SI 3), Shenmai (B 62) are used for epilepsy, mania, depression, hysteria and syringomyelia. In 1972, a middle aged woman became restless because of fright, accompanied with palpitation, insomnia, weakness of the lower extremities, failure in walking, pale tongue proper with thin white coating, and string-taut thready pulse. Differentiation: Deficient nourishment of the heart and mind and disharmony of the blood vessels. After one puncturing of Shenmai (B 62) and Houxi (SI 3), the patient felt strong on the lower extremities and could walk. After another three treatments in combination with needling of Shenmen (H 7) and Sanyinjiao (Sp 6), all the symptoms disappeared.

4) *Synchronous manipulation on the corresponding points in the front and on the back* According to the principle of combination of Front-Mu and Back-Shu points, the corresponding points on the chest, abdomen, waist and back, medical and lateral aspects of the four limbs are selected with rotation or sparrow-pecking method, which is applicable to sprain, contusion and local pain. For instance, in the summer of 1976, a boy had a lumbar sprain with severe pain. He had to walk with his hands supporting his waist. There was tenderness upon palpation around right Dachangshu (B 25). The pain was reduced greatly after synchronous manipulation was applied on Dachangshu (B 25) and its corresponding point on the abdomen for three minutes. After that, two more manipulations were taken with the retention of the needles, thirty minutes in all. The student could move his waist free from pain.

5) *Synchronous manipulation on the different regions* In accordance with the stimulating regions of scalp acupuncture in combination with the pathological conditions, synchronous manipulation on some regions or secondary regions is applied. The Motor Area is selected for paralysis of the extremities, and the Sensory Area used for sensory impairment. For instance, in the mid-spring of 1972, a male peasant suffered from motor impairment of the lower limbs for more than two years, which was diagnosed as cerebral

thrombosis in Western medicine. Having failed to respond to various treatments including twenty scalp acupuncture treatments, the synchronous manipulation on Motor Area and Sensory Area of the lower extremities was applied three times, five minutes each. The needles were retained for thirty minutes. After the treatment, the patient felt better. The next day when the patient had the treatment, he felt a stream of hot sensation going down directly to the toes and he could lift his leg 30 cm high. The patient became normal after another ten treatments.

2. Selection of pair points

The pair point refers to the combination of two points, which function in harmony of opening and closing, coordination of movement and tranquility, and interpromotion of ascending and descending. Under the guidance of giving treatment upon differentiation, make clear the etiology, determine the treatment principle, understand the point function and prescribe the points.

1) *Combination of Renzhong (Du 26) with Fengfu (Du 16) for resuscitation* Renzhong (Du 26) is able to dispel wind and subdue heat, regulate yin and yang, restore consciousness and induce resuscitation, restore yang from collapse, tranquilize and ease the mind, dredge the meridians and relieve the pain. Fengfu (Du 16), a meeting point of Du Meridian and Yangwei Meridian, functions to dispel wind and eliminate the pathogenic factors, restore consciousness and induce resuscitation, reduce heat and fire, tranquilize and calm the mind. Du Meridian, the commander of yang meridians, is known as the sea of yang meridians, running along the spinal cord and entering into the brain, pertaining to the kidney. The combination of the two points, in the front and at the back, is used to dispel wind and eliminate the pathogenic factors, restore consciousness and induce resuscitation, dredge the meridians and relieve the pain in cases of syncope, windstroke, deviation of the mouth and eyes, hemiplegia, and acute lumbar sprain. For instance, in the treatment of apoplexy, clenched jaws and loss of consciousness, reinforcing Renzhong (Du 26) can open the mouth, restore yang and calm the mind. Reducing Fengfu (Du 16) is able to dispel wind from the tongue, and needling the three Yang Meridians can induce resuscitation, restore speech and rescue the patient from danger. In addition, the deviation of mouth and eyes, and hemiplegia may be treated by using this method with good results although the different meridians or collaterals are involved because their etiologies are similar. For instance, in the early autumn morning of 1969, a young male doctor had a sudden coma with pallor and profuse sweating. Rapid needling of Fengfu (Du 16) and Renzhong (Du 26) with a short needle helped the patient recover. This method can also be applied to the treatment of acute lumbar sprain. At the end of 1975, a French merchant got a lumbar sprain with the tendons injured. The patient could hardly walk, due to the severe pain on the left side. The above method was applied, and the needles manipulated for one minute. The pain was somewhat checked and he could move his waist freely after three manipulations, once every ten minutes.

2) *Combination of Tanzhong (Ren 17) and Neiguan (P 6) for qi regulation and inducing resuscitation* Tanzhong (Ren 17), the sea of Zong qi (Pectoral qi), the Influential Point of qi, the Front-Mu point of pericardium and a crossing point of

Foot-Taiyin, Foot-Shaoyang, Hand-Taiyang, Hand-Shaoyang and the Ren Meridians, is able to regulate qi and check the adverse flow of qi, clear the lung-heat and resolve phlegm, check coughing and relieve asthma and stuffiness of the chest and is good at treating disorders of qi. Neiguan (P 6), the Luo-Connecting point of the Pericardium Meridian, diverging from the Sanjiao Meridian of Hand-Shaoyang, and one of the eight Confluent Points, connecting with Yinwei Meridian, is able to reduce heat from the pericardium, promote the water passage of Sanjiao, relieve the stuffiness of the chest, harmonize the stomach and lower the adverse flow of qi, calm the mind and relieve pain. It is effective for the treatment of various disorders of the stomach, heart and chest. Ren Meridian governs all the yin meridians of the body, and is the sea of all the yin meridians, crossing with the three Hand Yin Meridians, and closely related to pregnancy. The collateral of Hand Jueyin Meridian ascends along the Ren Meridian, connects with the pericardium, and ends at the heart. The combination of the two points functions in relieving stuffiness of the chest and removing masses, lowering the adverse flow of qi, and resolving the phlegm, tranquilizing the mind and inducing resuscitation in cases of syncope resulting from disorder of qi, hysteria, and functional aphasia. Tanzhong (Ren 17) is effective for those due to stagnation of qi, but not for those due to deficiency of qi. The chicken-claw method is applied on Tanzhong (Ren 17) with oblique needling in the four directions of the point, aiming at dispersing qi and removing stagnation. For instance, in the autumn of 1979, a boy had hysteric aphasia due to emotional factors and was treated by needling Yamen (Du 15), Lianquan (Ren 23), Shangwan (Ren 13), Qihai (Ren 6), Zusanli (S 36), and Yanglingquan (G 34), which were manipulated for four hours, but no effects were achieved. The next day the patient was treated again with dull complexion, aphasia, pale tongue, white coating and string-taut pulse. Tanzhong (Ren 17) and Neiguan (P 6) were needled and retained for forty-five minutes, and manipulated once every other ten minutes, each time rotating for five minutes. When manipulated for thirty minutes, the patient suddenly could speak. Later on, the patient had two attacks, but recovered with the above-mentioned treatment.

3) *Combination of Hegu (LI 4) with Quchi (LI 11) for relieving exterior symptoms and reducing heat* Hegu (LI 4), the Yuan-Source point is a place where the primary qi is retained and is closely related to Sanjiao and is also an important point for regulating qi, and is able to dredge the meridians, promote qi flow and induce resuscitation, to dispel wind and alleviate symptoms, to clear lung heat and reduce fever, to descend the gastro-intestinal qi, and to tranquilize and calm the mind.

Quchi (LI 11), the He-Sea point, is the place where the qi of the Large Intestine Meridian is infused. According to the principle that He-Sea points are able to treat disorders of fu organs, Quchi (LI 11) is able to promote qi flow of fu organs, to dispel wind and to relieve exterior symptoms, to harmonize qi and blood, to eliminate swelling and check pain.

These two points used in combination can dredge the meridians and promote qi flow and dispel wind and reduce heat. It is therefore an effective way to eliminate heat from the upper jiao. As said in *Compendium of Acupuncture*, "Quchi (LI 11) and Hegu (LI 4) are the principal points for the disorders of the head, face, ear, eye, mouth and nose." The head is the place where all the yang meridians meet, while the ear, eye, mouth, nose and throat are the openings to receive clear yang qi. The clear yang qi with its clearing and dispersing function passing all the openings on the head can sweep away all the pathogenic factors and regulate the qi activity of the whole body. It is frequently used for colds, headaches, toothaches, sorethroat, epistaxis due to the attack of wind and heat to the openings on the head, as well as motor impairment of the upper limbs, pain and numbness of the elbow and arm, contraction of the fingers, and urticaria. For instance, in the early spring of 1965, a middle aged woman caught a cold, accompanied with fever (39°C). She had aversion to cold, headache, general pain, thin and yellow tongue coating, superficial and slightly rapid pulse. Differentiation: Retention of heat with exposure to cold and wind. Principle of treatment: Dispel the wind and eliminate exterior symptoms and reduce heat. Prescription: Dazhui (Du 14), Quchi (LI 11) and Hegu (LI 4). Reducing is applied with the needles retained for thirty minutes. Manipulate the needles every ten minutes. After treatment, the patient felt free of pain, and the body temperature was reduced to 38°C. The next day, the fever was gone and the other symptoms disappeared.

4) *Combination of Dazhui (Du 14) with Shugu (B 65) for relieving the exterior symptoms and reducing fever* Dazhui (Du 14), a meeting point of three Hand and Foot yang meridians with Du Meridian, is able to promote the flow of yang qi all over the body, relieve exterior symptoms, dispel wind and eliminate cold, regulate qi and check adverse flow of qi, promote dispersing function of the lung, remove the heat from the heart and calm the mind. Shugu (B 65), a Shu-Stream point where the qi of Bladder Meridian is infused, functions to promote the qi flow of Taiyang Meridian, eliminate the wind and dispel cold, promote perspiration and relieve exterior symptoms.

The function of Dazhui (Du 14) lies stress on clearing while that of Shugu (B 65) on relieving. The two points used in combination can promote the free flow of qi, harmonize nutrient qi and defensive qi, reduce fever and relieve exterior symptoms, promote perspiration and expel pathogenic factors from the muscles. It is indicated in the common cold, influenza, and sprained neck. Common cold caused by wind-cold should be treated by both acupuncture and moxibustion or cupping after acupuncture, while that by wind-heat should be treated by acupuncture only with the reducing method or bleeding with a three-edged needle. For instance, in the mid-winter of 1968, a male patient caught cold when taking a shower, accompanied by the symptoms of chills and fever (38.5°C), nasal obstruction and running nose, headache and general pain, absence of sweating, pale tongue, thin white coating, superficial and tight pulse. Dazhui (Du 14) and Shugu (B 65) were needled with the reducing method and cupping. The patient felt a general burning sensation with sweating on the forehead after the arrival of qi. The symptoms of cold and heat disappeared and body temperature returned to normal after continuous treatments.

5) *Combination of Shaoshang (L 11) with Shangyang (LI 1) for reducing heat and detoxicating* Shaoshang (L 11) is a Jing-Well point of the Lung Meridian of Hand-Taiyin and is the place where its qi is infused. According to the theory of selecting Jing-Well points for Zang disorders, bloodletting on this point with a three-edged needle is able to dredge the meridians, promote the circulation of qi and blood, reduce the lung heat, dredge the collaterals, warm the cold hands and feet, soothe the throat, subdue swelling and relieve pain. Shangyang (LI 1), a Jing-Well (metal) point of the Large

Intestine Meridian of Hand-Yangming and the place where its meridian qi emerges, is able to induce resuscitation and clear the mind, relieve exterior symptoms and reduce heat, remove depression and resolve stagnation. The two points used in combination can remove the stagnation of qi and blood, reduce the heat from zang-fu organs, induce resuscitation and strengthen the closing and opening function. The Lung Meridian of Hand-Taiyin pertains to lung and connects with large intestine, while Large Intestine Meridian of Hand-Yangming pertains to the large intestine and connects with the lung. The lung is a zang organ pertaining to interior, and large intestine is a fu organ pertaining to exterior. Shaoshang (L 11) can disperse lung and relieve exterior symptoms, laying stress on relief, while Shangyang (LI 1) has the function to remove depression and resolve stagnation, stressing reduction. The two points used in combination can strengthen the function of both reducing heat and relieving exterior symptoms in cases of tonsillitis, acute laryngopharyngitis, acute tonsillitis, mumps, the common cold, influenza, heat-stroke, and tense-syndrome of windstroke. For instance, in the winter of 1965 when influenza was common, a boy got acute swelling and pain in the throat, accompanied with chills and fever, soreness of the limbs, irritability and no sweating, redness of the throat. Pricking Shaoshang (L 11) and Shangyang (LI 1) made the patient feel comfortable. The next day the patient was completely recovered.

6) *Combination of Zanzhu (B 2) with Sanjian (LI 3) for reducing heat and improving eyesight* Zanzhu (B 2) is the gathering place of all the yang qi and functions to disperse and regulate qi of Taiyang Meridian, dispel wind and expel pathogenic factors, reduce heat and improve eyesight, dredge the meridians and relieve pain. Sanjian (LI 3) is the place where the qi of the Large Intestine Meridian of Hand-Yangming is infused and is able to regulate qi of the large intestine, reduce heat and soothe the throat, subdue swelling and relieve pain. Zanzhu (B 2) is characterized by ascending the clarity, functions in relieving the exterior symptoms, while Sanjian (LI 3) is characterized by descending the turbidity, functions in reducing interior heat. Those two points used in combination can help each other for reducing heat and detoxicating, to subdue swell and check pain. They are suitable for the treatment of red, swollen and painful eyes (acute conjunctivitis), blurring vision due to hyperactivity of the liver and gallbladder fire. For instance, in the summer of 1955, a male patient suffered from red, swollen and painful eyes for three days, accompanied with aversion to light, lacrimation, blurred vision, thin yellow tongue coating, and string-taut rapid pulse. Differentiation: Hyperactivity of liver and gallbladder fire affecting the eyes. Principle of treatment: Reduce the heat and cool the blood, subdue the swelling and check pain. Prescription: Bloodletting at Zanzhu (B 2) and Sanjian (LI 3) with a three-edged needle is applied. Immediately after the treatment, the vision became clear and pain relieved. After being treated continuously three times, the fever was reduced, swelling disappeared and the pain checked.

7) *Combination of Hegu (LI 4) with Guangming (G 37) for reducing heat and improving eyesight* Hegu (LI 4), the Yuan-Source point of Hand Yangming Meridian, has the functions of dredging the meridian, dispelling wind and relieving exterior symptoms, reducing the lung heat, promoting the descending function of intestines and stomach, calming the mind and checking the pain. Guangming (G 37), the Luo-Connecting point of Gallbladder Meridian of Foot-Shaoyang and the place where its qi

converges, has the functions of reducing liver and gallbladder fire, expelling wind and improving eyesight, dredging the meridians and checking pain. Hegu (LI 4) can disperse clarity and descend turbidity, while Guangming (G 37) can ascend clarity and reduce fire. The two points used in combination can help each other in descending and ascending functions so as to reduce heat, dispel wind and improve eyesight in cases of red, swollen and painful eyes due to hyperactivity of liver and gallbladder fire, pseudomyopia, night blindness, optic atrophy, and the disorders of both inner canthus and outer canthus. The reducing method is applied for those due to hyperactivity of liver and gallbladder fire or dryness and heat of Yangming Meridian, and even-movement applied for those with the mixed deficiency and excess. In recent years juvenile pseudomyopia was treated with satisfactory short-term effects and average improvement of the eyesight 0.3 to 0.5. For instance, a female patient aged eighteen came to the clinic on March 10, 1981, complaining of being unable to read the blackboard clearly for half a year, accompanied with dizziness and headache. Diagnosis: Myopia with eyesight vision 0.5 and 210 diopter on the left, and 0.3 and 275 diopter on the right. Prescription: Hegu (LI 4) and Guangming (G 37). Ten minutes after the needles were inserted, the patient had clear vision. After another five treatments, the vision improved to 1.0 on the left and 0.8 on the right.

8) *Combination of Shangxing (Du 23) with Heliao (LI 19) for reducing heat and checking bleeding* Shangxing (Du 23) is able to activate the qi of the meridians, dispel wind and improve eyesight, reduce heat and check bleeding, expel the pathogenic factors and promote the free flow of the nose. Heliao (LI 19) is able to eliminate the heat of the meridian, promote qi flow of the nose, cool the blood and check bleeding, invigorate blood circulation and remove stagnation. These two points, one above, two below, used in combination, function in dredging the meridians, promoting blood circulation and removing stagnation, reducing heat, and checking bleeding in cases of nasal bleeding and chronic rhinitis. For instance, in the summer of 1982, a female patient suffered from nasal bleeding for three days, the severity of the condition varying from time to time, accompanied with dizziness, dim vision, lassitude, pallor, pale tongue, thin white coating, thready and rapid pulse. Differentiation: Excessive heat of Yangming Meridians. Turning into fire, attacking upward to injure the yang collaterals. Principle of treatment: Reduce heat and cool blood. Shangxing (Du 23) and Heliao (LI 19) were needled with reducing method and the needles were retained for twenty-five minutes. There was no bleeding until the next day when she came for the treatment. Two more treatments were given to strengthen the effects. Erjian (LI 2), Neiting (S 44) and Zusanli (S 36) were added to strengthen the function of the spleen and stomach, and to supplement qi and produce blood. The patient received five treatments based on this prescription and recovered. The follow-up visit two years later found no relapse.

9) *Combination of Yuji (L 10) with Taixi (K 3) for nourishing yin and reducing fire* Yuji (L 10), the Ying-Spring point of the Lung Meridian of Hand-Taiyin where its qi flows copiously, can promote the dispersing function of the lung and stop coughing, reduce heat and fire, benefit the throat, subdue swelling and relieve pain, and promote the stomach function to descend turbidity. Taixi (K 3), the Shu-Stream and Yuan-Source point, where the qi is infused, can nourish the kidney yin, reduce deficiency heat, strengthen the primary yang, promote deuresis of the three jiao, reinforce the Mingmen

fire, nourish brain, supplement liver and kidney, and strengthen the lower back and the knee. Yuji (L 10) is characterized by reducing fire, while Taixi (K 3) is characterized by nourishing yin. These two points used in combination, one for reducing, another for nourishing, can nourish yin and moisten dryness, reduce heat and fever, stop coughing and check bleeding in cases of asthenia, dryness of the lung and soreness and swelling of the throat due to yin deficiency leading to hyperactivity of fire. Asthenia is mainly caused by the deficiency of the spleen and kidney leading to dryness of yin fluid which fails to ascend to nourish the heart and lung, causing the consumptive lung diseases. Principle of treatment: Reduce heat and moisten the lung dryness by nourishing yin. Once a male patient suffered from a dry and sore throat for two years with the severity varying from time to time, accompanied with red tongue with scanty coating, thready and rapid pulse. Reducing method on Yuji (L 10) and reinforcing on Taixi (K 3) were applied ten times, then the swelling disappeared and the pain was checked.

10) *Combination of Zhigou (SJ 8) with Yanglingquan (G 34) for harmonizing Shaoyang* Zhigou (SJ 8), a metal (fire) point, has the functions to regulate zang-fu organs, dredge the meridians and remove stagnation, promote qi flow and check pain, clear Sanjiao, and regulate the qi of the fu organs, drop the perverted qi and reduce fire. Yanglingquan (G 34), an influential point of tendon, where the qi is infused, is able to regulate Shaoyang, promote the depressed liver and gallbladder qi, reduce dampness and heat, eliminate wind, relax the tendon and dredge the meridians, and relieve pain. Zhigou (SJ 8) is mainly used to clear the qi of Sanjiao, while Yanglingquan (G 34) is mainly used to promote the free flow of liver and gallbladder qi. The two points, one above, one below, pertaining to the meridian with the same name, can eliminate stagnation and regulate Shaoyang in the treatment of Shaoyang disease, cholycistitis, hyperchondriac pain due to chronic hepatitis, intercostal neuralgia, habitual constipation, constipation during pregnancy, distension of breasts during menstruation, and irregular menstruation. For instance, a male patient suffered from dizziness and blurred vision due to not being treated after being attacked by wind-cold. Zhigou (SJ 8) and Yanglingquan (G 34) were punctured with manipulation and qi regulation for twenty minutes. After that, the patient felt relieved. The next day, he recovered.

11) *Combination of Jianli (Ren 11) with Zusanli (S 36) for strengthening the spleen and stomach* Jianli (Ren 11) has the functions of strengthening the spleen and stomach and promoting digestion. Zusanli (S 36), a He-Sea point of Stomach Meridian, can regulate the spleen and stomach, regulate qi, remove retention and distension, promote qi flow and check pain, and strengthen the constitution. Jianli (Ren 11) is characterized by strengthening the Middle Jiao, raising yang and lowering the perverted qi, while Zusanli (S 36) is characterized by reinforcing the spleen and stomach, regulating the Middle Jiao and descending turbidity. The combination of the two points, one for ascending, one for descending, is able to strengthen the spleen and stomach, reinforce qi of the Middle Jiao, treat deficiency, improve appetite and promote digestion, and check diarrhoea, which is mainly indicated in annorexia, indigestion, epigastric pain, chronic diarrhoea due to deficiency of the spleen and stomach, spontaneous sweating, and lassitude. The reinforcing method is applied in most cases in combination with moxibustion. A middle aged male patient suffered from chronic diarrhoea for eight years, with

loose stools four or five times a day, annorexia, lassitude, abdominal distention, flat and soft abdomen, pale tongue, white coating, thready and weak pulse (especially at the *guan* and *chi* regions on the right side.) Differentiation: Yang deficiency of the spleen and kidney leading to weakness of digestive function and sinking of the qi. Prescription: Both acupuncture (reinforcing) and moxibustion were applied on Jianli (Ren 11) and Zusanli (S 36). After being treated continuously ten times, the condition greatly improved, appetite increased, the frequency of bowel movements reduced to three or four times each day. Another ten treatments were given with the same prescription and the patient recovered with formed stools once or twice a day.

12) *Combination of Hegu (LI 4) with Zusanli (S 36) for ascending the clarity and discending the turbidity* Hegu (LI 4), the Yuan-Source point of the Large Intestine Meridian of Hand-Yangming, is able not only to dredge the meridians, promote qi flow, dispel wind and relieve exterior symptoms, reduce heat, promote the descending function of the stomach and intestine, tranquilize and calm the mind, regulate the general function of the human body, but also to regulate the function of the intestines and stomach. The present studies have proved that this point can weaken the peristalsis of the stomach, relieve spasm and loosen the pyloric spasm. Zusanli (S 36), a He-Sea and earth point of the Stomach Meridian, is able to regulate the stomach and intestines, regulate qi and relieve distension, eliminate stagnation and dispel fullness, descend the turbidity and promote bowel movement, regulate the function of the intestines and check diarrhoea. According to a study, Zusanli (S 36) can strengthen peristalsis of the stomach in cases of hypofunction and weaken peristalsis in case of hyperactivity and normalize the gastric acid. According to the theory of Five Elements, Hegu (LI 4) pertains to fire, while Zusanli (S 36) pertains to earth. These two points used in combination can promote each other. The former is characterized by ascending and dispersing, while the latter is characterized by heaviness and descending. They have the functions in ascending clarity and descending turbidity, regulating qi flow and relieving pain, eliminating distension, promoting bowel movement and checking diarrhoea, which are mainly indicated in descending dysfunction of the spleen and stomach such as indigestion, annorexia, epigastric and abdominal distension, constipation, or first dry and then loose stools, chronic and acute diarrhoea. In recent years, this method has been applied in the treatment of the common cold, influenza (stomach and intestinal) and retention of heat of Yangming Meridian. In March, 1985, a male patient over sixty came for treatment of gastrointestinal neurosis, complaining of dizziness, a stuffy sensation of the head, annorexia, indigestion, gastric distension, frequent belching, first dry and then loose stools, pallor, pale tongue, thin white coating, thready and string-taut pulse. The above points were needled once every other day ten times. After that, dizziness and stuffiness were relieved, and stools became normal. After another ten treatments, the patient had a normal appetite and felt strong and all the symptoms disappeared.

13) *Combination of Xinshu (B 15) with Shenshu (B 23) for harmonization between the heart and kidney* Xinshu (B 15), a point where the heart qi is converged, has the functions of dredging the heart collaterals, regulating qi and blood, nourishing the heart and calming the mind, clearing away the heart-fire and tranquilizing. Shenshu (B 23), a point where the kidney qi is converged, is able to nourish the kidney yin, strengthen the

brain and nourish water to reduce fire, promote eyesight and hearing, facilitate qi activity and eliminate dampness, and strengthen the lumbar function. The use of Xinshu (B 15) and Shenshu (B 23) can be traced back to *Song of the Jade Dragon*, in which it said, "Xinshu and Shenshu are for seminal emission due to deficiency of kidney." That is because the heart, which is located in the Upper Jiao, pertaining to yang, controls fire and stores the spirit, while the kidney, which is located in the Lower Jiao, pertaining to yin, controls water and stores essence. Xinshu (B 15) clears away the heart fire, while Shenshu (B 23) nourishs the kidney yin. These two points, used in combination, can help each other to nourish yin, subdue fire, harmonize the heart and kidney, and balance yin and yang, effective for palpitation, anxiety, irritability, insomnia, excessive dreams, seminal emission and premature ejaculation due to disharmony and dysfunction of the heart and kidney. In the winter of 1966, a young man complained of erection of peis but not firm, and seminal emission after marriage for one year, accompanied with dizziness, tinnitus, insomnia, excessive dreams, poor appetite, lassitude, hypomnesia, red tongue tip, thin white tongue coating, string-taut and thready pulse. Differentiation: Loss of yin affects yang, deficiency of both yin and yang results in the failure of the kidney in its storing ability. Principle of treatment: Warm and strengthen the kidney, nourish heart and calm the mind, restore the harmonious relations between the heart and the kidney. Prescription: Xinshu (B 15), Shenshu (B 23), Shenmen (H 7) and Sanyinjiao (Sp 6). Treat once daily. After being treated for 7 days, insomnia and excessive dreams were relieved, the patient felt strong and the appetite improved. After another five treatments by needling Qihai (Ren 6) instead of Shenmen (H 7), spontaneous sweating disappeared. The treatment continued for more than one month and the patient recovered. In order to consolidate the effect, treatment was given one or two times a week and the patient was advised not to have any sexual intercourse within three months. The follow-up visit after one year found no relapse.

14) *Combination of Hegu (LI 4) with Taichong (Liv 3) for calming the liver to stop the wind* Hegu (LI 4), the Yuan-Source point of the Large Intestine Meridian of Hand-Yangming, is able to regulate the meridians and dredge the collaterals, promote qi flow, dispel the wind, relieve the exterior symptoms, clear away heat, reduce fever, free the intestinal passage and stomach, tranquilize and calm the mind. Taichong (Liv 3), the Yuan-Source point of the Liver Meridian of Foot-Jueyin, can regulate qi and blood, dredge the meridians, regulate the liver qi flow, calm the liver and subdue the wind, clear away heat and dampness. Hegu (LI 4) and Taichong (Liv 3) known as "the four gate points," come from the *Compendium of Acupuncture*, which said that "in case of pain radiating from hand to shoulder, Hegu (LI 4) and Taichong (Liv 3) should be punctured. In case of nasal obstruction and boils, rhinitis—puncture Hegu (LI 4) and Taichong (Liv 3)." Hegu, pertaining to yang, dominates qi and is characterized by lifting and ascending, while Taichong (Liv 3), pertaining to yin, controls blood and is characterized by heaviness and descending. The two points used in combination help each other promote qi flow and activate the blood circulation, calm the liver and subdue the wind. Hegu (LI 4) is a representative Yuan-Source point of the Yang Meridian, while Taichong (Liv 3) is a representative Yuan-Source point of Yin Meridian. They are used to treat headache, dizziness, hypertension due to hyperactivity of Liver Yang, tense-type windstroke,

syncope resulting from qi disorder, epilepsy, mania, infantile convulsion, insomnia, nasal obstruction, chronic rhinitis and atrophic rhinitis and bi syndrome. For instance, a middle-aged woman had coma due to perversion and disorder of qi causing blood going upward together with qi, accompanied with loss of consciousness, cold extremities, convulsion, clenched jaws, thready and string-taut pulse on both hands. Synchronous manipulation was applied at Taichong (Liv 3) and Hegu (LI 4) for one minute, and the patient regained consciousness.

15) *Combination of Taixi (K 3) with Taichong (Liv 3) for nourishing the kidney and subduing the liver* Taixi (K 3), the Yuan-Source point of Kidney Meridian of Foot-Shaoyin, has the function of nourishing the kidney yin and reducing deficiency heat, strengthening the primary yang, to support the lumbur and knee functions. Taichong (Liv 3), the Yuan-Source point of the Liver Meridian of Foot-Jueyin, can promote the liver qi flow, activate the blood circulation, dredge the meridians, calm the liver and subdue wind, clear away heat and dampness. Taixi (K 3) is characterized by reinforcing, while Taichong (Liv 3) is characterized by reducing. The two points are able to nourish the kidney and calm the liver, remove the excess and reinforce the deficiency, clear the upper body and stabilize the lower part, and drop the blood pressure. They are used to treat hypertension, headache and dizziness due to hyperactivity of fire resulting from yin deficiency and stirring-up of liver yang, insomnia, excessive dreams, disturbed sleep due to hyperactivity of fire resulting from yin deficiency and disharmony between the heart and kidney, irregular menstruation and uterine bleeding due to hyperactivity of fire resulted from yin deficiency causing extravasation of the blood, or the symptom of feeling qi rushing up through the thorax to the throat from the lower abdomen. For instance, in the summer of 1965, a female patient, who for the last five years suffered from frequent headache, dizziness, tinnitus, soreness of the lower back, weakness of the lower extremities, disturbed sleep with excessive dreams, pale tongue, thin white coating, deep thready and weak pulse. BP: 170/120 mmHg. Differentiation: Deficiency of liver and kidney leading to the hyperactivity of fire and stirring up of the liver yang. Principle of treatment: Nourish yin to subdue fire, clear the upper and stabilize the lower. Prescription: Taixi (K 3) was reinforced and Taichong (Liv 3) reduced, retaining the needles for thirty minutes with manipulation every ten minutes. The patient felt much better after the third treatment and recovered after another five treatments, blood pressure being 140/100 mmHg.

16) *Combination of Renzhong (Du 26) with Weizhong (B 40) for activating the blood circulation to remove obstructions from the meridians* Renzhong (Du 26), located between the mouth and nose, is able to dispel wind, eliminate internal heat, dredge the meridians, clear the head, calm the mind, regulate yin and yang, and check pain. Weizhong (B 40), the earth and Lower He-Sea point where its qi is infused, is able to relax the tendons, promote qi flow and activate blood circulation, clear away heat and detoxicate, and regulate yin and yang. Renzhong (Du 26) is located in the upper and characterized by ascending, while Weizhong (B 40) is located in the lower and characterized by descending. The combination of the two points is able to regulate yin and yang, relax tendons, promote qi flow and check pain, suitable for the treatment of the febrile disease. As for lumbago, apply the reducing method for acute cases and bloodletting with

a 3-edged needle for chronic cases. For instance, in 1965, a male patient got lumbago and motor impairment due to the lumbar sprain during physical labour, the condition got worse the next morning and he had been treated for two months, but failed to improve. Examination: Obvious tenderness at Mingmen (Du 4) and Dachangshu (B 25) points, dark tongue proper, thin white coating, string-taut and choppy pulse. Reducing Renzhong (Du 26) and bleeding at Weizhong (B 40) relieved the pain. Another two treatments were given and the pain disappeared.

17) *Combination of Yanglingquan (G 34) with Taichong (Liv 3) for relaxing the tendons and muscles and activating the flow of qi and blood* Yanglingquan (G 34), the Earth He-Sea point and Influential point of tendon, is able to clear away the heat from the liver and gallbladder, eliminate dampness, relax muscles and tendons, activate the flow of qi and blood, relieve and check pain. Taichong (Liv 3), the Earth Shu-Stream point where the Liver Meridian qi is infused, is able to promote the flow of liver qi, activate blood circulation and dredge the meridians, calm the liver to subdue wind, eliminate heat and dampness. The gallbladder is a fu organ, pertaining to yang, while the liver, a zang organ, pertains to yin. The combination of these two points can regulate and harmonize liver and gallbladder, promote qi flow and check pain, promote the earth to inhibit wood, eliminate distension and fullness, activate blood circulation and remove stagnation, and relax the tendons and muscles, suitable for periarthritis of the shoulders, shoulder pain due to sprain, hyperchondriac pain, dizziness, motor impairment of the lower limbs and painful knees and foot, especially effective for acute shoulder pain. Method: When the needling sensation is obtained, apply the manipulation and at the same time ask the patient to move shoulder joint with the range of movement increasing. For instance, in July, 1980, a train attendant got pain and motor impairment of the right shoulder after sleeping in exposure to wind, the treatment was given as mentioned above, and the pain was relieved and motor ability restored.

18) *Combination of Guilai (S 29) with Taichong (Liv 3) for elevating yang to check sinking* Guilai (S 29), located in the lower abdomen, pertaining to lower jiao, is able to regulate the flow of qi, receive qi, activate the flow of qi, relieve pain, warm the meridians to dispel cold, and lift yang to check sinking. Taichong (Liv 3) is able to promote the flow of liver qi, activate blood circulation and dredge meridians, calm liver to subdue yang, and tranquilize the liver wind, eliminate heat and dampness. Guilai (S 29) is mainly used to ascend the clarity and characterized by reinforcing, while Taichong (Liv 3) mainly used to clear the turbidity and characterized by reducing. The combination of the two points functions to elevate yang to check sinking, clear away heat and dampness, check pain and relieve swelling, effective for the treatment of swelling and pain in testis, pain caused by flatulence of the small intestine, hernia, prolapse of the uterus, especially effective for various disorders of the anterior orifice. Oblique needling is applied at Guilai (S 29) with the needle directing to the anterior orifice and the needling sensation reaching the focus affected area. The effect will be better in case of appearance of contraction. For instance, in the autumn of 1968, a female patient suffered from prolapse of the uterus for more than one year and complained of shortness of breath, lassitude, distension in the lower abdomen in standing which may be aggravated in standing and relieved in a lying position, weakness and soreness of the lower back and

knees, pale complexion, pale tongue with a thin white coating, weak and thready pulse. Differentiation: Deficiency of the kidney and sinking of the spleen qi. Principle of treatment: Reinforce qi to check sinking, strengthen the functions of the liver and kidney. Prescription: Guilai (S 29) and Taichong (Liv 3) were punctured with the reinforcing method. Ten treatments in all were given and II degree prolapse of the uterus was cured. No relapse was found in the follow-up visit one year later.

19) *Combination of Yintang (Extra 1) with Shangwan (Ren 13) for calming the mind and checking vomiting* Yintang (Extra 1) is able to dispel wind and activate the flow of qi and blood in meridians, tranquilize and calm the mind. Shangwan (Ren 13) is able to descend the perverted qi and promote the stomach function to check vomiting, and calm the mind. Yintang (Extra 1) is used mainly for clearing and calming the mind, while Shangwan (Ren 13) is used mainly for descending the turbid qi and promoting the stomach function. The combination of the two points is applied to the treatment of car-sickness and sea-sickness due to dysfunction of ascending and descending. Thirty years ago, Dr. Lu himself suffered from car-sickness, with foam at the mouth, dizziness, vertigo, nausea and vomiting due to perversion of stomach qi in each attack. Yintang (Extra 1) was punctured and he felt relieved, then Shangwan (Ren 13) was followed and it was effective.

II. Case Analysis

Case 1: Hysteria

Name, Jiao x x; sex, female; age, 32; date of the first visit, October 15, 1979.

Complaints Mental confusion and convulsion for one hour. The patient was generally depressive. One hour before a woman screaming brought about her loss of consciousness, accompanied with clenched jaws, fullness of the chest and convulsion. Examination: Pinkish complexion, coarse breath, pale dark tongue proper, white and sticky coating, string-taut and rolling pulse, rigidity and cold of the limbs, the pupillary light reflex present. Differentiation: The depression of liver qi leading to qi going upward to obstruct the heart and chest and mist the mind, thus appeared coma, clenched jaws and fists. The obstruction of qi resulted in fullness of the chest and coarse breath. The depression of yang qi which failed to reach the four limbs, the muscles and tendons became short of nourishment, then cold limbs and convulsions took place. Principle of treatment: Promote qi flow and disperse stagnation, induce resuscitation and relieve the symptoms.

Prescription Tanzhong (Ren 17) and Neiguan (P 6)

Treatment procedure Quickly insert the needle into Tanzhong (Ren 17) with reducing method, the patient restored the consciousness after manipulation for thirty seconds. Then puncture Neiguan (P 6) and apply synchronous manipulation after qi arrival. The patient felt relief from the stuffy chest. The needles were retained for thirty minutes and manipulated three times. The follow-up visit six years later found no relapse.

Remarks After recovery the patient said: "When I heard the screaming, I felt palpitation and then got a hot sensation in the chest, as if a stream of hot air rushed to the throat from the epigastric region. After that, I could see nothing and lost consciousness."

Case 2: Aphasia

Name, x x x; sex, male; age, 30; date of the first visit, June 3, 1976.

Complaints Aphasia for seventeen days. The patient was depressive all the time. One day at work he burst into tears. Though clear in his mind, he could no longer speak, associated with distension of the chest, excessive dreams, poor appetite, normal stool and urine. He was treated with some Western drugs and by spraying the throat with medical powder, but he failed to respond to the treatment. Then he was sent to a private clinic and was treated with herbal medicine, but still with no improvement, coughing blood resulted. Examination: Nothing was wrong with the throat, pale tongue proper, white and sticky coating, string-taut and retarded pulse. Differentiation: Wood-fire impairing the metal (lung), affection of pectoral qi misting the mind, aphasia resulted; disorder of the lung leads to deficiency of the heart qi, failing to nourish the heart, thus appeared stuffy chest, insomnia and excessive dreams; liver depression attacking the stomach, so annorexia happened. Principle of treatment: Promote qi flow, remove the depression and promote mental clearness, then regulate the heart and spleen.

Prescription 1. Tanzhong (Ren 17), Neiguan (P 6). 2. Hegu (LI 4), Zusanli (S 36), Neiguan (P 6), Sanyinjiao (SP 6).

Treatment procedure Quick insertion of Tanzhong (Ren 17). Induce strong stimulation with quick and continuous rotation after appearance of needling sensation. When manipulation was done for five minutes, air gushed out from the throat. The patient could say and felt relieved after removing the needles. The next day, apart from poor sleep, dizziness and poor appetite, he could respond to whatever was asked. Another five treatments were given, and the patient recovered.

Explanation Tanzhong (Ren 17) and Neiguan (P 6) used in combination may regulate qi and promote mental clearness. The above two cases are both of qi stagnation obstructing the mind. Different diseases were treated with the same treatment. Tanzhong (Ren 17) is for free flow of qi and opening the chest, and resolving stagnation. Neiguan (P 6) is to help open the chest and promote qi flow, regulate stomach and descend perverted qi and calm the mind. The two points used together can achieve better results.

Case 3: Arthralgia due to qi stagnation

Name, Fu x x; sex, male; age, 47; date of the first visit, June 9, 1980.

Complaints Pulling pain on the left leg for sixteen hours. The patient normally had lower back pain, which got worse on anger or exertion with pulling pain radiating to the left leg. Recently being frustrated, there appeared pulling pain on the left hip and on the anterior-lateral side of the foot, radiating even to the toes. The accompanying symptoms were: weakness of the lower limbs with difficulties standing and walking, annorexia, dry mouth, preference for hot water, unsmooth throat, stuffy chest, occasionally with mental confusion, dry stools and profuse clear urine ten times a day. Examination: Red tongue, thin yellow coating, string-taut pulse, clear mind with suffering look, failure in flexion and raising the affected leg, BP. 100/70 mmHg. Differentiation: Arthralgia. Liver, a zang organ of wood characterized by yin nature, but with the use of yang, stores the blood and controls tendons, the liver qi is often depressed, the depression of the liver may affect the collateral passage and obstruct qi circulation, then the leg pain happened; malnourishment of tendons and muscles may weaken the limbs. Principle of treatment: Open the chest and promote qi flow, dredge the obstructed meridians.

Prescription Tanzhong (Ren 17) and Yanglingquan (G 34).

Treatment procedure Insert the needle quickly into Tanzhong (Ren 17) and apply the reducing method after qi arrival. After manipulation for half a minute, the area around the point (3 x 3 cm) was congested, and the patient felt stuffy chest relieved and pain on the left leg reduced. After manipulation for another half a minute, the pain on the hip and thigh disappeared except for the lateral side of the lower leg. Yanglingquan (G 34) on the left side was punctured and the needling sensation conducted along the lateral side of the leg to the toes, then the pain immediately disappeared. After withdrawal of the needles, apart from the weakness of the leg, he could walk. The next day, the patient came all the way by himself because there had been much improvement, and the affected leg could be raised. Acupuncture treatment was given, based on the same prescription. The congestion around the point dwindled when Tanzhong (Ren 17) was punctured. On the third day, the left leg could be moved flexibly and the pain was eliminated. However, the patient still felt cloudy-headed, poor appetite, dry mouth, dry stool, pale tongue with thin yellow coating, then Zhongwan (Ren 12), Tianshu (S 25), Zusanli (S 36), Sanyinjiao (Sp 6) were needled.

Explanation Arthralgia is caused by disturbance of seven emotions affecting the muscles and tendons with the manifestation of pain on the limbs.

Case 4: Neck pain (spasm of the sternocleidomastoid muscle)

Name, Deng x x; sex, female; age, 12; date of the first visit, August 10, 1979.

Complaints Paraxysmal neck pain on the left side. For many years, this condition attacked her every afternoon at one o'clock, and her head turned to the left side. She had been treated for a long time, but with no positive results. Examination: Malnutrition with lustreless complexion and thin constitution, spasm of the sternocleidomastoid muscle, pale tongue, thin white coating, string-taut and thready pulse. Differentiation: Deficiency of qi and blood, obstruction of wind in the collaterals, disharmony of blood vessels, and spasm of the tendons. Principle of treatment: Promote qi flow, dredge the collaterals to relieve spasm.

Prescription Lieque (L 7) and Houxi (SI 3).

Treatment procedure The needles were inserted synchronous manipulation was applied for one minute after the needling sensation was obtained, the patient felt the pain relieved. The needles were retained for thirty minutes with three manipulations during retention. The patient was advised against being attacked by cold during sleep at night. The next day, the patient's condition remained stable. The patient was asked to have treatment the next day. After the third treatment, there was no relapse. Later another two treatments were given. The follow-up visit for five years found no relapse.

Explanation Lieque (L 7) and Houxi (SI 3) are especially effective for nape pain. Lieque (L 7), a Luo-Connecting point and also one of the Eight Confluent points communicating with the Ren Meridian and one of the four general points, is able to dispel wind and relieve the exterior symptoms, promote the dispersing function of the lung and check asthma, dredge the meridians and relieve pain. Houxi (SI 3), an earth point where its qi infuses, also one of the Eight Confluent points connecting with the Du Meridian, is able to activate circulation of yang qi, calm and tranquilize the mind, eliminate dampness and heat, dredge the collateral and check pain. The two points used together can double the effects to dredge Du and Ren Meridians, promote qi flow in Taiyang Meridian, activate the flow of the collaterals and check pain.

Case 5: Shoulder pain (frozen shoulder)

Name, Yang x x; sex, female; age, 60; date of the first visit, May 2, 1965.

Complaints Shoulder pain on both sides for four years. In the winter of 1961, she began to feel pain, soreness, stiffness and heavy sensation on both shoulders, and difficulty in lifting, the pain became aggravated on exertion or in cold and rainy days and became relieved on warmth. The right side was more affected. She was treated by herbal medicine but with no effect. Examination: Appearance of the both shoulders normal, abduction 60° and lifting 100°, pale tongue, thin white coating, deep and string-taut pulse. Differentiation: Damage to tendons and meridians by cold and wind, resulting in stagnation of qi and blood.

Prescription Yanglingquan (G 34), Taichong (Liv 3).

Treatment procedure After the first treatment, the pain was relieved and the amplitude of the shoulder movement increased with abduction 80° and lifting 120°. After the second treatment, the pain was eliminated, but soreness was left. Abduction and lifting both 150°. Another two treatments were given and all the remaining symptoms disappeared and the shoulder could move flexibly.

Explanation Shoulder pain is mostly related to wind and cold (also caused by stagnation resulted from tendon injury and disharmony of qi and blood). According to the theory of puncturing the points on the lower part of the body for the diseases on the upper part, Yanglingquan (G 34), the influential point of tendon, is selected and is especially effective for the newly acquired conditions due to sprain or contusion. And its effects will be doubled if used in combination with Taichong (Liv 3) because Taichong (Liv 3) is the Yuan-Source point of the liver and functions to store blood, control tendons, regulate qi flow of the Liver Meridian, relax tendons and activate the flow of qi of the collaterals, promote blood circulation and check pain.

Case 6: Sprain in the lumbar region

Name, x x x, sex, male; age, 51; date of the first visit, July 15, 1976.

Complaints Sprain on the lumbar region for three days. The condition was so severe that he could not bow his back, neither could he put on or take off his shoes or socks. He could only walk with back straight and the pain got worse during coughing. He came here with the help of his wife. Examination: Tenderness around Mingmen (Du 4), inability to bend forward or backward or to both sides, or to squat, pain became severe upon coughing, pale tongue, thin white coating, string-taut pulse. Differentiation: Injury of the tendons and meridians due to contusion, and obstruction of the collaterals.

Principle of treatment: Dredge the meridians, activate the flow of the collateral and check pain.

Prescription Renzhong (Du 26) and Yamen (Du 15).

Treatment procedure Quickly insert the needles about 0.3 to 0.5 cun in depth. Apply synchronous manipulation with the sparrow-pecking method for one minute, the pain was half reduced. The needles were retained for thirty minutes with another two manipulations in between, then the patient recovered and could move his lower back flexibly.

Explanation The combination of Renzhong (Du 26) and Yamen (Du 15) is for acute sprain in the lumbar region and contusion. Renzhong (Du 26) is located between the nose and mouth, and able to dispel wind and eliminate heat, regulate yin and yang, induce resuscitation, rescue yang from collapse, calm the mind, activate the flow of the collaterals and check pain. Yamen (Du 15) is located on the occipital head and is able to dredge the meridians, clear the mind, and treat aphasia. The two points, one in the front, another at the back, correspond with each other and are able to regulate and dredge the Du Meridian and promote qi flow, resolve stagnation and check pain.

PROFICIENT IN APPLYING THE NEEDLING, PRICKING, SCRAPING AND CUPPING TECHNIQUES

—Qu Zuyi's Clinical Experience

Qu Zuyi, born in Beijing in 1914, started to learn traditional Chinese medicine in his childhood, because his mother had suffered from many kinds of diseases. He learned the internal medicine, acupuncture, surgery, and pediatric massage from the famous traditional Chinese medical doctors Wang Mingrui, Zhang Jiantang, and Qi Futing. In 1930, he learned *Treatise on Febrile Diseases Caused by Cold* from a famous doctor Zhang Xichun, and joined the Chinese Acupuncture Research Association for further study of acupuncture from a famous doctor, Chen Dan'an. In 1933, he passed the examination as a qualified acupuncturist and in 1936, he passed the examination as a TCM doctor. In 1950, after he graduated from the First Course of Traditional Chinese Medicine Postgraduated School sponsored by the Ministry of Public Health of the Central Government, he worked in the Acupuncture Research Department of the Central Health Academy. In 1954, he transferred to work in the Academy of Traditional Chinese Medicine, and in 1956, he was engaged in teaching in the Acupuncture Department of the Beijing College of Traditional Chinese Medicine. In 1974, he transferred to Lanzhou City, where he was the chief editor of *Acupuncturist Huang Fuyi of the Jin Dynasty*, and he also published some papers on acupuncture and moxibustion, external treatment, massage, breathing exercise, food therapy, etc. Now, he is the chief and associate professor and associate research fellow of the Acupuncture Office of the Institute of New Medicine and Pharmacology of Gansu Province.

I. Academic Characteristics and Medical Specialities

1. The improvement of cupping method

The traditional cupping refers to the cupping of blood stasis, in which cupping is performed on the face, and the purplish petechia remains. It is therefore not convenient for the professional actors, singers and teachers. Dr. Qu improved this therapy into congestion cupping, and the fixed cupping into continuous flashing cupping method, which is not only beneficial for the patient, but also good for increasing the therapeutic effect. For many years, it has been welcomed by the people.

2. Eruptive disease and pricking therapy

From the view of the symptoms, eruptive disease includes sunstroke, acute gastroenteritis, dry cholera, eruptions and food poisoning, which mostly occur in the period between summer and autumn. In the summer of 1930, cholera was epidemic in Yantai of Shandong Province. In clinic, most patients suffered from eruptive disease due to sunstroke. For the mild cases, Eruptive Disease Drug and Health Epidemic Prophylactic Pills made by Tongren Pharmacy were administered, and for the severe cases, acupuncture was applied in combination with moxibustion. The first-aid restoring yang drug of Radix Codonopsis Pilosulae, Rhizoma Dioscoreae, Fructus Corni and Rhizoma Zingiberis were orally administered for dehydration due to vomiting and diarrhoea. More than sixteen hundred cases were cured within three months, but some difficult cases failed in treatment with simple filiform needles. For example: Guo x x, a male worker of twenty-four years old, suffered from chills, spasm of the legs, repeated vomiting, and palpitation after intake of bad food and catching cold in sleeping at night. Examination: Emaciation and dullness, unstable walking, pallor, vomiting, gastric pain, and palpitation, deep and hesitant pulse, cold fingers, dry tongue with white coating, and collapsed fingers. The diagnosis was eruptive disease. According to the pulse, since the toxic was stagnated in the blood vessels, the pulse was deep and hesitant and lassitude appeared. Because the gastric region was obstructed, vomiting and gastric pain happened. In case the defensive qi was injured, profuse sweating and cold fingers occurred. Dr. Qu treated this case by dredging the eruption to support the antipathogenic factors, and to eliminate the pathogenic factors by needling Dazhui (Du 14) with a filiform needle, then by needling Quchi (LI 11), Hegu (LI 4) and Zusanli (S 36) to regulate the spleen and stomach and check vomiting, in combination with moxibustion at Guanyuan (Ren 4) to support yang and eliminate the pathogenic factors. But the patient's condition was just the same after treatment, and vomiting continued after taking herbs. This confused Dr. Qu, then he invited Dr. Liu to treat the patient with pricking therapy, in which the patient's anterior and posterior intercostal space was tapped with the tip of the middle finger of the right hand. Small lumps were formed on the tapping place. Dr. Liu pricked them immediately after tapping, nearly a hundred lumps in all. The vomiting stopped after disappearance of the lumps. The patient felt comfortable immediately. Dr. Liu said: "The disease is called eruption, and the method is called pricking, but these points were unknown. There are so many kinds of needling methods, but the simple use of the filiform needle cannot treat the disease, otherwise you'll make mistakes." After that, again no response was found in another three cases after needling with the filiform needles. Dr. Qu applied Dr. Liu's pricking method, pricking immediately followed tapping, vomiting stopped, and the symptoms were all relieved.

Eruptive syndrome in popular terms is known as "disease in summer with severe digestive symptoms." Pricking the eruption is also called "releasing the eruption." For example, sunstroke, dry cholera, eruption or food poisoning may have this symptom. Tapping may produce a lump, easy to diminish by pricking. It is named "pricking the monkey," and falls into the category of pestilence.

There are many methods for discharging the eruption. In the folk, the commonly used are scraping the eruption, twisting the eruption, pulling the eruption, tapping the eruption, and pricking the eruption.

The traditionally used needle for pricking the eruption is a coarse needle, thus the wound is big, and can be easily infected in case of a large area of eruption for pricking. A one-inch-long No. 32 filiform needle is applied with very light manipulation, which ensures a quick effect and a safe manipulation.

3. Scraping to eliminate the neonatal tetanus

Neonatal tetanus is an infection of the umbilical cord by the Bacilius tetani, which falls into the category of convulsive disease in traditional Chinese medicine. It may appear immediately after birth, or at the neonatum period.

In the spring of 1963, Dr. Qu worked in a medical team. Once he treated a male infant, who had a high fever four days after birth, followed by convulsions. Examination: Purplish complexion, cold hands and feet, closed eyes and jaws, paroxysmal convulsion, burning feeling of the skin, the axillary temperature 41.6°C, and cyanosis of the finger print. No response by pinching Zhongchong (P 9) point. The large area of scraping manipulation was used instead of needling to support the body resistance and eliminate the pathogenic factors. Dr. Qu put a handkerchief on the back of the infant, and scraped over the bilateral Huatuojiaji points rapidly up and down twenty times with an organic glass piece (1 x 6 cm) to support the body resistance and eliminate the toxins, then scraped Dazhui (Du 14), Feishu (B 13), Kunlun (B 60), Taixi (K 3) a hundred times each to reduce heat and resolve the phlegm, and tapped the finger and toes crease with the thumb twenty times respectively to control the convulsion and diminish the wind, then scraped Laogong (P 8) and Yongquan (K 1) a hundred times each to stimulate the heart and kidney to restore Yang, and then again scraped Guanyuan (Ren 4) and Mingmen (Du 4) a hundred times respectively. He repeated the above procedure after resting for five minutes. The convulsion stopped, but the baby's eyes were still closed. Dr. Qu heavily pressed the internal margin of the infant's orbit and bilateral Jingming (B 1) points, the infant opened his eyes and was conscious, and the temperature dropped to 37.2°C, the fever subsided and there were no more convulsions.

4. The combination of the finger pressure with cupping in the treatment of infantile toxic indigestion

In 1972, a toxic indigestion infant, accompanied with dehydration and even venous collapse, was treated by fluid infusion, but the treatment failed. The patient had a coma and severe abdominal distension. Dr. Qu treated him by pinching the Zhongchong (P 9) point, but with no response. The fingerprint already reached Mingguan, the abdomen was highly distended, and the infant was in a critical stage. He had to be treated quickly to support yang and to protect yin, to dredge the exterior to promote the interior. Dr. Qu pressed the infant's bilateral Jingming (B 1), Laogong (P 8), Yongquan (K 1) points with his fingers, and also pinched the both finger prints to consolidate qi to prevent collapse. Dr. Qu immediately used the glass cup No. 3 which was dipped previously in warm ginger water, pushing quickly up and down thirty times on bilateral Huatuojiaji points, then moving the cupping surrounding Zhongwan (Ren 12), Tianshu (S 25) (bilateral), and Guanyuan (Ren 4) sixty times in order to activate zang-fu organs. The infant had peristalsis in his abdomen after moving twenty times, and passed flatus frequently after another sixty times. Abdominal distention was gradually alleviated, and the abdomen became flat after the same procedures were repeated once more. For consolidation of the effect, the finger pressure method was applied at Laogong (P 8), and Yongquan (K 1) and at twenty-eight junctions of both fingers for twenty times, all the symptoms were relieved.

5. Water cupping in treating asthma

In the autumn of 1978, Dr. Qu used the water cupping method to treat several asthma patients at Yuzhong of Gansu Province with satisfactory results. Treatment procedure: In a warm room, a burned piece of paper was put into a No. 1 large glass cup containing half warm water and then quickly put on the Feishu (B 13) point (1.5 cun lateral to the T3), first at the left side, then at the right side, retained for three minutes, numerous bubbles were produced in the cup. The cup was left there for fifteen minutes and then was removed by sliding the cup slowly to one side with the opening of the cup facing upward to avoid leaking of the water. Apply four to five cuppings for the mild cases, and five to six cuppings for severe cases. Wuyi (S 15) point in the front of the chest is added bilaterally for persistant cases (3 cun superior to the nipple).

Asthma is divided into excess and deficiency type. The excess asthma is due to either wind-cold or wind-heat invading the lung, or phlegm obstructing the respiratory tract. Dr. Qu experienced that water cupping is able to disperse the inhibited lung qi, regulate the lung-qi and resolve the phlegm, therefore, it is effective for asthma. The deficiency asthma occurs mostly in elderly and weak patients with a long duration of disease, due to failure of lung qi in descending, failure of the spleen in transportation and transformation, resulting in dyspnea and palpitation, failure of the kidney qi in receiving qi, and insufficiency of kidney yang and kidney yin, resulting in sweating on exertion and upward flowing of phlegm-dampness. The treatment must support yang and protect yin. Marvellous effects will be obtained in combination with water cupping with herbs.

II. Case Analysis

Case 1: Migraine

Name, Liang x x; sex, male; date of the first visit, August, 1977.

Complaints He had general weakness before illness. Recently he caught cold and had a cough, and migraine on the right side, radiating to the vertex and the right canthus. He administered the drugs for promoting sweating to relieve the exterior symptoms and then the cough stopped, but the headache was aggravated. Nervous headache was diagnosed. The headache was prolonged and more serious, accompanied by palpitation and dyspnea during attacks. Examination: Thin body, internal sinking of the eyeball socket, lassitude, poor appetite, insomnia, right migraine aggravated on pressure, sweating on exertion, palpitation, soft abdomen, liver and spleen (-), string-taut and weak pulse, and thin white coating. Differentiation: General weakness, repeated attacks of cold, overadministering of the drugs for clearing away heat injured yin fluid and defensive qi, which failed to protect the body surface, thus sweating appeared. The nutrient blood fails to nourish the interior, so palpitation results. In case of obstruction of qi flow, and stagnation of qi and blood, headache takes place. According to the location of the headache, the left and right sides pertain to Yangming and Shaoyang Meridians. For chronic weakness, too much needling is avoided. So needling a few points is used to dredge these two meridians and to eliminate the pathogenic factors, and massage is applied to regulate qi.

Prescriptions Zanzhu (B 2), Toulinqi (G 15), Shuaigu (G 8) and Tianyou (SJ 16).

Treatment procedure Filiform needles No. 30 were applied to puncture Zanzhu (B 2) 1 cun upward, Shuaigu (G 8) 1 cun posterior horizontally, Toulinqi (G 15) 1 cun upward, and Tianyou (SJ 16) horizontally 0.8 cun deep. When needling Tianyou (SJ 16), after deqi, twist the needle quickly for one cycle and let the needle sensation reach the base of the eye and radiate to the vertex. After needling, the patient was asked to use eight tips of the bilateral index, middle, ring and small fingers to massage quickly a hundred times. The headache disappeared after twenty-four treatments. No relapse was found after the follow-up visit for one year.

Explanation Headache originated from cold and weakness of the constitution, and wrong intake of too many drugs for perspiration. So the body became weaker, thus derangement of meridian qi, obstruction of the meridian with the result of a headache. Not too many needles are advisable due to weakness, only four points are selected. And massage is combined to activate the blood circulation, dredge the obstructed qi and promote the meridians. Thus pain stopped due to smooth flow of the meridians.

Case 2: Enuresis

Name, Li x x; sex, female; age, 19; date of the first visit, January 24, 1960.

Complaints She suffered from enuresis since childhood. She dared not to drink at night and ate congee during the day, but enuresis still took place. She was treated with acupuncture and physiotherapy in other hospitals, but with no response. The body constitution was weak, the pulse at two "cun" region was deep and weak, and that at "chi" region was deep and string-taut, the tongue with a thin white coating and normal tongue proper. The pulse indicates the evident deficiency of the kidney qi. Since the bladder and kidney are externally-internally related, deficiency of kidney qi will cause deficiency of the bladder, which fails in controlling urine, then enuresis results.

Prescriptions Pangguangshu (B 28), Shenshu (B 23), and Duiduan (Du 27).

Treatment procedure Finger pressure. Heavy stimulation was used at Pangguangshu (B 28) to reduce the depressed heat from the urinary bladder, while light stimulation at Duiduan (Du 27) and Shenshu (B 23) to reinforce the kidney qi and strengthen the function of the Du Meridian. Five treatments in all with finger pressure method were applied since January 24 to February 1, 1960. Good therapeutic effect was obtained during treatment, no more enuresis happened.

Explanation Dr. Qu experienced that the pulse at two "cun" region not only dominates the heart and lung, but is also closely related to the heart and kidney. Deficiency of the kidney qi will cause weakness of the pulse at "cun" region, because the meridian qi is too weak to circulate to the distal end. Now the patient's pulse was deep and weak, yet she had no dyspnea, palpitation and the symptoms showing sinking of qi in the middle jiao; however, enuresis was frequent. Dr. Qu suggests that this symptom was due to deficiency of the kidney qi. As to the reinforcing or reducing with finger pressure, light pinching with the thumb tips of both hands is called reinforcing, while heavy pressing and anterior-posterior moving is reducing. Reducing first and reinforcing later means to dispel the pathogenic factors and to support the body resistance.

Case 3: Facial paralysis (bell's palsy)

Name, Zhang x x; sex, female; date of the first visit, September 26, 1983.

Complaints She had heat pain around her left head and ear on September 18, 1983. She found numbness and stiffness of the left side of the face after she got up in the morning and the next day during washing her face. Failure in closing the eyes, lacrimation, slurred speech, leaking of the mouth in speaking, water leaking in brushing teeth, food residues remained between the cheeks during eating, numbness of the tongue, and ageusia. Examination: Inability in wrinkling the eyebrow, and blowing the cheeks, disappearance of the frontal wrinkle, incomplete closing of the eye on the affected area, flat naso-labial fissure, loose facial muscle, dropping and deviation of the mouth corner to the healthy side, especially aggravated during laughing, pale red tongue, thin white coating, and weak pulse. The above manifestations indicated the internal stagnation of heat, attacking by wind-cold, wind invading the meridians, thus facial paralysis.

Treatment procedure She felt alleviated after four treatments with continuous quick flashing cupping method. The frontal wrinkles 3 cm extended to the healthy side and her eyes could be basically closed. The frontal wrinkle and naso-labial fissure were basically recovered after seven treatments, and the deviation of the mouth corner was chiefly checked. Numbness of the tongue disappeared and taste sensation restored. After another five treatments for consolidation, the symptoms completely disappeared. She was totally recovered after twelve treatments. No relapse was found after the follow-up visit one year later.

PRINCIPLE BASED ON DIFFERENTIATION, PRESCRIPTION ACCORDING TO PRINCIPLE

—Liu Guanjun's Clinical Experience

Liu Guanjun, a native of Huinan, Jilin Province, was born in 1929. He first followed his uncle, Dr. Tian Runzhou in the early years, and later on learned from Dr. Hong Zheming, an expert in febrile diseases caused by cold, for six years. In 1956, he was invited to give lectures in Changchun on *Golden Chamber, Diagnosis, Febrile Diseases, Doctrines of Various Historical Schools, Prescription,* and *Acupuncture*. He advocates combining the advantages of both herbal medicine and acupuncture, absorbing good points of various schools, and following the creative style of one's own. His works include *Pulse Diagnose, Simplified Version of Ziwuliuzhu, Selections of Medical Cases in Modern Acupuncture, The Understanding of Acupuncture, Collection of Needling Techniques in TCM, Explanation to Nomenclature of Acupoints, Pricking Therapy*. With the help of Dr. Jin Boshu, he made a model of meridians and collaterals, which was sent to Japan to be shown on the International Scientific Exhibition. He is now a council member of the All-China Society of Traditional Chinese Medicine and the China Society of Acupuncture and Moxibustion, deputy council director of the Jilin Society of Traditional Chinese Medicine, director member of the Jilin Society of Acupuncture and Moxibustion, professor of the Changchun College of Traditional Chinese Medicine, and president of its affiliated hospital.

I. Academic Characteristics and Medical Specialities

1. Considering of both the root cause and the symptoms, treatment of gastroptosis with "Weishangxue"

According to the explanation from *Internal Classic*, gastroptosis results from a delicate constitution, deficiency of the body resistance, sinking of the spleen qi, and weakness of the stomach failing in contraction, then appeared symptoms such as distension, pain and constipation. To treat such condition, the gastrohepatic ligament and the contraction and intensity of the abdominal muscle should be first strengthened, and then the spleen qi reinforced, the body resistance supported. Weishangxue, 2 cun superior to the umbilicus and 4 cun lateral to Xiawan (Ren 10), is selected to raise the tension of the smooth muscle of the digestive tract, and strengthen the movement to lift the stomach. Since Weishang is the branch collateral of Spleen Meridian, needling is able to strengthen the spleen qi. The addition of Zhongwan (Ren 12) and Qihai (Ren 6) can strengthen the body resistance, and the use of Baihui (Du 20), Pishu (B 20), Weishu (B 21) and Shenshu (B 23) can support yang and strengthen the spleen. Procedure: Ask the patient to lie in prone position with knee flexed. One hand pressing on the other, the doctor massages the abdomen clockwise from right to left fifty times, then presses lightly with the thumb the soft tissue of the upper margin of public bone and tries to find the lowest part of stomach, then pushes the stomach with the palm slowly upward to the umbilicus and remains there for five minutes. Another doctor (or the doctor himself) punctures Weishangxue with a 6-cun needle through the muscle layer to the umbilicus, with large amplitude of rotation, lifting and thrusting until the warm distension and contraction on the stomach appears, then needles Zhongwan (Ren 12), Qihai (Ren 6) (warming method), and Baihui (Du 20) with electric stimulation on Weishangxue. Increase the intensity of the stimulation until the patient cannot withstand the tolerance. Retain the needles for fifteen minutes. In order to strengthen the effect, the patient can lie in a supine position with hips joint flexed and head lowered to do the abdominal muscle exercise, in which inhale three times to Dantian and hold the breath as long as possible and then exhale three times. Repeat the procedure thirty times. After exercise, moxibustion is applied on Weishu (B 21), Pishu (B 20) and Shenshu (B 23) five cones each. In case of liver qi depression, puncturing of Taichong (Liv 3) and Qimen (Liv 14) is added to pacify the liver. In case of deficiency-cold, apply moxibustion on Guanyuan (Ren 4) and Mingmen (Du 4) to dispel cold. In case of dampness, Sanjiaoshu (B 22) is added to eliminate damp. In case of blood stagnation, Geshu (B 17) is added. In case of stomach heat, Neiting (S 44) and Jiexi (S 41) are added to eliminate the stomach fire.

When the stomach has returned to the original position, reinforce the spleen qi to treat the root cause, which is performed by applying moxibustion on Baihui (Du 20), Shenque (Ren 8), Yongquan (K 1), Weishu (B 21), Pishu (B 20) and Shenshu (B 23). Herbal remedies to strengthen the spleen and stomach, helping to eliminate damp and distension can be used in addition to moxibustion. The prescription is as follows: Astragalus root, Ciminifuga, Bupleurum, Fructur aurantii, Chinese angelica. For external use, 50 g of powder of Castor seed and 20 g of Chinese gall are mixed with venegar into paste, which is applied at Baihui (Du 20) and Shenque (Ren 8), and covered with a hot thermos bottle for warming. Treat once a day, thirty minutes each, continuously for seven days. During the treatment, the patient is advised not to eat too much, and to wrap the lower abdomen with a piece of cloth to prevent transverse attacks of the liver qi and failure of the spleen qi in descending.

2. The use of Jinsuo (Du 8) in the treatment of epigastric pain

A patient had epigastric pain resulting from a long journey and cold and greasy diet, accompanied with distension, acid regurgitation, belching, deep and tense pulse and a white sticky tongue coating. Muscle spasm could be seen on the epigastric region. It felt hard but free of tenderness. He was first diagnosed as having epigastric pain of deficiency cold type due to dysfunction of the stomach, and failure of the spleen in transportation and transformation. However, acupuncture on Zhongwan (Ren 12), Liangqiu (S 34) and Neiguan (P 6) made the spasm and pain even worse. Further examination found that though suffering from stomachache, the main problem was spasm. As the liver controls tendons, and the stomachache caused spasm. Jinsuo (Du 8), which has the function of checking pain and relieving spasm, was used based on the theory of inducing yin from yang mentioned in the *Internal Classic*. The pain was checked and spasm disappeared immediately after needling. Dr. Liu holds that though it was a case of epigastric pain, the main problem was spasm, Zhongwan (Ren 12), Liangqiu (S 34) and Neiguan (P 6) could not check the spasm but make it worse. This is the change in general. Therefore, careful diagnosis should be made to distinguish the primary from the secondary.

3. Making the principle based on differentiation, simultaneous use of acupuncture and herbal medicine

Dr. Liu attaches great importance to the principle of treatment according to the differentiations and prefers to the application of both acupuncture and herbal medicine. For instance, a patient had an obese body, lassitude and closing his eyes like sleeping, a lustreless complexion, string-taut and rolling pulse, pale tongue with white sticky coating, fullness and distension in the chest and diaphragm, nausea and vomiting. Differentiation: The phlegm and dampness obstructing the middle jiao, leading to dysfunction of the spleen in transportation and transformation, resulting in the failure of yang qi in ascending, thus appeared dizziness. The treatment was given based on the principle of strengthening the spleen and stomach for phlegm elimination, and subduing the wind for relieving dizziness. Prescription: Zhongwan (Ren 12), Fengchi (G 20), Baihui (Du 20), and Zusanli (S 36), and decoction for checking dizziness was also prescribed (Gastrodia, Hooked Uncaria, Pinellia Tuber, Ligustici Chuanxiong, Tribulus Fruit, Tangerine Peel, Chrysanthemum, Caulis Bambusae in Taeniam with Poria, Haematitum and Ginger juice.) The patient recovered after twelve acupuncture treatments and six herbal remedies. Another patient was weak and looked tired, with dizziness, blurred vision, pallor, palpitation, insomnia, poor appetite and sore lower back, soft and weak pulse, thready at two *chi* regions, and a pale and moist tongue. Differentiation: Insufficient marrow and weakness of Kidney Meridian resulting in dizziness. He was cured after taking twenty-four remedies for checking dizziness with additional herbs, such as Aconiti Praeparata, Poria, Cassia, Date core, Yuan rou, Ginsen, Powder of antler. Patient C was strong and had dizziness and redness of the eye, aggravated by excitement, accompanied by headache, tremor, string-taut and rapid pulse, red tongue edge with thin yellow coating, BP 130/80 mmHg. Differentiation: Deficiency of nutrient yin and predominance of liver qi. He was cured after thirteen decoctions for checking dizziness with additional herbs, such as Achyranthis, Spica Prunellae, Plastrom Testudinis, Fructus ligustri lucidi, white peony, Polygonati Odorati, in combination with sixteen acupuncture treatments on Taichong (Liv 3), Taixi (K 3), Fengchi (G 20), and Hegu (LI 4). Among these three cases of dizziness, the first was due to obstruction of phlegm in the middle jiao, the focus was on phlegm elimination, the second resulting from the deficiency of kidney yin, the principle was to nourish the kidney, the third was caused by hyperactivity of liver yang, the stress was to pacify the liver. Three cases were treated with remedies for checking dizziness but with additional herbs according to the differentiations.

4. Reinforcing the stomach and spleen for the treatment of deafness and deviation of mouth

In the light of the theory mentioned in *Internal Classic*, "Stomach and spleen are the causes for headache, tinnitus and other problems related to organs on the face." It has been applied to treat various kinds of diseases in practice and has been proved very effective. For instance, a construction worker slept on the wet ground after physical work and then poor appetite, loose stools and borborygmus appeared. Gradually he felt distension and stuffiness in the left ear and hearing was decreasing drastically. He was thin and emaciated, depressive and looked tired, slight sallow complexion, pale tongue with thin white coating, deep slow and forceless pulse. He was cured after two weeks treatment by needling Zusanli (S 36), Pishu (B 20), Tinghui (G 2) (left), Yifeng (SJ 17) (left) for sixteen times and applying moxibustion with Xanthium in the left ear four times. The follow-up visit was given for three months and no relapse was found. Treatment should be focused on strengthening the stomach and spleen for the cases of tinnitus and deafness due to dysfunction of the stomach and spleen. Zusanli (S 36) and Pishu (B 20) can regulate and strengthen the stomach and spleen, reinforce the qi in the Middle Jiao and lift clear yang qi. Tinghui (G 2) and Yifeng (SJ 17) are needled to activate the qi flow in the ear. The most wonderful point is the moxibustion with Xanthium, which contains a large amount of vitamin and is able to strengthen the spleen and eliminate dampness, and improve the blood circulation of the internal ear. Though the nine orifices are respectively dominated by the zang organs, they should be nourished by the stomach qi, and dependent upon the ascending of the spleen qi, then they can function well.

As to the treatment of deviation of mouth, many doctors would like to dispel wind and dredge the collaterals. But Dr. Liu experienced that deviation of mouth may also be caused by malnourishment of tendons and muscles due to deficiency of stomach fluid and failure in descending of clear yang qi resulting from excessive fire in the stomach leading to consumption of stomach fluid by hot and dry diet. For instance, a male patient had spontaneous sweating, lassitude, and numbness on the right side of the face and the mouth deviated to the left, inability to blow the mouth, and salivation. Examination: Flush face, yellow tongue coating, deep rapid and forceful pulse, dark yellow urine, constipation for three days. All these indicate that the exogenous pathogenic factors turned into heat and entered the body leading to accumulation of stomach heat, then the pathogenic wind attacked the tendons and vessels on the face, resulting in deviation of the mouth. Decoction for yang ascending was used together with some additional herbs, such as Puerariae, Dendrobii, Glehniae, Yuanshen, to nourish the stomach yin and reduce the stomach heat. Cimicifugae was added to lift yang and dispel fire. Toasted astragalus was for reinforcing qi and checking perspiration. Chinese angelica, Cassia twig, Flos carthami, Lignum sappan were added to activate the qi flow of the meridians and nourish the blood. Moxibustion on the face was used to remove the local obstruction. The patient was treated for five days and cured. The above diseases were all treated by strengthening the stomach and spleen because if the spleen and stomach qi are damaged, the source qi can not be replenished and all kinds of diseases may occur therefrom.

5. Differentiation according to the meridians and selection of points along the meridians

Dr. Liu holds that there exist the interrelation and interaffection between the meridians and zang-fu organs and between the internal organs and the sense organs. For instance, a worker suffered from weakness and soreness of the four limbs, lassitude and poor appetite due to sexual indulgence. Dr. Liu thinks that the spleen controls the four limbs. "The essential part of yang qi can nourish the mind, while the gentle part can nourish the tendon." The warming needle was first used on Baihui (Du 20), Pishu (B 20) and Zusanli (S 36), adding Dazhu (B 11), Dabao (Sp 21) and Yanglingquan (G 34), and then Radix Astragali seu Hedysari, Rhizoma Cimicifugae, Rhizoma Atractylodis Macrocephalae, Radix Bupleuri were prescribed. The patient was cured after nine treatments. Dr. Liu attaches great importance to the theory of contralateral puncture—puncture the points on the right side to treat the disease on the left side. He holds that under the normal condition, qi and blood circulate along the meridians to nourish zang-fu organs and the whole body. Once the imbalance (predominance or discomfiture) of the meridians occurs, the measures should be taken to restore the balance. According to the theory of the meridians which are connected from up to bottom, from left to right, needle the points on the upper portion to regulate the lower, and puncture the points on the left to treat the disease on the right. For instance, a male patient had upper toothache on the left side, chewing limitation, which was aggravated in inhalation, and insomnia. Examination: Slightly red and swelling of the upper gum, pink tongue proper with yellow coating, deep rapid pulse, constipation for three days. Differentiation: Stomach heat. Jiexi (S 41) on the right side was punctured to reduce the stomach fire, Jiache (S 7) on the affected side was needled to check pain, and bloodletting was applied on the affected gum with a sharp needle. The patient was cured after one treatment. Another patient had lumbar sprain pain which radiated to the hyperchondrium, contracture and stiffness of the back and neck, clear tenderness on both Shenshu (B 23) and congestion of the superficial venules around both Weizhong (B 40). Bleeding on Weizhong (B 40) was applied to resolve stagnation. Prick the tenderness of both Shenshu (B 23) in combination with cupping. After two treatments, the patient was cured.

6. Selection of points according to the different times

Dr. Liu attaches importance to the pathological development of a disease "relieved in the early morning, good at day, aggravated in the evening, and worsened at night" recorded in *Internal Classic* in selection of points. Since the human body is an organic whole adapted to the environment, there exists a very close relationship between weather and the physiological activities of zang-fu organs. As to the influence of the climate of the four seasons to zang-fu activity, it is said in *Plain Questions* that the heart is in communication with the summer qi, the lung in communication with the autumn qi, the kidney in communication with the winter qi, the liver in communication with the spring qi, and the spleen in communication with the earth qi. Therefore, it is said again in *Plain Questions* that "runny nose and nosebleed are the most likely symptoms in spring; chest and ribs are the most likely symptoms in summer, diarrhoea of dampness and internal cold are the most likely symptoms in prolonged summer; malaria of wind is the most likely symptoms in autumn; rheumatism and cold limbs are the most likely symptoms in winter." Some diseases may have biologically periodical changes within a day. For instance, asthma mostly occurs at 3 to 5 o'clock, the morning diarrhoea mostly takes place at dawn. So the doctors must observe the periodical regulation of six cycles of heaven and nine divisions of the earth. It is therefore pointed out in *Miraculous Pivot* that "the qi of the four seasons attack different regions of the body, so that the essentials of acupuncture and moxibustion involve the acupuncture points to be applied." In the *Plain Questions*, it is further pointed out: "The method of acupuncture is such that the doctor should await the right moments regarding the movements of the sun, the moon, the stars, and the qi of the four seasons and the eight seasonal dates, and as soon as right movements arrive relative to the stable state of qi, acupuncture treatment should begin." Dr. Liu has simplified and standardized the method of Mid-Night Ebb-Flow and achieved good results in clinic. For instance, a patient had attack of stomach pain at 1 to 3 o'clock every day, with deep and string-taut pulse at "guan" region. Examination of the Yuan-Source points with electric instrument showed liver hyperactivity and spleen weakness.

Stomachache was due to the attack of stomach by liver qi. According to the Midnight-noon Ebb-flow, at 1 to 3 o'clock, qi and blood flow to liver, predominant liver attacks the stomach transversely, leading to spleen weakness and liver hyperactivity. Since deficient spleen was too weak to help, the lung was also too deficient to control the liver (wood). At night about 1 to 3 o'clock, when the liver overattacked earth, increasing epigastric pain resulted. Reduce Taichong (Liv 3) to calm transverse liver qi, reinforce Gongsun (Sp 4) to strengthen spleen, and reinforce the mother point Taiyuan (L 9) to activate the lung qi so that metal would be strong enough to control wood. After being treated seven times, the epigastric pain stopped. The patient only felt hypochondriac distension occasionally. To this, Taichong (Liv 3) was punctured to calm the liver, Zhangmen (Liv 13) was needled to resolve local stagnation. The treatment proved satisfactory. Another patient vomited the deep, string-taut *guan* pulse on the left side suggested that it was due to liver qi attacking the stomach, Dadun (Liv 1), Taichong (Liv 3), Ququan (Liv 8) were punctured to relieve depression and calm the liver at the time when the liver is abundant in qi and blood. This method worked very well.

II. Case Analysis

Case 1: Tic pain of the fingers

Name, Liu x x; sex, male; age, 13; date of the first visit, April 19, 1975.

Complaints On April 14, the patient caught a cold and had fever, cough and sore throat which were relieved after treatment. In the evening of April 17, he suddenly had a chilling sensation, followed by convulsion and pain of the right arm. During the attack, the right index finger felt cold. The tic pain radiated to the neck along the index finger in a band state. Pain referred to the nape and back, accompanied with nasal obstruction and sore throat. Herbal medicine failed to relieve the problem. The pain attacked two to four times a day, each time for five minutes. The index finger has preference for warmth, but disliked cold, the patient often wrapped it with the left hand for more warmth to prevent the attack. Examination: The patient was of medium size, thin body, pale complexion, two nodules the same size as date core at the right neck, no pain, slightly congested throat, temperature 36.8°C, deep, weak and forceless pulse, thin white tongue coating. The pain happened to attack him during the examination, the right arm flexed inside, with motor hindrance. According to the patient's complaints, the pain started from the medial side of the index finger with a cold sensation, along the second metacarpal bone, through Hegu (LI 4), Quchi (LI 11), upward to Jianyu (LI 15), and Tianding (LI 17), and then to Dazhui (Du 14). The tic pain was like a band, downward narrow, and upward wide, the widest was about 1.5 cm. The pain radiated to all directions about 3 cm on the elbow and shoulder. Obvious tenderness was found on Hegu (LI 4), Quchi (LI 11), and Jianyu (LI 15), but not obvious on Dazhui (Du 14) by percussion. The skin resistance on Shangyang (LI 1) was 9 uA (left) and 4 uA (right), that of Hegu (LI 4) was 12 uA (left) and 7 uA (right). The skin resistance on the affected side (Quchi (LI 11), Jianyu (LI 15)) was 3 to 6 uA higher than that on the healthy side. No symptoms such as upward staring eyes or salivation occurred during the attack. Differentiation: Tic pain due to cold and deficiency of the Large Intestine Meridian. Principle of treatment: Warm Large Intestine Meridian to remove obstruction.

Prescription Hegu (LI 4), Quchi (LI 11), and Jianyu (LI 15) on the affected side.

Treatment procedure The needling sensation (numbness and distension) went upward slowly to Tianding (LI 17), and then radiated to Dazhui (Du 14). Where the needling sensation went, the tic pain was checked and tenderness disappeared. The needles were retained for fifteen minutes. Warming needling was applied at Quchi (LI 11), the pain disappeared after the treatment. The next day, except for cold sensation of the arm at night, the pain did not attack. Examination: Skin resistance at Shangyang (LI 1) 9 (left) and 7 (right), that at Hegu (LI 4) 17 (left), and 15 (right). There was no significant difference between the skin resistance of the affected and healthy side. Only Hegu (LI 4) was punctured with the needle counterclockwise rotating to radiate the needling sensation along the Large Intestine Meridian upward to Dazhui (Du 14), 1 cm wide in band state. Then, puncture Yingxiang (LI 20) with the needling sensation going to Tianding (LI 17) 3 cm away from the numb band of Dazhui (Du 14). The third day, he recovered. The pain did not attack even when the index finger was exposed to cold. Examination: The skin resistance of both sides was quite close, Jing-Well point, left 9, right 9; Yuan-Source point, left 17, right 16. Qi and blood 47 Am. The follow-up visit was given two weeks later and no relapse was found.

Explanation The fact that the patient caught cold and then was followed by tic pain along the Large Intestine Meridian indicates that the patient had a weak constitution deficient of meridian qi. The exogenous pathogenic factors turned into interior. As the Lung Meridian travels through Lieque (L 7) to the medial side of the index finger and connects with the Large Intestine Meridian, which goes downward to Quepen (S 12) and connects with the lung. The patient caught cold, followed by a cough, sore throat and fever, indicating the lung affected first. And then cold sensation and tic pain along the meridian appeared, showing deficiency of qi of the Large Intestine Meridian. Since the lung and large intestine are related, the pathogenic factors transferred from the lung to the large intestine. The qi of the Large Intestine Meridian is deficient. A cold feeling appeared along the meridian and travelled upward demonstrating the existence of the meridians.

Case 2: Cough

Name, Song x x; sex, female; age, 33; date of the first visit, March, 1974.

Complaints The patient had general weakness, poor appetite and gastric distension. Recently she caught cold and had a cough, which was aggravated after wrong intake of herbal decoction cool in nature. She had white sputum and lassitude and weak limbs. Examination: Slight sallow complexion, mild edema of the face, pale tongue proper, thin white coating, soft and rolling pulse, but thready at "guan" region on the right side. Differentiation: Deficiency of the spleen yang, attacked by the exogenous pathogenic factors, leading to turbid phlegm in the lung and affecting the lung dispersing function. Principle of treatment: Nourish the spleen to strengthen the lung and to check cough.

Prescription Taiyuan (L 9), Feishu (B 13), Lieque (L 7), Fenglong (S 40), Pishu (B 20) and Zusanli (S 36).

Treatment procedure Reinforce Taiyuan (L 9), reduce Feishu (B 13), Lieque (L 7) and Fenglong (S 40), apply moxibustion at Pishu (B 20), and Zusanli (S 36). Treat once a day. The patient recovered after being treated for seven days.

Explanation This condition is due to constitutional deficiency of spleen yang with the attack of exogenous pathogenic factors, and wrong intake of herbal medicine of a cool nature, which in turn, made the spleen yang more deficient. It is the cold cough due to yang deficiency. Reinforce Taiyuan (L 9), reduce Lieque (L 7) and Feishu (B 13) to promote lung qi. Fenglong (S 40), the Luo-Connecting point of Stomach Meridian and divergent from Spleen Meridian, reducing can resolve phlegm and descend the turbidity. Moxibustion on Pishu (B 20) and Zusanli (S 36) can strengthen the spleen and reinforce qi, dispel humor and check cough.

Case 3: Low fever

Name, Qiu x x; sex, male; age, 46; date of the first visit, September, 1974.

Complaints The patient had general weakness and poor appetite. Recently, due to overstress and attack by exogenous pathogenic factors, he had headache and fever. Treatment made him better, but failed to reduce the low fever (37 to 38°C). Even the continuous use of Penicillin, Streptomycin and Tetracyline failed to resolve the problem. More than twenty decoctions prescribed by one hospital with the herbs of R. Rehamaniae, R. Scutellariae, Hb. Artemisiae Chinghao, Hb. Artemisiae, Carapax Trychycis, Cortex Lycii Radicis of cold nature led to cold limbs, lassitude, poor appetite, aversion to cold, spontaneous sweating, palpitation, loose stools and borborygmus. Examination: Weak constitution, lassitude, slight sallow complexion, pale lips, thin white coating, deep thready and forceless pulse, BP 130/90 mmHg, white cell totalled 5500/mm^3, neutrality 74 percent. Differentiation: Deficiency of the spleen and primary qi leading to hyperactivity of yin fire, thus the low fever. Principle of treatment: Strengthen the spleen and raise yang to eliminate heat.

Prescription Zhongwan (Ren 12), Zusanli (S 36), Pishu (B 20), Qihai (Ren 6), Dazhui (Du 14), Yangchi (SJ 4) (moxibustion).

Treatment procedure Apply moxibustion on Zhongwan (Ren 12), Qihai (Ren 6), Dazhui (Du 14) and Yangchi (SJ 4) respectively for five cones, and on Zusanli (S 36) and Pishu (B 20) for seven cones. Treat once a day. After seven continuous treatments, low fever was reduced and pulse became normal. White cell totalled 6800/mm^3. Another seven treatments were given to consolidate the effect.

Explanation The low fever was due to constitutional weakness with low body resistance. The herbal medicine of a cold nature made the deficient spleen even worse. Zhongwan (Ren 12), Pishu (B 20), and Zusanli (S 36) are essential points to strengthen the spleen and stomach. Moxibustion on them can reinforce the spleen and stomach qi and reduce heat. Qihai (Ren 6) is the origin of primary qi. Performing moxibustion on it can strengthen the body and nourish the vessels. Moxibustion on Dazhui (Du 14), the crossing point of all the yang meridians, can reduce heat from the yang meridians. Yangchi (SJ 4) can free the qi of the three Jiao.

Case 4: The fixed bi syndrome

Name, Chen x x; sex, female; age, 47; date of the first visit, August, 1973.

Complaints The patient had painful knee joints, diarrhoea and poor appetite due to being drenched in the rain. After taking some herbal pills, he felt a little better, still he had a heavy sensation, and numbness and pain of the knee joints. Examination: Slight sallow complexion, thin white coating, deep, retarded and forceless pulse, both knees slightly swollen with tenderness and motor limitation. Differentiation: Weak constitution and spleen deficiency in combination with dampness and cold damaging yang qi. Principle of treatment: Warm yang, strengthen the spleen, eliminate dampness to check pain.

Prescription Yangguan (Du 3), Yangfu (G 38), Yanglingquan (G 34), Yinlingquan (Sp 9). Warming needling on Zusanli (S 36), Yangguan (Du 3) (lumbar) and Pishu (B 20).

Treatment procedure Seven treatments relieved the pain and diarrhoea. Another seven treatments of warming the needle on Mingmen (Du 4) eliminated all the symptoms.

Case 5: Intestinal tuberculosis

Name, Wang x x; sex, male; age, 49; date of the first visit, July 20, 1976.

Complaints He suffered from impairment of the lung for many years, which improved after treatment. Two years before, he occasionally had diarrhoea. In recent months, he had borborygmus, abdominal pain and then diarrhoea occurred every day at 6 to 7 o'clock in the evening. The stools were free from blood and pus, the urine was clear in increased volume. Diagnosis was made as "intestinal tuberculosis." He was treated by antituberculosis medications and herbal medicine, but with no marked improvement. Examination: Normal body build, malnutrition, slight sallow complexion, thin white tongue coating, deep, weak and forceless pulse at both "chi" region. Nothing abnormal in heart or lung, abdomen was flat without tender point, uncomfortable upon pressure. Differentiation: Diarrhoea due to kidney deficiency. Principle of treatment: Warm and reinforce the spleen and kidney.

Prescription 1. Mingmen (Du 4), Dadu (Sp 2), Tianshu (S 25). 2. Taixi (K 3), Dadun (Liv 1), Lingdao (H 4).

Treatment procedure Warm and reinforce the spleen and kidney. Apply moxibustion at Mingmen (Du 4) to reinforce the kidney yang, and that at Dadu (Sp 2), Tianshu (S 25) to regulate the stomach and intestines and support the spleen qi. The patient remained in the same condition after four treatments. Between 5 to 7 o'clock in the evening, qi and blood circulate in the Kidney Meridian, so diarrhoea is caused by incomplete closing due to failure of deficient kidney yang in nourishing the spleen (earth). Examination: Taixi (K 3) value 16 uA on the left and 7 uA on the right. At 1 to 3 p.m. of Day Ji, Taixi (K 3) is on value, reinforce Taixi (K 3) for fifteen minutes in combination with Mingmen (Du 4), Dadu (Sp 2), and Tianshu (S 25). The next day, he had a bowel movement two hours before the usual time. At 3 to 5 p.m. of Day Geng, no point is open for acupuncture, reinforce Dadun (Liv 1) instead. At 5 to 7 p.m. of Day Xin, Lingdao (H 4) is open. At 9 to 11 p.m. of Day Ren, again no point is open. Reinforce Dadu (Sp 2) instead. After three days interval, the diarrhoea was checked. Bowel movement occurred at 9 o'clock in the morning with formed stools. Then examination showed Taixi (K 3) was 27 uA on the left and 28 uA on the right.

Explanation For the first four treatments, the routine selection of points was applied, but with no improvement, for the later four treatments, the selection of points made according to the time and good results obtained.

Case 6: Dizziness (hypertension)

Name, Chi x x; sex, female; age, 47; occupation, shop assistant; date of the first visit, August 15, 1976.

Complaints Intermittent headache, dizziness with tinnitus (left) for two weeks, difficulty in falling asleep after slight fright, sleep with dreams and easily frightened, profuse urine, bowel movement once every other day, menopause for three months. Diagnosis: Primary hypertension. Treat with verticil, she didn't have any marked improvement. Examination: Normal body build, flushed face, obese body, red tongue with sticky coating, deep, tight and forceful pulse, but weak at two "chi" regions, BP 200/120 mmHg. Differentiation: Deficiency of the kidney, and hyperactivity of liver yang. Principle of treatment: Nourish the kidney (water) to control and pacify the liver. Prescription: (Selected according to different times) Taixi (K 3), Taichong (Liv 3), Fengchi (G 20), Shenmen (H 7), Rangu (K 2), Ququan (Liv 8). Treatment procedure: Dizziness, headache, flushed face, tinnitus, insomnia and irritability, deep, tight and forceful pulse indicated the hyperactivity of the liver leading to failure to store the mind, weak "chi" pulse explained the cause for liver hyperactivity—deficiency of kidney water. The treatment is to nourish the kidney water and calm the liver. So acupuncture was employed at different times. The first time, reinforce Taixi (K 3) at 1 to 3 a.m. to nourish the kidney water and liver wood, in combination with Taichong (Liv 3) for reducing the hyperactive liver yang, and then with Fengchi (G 20) for checking dizziness. The second time, puncture Taixi (K 3) at 1 to 3 p.m. and Shenmen (H 7) to calm the mind. The third time, puncture Rangu (K 2), the Ying-Spring and fire point of the Kidney Meridian at 5 to 7 a.m. and Fengchi (G 20). The fourth time, puncture Ququan (Liv 8), the He-Sea and water point of the Liver Meridian at 9 to 11 a.m. and Fengchi (G 20). After the fourth treatment, blood pressure was reduced to 160/100 mmHg, dizziness was checked and sleep improved. A follow-up visit half a year later found blood pressure basically stable.

Case 7: Neurotic vomiting

Name, Li x x; sex, female; age, 23; occupation, shop assistant; date of the first visit, April 2, 1977.

Complaints In February of the year, the patient quarrelled with somebody, then she went to sleep and had meal after awaking. Half an hour after meal, vomiting occurred with food she had just taken. Diagnosis: Neurotic vomiting. Treated with antivomiting and sedative pills, her condition remained the same. Examination: Normal body build, malnutrition, slightly red face, healthy, clear mind, red tongue with sticky coating, left "guan" pulse deep and string-taut, flat abdomen, lung, heart, liver and spleen normal, BP 94/65 mmHg. Differentiation: Vomiting due to liver qi attacking stomach. Principle of treatment: Promote the liver qi flow and regulate the stomach to descend the perverted qi. Prescription: (Selected according to different times) Zhongwan (Ren 12), Zusanli (S 36), Taichong (Liv 3), Dadun (Liv 1), Neiguan (P 6), Ququan (Liv 8).

Treatment procedure First puncture Zhongwan (Ren 12), the Mu-Front point of the stomach, and Zusanli (S 36) to regulate the stomach, and Taichong (Liv 3) to promote liver qi flow. The treatment was given continuously eight times, vomiting was still present as usual. Then, apply acupuncture according to the different times. The first time, puncture Dadun (Liv 1) at 3 to 5 a.m. to calm the liver, Neiguan (P 6) for vomiting, Zusanli (S 36) to descend the perverted qi. The second time, puncture Taichong (Liv 3) at 5 to 7 a.m. to calm the liver qi and the same points used as the previous day. The third time, puncture Ququan (Liv 8) at 9 to 11 a.m. to resolve liver depression, in combination with Taichong (Liv 3) to calm the liver, and Neiguan (P 6) to check vomiting. Altogether four treatments were given and she was cured.

Explanation The vomiting is due to liver qi depression attacking stomach, so treatment is given at the time (day hour) when the Liver Meridian is predominant with puncturing of Dadun (Liv 1), Taichong (Liv 3), Ququan (Liv 8) to calm the liver, resolve depression and prevent the transverse attack.

THE REINFORCING AND REDUCING METHOD, APPLICATION OF BACK-SHU POINTS AND CROSSING COMBINATION OF ACUPOINTS

—Yan Runming's Clinical Experience

Born in Wuqing County of Tianjin in 1921, Dr. Yan Runming studied in Beijing Huabei College of Traditional Chinese Medicine in 1938. After graduation she followed the famous doctors Zhao Shuping and Li Chunxuan. She began to practice medicine after she passed the examination of the Nanjing Academy of Examination in 1947. From 1952 to 1957, she studied in the Medical Department of Beijing Medical College (the present Beijing Medical University). From 1958 to 1963, she worked in the Acupuncture Department of the Sino-Mongolian Friendship Hospital in the People's Republic of Mongol, where she was awarded the title of Hero of Labour Decoration. Since 1966, she has been invited to give lectures and treatments in Pakistan, Japan, and India, and other countries. Her works *Miraculous Pivot Teaching Materials* and *Gynecology Teaching Materials* have been published. She is now chief of the Acupuncture Department, Xiyuan Hospital, China Academy of Traditional Chinese Medicine, and a council member of the Chinese Acupuncture Association.

I. Academic Characteristics and Medical Specialities

1. Emphasis on the reinforcing and reducing method, and proficient application of the Back-Shu points

Dr. Yan has been attaching great importance to the acupuncture manipulations. She holds that each Shu point has its specific effect, and at the same time, provides the bilateral function of regulation, which depends mainly on the change of the needling manipulation—reinforcing or reducing method. What she has been using is a combined method, i.e. the combination of twisting, rotating, lifting and thrusting, and the open-close reinforcing-reducing method. When the needle is inserted, hold the needle with the right hand, deepen it downwards with the thumb rotating the handle of the needle clockwise, from shallow to deep until the qi reaches the diseased area, and then insert the needle 0.1 cun deep. If the needle is withdrawn quickly and the punctured hole is pressed closely, it is the reinforcing method. When the needle is inserted to the required depth, lift the needle with the thumb rotating the handle counterclockwise, from deep to shallow, and when the qi reaches the diseased area, lift the needle about 0.1 cun. If the needle is withdrawn slowly, and the punctured hole is not pressed, this is the reducing method.

Clinically, Dr. Yan is good at using the Back-Shu points. According to the theory of "as soon as the qi arrives, withdraw the needle immediately" recorded in *Internal Classic*, the Back-Shu points are not only able to treat the diseases corresponding to zang-fu organs, but also to the diseases of the five sense organs, nine orifices, skin, tendon and bone, which are related to zang-fu organs. For example, reducing Ganshu (B 18) may reduce the excess fire of the Liver Meridian and clear away the damp-heat, which is similar to the function of Radix Gentianae, and an important point to treat female hysteria, and tinnitus and dizziness resulted from dominant heat of the Liver Meridian. Reinforcing Ganshu (B 18) may nourish the blood and soften the liver, which is similar to the function of Radix Paeoniae Alba, and is an important point to treat eye diseases, such as glycoma and senile cateract. Dr. Yan is experienced in treating menstrual problems. She has summarized the following experience: Mainly nourishing the kidney for girls of puberty age, regulating chiefly the liver for those of child-bearing age; and regulating the acquired spleen and stomach for menopausal women, because of the gradual exhaustion of menstruation due to the deficiency of Taichong Meridian. In treating gynecological diseases based on differentiation according to the theory of meridians, Dr. Yan is good at using Shenshu (B 23), Ganshu (B 18), Pishu (B 20) to treat the root cause. For example, she treated a middle-aged woman who had endless dripping of blood of an indefinite amount for four months caused by anger during menstruation. The pulse was string-taut and thready, especially at the left "guan" region. As the disease was resulted from the liver qi and the injury of the Chong and Ren Meridians, endless dripping of the blood appeared. The bleeding was stopped after three treatments by reducing Ganshu (B 18) and reinforcing Qihai (Ren 6).

2. Application of crossing combination of points

Whenever the Shu points on the extremities are selected from the two meridians, Dr. Yan used to select the points crossly on the left and right sides. For example, in case of Neiguan (P 6) combining with Gongsun (Sp 4), she selects either left Neiguan (P 6) in combination with right Gongsun (Sp 4) or right Neiguan (P 6) in combination with left Gongsun (Sp 4). Similarly, one is on the left and the other is no the right for selecting Hegu (LI 4) and Taichong (Liv 3). Dr. Yan considers that this method has the following advantages: First, the application of less points can minimize the patient's sufferings; second, it can elaborate the special action of the meridian and Shu points can be elaborated; and third, better therapeutic effect obtained. For example, the needling of Hegu (LI 4) on one side in combination with Fuliu (K 7) on the opposite side with the reinforcing method can check spontaneous sweating due to heat for the climacteric women. Hegu (LI 4) is the Yuan-Source point of the Hand-Yangming, and reinforcing it can reinforce qi and strengthen the body surface to prevent diseases. Fuliu (K 7) is the point of Foot-Shaoyin Meridian and reinforcing it can warm yang of the kidney, and elevate qi of the urinary bladder to the whole body. Needling Ximen (P 4) and Shenmen (H 7) on one side in combination with Sanyinjiao (Sp 6) on the opposite side with the reinforcing method can treat palpitation and short breath. Ximen (P 4) is the Xi-Cleft point of the Hand-Jueyin Meridian, Shenmen (H 7) is the Yuan-Source point of the Hand-Shaoyin Meridian, and Sanyinjiao (Sp 6) is the crossing point of the three yin meridians. The three points in combination can promote the heart yang, reduce the heart heat, nourish the yin blood, and calm the mind, thus palpitation treated. Paroxysmal atrial premature, paroxysmal tachycardia and auricular fibrillation have been treated with this method. Usually the heart rate can be reduced or gradually restored to normal after needling for 20 to 30 minutes.

II. Case Analysis

Case 1: Aphasia

Name, Dalgon; sex, male; age, 45; date of the first visit, October 14, 1959.

Complaints He fell down from a running horse, and lost consciousness for about an hour twenty years ago. After he woke up, dizziness, vertigo, occipital headache, and aphasia appeared, and the tongue could make left-right movement in the mouth. After three treatments, the tongue could move freely and pronunciation was restored to normal.

Explanation For stiffness of the tongue and aphasia, the disease lies in the tongue. However, the tongue is the opening of the heart, if the qi of the heart fails to reach the tongue, stiffness of the tongue will result. Reducing Yamen (Du 15) and Lianquan (Ren 23) is regarded as the paired needling method and is able to regulate the local meridian qi. Tongli (H 5) is the Luo-connecting point of the Heart Meridian. "Aphasia" is the illness on the collateral. Reducing this point can reduce the heat from the Heart Meridian, and induce resuscitation. At the same time, the point Zhaohai (K 6) on the opposite side is crossly combined. Zhaohai (K 6) originates from the Yinqiao Meridian, and dominates the phlegm from the chest, larynx and pharynx, and is also a Shu point of the Foot-Shaoyin Meridian. Since the origin and exterior of the Foot-Shaoyin Meridian are situated at Lianquan (Ren 23), reinforcing can induce the yin qi to ascend and to coordinate the function. Bloodletting on Jinjin and Yuye (Extra) can promote resuscitation. Although headache and dizziness gradually subsided after various treatments, aphasia and stiffness of the tongue had not been improved. He had to communicate with his family with gestures or simple language. The tongue still couldn't protrude out of his lips. The tip of the tongue was red, with thick and greasy tongue coating. The pulse was deep and string-taut.

Differentiation Stagnation of qi obstructing the mind. The principle of treatment was to restore the flow of qi and regulate the mind.

Prescription Yamen (Du 15), Lianquan (Ren 23), Tongli (H 5), Zhaohai (K 6), Jinjin and Yuye (Extra 10) for bloodletting.

Treatment procedure Yamen (Du 15), Lianquan (Ren 23) and left Tongli (H 5) were needled with reducing method, and the right Zhaohai (K 6) needled with reinforcing method. The needles were retained for half an hour. After withdrawing the needles, pricking blood therapy was applied on Jinjin and Yuye (Extra 10) points. After the treatment, the stiff tongue was alleviated, Yamen (Du 15) and Lianquan (Ren 23) can make the tongue contract and relax freely, thus aphasia is cured.

Case 2: Abdominal mass

Name, Hu x x; sex, female; age, 45; date of the first visit, February 18, 1979.

Complaints In recent years menstruation came always ahead of time with a cycle of about twenty to twenty-three days. During menstruation, she had sore pain of the lower back and legs, and difficulty in backward bending due to abdominal distension. The last period came on February 10. The bleeding was abundant and the colour dark red with clots. She had dizziness, vertigo, and fatigue after the menstruation. Myoma of the uterus was diagnosed after a gynecological examination. The examination also showed the flabby tongue with tooth prints, thin white coating, deep and thready pulse.

Differentiation Deficiency of both spleen and kidney, and derangement of Chong and Ren Meridians. The principle of treatment is to strengthen the spleen, benefit the kidney and adjust the Chong and Ren Meridians.

Prescription Pishu (B 20), Shenshu (B 23), Dazhui (Du 14), Guanyuan (Ren 4), Zusanli (S 36) and Sanyinjiao (Sp 6) with reinforcing method.

Treatment procedure Needling was given eight to ten times after the end of menstruation every month. Zusanli (S 36) and Sanyinjiao (Sp 6) were needled alternately from left to right. After being treated continuously for four months, the cycle and amount of the menstruation were both recovered to normal, and the rest symptoms were also relieved. A follow-up gynecological examination in June showed that the size of the uterus was a little large with soft consistency.

Explanation Abdominal mass is a disease of Ren Meridian according to the differentiation based on the eight extra-meridians. When the qi of the lower abdomen goes upward to the Chong Meridian, the patient will be unable to bend backward. Therefore, this is a combined disease of the Chong, Ren and Du Meridians, which is the origin of the disease. Dizziness and vertigo are due to the deficiency of both qi and yin after the excessive loss of blood at the menstruation period. This is in fact a state of weak body resistance and excessive pathogenic factors. Dr. Yan used the method of supporting the body resistance and eliminating the pathogenic factors by reducing Dazhui (Du 14) and Guanyuan (Ren 4) and reinforcing Sanyinjiao (Sp 6) to regulate the Du, Chong and Ren Meridians; reinforcing Pishu (B 20), Shenshu (B 23) and Zusanli (S 36) to strengthen the spleen and stomach and benefit the kidney qi to support the body resistance. The patient was cured because the body resistance was supported and the pathogenic factors were eliminated.

Case 3: Omalgia

Name, Wang x x; sex, female; age, 61; date of the first visit, August 12, 1980.

Complaints She had pain on the left arm after being exposed to cold half a year ago. The disease became aggravated in recent two weeks, especially at night, aversion to cold of the shoulders, numbness of the left thumb and index finger, pain exaggerated in raising the left arm and motor limitation. Examination: Absence of red swelling on the left shoulder, the left arm raising 110°, abduction 70°, and posterior extension to L2, thin white coating, deep and string-taut pulse.

Differentiation Cold affecting the meridian and obstruction of both qi and blood.

Principle of treatment Warm the meridian to dispel the cold and dredge the collaterals to stop pain.

Prescription Tianzong (SI 11), Jianwaishu (SI 14), Jianyu (LI 15), Quchi (LI 11), Hegu (LI 4), Tiaokou (S 38) penetrating towards Chengshan (B 57), moxibustion on the shoulder.

Treatment procedure Pain on the shoulder and arm disappeared after ten treatments. The left arm could be lifted 180°, and abduction 90°, and all the symptoms vanished. No relapse was found in the follow-up visit for half a year.

Explanation Hand Taiyang and Yangming Meridian travel along the lateral aspect of the shoulder and arm. Pain and numbness will appear along the running course of these two meridians when attacked by wind and cold. Reducing Tianzong (SI 11) and Jianwaishu (SI 14) points can dispel the wind from the Hand-Taiyang Meridian and needling Jianyu (LI 15) and Quchi (LI 11) in combination may activate the circulation of qi and blood, and expel the wind. At the same time, penetrating Tiaokou (S 38) towards Chengshan (B 57) on the healthy side is a method of treating the disease in the upper part by selecting the points in the lower. Moxibustion is added locally to expel the wind and cold, and to dredge the meridians, thus pain stopped.

Case 4: Glaucoma

Name, Wang x x; sex, female; age, 51; date of the first visit, March 20, 1984.

Complaints She had temporal pain on both sides ten years ago with gradual hypopsia, occasionally, she could see the coloured circle around the light. The symptoms became aggravated in the last two years. She had blurred vision, and often saw black spots. Examination: Elevation of intraocular pressure of both eyes. Diagnosis: Glaucoma. No obvious effect was achieved after long-term treatment. In the last two weeks she had severe headache, dry and swelling pain of both eyes, and photophobia, dark red tongue, thin white coating, and deep pulse, and thready at the "chi" region.

Differentiation Deficiency of both liver and kidney, and failure of blood to nourish the eyes.

Principle of treatment Nourish the liver and kidney to improve the eyesight and relieve the pain.

Prescription Ganshu (B 18), Shenshu (B 23), Fengchi (B 20), Taiyang (Extra 2), Jingming (B 1), Hegu (LI 4) and Sanyinjiao (Sp 6).

Treatment procedure Remarkable alleviation was achieved for the headache and other symptoms after six treatments. The intraocular pressure of both eyes was found normal in reexamination. Six more treatments were given to consolidate the therapeutic effects. No relapse was noticed in the follow-up visit for half a year.

Explanation Blurred vision is the disease of the Foot-Shaoyin and Foot-Jueyin Meridians. The eyes are the openings of the liver, and the kidney essence goes upward to nourish the eyes. The deficiency of the kidney essence and insufficiency of blood in the liver will cause yin deficiency of liver and kidney and exhaustion of the essence and blood. Since the essence and qi fail to ascend to nourish the eyes, the short nourishment of the eyes brings about dry eyes and blurred vision. Therefore, the disease lies in the Liver and Kidney Meridians. Reinforcing of Ganshu (B 18) and Shenshu (B 23) can treat the root cause, while reducing Fengchi (B 20) and Taiyang (Extra) can expel the wind and relieve the pain. Being a crossing point of the Hand and Foot-Taiyang, and Yangming and Yinqiao and Yangqiao Meridians, Jingming (B 1) has the function to dredge the meridian, improve the vision and stop the pain, and is an essential point in treating glaucoma. Reinforcing Hegu (LI 4) and Sanyinjiao (Sp 6) with crossing method is not only able to supplement the qi and nourish the blood, but also to dredge the meridians and collaterals. Thus the pain is relieved and the visual acuity restored.

Case 5: Migraine

Name, Chen x x; sex, female; age, 35; date of the first visit, April 12, 1984.

Complaints She began to have left migraine ten years before because of great anger. The pain was intermittent and attacked after overwork or emotional stress. In the last two weeks, the headache attacked more frequently and more severe at night, especially at the parietal and left temporal region, accompanied by dizziness, vertigo, nausea and vomiting. No response was found by medication of analgesics. The tongue tip was red, the coating was thin and yellow, the pulse was string-taut and rapid.

Differentiation Upward disturbance by wind-heat.

Principle of treatment Expel the wind, reduce the heat and kill the pain.

Prescription Fengchi (B 20), Baihui (Du 20), Taiyang (Extra 2), Shuaigu (B 8) and Taichong (Liv 3).

Treatment procedure The headache was diminished after one treatment with the reducing method on the above mentioned points. The pain at night stopped and the other symptoms were alleviated after three treatments. Only slight distension of the head and lassitude remained. The needling was stopped after five treatments. No relapse was noticed in the follow-up visit after one year.

Explanation The disease is caused by the wind-heat of the liver and gallbladder, which goes upward along the meridian to disturb the head. The derangement of qi and blood leads to obstruction of the meridians and collaterals. The Liver and Gallbladder Meridians are obstructed at midnight, so the pain is exaggerated at that time. Reducing of Baihui (Du 20) and Fengchi (B 20) can clear the wind-heat and remove the stagnation of qi from the liver and gallbladder. The combination of Taiyang (Extra) with Shuaigu (B 8) can clear the heat, diminish the wind and check pain. Reducing the opposite Taichong can pacify the liver, dispel the wind, and induce the heat to go downward. It is a method to treat the disease in the upper part by selecting the points in the lower.

ADVOCATING ACUPUNCTURE TREATMENT BASED ON DIFFERENTIATION OF SYNDROMES ACCORDING TO THE THEORY OF JINGJIN AND EMPHASIS ON THE RESEARCH OF NEEDLING TECHNIQUE

—Dr. Guan Jiduo's Clinical Experience

Guan Jiduo was born in Liaoyang, Liaoning Province in 1916. In 1932, he entered the Tianjin School of Chinese Medicine and followed Mr. Chen Zedong, a famous doctor in Tianjin. Two years later he entered the Huabei College of Chinese Medicine in Beijing where he learned acupuncture from Dr. Wu Caiyi for two years. In 1937, he moved to Chengdu and practised medicine there, adopting the combination of acupuncture and herbal medicine, and came to be known with his excellent acupuncture treatment. In 1957, he was transferred to the Chengdu College of Traditional Chinese Medicine to work as a teacher. He has carefully performed the textual research on acupoints, advocating the reinforcing and reducing technique based on differentiation according to Jingjin (muscle regions along the twelve regular meridians). He is good at treating various pain syndromes by using finger acupuncture therapy. During the last thirteen years he has treated over fifteen hundred cases of epilepsy with the combination of acupuncture and herbal medicine, the effective rate of which reached 83 percent. He designed and created nonsmoking moxa sticks, which have raised the therapeutic effect of the original moxa sticks and eliminated the smoke and ash. He helped compile *Acupuncture* and *Acupuncture Points*. He is now a professor of the Acupuncture Teaching and Research Group of the Chengdu College of Traditional Chinese Medicine.

I. Academic Characteristics and Medical Specialities

1. Treatment based on differentiation of syndromes according to the theory of Jingjin

Dr. Guan considers that acupuncture is a kind of external treatment. In addition to the treatments of zang-fu disorders which are based on the differentiation of syndromes according to the theory of zang-fu, all the pathological changes of the trunk and limbs should be treated by differentiating syndromes according to the theory of Jingjin. The muscle regions along the twelve regular meridians are the important component of the meridian system. Their distributions follow those of the twelve regular meridians and they are nourished by the qi and blood from the meridians. However, Jingjin and Meridians have different functions. Jingjin involves muscles, tendons, ligaments, and fasciae, etc. which link the bones dominating movement of the body. Therefore, they are mainly distributed in the four limbs, joints and trunk, but not pertaining to the internal organs. They meet and connect with each other at the joints and the places where muscles are thick. When the function of Jingjin is normal, the muscles and tendons are forceful and they flex and extend freely, otherwise, the muscles and tendons will be diseased, leading to dysfunction of joints and giving rise to spasm, convulsion or flaccidity. The manifestations of Jingjin diseases are actually the symptom complex of the muscular tissues along the twelve regular meridians. In clinic, most of the pathological changes of the muscles, nerves, joints and ligaments such as shoulder pain, facial spasm, sciatica, prolapse of eyelids, facial paralysis, and bi syndrome, fall within the aspect of Jingjin disease.

1) *Differentiation of syndromes according to the theory of Jingjin* The Jingjin of the twelve regular meridians have their own running courses and distributions, and physiological functions. Once they are changed pathologically, there will appear specific diseases, which are generally characterized by such manifestations as spasm of gastrocnemius muscle, convulsion, flaccidity, pain, and palpable mass in the area of the distributions. The pathological changes are nothing more than spasm and flaccidity. Spasm pertains to cold and flaccidity to heat. Their manifestations are as mentioned in the book of *Plain Questions*: "Cold syndrome of Jingjin gives rise to spasm of the tendons and pain of the bones, while heat syndrome of Jingjin leads to flaccidity of the tendons and weakness of the bone." Based on the affected areas, there are spasms of the yang Jingjin and that of the yin Jingjin. The book *Miraculous Pivot* states, "Yang spasm gives rise to opisthotonus and yin spasm to folded body with difficulty to extend." The spasm of the muscle regions distributed on the yin aspect is known as yin spasm and that of the muscle regions distributed on the yang aspect as yang spasm. In addition, it also needs to inspect the diseased area to determine to which meridian it belongs. Generally, differentiation of syndromes according to Jingjin lays emphasis on differentiating spasm or flaccidity and yin or yang. When the eye is diseased, "spasm leads to difficulty in closing the eye and heat leads to flaccidity which makes the eye fail to open." When the lumbus is diseased, "yang disease leads to opisthotonos and yin disease leads to difficulty in extending the body." In August, 1982, there was a middle-aged female patient who suffered from chest pain for seven days. The pain was aggravated by movement, breathing and swallowing. The Western diagnosis was esophagitis. Examination: The chest was flat and two sides symmetrical. The skin colour was normal and she had no history of traumatic injury. Palpation found a slip-like subcutaneous node with obvious tenderness which radiated to the hypochondriac region, axillary fold and elbow. Therefore it was a disorder of Jingjin. According to the theory of Jingjin, the muscle region along the Pericardium Meridian "gathers at the medial aspect of the elbow joints. It goes upward along the medial aspect of the upper arm and again gathers at the axillary fold. Its branch enters the axillary fold, distributes on the chest and gathers at the shoulder." (From the chapter Jingjin of *Plain Questions*). Along the affected area, there appeared spasm of the muscle and anteriorly it affected the chest and caused chest pain. Neiguan (P 6) was therefore selected to eliminate the pain caused by spasm. A filiform needle was used obliquely towards the shoulder. Five minutes after insertion the needle was manipulated for one minute and at the same time Ashi point on the chest was pressed. The pain was immediately alleviated and the chest relaxed. The needle was retained for thirty minutes. After three treatments the chest pain was controlled.

2) *Treatment based on differentiation of Jingjin* The muscle regions not only exactly follow the running courses of the twelve regular meridians, but also reach the area where the twelve regular meridians do not reach. For example, the Bladder Meridian of Foot-Taiyang doesn't reach the shoulder region while one branch of the corresponding muscle region does and accumulates at Jianyu (LI 15). In addition, Jingjin distributes crisscross at ankle, elbow, wrist, thigh, poplitea, gluteus and shoulder, etc. Pathological changes in these areas directly relate to the muscle regions and hence are treated based on differentiation according to the theory of Jingjin with especially good results. As mentioned in the book *Plain Questions*, "When the muscle is diseased, it should be adjusted, and treatment should be given to the diseased area." When treating diseases of Jingjin, the method that takes the painful spots as the points combined with meridian points is mainly adopted. Diseases of Jingjin are mostly due to invasion of exogenous pathogenic wind, cold and damp, or stagnation of qi and blood caused by traumatic injury, giving rise to swelling, pain and contraction of muscles along the meridian which indicate the stagnation of qi and blood, obstruction of the meridian and malnourishment of the muscles along the meridian. The emphasis of treatment is therefore on regulating the contraction or flaccidity, yin and yang, so as to remain the integral balance. The main therapeutic method is to tap the diseased area with a cutaneous needle. In May, 1986, there was a male patient suffering from wandering redness, swelling and hot pain of joints on the four extremities with dysfunction of flexion and extension. Since the disease was located in Jingjin, Ashi points were selected and tapped to cause bleeding with cutaneous needles. The swelling and pain were eliminated after three treatments and the patient was cured. It is rigid to simply use the fire needle with the selection of painful spot as therapeutic point for the disorders of Jingjin, as its indications are limited. The book *Miraculous Pivot* therefore points out, "Fire needling is used for cold syndromes." According to the theory of meridians and collaterals, the muscle regions of the twelve regular meridians are distributed and nourished by the qi and blood of these meridians. The meridians are distributed among the muscle regions. The two systems are related to and complement each other. Therefore the points of the meridians are indicated in the diseases of the muscle regions along the meridians. Besides, filiform needling also has the function to adjust the functions of the muscle regions.

3) *Success on treating various diseases according to the differentiation of Jingjin*

a. Shoulder disorders: Shoulder joints are the places where the muscle regions of the three yin and yang meridians of hand and those of part foot meridians accumulate. The disorders of the shoulder are characterized by dysfunction of the joints in movement and pain, such as frozen shoulder, the shoulder pain caused by degeneration of cervical vertebra, bi syndrome, etc. Such local points as Jianyu (LI 15), Tianzong (SI 11), and Jianzhen (SI 9) should be selected to adjust the tendons and arrest pain. In addition, we can also select Houxi (SI 3) from the Meridian of Hand-Taiyang and Waiguan (SJ 5) from the Meridian of Hand-Shaoyang in combination. Since the muscle region of Hand-Taiyang runs upward through the shoulder and neck, and that of Hand-Shaoyang accumulates in the shoulder, all joining the Meridian of Hand-Taiyang, the selection of points from both may strengthen the therapeutic effect. In treating diseases of Jingjin, the key is to select the points near the joints, such as Quchi (LI 11) from the Meridian of Hand-Yangming, Liangqiu (S 34) from the Meridian of Foot-Yangming and the Influential Point of the tendons Yanglingquan (G 34), all which have good therapeutic effects for disorders of the shoulder joints. Particularly, ask the patient to raise, abduct and dosiflex the arm fifty times when needling Yanglingquan (G 34) and this mostly obtains immediate effect. The synchronisity of needling and movement may activate circulation of qi and blood, relax the tendons and remove the obstructions from the meridians. In May 1986, there was an elderly patient who had suffered from right shoulder pain with limitation of movement for two months. Examination: Normal appearance of the right shoulder, pain radiating to the anterior aspect of the shoulder during joint movement; elevation 180°, abduction 70° and dosiflexion touching the sacral region only. Diagnosis: Frozen shoulder. Since the case was characterized by dysfunction of the shoulder in movement and pain, the disease was located in the muscle regions and treatment should be given according to the differentiation of Jingjin. Yanglingquan (G 34) was needled first and the patient was advised to have some movement of the shoulder joint in elevation, abduction and dosiflexion fifty times each. Then Jianyu (LI 15), Jianneiling (Extra) and Jianzhen (SI 9) were needled with even method and the pain was immediately alleviated and the amplitude of the shoulder joint movement enlarged. The patient was cured after six treatments.

b. Diseases of the face: The muscle regions of the three yang meridians of foot go upward to meet at the cheek, the area beside the nose around the zygoma. In such cases as facial paralysis, facial spasm, it is very important to select points to regulate the tendons and muscles so as to restore the functions of the muscles and nerves. When treating such diseases, therefore, local points are mainly selected, Quanliao (SI 18) in particular, and distal points along the meridians in combination such as the points from the three yang meridians of the foot Zusanli (S 36), Yanglingquan (G 34) and Xuanzhong (G 39). Prolapse of the eyelids is commonly seen in the clinic. The upper and lower eyelids are covered by Taiyang and Yangming Meridians. The book *Miraculous Pivot* says, "Taiyang Meridian covers the upper eyelid and Yangming Meridian covers the lower eyelid." The book *Internal Classic* also states, "The eyelids dominate the eye and eyelash, and govern the opening and closing of the eye." When the eyelids are diseased, the muscle regions following the Taiyang and Yangming Meridians must be dealt with. In July of 1986, there was a female patient who had suffered from left facial spasm for over a year. The left facial muscle continuously had a tic and the left canthus and mouth angle in particular. She had blurred vision of the left eye and unclear speech. She was treated with various methods but with little effect. Diagnosis: facial spasm. This disease was characterized by spasm of the muscle, it is therefore the spasm of Jingjin. The face is the area where the muscle regions of the three yang meridians meet, Quanliao (SI 18) on the face was first selected, which not only has the therapeutic function of the local area, but also has the regulatory function to the adjacent area. Then Zanzhu (B 2), Tongziliao (G 1), Shuaigu (G 8) and Sizhukong (SJ 23) were selected to regulate the muscle regions along the Taiyang and Yangming Meridians and alleviate the spasm. The points were punctured with even method and the needles were retained for thirty minutes. Treatment was given once a day and twelve treatments were taken as a course. The patient received three courses of treatment which made the attacks sparse. Each attack shortened in duration, vision and speech were clear.

c. Diseases of the neck: The neck is also the area where the tendons and muscles meet. Rigidity, pain and dysfunction in movement of the neck are all pathological changes of Jingjin. The muscle regions of the three yang meridians of the hand and foot go upward to meet at the neck. Therefore, selection of Shousanli (LI 10), Waiguan (SJ 5), Jianyu (LI 15) and Jianjing (G 21) of the three yang meridians of Hand, and Yanglingquan (G 34) and Xuanzhong (G 39) of the three yang meridians of foot may obtain a good therapeutic result. In June of 1986, there was a male patient who suffered a lot from rigidity and pain of the neck which affected the movement in the left and right turn. Shousanli (LI 10) was needled first with the movement of the neck in left and right turn for one minute, and then local points Fengchi (G 20) and Jianjing (G 21) were punctured with even method. The needles were retained for thirty minutes. Three treatments cured the patient.

d. Diseases of the lumbus and legs: The muscle regions of the three Yang Meridians of Foot run along the legs and lumbus, and those of the three Yin Meridians of Foot run along the medial aspect of the legs, and pubic and abdominal regions. When treating the diseases of the lumbus and legs, local points and Ciliao (B 32), Huantiao (B 30), Zusanli (S 36) and Yanglingquan (G 34) are mostly selected to stimulate the muscles and tendons so as to alleviate spasm and arrest pain. Filiform needles are applied with an even method. Needles are retained for thirty minutes.

2. The importance of research on the various related therapeutic methods

1) *Direction of insertion and the propagated sensation along the meridians* The needling direction usually indicates the direction of the propagated sensation along the meridian. It is the key point of treatment to guide the qi to the affected area after qi arrives. The direction of insertion, therefore, should be determined according to the location of the disease and the points selected. The needles should be inserted directing the affected area, otherwise, the therapeutic result would be poor. Dr. Guan punctures Fengchi (G 20) with four different directions respectively for different headaches. In case of Yangming headache, the needle is inserted into the point a little obliquely upward towards the eyeball on the same side; in the case of Jueyin headache, the needle is inserted a little obliquely upward towards the midline of the scalp; in case of Shaoyang headache, the needle is inserted obliquely towards the outer canthus of the eye on the same side; and, in case of Taiyang headache in which the head and neck are rigid and painful, the needle on each side is inserted horizontally towards the other. With proper application of the four methods, a marked effect can be expected in treating various kinds of headache. The needle is inserted 0.5 to 0.8 cun. It is advisable to rotate the needle gently, avoiding rough lifting and thrusting. In the spring of 1978, there was a female patient suffering from prolapse of the eyelids for two years. General lassitude and difficulty in opening of the eyes first appeared after catching cold. The condition became so bad one year later that she could only open her eyes a little. West diagnosis: Neurosis. Differentiation: Deficiency of both qi and yin. Qiaoyin (G 11) was needled obliquely upward with the depth of 0.5 cun. When the qi arrived the needle was rotated to guide

the qi to the affected area. When the qi reached the forehead, the left eye opened suddenly normally. The point on the right side was punctured by another doctor, there was no propagation after the qi arrived, the eye still could not open. Then the needling direction was adjusted and rotation was done to guide the qi towards the affected area. Both eyes opened at once.

2) *The close relation between depth of insertion and therapeutic effect* a: Location and nature of a disease determine the depth of insertion. Dr. Guan emphasizes the depth of insertion since the muscle regions could be either thin or thick. When a disease is deeply located, points should be punctured deeply, and vice versa. The patient will be possibly injured due to carelessness. b: Body build and age determine the depth of insertion. Shallow insertion is advisable for the elderly, weak and children, while deep insertion is advisable to the strong patient with ample qi and blood. Besides, shallow insertion is suitable for the emaciated patients and those who are sensitive to acupuncture, and deep insertion for the patients with a big body build and sluggish response to acupuncture.

3) *Retention of needles and therapeutic effect* Dr. Guan considers that various motions of matters in the universe are fulfilled in certain period of time. The treatment of disease is therefore closely related to the time as well. a. Time for retention of needles: The time for the needles retained in the points is mainly related to the intensity of stimulation. Dr. Guan considers that, for pain syndromes, needles are usually retained for thirty minutes, or even one or two hours. For some deficiency or heat syndromes, needles are retained for short, generally one or two minutes. b. Acupuncture time: Points should be selected according to the periodic changes of zang-fu, meridians and collaterals, and qi and blood—Midnight-noon Ebb-flow (Ziwuliuzhu). Points may also be selected according to the time of attacks. For some diseases such as malaria, Yangming headache and Yangming afternoon fever with regular attacks at certain time. Dr. Guan mostly gives treatment one or two hours prior to the attack. In May of 1986, there was a male patient suffering from frontal headache which became worse in the afternoon. Each attack lasted for two hours and subsided spontaneously. Treatment was given one hour before the attack with selections of Fengchi (G 20), Hegu (LI 4), Zanzhu (G 2) and Shuaigu (B 8). Fengchi (G 20) was punctured with the needle slightly oblique towards the eyeball on the same side. The other points were all punctured with the needles towards the affected area. Needles were retained for one hour and the pain was markedly alleviated. The case was cured after three courses of treatments.

4) *Combination of acupuncture and herbal medicine* Dr. Guan holds that acupuncture and herbal medicine have the same theoretical foundation. He has therefore taken the combination of acupuncture and herbal medicine to treat epilepsy and achieved comparatively good results. He considers that epilepsy is caused by phlegm, fire, fright and fear, and is mostly related to the Meridian of Foot-Shaoyin, Du Meridian and Yangqiao and Yinqiao Meridians. The book *Miraculous Pivot* says, "When the muscle regions along the Meridian of Foot-Shaoyin are diseased, epilepsy and convulsion may result." The advisable points are Baihui (Du 20), Dazhui (Du 14), Zhaohai (K 6), Taodao (Du 13), Yaoqi (Extra 20) and Shenmen (H 7). The general effective rate (of the fifteen hundred cases treated) was 83 percent.

II. Case Analysis

Case 1: Frozen shoulder

Name, Hu x x; age, 61; date of the first visit, September 5, 1986.

Complaints He had suffered from soreness and pain of the left shoulder with limitation of movement for more than two months. Examination: Normal appearance of the left shoulder, apparent tenderness at Tianzong (SI 11) and referring pain on the anterior aspect of the shoulder and upper arm during movement. Amplitude of the movement of the left arm: Elevation 180°, abduction 70° and dosiflexion touching the sacral region. The disease was located in Jingjin and treatment was given according to the differentiation of Jingjin.

Prescription Liangqiu (S 34), Yanglingquan (G 34).

Treatment procedure The points were punctured with even method. Needles were retained for thirty minutes. Treatment was given once every other day and twelve treatments were taken as a course. Yanglingquan (G 34) is the influential point of the tendons, which can regulate the muscle regions along the twelve regular meridians. Liangqiu (S 34) is a point of the Stomach Meridian of Foot-Yangming with which Shaoyang and Taiyang Meridians are all connected. The muscle regions of this meridian goes upward to the neck and winds around the shoulder. Therefore Yanglingquan (G 34) of this meridian has distal therapeutic function to the shoulder. The pain was immediately alleviated right after it was needled and the movement was markedly improved. After one course of treatment, the pain basically disappeared and the movement of the shoulder joints was markedly improved with normal elevation, abduction and dosiflexion.

Case 2: Facial spasm

Name, Chen x x; age, 54; date of the first visit, September, 1986.

Complaints She had suffered a lot from persistent twitching of the facial muscle, the left canthus and mouth angle in particular, which disturbed the vision and speech. She had received different kinds of treatment with no apparent effect and finally came to our department.

Differentiation Pathological changes of muscle regions along the meridian.

Prescription Quanliao (SI 18), Tongziliao (G 15), Shuaigu (G 8), Sizhukong (SJ 23).

Treatment procedure The face is the area where the three yin meridians of the foot meet. Quanliao (SI 18) was first selected, which not only has the therapeutic function to the local area, but also regulates the adjacent muscle regions of the three meridians. Therefore it functions very well for the disease of the facial muscle. "Taiyang Meridian dominates the upper eyelid and Yangming Meridian dominates the lower eyelid." Selection of Zanzhu (B 2), Tongziliao (G 1), Shuaigu (G 8) and Sizhukong (SJ 23) may regulate the muscle regions of the Taiyang and Yangming Meridians to alleviate the twitching. Filiform needling was applied with even method. Needles were retained for thirty minutes after the qi arrived. Treatment was given once a day or every other day. Twelve treatments were taken as a course. After three courses of treatment, the attacks dispersed and the duration of each attack shortened. The patient had no difficulty to speak and see objects, sometimes as normal as a healthy person.

Case 3: Bi syndrome (sciatica)

Name, Feng x x; age, 59; date of the first visit, September 1, 1986.

Complaints The patient had a pulling pain on the right leg, which was aggravated by movement and a little alleviated with the lower extremities flexed. Examination: Tenderness on the gluteal fold, popliteal fossa and malleous. Test with the leg raising straight: (+).

Diagnosis Sciatica. The disease was located in the muscle regions. Treatment should be given according to the differentiation of Jingjin.

Prescription Ciliao (B 32), Huantiao (G 30), Zusanli (S 36), and Yanglingquan (G 34). Filiform needling was applied with even method and the needles were retained for thirty minutes. Treatment was given once a day and after two months the symptoms were greatly alleviated and the pulling pain disappeared with the remaining of slight tenderness only. Walk and other movement became free.

Case 4: Hiccup (spasm of diaphragm)

Name, Feng x x; age, 61; date of the first visit, March 28, 1986.

Complaints He first suffered from hiccup after eating eggs when he was hospitalized due to hypertension seven years ago. The application of diazepam and the calyx and receptacle of persimmon didn't stop the persistent hiccup. It stopped spontaneously two weeks later. However, it had attacked intermittently since then with the frequency of once every four or five days and each attack lasted for one to three days. After being treated with various methods, no apparent effect was obtained. It became worse half a year ago with frequent attacks day and night and each attack lasting from four to six days with an interval of one or two days between attacks. It is known in TCM as hiccup, which is mostly caused by rebellious qi. The essence of this disease is spasm of the diaphragm which pertains to Jingjin. Therefore, treatment should be given according to the differentiation of Jingjin.

Prescription Neiguan (P 6), Tanzhong (Ren 17).

Treatment procedure Filiform needling was applied with the needles retained for thirty minutes after qi arrived. Treatment was given once a day and twelve treatments were taken as a course. The duration of each attack was obviously shortened after the first course of treatment and the hiccup stopped after three courses. No more attacks occurred during the follow-up visit for three weeks.

Case 5: Headache

Name, Deng x x; age, 30; date of the first visit, May 19, 1986.

Complaints The patient had the first attack of right temporal headache which referred to the whole right side and front of the head without the obvious inducing factor seven years ago. The pain was alleviated by the intake of analgesic tablets. Since then, it had attacked every afternoon with the symptoms not alleviated after the application of the tablets and Tianma (Rhizoma Gastrodiae) Injection. It was worse during the period between January and June. Since May of 1986, it attacked from 3 to 4 o'clock every afternoon with such manifestations as severe intolerable headache, distending pain in the orbital frame and lacrimation. The patient was examined in the Five Sense Organs Department and Ophthalmological Department of our hospital and no abnormal changes were found. It was considered as the disease of Jingjin, and must be treated according to differentiation of Jingjin.

Prescription Fengchi (G 20), Shuaigu (G 8), Zanzhu (B 2), Yangbai (G 14).

Treatment procedure Fengchi (G 20) and Shuaigu (G 8) of Shaoyang Meridian were first selected to regulate tendons and arrest pain. Zanzhu (B 2) was needled to eliminate distention in the eye and lacrimation. The local point Yangbai (G 14) was tapped with a plum-blossom needle to cause slight bleeding so as to remove stagnation. It is also an effective method for treating diseases of Jingjin. The other points were all punctured with even method. The needles were retained for one hour after qi arrived. Treatment was given once a day and twelve treatments were taken as a course. The headache was basically eliminated after treatment for over a month.

FINGER PRESSURE AND WARM REINFORCEMENT

—Xu Shiqian's Clinical Experience

Xu Shiqian was born in Shexian County, Hebei Province, in 1921. He learned traditional Chinese medicine from his father when he was young. In 1964, he studied at the Shanxi-Hebei-Shandong-Henan Border Region Health School, where he learned acupuncture from a famous acupuncturist, Zhu Lian. From 1960 to 1962, he attended the "Course of Traditional Chinese Medicine for Western Medical Doctors" in Beijing College of Traditional Chinese Medicine. At the end of 1962, he was appointed as the deputy director of the Acupuncture Department of Friendship Hospital in the People's Republic of Mongolia. He directed the research on "Clinical Observation of the Therapeutic Effects on Fifty Cases of Coronary Heart Disease Treated by Acupuncture, and the Observation of the Difference of Main Acupoints for Treating Coronary Heart Disease," "Clinical Observation of the Therapeutic Effects on Fifty-one Cases of Cardiovascular Diseases and Hyperlipoidemia Treated by Acupuncture," "Observation of the Influence on the Left Heart Function in 106 Normal Subjects and A Hundred Heart Disease Patients After the Needling of Hegu Point." Now he is an associate professor and director of the Nanning Institute of Acupuncture and Moxibustion, Guangxi Zhuang Nationality Autonomous Regions, the member of Chinese Acupuncture Association, and the member of the standing committee of the Guangxi Branch of Chinese Association of Traditional Chinese Medicine.

I. Academic Characteristics and Medical Specialities

1. Multiple use of one point

In selecting the point, Dr. Xu adopted the principle of less but effective points. In addition to the commonly used penetrating points such as Waiguan (SJ 5) penetrating towards Neiguan (P 6), Zhigou (SJ 6) towards Jianshi (P 5), Quchi (LI 11) towards Shaohai (H 3), Yinlingquan (Sp 9) towards Yanglingquan (B 34), Jiache (S 6) towards Dicang (S 4), he also put forward using one point for multiple purposes.

1) *Needling Futu (LI 18) point* Dr. Xu treats such diseases as humeroscapularis periarthritis, shoulder and back pain, and chest pain by adjusting the needling direction. For example, the needle tip directs to the cervical vertebra to radiate the needling sensation to the fingers in case of humeroscapularis periarthritis and shoulder-arm pain; the tip directs slightly to the posterior neck to radiate the needling sensation to the back in case of shoulder and back pain; the needle is penetrated to the anterior part of the neck, and the needling sensation is referred to the thoracic region in case of chest pain.

2) *Needling Jianjing (G 21) point* For treating pain of the neck, shoulder chest, and back as well as mastitis, its therapeutic action is also carried out through the control of

the needling sensation or through the direction of the propagated sensation.

3) *Needling Guanyuan (Ren 4) or Zhongji (Ren 3) point* The gastrointestinal and urogenital diseases can also be treated by controlling the direction of the propagated sensation. For example, a patient with endometriosis was found to have a mass of 4.7 x 3.0 cm at the place close to the urethra at the cervix and the public symphysis in B ultrasonic wave examination. She suffered pain before and after menstruation, which failed to be relieved by analgesics. However, the pain was immediately relieved after Zhongji (Ren 3) point was needled by directing the needling sensation to the painful region through Henggu (K 11) point.

2. Selecting points by finger pressure method

In 1947, when he was working at Shanxi-Hebei-Shandong-Henan Border Region Hospital, there was a female patient in the hospital who had frequent hysterical attacks. Before each attack, her tongue would contract backward and failed to protrude out. Dr. Xu stopped the attack effectively by pressing his fingers on Baihui (Du 20) and Fengfu (Du 16) points when the patient had a premonition, and Dr. Xu cured this case later by needling Baihui (Du 20) and Fengfu (Du 16). In another case, an artist who suffered from a facial spasm on the right side, could not work because his vision affected by the spasm. Dr. Xu found that the left Quanliao (SI 18) was an effective point. Later on, whenever the spasm on the left side occurred, the patient was told to press the left Quanliao (SI 18) himself and then he could go on with his work. Dr. Xu would select the points by using the finger pressing method to treat acute pain or some evident signs.

3. The simplified warm reinforcing method

Warm reinforcing manipulation is often used for cold syndrome. That is to say, the needle is inserted progressively, slowly and with pressure. When the patient had a distension, the needle should be twisted to increase the distension (the needle can be turned clockwise or counterclockwise). Most patients will feel a warm sensation after a few seconds. For example, Dr. Xu cured a female patient who had suffered from vegetative nerve disturbance, accompanied with fear of cold and aversion to wind. She had to wear thick clothes in the summer when the room temperature was 36°C. A thick cotton-padded quilt had to be used to cover her during the acupuncture treatment. She felt warm over the whole body, took off all the thick clothes and removed the quilt after the warm reinforcing method was applied at Zusanli (S 36) and Waiguan (SJ 5).

4. Observation of "qi reaching the diseased area" in needling Neiguan (P 6)

In general, many acupuncturists are thinking that "qi reaching the affected area" means the needling sensation should transmit to the diseased area. However, the propagated sensation along the meridian includes recessive propagation. Sometimes though the needling sensation is not transmitted to the diseased area, it does not mean that "qi has not reached the affected area." The "multiple use of one point" is a method to direct "the needling sensation to reach to the diseased area." Dr. Xu considered that for certain diseases, so long as qi arrives, the symptoms can be relieved, so it is not necessary to have the needling sensation reach the diseased area. Otherwise, the intensity of stimulation has to be increased which may influence the therapeutic effects. With a cardiomyograph with electro-physiological recorder, Dr. Xu has found that the contractive function of the left heart was improved no matter whether the needling sensation was transmitted to the diseased area or not. Altogether ninety-eight patients were observed, among them, if the needling sensation reached above the elbow and to the precardial area, it is regarded as "qi reaching the affected area," and "qi not reaching the affected area" if the sensation is only transmitted to the palm or fingers. Both groups had some improvement in the changes of the cardiomyography after the needling. The difference is not significant. On the contrary, the cardiac function of some individuals didn't show any improvement when the qi was forced to reach the affected area.

II. Case Analysis

Case 1: Aphasia (sequelae of encephalitis B)

Name, Zhu x x; sex, male; age, 10; date of the first visit, February, 1977.

Complaints The patient suffered from encephalitis B in August, 1976. He had fever, convulsions and coma, and remained aphasia and mentally retarded after first aid treatment in the local hospital. No improvement had been revealed after numerous treatments. Examination: Aphasia, restlessness, mental retardation, red tongue, thin white coating and a little rapid pulse. No positive findings had been found on examination.

Differentiation Heat attacking the mind.

Principle of treatment Regulate the spirit and benefit the mental function.

Prescription Baihui (Du 20), Renzhong (Du 26) and Hegu (LI 4).

Treatment procedure He could mimic the speech of an adult after the first treatment when the above-mentioned points were needled. The needles were retained for twenty minutes. He could reply to simple questions after the second treatment, but couldn't speak freely. After ten treatments (the needling was given every other day) with the same method, his speech was completely recovered.

Explanation In this case, instead of stimulation, inhibition method was adopted (even reinforcing and even reducing) because of irritability. The brain is regarded as the room of the spirit in traditional Chinese medicine. Baihui (Du 20) and Renzhong (Du 26) all belong to the Du Meridian, which goes through the brain. So these two points have the function of "regulating the spirit and benefiting the mental power." Hegu (LI 4) is the Yuan-Source point of the Large Intestine Meridian of Hand-Yangming. These meridians curve around the mouth and cross at Renzhong. According to the principle of "where the meridians pass through, the disease there will be cured," the satisfactory results are obtained in the combination of these three points.

Case 2: Convulsion (sequelae of concussion of brain)

Name, Zeng x x; sex, male; age, 14; date of the first visit, March 12, 1975.

Complaints He was beaten on his head and the right side of the neck on March 4, 1975, and then he lost consciousness for two hours. He was admitted to the hospital because of repeated convulsions and speech disturbance. He suffered from vague headache and repeated convulsions. He couldn't speak during the convulsions and had difficulty walking. Examination: Clear mind, general condition normal, convulsions every few minutes, speech not fluent, no motor disturbance and normal patella tendon reflex. Differentiation: Fright invading the mental activity. The principle of treatment was to tranquilize and ease the mind.

Prescription Renzhong (Du 26) and Chenjiang (Ren 24).

Treatment procedure The above-mentioned two points were needled as soon as the patient was admitted and the needles were retained for one and a half hours. After the needling, the convulsion was stopped, and he could speak fluently. He had no convulsion at night, but his sleep was not sound because of the headache. Again these two points were needled. The needles were retained for two and a half hours, and Zusanli (S 36) was needled with the inhibition method before the patient went to bed. On the third day, he had a sound sleep and the headache was alleviated. He could take a walk in the garden. According to the above prescription, the needles were retained for three hours in the evening, and the symptoms completely disappeared on the fifth day and the patient was discharged. No relapse was found in the follow-up visit a month later.

Case 3: Costalgia (biliary ascariasis)

Name, Yue x x; sex, male; age, 34; date of the first visit, August 1985.

Complaints The patient had right epigastric cholic pain last night and no response was found after injection of atropine. Examination: Lassitude, yellow complexion, right epigastric cholic pain, slight red tongue proper, white yellow thick coating, string-taut pulse, tenderness at the biliary area of the abdomen, Murphy's sign positive, and tenderness at the right Gaohuang (B 34) point on the back. Stool test: Ova (+++). Differentiation: Disturbance of the middle jiao by worms. The principle of treatment was to soothe the liver and gallbladder, and to dispel the ascariasis to check pain.

Prescription Gaohuang (B 34) penetrating towards Geguan (B 46) on the right side.

Treatment procedure A filiform needle gauge No. 32 was inserted from Gaohuang (B 34) point horizontally along the subcutaneous tissue to Geguan (B 46) point. The pain was stopped three minutes after the needling. The needle was retained for one hour and he was cured only by one treatment.

Explanation Gaohuang (B 43) and Geguan (B 46) are both pertaining to the Bladder Meridian. As the liver and gallbladder are all situated at the right epigastric region, the points on the right side are selected based on the principle of "when the illness situates in the front, the points on the back should be chosen." Right back points are often selected by Dr. Xu for biliary diseases, and good effects are often achieved.

Case 4: Apoplexy (cerebral vascular spasm)

Name, Liu x x; sex, female; age, 86; date of the first visit, June 15, 1964.

Complaints She had headache, dizziness and weakness of the right extremities in the last ten days. She had sudden right hemiplegia in the morning before she came to the doctor, accompanied by lassitude, pallor, white thick sticky tongue coating and string-taut pulse. Examination: Clear consciousness, clear speech, free of tongue deviation, heart, lung, liver and spleen normal, blood pressure 170/100 mmHg, cranial nerve examination normal, the muscle strength of the right upper and lower limbs grade II, and the muscle tonicity poor, the right biceps, triceps and pattelar tendon reflex, byeractive, Hoffmann sign (+), Babinski sign on the right side (+). Differentiation: Obstruction of qi and blood leading to short nourishment of the meridians and vessels. The principle of treatment is to dredge the meridians and activate the blood circulation.

Prescription Zusanli (S 36) bilaterally, Quchi (LI 11) bilaterally.

Treatment procedure The blood pressure was lowered down to 150/90 mmHg after the needling. The right limbs could move with the muscle strength of grade IV. She could walk on crutches the next day. She recovered after the above points were needled again. No relapse was found in the follow-up visit ten days later.

Case 5: Fever and vomiting (cold of epidemic gastro-intestinal cold)

Name, Li x x; sex, male; age, 39; date of the first visit, March 25, 1963.

Complaints He felt general discomfort for two days and the symptoms were worse in the afternoon. When he came to the hospital, he had aversion to cold and fever, yellow complexion without lustre, general soreness, frequent vomiting, abdominal and epigastric pain, loose stool, white thick tongue coating, and rapid pulse. Physical examination: Body temperature 39.5°C, pulse 100/min., slightly distended abdomen, and tyinpany heard during percussion. Differentiation: Wind and cold restraining the body surface and internal compressing of Yangming Meridian. The principle of the treatment is to reduce the heat and descend the perverted qi.

Prescription Jinjin (Extra 9), Yuye (Extra 10), Quze (P 3) and Weizhong (B 40).

Treatment procedure Round and sharp needles were pricked to cause bleeding on these four points. No vomiting occurred after bloodletting. The temperature dropped to 38°C and was restored to normal on the second day. All the symptoms except fatigue disappeared.

SUPPURATING MOXIBUSTION

—Yan Dingliang's Clinical Experience

Yan Dingliang, a native of Pinghu County, Zhejiang Province, was born in a famous acupuncturist family in September 1924. From 1941 to 1944, he studied in the Shanghai School of Chinese Medicine. After graduation he began his private practice following his father in Pinghu County. In 1954, he opened an acupuncture department in the Provincial Hangzhou Hospital (the former Provincial Chinese Medical Hospital). In 1958, he was transferred to undertake acupuncture education in the Medical Cadre Training School of Jiaxing District. In 1962 he was transferred to Jiaxing Second Hospital. He has compiled *Brief Introduction of Yan's Suppurating Moxibustion in Pinghu, Acupoint Selection and Application of Acupuncture Tonic Therapy, A Talk on Moxibustion, Twelve Principles of Penetrating Puncture, Reading Notes on Yang's Moxibustion* and other theses. At present he is a deputy-chief doctor of the Acupuncture Department in the Chinese Medical Hospital of Zhejiang Province and in the Hospital Affiliated to the Zhejiang College of Traditional Chinese Medicine.

I. Academic Characteristics and Medical Specialities

1. To select precise acupoints in moxibustion

Yan's family-inheritance of suppurating moxibustion has prevailed for more than a hundred years. There are strict laws regarding the time of moxibustion and location of acupoints. There are special ways to select acupoints. Because of the scar left by suppurating moxibustion, this therapy is limited to only a few points on the body and head. The standard acupoints should be located in advance: a. First of all, Baihui (Du 20) is located as a standard point on head (the central concave on top of cranium as standard, acupoints on head can be done only with three moxa cones and no more are permitted). b. Shenque (Ren 8) is taken as the standard point on chest and abdominal region. c. Dazhui (Du 14) is taken as the standard point on the back. And the other points are located analogously. Dr. Yan holds that on back Dazhui (Du 14) must be located in a sitting position with head downwards and elbows flexed. By this position the cervical vertebrae are shown. Dazhui (Du 14) is exactly below the biggest cervical vertebra. In the thoracic vertebrae, the points are just below the spinous processes. The transverse level of Jugu (LI 16) is taken as the landmark. Dazhui (Du 14) is located first and then the others are located analogically. For example, Shenzhu (Du 12) is three vertebrae below, i.e. below the third thoracic vertebra where Feishu (B 13) is 1.5 cun lateral to its Huatuojiaji (Extra). The method of localizing Feishu (B 13): Dazhui (Du 14) is localized first and then Feishu (B 13) is localized three vertebrae below and 1.5 cun lateral to

Huatuojiaji (Extra). If the left Feishu (B 13) is localized, the patient's right hand should be put across the neck in the front, and the palm should be put on the upper back, the point is just where the middle finger touches. The method of localizing Gaohuang (B 43): It is 3 cun lateral to Huatuojiaji (Extra) where the depression is four vertebrae below Dazhui (Du 14). Try to take the patient's arm backwards and then to put Yangchi (SJ 4) between Shenshu (B 23) and Zhishi (B 52) on the same side, which makes the scapula move and project. Gaohuang (B 43) is in the depression between the two ribs about 0.5 cun to 1.0 cun medioinferior to the scapular angle. It is just where there is a sensitive soreness if pressed. It is proved that in terms of its effectiveness, Gaohuang (B 43) is juxtaposed with Guanyuan (Ren 4) and Zusanli (S 36), one of the three major tonic points. It is difficult to choose the correct acupoints.

2. Treatment of asthma with acupuncture first and moxibustion afterwards

1) *Acupuncture* When asthma attacks, it is necessary to puncture first to descend qi and relieve wheezing in order to control the symptoms. These must be tenacious sputum in repeated attacks and therefore it is beneficial to disperse phlegm and remove dampness, and to promote lung qi in its dispersing function. Its prescription: a. Feishu (B 13), Dingchuan (Extra), Neiguan (P 6), Hegu (LI 4), Fenglong (S 40), Lieque (L 7) towards Taiyuan (L 9). In a prone sitting position, first Feishu (B 13) is punctured 0.1 to 0.2 inch and then the needle is inserted transversely all the way to Pohu (B 42). When Dingchuan (Extra) is penetrated and a needling sensation is obtained, the needle should be manipulated further and then be lifted to a superficial area and afterwards the needle should be inserted subcutaneously downwards along Huatuojiaji (Extra) for one inch in depth and thirty minutes' retention. In a lying position with a high pillow, Neiguan (P 6), Hegu (LI 4) and Fenglong (S 40) are punctured and retained. Lieque (L 7) is punctured to reach Taiyuan (L 9). Here Lieque (L 7) must be punctured carefully and slowly to cross Jingqu (L 8) and reach Taiyuan (L 9). The needle is retained for twenty to thirty minutes. The effectiveness can only be obtained by retaining the needle until the wheezing decreases. b. Fengmen (B 12), Dingchuan (Extra), Chize (L 5), Kongzui (L 6), Quchi (LI 11), Tanzhong (Ren 17) to Zhongting (Ren 16), Fenglong (S 40). In a prone sitting position first, Fengmen (B 12) is punctured towards Fufen (B 41). Dingchuan (Extra) is punctured as the above. And then in lying position with a high pillow, Tanzhong (Ren 17) is punctured downwards to reach Zhongting (Ren 16) and towards Jiuwei (Ren 15). Chize (L 5), Kongzui (L 6), Quchi (LI 11) and Fenglong (S 40) are punctured and retained as indicated above.

It is said in *Classics on Medical Problems* that the points on the yang side are chosen for healing diseases on the yin side and vice versa. Thereafter the Back-Shu points are often used for relieving zang problems and the Front-Mu points are used for eliminating fu diseases in both acupuncture and moxibustion. Feishu (B 13) is the main point, the prescription (b) is suitable for excess-heat syndromes, in which Fengmen (B 12), Chize (L 5) and Kongzui (L 6) are supposed to clarify heat, to promote lung qi in dispersing function and to relieve wheezing, and they are used to relieve acute symptoms on their own meridian. The treatments are given twice per day with reducing technique for the recurrent patient.

2) *Moxibustion* Xu Lingtai said: "Without moxibustion asthma can not be cured completely. It strengthens the body's resistance emphatically for the patient without attack, and it dispels pathogenic factors for the patient undergoing an attack." Therefore suppurating moxibustion is in summer (from the eleventh solar term to fifteenth solar term), when there are no acute symptoms. It is important to strengthen and tonify the body's resistance emphatically in order to dispel cold and disperse phlegm dampness additionally. Qi and blood in the body need to flow freely and normally. When blood does not flow normally, it will be stagnant and form phlegm. When qi does not circulate, it will make dampness accumulate. Therefore it is important in the treatment of asthma to warm up yang and benefit qi for dispelling phlegm and dampness. Prescription: a. First year, Dazhui (Du 14) (nine moxa cones), Feishu (B 13) (nine moxa cones). For teenagers and adults with a mild condition and a short course of disease (within three years), three moxa cones on these two points are enough. For the patient with a long course of disease and a severe condition, moxibustion must be repeated next year, or the other point should be added accordingly. The commonly chosen point is either Lingtai (Du 10) or Tiantu (Ren 22). b. Second year, Fengmen (B 12) (nine moxa cones), Lingtai (Du 10) (nine moxa cones), or Tanzhong (Ren 17) (seven moxa cones). c. Third year, Gaohuang (B 43) (nine moxa cones), Dazhu (B 11) (nine moxa cones).

For those with a weak constitution and a serious condition, who have some improvement and also have occasional slight attacks, they are recommended to have moxibustion on the above two points in the third year. For those who have serious wheezing and gasp for breath, Lingtai (Du 10) should be added with nine moxa cones in the first year. Tiantu (Ren 22) should be added with five moxa cones in excessive phlegm. Gaohuang (B 43) must be added with nine moxa cones for those who are weak and thin. Qihai (Ren 6) should be added with nine moxa cones for those who have wheezing caused by kidney deficiency and reverse-going qi. Zhongwan (Ren 12) is added with nine moxa cones for those with excessive phlegm and dampness. Taodao (Du 13) is added with nine moxa cones for those with spontaneous and night sweating. In the above additional points, just one point is to be added accordingly in the first and second year respectively.

In suppurating moxibustion, a moxa cone is large and fire is strong and quick and it takes long time to suppurate (forty to fifty days). Generally it is suitable to do moxibustion on two or three acupoints and three to four sites every year. It is not advisable to choose more acupoints. The moxa cones are made with the specially manufactured copper mound. Every cone is about 0.1 g in weight, and 0.7 cm in diameter in bottom. Every nine cones are made of pure white and fine moxa should be added with 0.15 g of musk which is fragrant and able to warm up yang. Suppurating moxibustion is not permitted to be done on those who have hemoptysis due to yin deficiency and consumption of fluid. In autumn, dampness goes and dryness comes. It is dry and hot in early autumn, and it is dry and cold in late autumn. Lung likes moisture and dislikes dryness. This is the reason why moxibustion is not to be continued after autumn, and therefore suppurating moxibustion should stop in the fifteenth solar term.

3. To do moxibustion necessarily in chronic diarrhoea

1) *Causes of chronic diarrhoea* Primarily chronic diarrhoea is due to qi deficiency in spleen and stomach, dysfunction in transportation and transformation and due to disturbance in gastrointestinal capacities. As time passes, spleen yang declines every day and damages kidney yang, which would decrease the spleen function of transformation further, resulting in poor appetite, lassitude, pallor, cold limbs and loss of weight. Loose stool is often seen with undigested food. The prolonged existence of disease makes the constitution weaken further. The syndrome belongs to deficiency and cold, and spleen and kidney are responsible for this condition. It is suitable to be treated with moxibustion for tonifying the resource of fire in order to dispel pathogenic cold and deficiency. This is one of the expressions. It was mentioned in *The Supplement to the Golden Chamber* that "in prolonged diarrhoea which is unable to be eliminated by medication, there must be retention in the stomach and intestines; chronic diarrhoea lasted until the retention is removed; and it is beneficial and necessary to remove retention first and afterwards to tonify the constitution." The retention in the above expression does not refer to ordinary retained food. That can be palpated in mass with complaints of progressive pain in the abdominal region, or of loose stool in purulent and bloody mucus. This is similar to ulcerative enteritis. The patient with prolonged illness would have symptoms of yang deficiency at the same time, but with no obvious emaciation. The above is the another expression.

2) *Prescription for suppurative moxibustion* a. Guanyuan (Ren 4): To tonify kidney, to strengthen the constitution, and to warm yang and regulate qi. This is the Front-Mu point of the small intestine. Tianshu (S 25): To improve intestines and regulate qi and remove retention. This point is often indicated in abdominal pain, diarrhoea and dysentery. b. Dazhui (Du 14), Gaohuang (B 43): These are the main tonic points and should be done with moxibustion in the second year. In this prescription, Guanyuan (Ren 4) and Tianshu (S 25), the Front-Mu points of small and large intestines respectively, are chosen as the major acupoints to warm up yang and benefit qi for regulating gastrointestinal organs. Guanyuan (Ren 4), the original site of three extra meridians, i.e. Ren Meridian, Du Meridian and Chong Meridian, locates just where there is the motive force of qi in kidney. Tianshu (S 25) implies an axis of transmission between heavenly qi and earthly qi, and its therapeutical significance cannot be limited on its own fu organ only. As for Gaohuang (B 43) and Dazhui (Du 14), moxibustion on these two tonic points are indicated for various deficient syndromes. For the treatment of prolonged chronic diarrhoea, the symptoms can be eliminated after moxibustion, but the weakness in the constitution cannot be corrected and recovered in a short time. Therefore, it is very important to apply moxibustion on tonic points next year which are able to consolidate therapeutical results and support the constitution. One moxa cone in suppurating moxibustion works as ten moxa cones and nine moxa cones can equal the power of one hundred moxa cones. After the moxibustion, deep burn is formed locally for suppuration. The moxibustion must be done with the demanded moxa cones. In the preparation of moxa cones, powder of cassia bark and musk can be added accordingly in order to assist the function of warming up yang. In application of moxibustion on the abdomen, manual

manipulation should be soft, gentle and efficient. And after moxibustion, all the medications should be stopped.

II. Case Analysis

Case 1: Asthma

Name, Wang x x; sex, male; age, 17.

Complaints He has had asthma since childhood, often accompanied by shortness of breath, scratchy throat, gasping for breath, difficulty in expectoration and in lying flat. The symptoms could be decreased with medication, but were unable to be cured. In recent years, the disease reoccurred frequently and continuously without interval even in summer. The condition turned worse in autumn and winter with lassitude, emaciation, susceptibility of external pathogens and retardation in development. Having been hospitalized several times, the patient started to be treated with acupuncture in cooperation for relieving the symptoms and preventing attacks. The condition was differentiated as dysfunction of the lung in dispersing and ascending abilities, and the accumulation of turbid phlegm in the lungs. The treatment was designed to strengthen the constitution, to improve the lung's dispersing ability and to dispel phlegm and dampness. In the summer of 1982, the patient was asked to undergo suppurating moxibustion.

Prescription Dazhui (Du 14), Feishu (B 13), Lingtai (Du 10).

Treatment procedure The above acupoints were done with nine moxa cones respectively. Under the treatment, asthma did not recur that year and afterwards his constitution became gradually stronger and his appetite increased. Up to now, there has been no asthma attack for three years with good development of body structure.

Case 2: Chronic diarrhoea

Name, An x x; sex, female; age, 35.

Complaints Diarrhoea for seven to eight years. At the very beginning, it was caused by improper food intake. The condition could be eliminated with medication in the early stage. Several attacks later, it turned into chronic diarrhoea, with two or three bowel movements at least and seven to eight times maximum every day. Medication was unable to decrease and eliminate the symptoms. Body weight decreased from 60 kg to 35 kg, accompanied by yellow complexion, poor appetite, a distending sensation after slight overeating, lassitude, cold sensation in the four limbs, lumbar soreness, back pain, undigested food in stool, abdominal pain in the early morning which decreased after diarrhoea, scanty urine, scanty sweating in summer. The tongue coating was slightly white and pulse was soft and weak. The condition was differentiated as chronic diarrhoea caused by yang deficiency in spleen and kidney. It was treated by warming and toning the spleen and kidney.

Prescription Tianshu (S 25), Guanyuan (Ren 4).

Treatment procedure After nine moxa cones on the respective points, there was a warm and comfortable sensation in the abdominal region. Diarrhoea decreased and abdominal pain was gradually relieved. Several months later, there was one or two bowel movements per day and stool started to form. Appetite became good and spirits improved. Next year Dazhui (Du 14) and Gaohuang (B 43) were added as tonic points. Afterwards the gastrointestinal functions returned to normal. Physical strength returned and the patient was able to work. Her weight increased to about 55 kg.

Case 3: Diarrhoea (Chronic nonspecific ulcerative colitis)

Name, Qian x x; sex, male; age, 35.

Complaints The condition started in the spring of 1965 with paste stool, two to six bowel movements per day. The condition got worse in spring and autumn with symptoms of abdominal pain before bowel movement which produced bloody stool with mucus in purplish dark colour. The patient sill wanted to move the bowels after diarrhoea. Hospitalized in Shanghai for more than one month, the patient was suspected to have amebic dysentery, as well as schistosomiasis. But negative results were shown in several stool cultures and incubation. Sigmoidoscopy indicated that there was slight chronic inflammation in rectal mucus. The diagnosis by photography of barium enema was scanty and coarse mucus in transverse and descending colon sigmoideum, which conformed to ulcerative colitis. The clinical diagnosis was chronic nonspecific ulcerative colitis. The patient was discharged when clinical symptoms decreased with the application of Western medication and rivanol solution for more than ten days. Afterwards the reoccurrence of the disease was treated with Western medications again, but the condition was as bad as before if the dosage was decreased. The condition lasted for many years with lassitude, cold sensation in limbs and poor appetite, all of which were treated with Chinese and Western medicine in alternation. All the therapies failed. In the autumn of 1973, the patient asked to be treated with moxibustion. The condition was differentiated as yang deficiency in both spleen and kidney, i.e. fire failing to produce earth. Treatment was to warm and tone the spleen and kidney and to benefit fire resource.

Prescription Moxibustion on Guanyuan (Ren 4) and Tianshu (S 25).

Treatment procedure During suppuration it was necessary to have proper food intake. After moxibustion the condition improved gradually, symptoms disappeared and appetite as well as bowel movement became normal. The patient recovered and there was no further moxibustion.

Case 4: Dismenorrhea

Name, Ge x x; sex, female; age, 22.

Complaints Supported by other people, the patient was transferred from the gynecological department and had severe pain, hands pressed on abdomen, wailing and yelling, pale complexion, profuse sweating and cold limbs. The pulse was deep, thready and string-taut. Upon inquiry, the history showed that dysmenorrhea started in the summer of 1983. A twenty-eight day cycle of menstruation lasted for one week, accompanied by a large volume of blood with abdominal pain and blood clots. The colour of menses became red when blood flowed freely. Nausea and vomiting appeared with severe pain. The patient was sent to hospital for emergency treatment five times before due to dysmenorrhea. Previous attacks were not so severe. The condition was differentiated as the accumulation of coldness and blood stagnation. It was treated by warming up the meridians.

Prescription Shiqizhuixia (Extra), Guanyuan (Ren 4), Sanyinjiao (Sp 6), Tianshu (S 25), Shenque (Ren 8).

Treatment procedure Pain decreased a little bit when the needle was manipulated by the reducing technique on Shiqizhuixia (Extra). Then a warm-needle technique was added on Guanyuan (Ren 4) and Sanyinjiao (Sp 6). Simultaneously moxibustion with moxa rolls were applied for twenty minutes on bilateral Tianshu (S 25), Shenque (Ren 8) and Guanyuan (Ren 4). Afterwards pain was eliminated and complexion became normal.

PRIMARY AND SECONDARY PRESCRIPTIONS AND NEW ADVANCES IN SELECTING LOCAL POINTS

—Li Zhuanjie's Clinical Experience

Li Zhuanjie was born in Tongyu County, Jilin Province in 1928. He learned Western internal medicine for five years after he graduated from the Harbin Medical College in 1950. Afterwards, he attended a TCM class for Western-trained doctors. He first followed the famous Dr. Sun Zhenhuan for four years to study acupuncture, and then professor Wei Rushu to research the action of acupuncture on the digestive system. He learned to treat malaria with needling in 1969. Since 1974, he has been the chief of the Department of Circulatory System in the Acupuncture Institute and has researched acupuncture for treating coronary heart disease and myocardial infarction. This subject, in cooperation with the research division of the basic science, was awarded the second class prize of the Ministry of Public Health. He helped compile the book *Simplified Acupuncture* and had more than twenty papers published in magazines and newspapers in China and abroad. He is now the professor of the Acupuncture Institute of China Academy of Traditional Chinese Medicine, and an executive member of both the Chinese Medical Association and the Clinical Research Society of China Acupuncture Association.

I. Academic Characteristics and Medical Specialities

1. Selection of chief and secondary points basically according to the etiology and location of disease

Dr. Li advocates that the chief and secondary points should be selected according to the etiology and location of the disease. Taking angina pectoris of coronary heart disease as an example, according to the records in *Internal Classic*, this disease belongs to the range of "precordial pain with cold limbs" and "angina pectoris," so the location lies chiefly in the heart. The chief points are related to the heart and pericardium. These points can be divided into two groups—the first group: Xinshu (B 15) (now it has been changed to Jiaji point which is located laterally to Xinshu for the sake of safety and convenience to be popularized), Juque (Ren 14), and Xinpingshu (on the Heart Meridern of Hand-Shaoyin and 3 cun inferior to the transverse crease of the elbow), and the second group: Jueyinshu (B 14) (now it has been replaced by the interior Jiaji point), Tanzhong (Ren 17) and Neiguan (P 6). The secondary points, which consist of five types, are selected according to such symptoms as palpitation, dyspnea, oppressed feeling of the chest, fatigue, aversion to cold, heat in the palms and soles, night sweating, and the attacking times of pain, the predisposing factors of the attack, tongue coating and the pulse condition. For yin deficiency, Sanyinjiao (Sp 6) and Taixi (K 3) are added; for deficiency of yang, Dazhui (Du 14) and Guanyuan (Ren 4) are added; for deficiency of qi, Qihai (Ren 6) and Zusanli (S 36) are added; for obstruction of phlegm, Pishu (B 20) and Fenglong (S 40) are added; and for blood stagnation, Geshu (B 17) and Xuehai (Sp 10) are added. Dr. Li once treated a forty-year old woman who suffered from precordial pain of a compressive nature. The pain radiated to her back. She had three or four attacks daily, ten minutes long, accompanied by a depressed feeling of the chest, palpitation, short breath, aversion to cold, loose stool, white tongue coating and thready pulse. ECG: S-T segment: Low horizontal position of V_5; T wave: Low voltage and flatness II. She was diagnosed as having angina pectoris of coronary heart diseases. Differentiation: Yang deficiency. She was treated with the chief and secondary points selected on the above-mentioned principle. All the symptoms disappeared and ECG was normal after the ninth treatment. Another twenty treatments were given to consolidate the therapeutic results. Altogether 140 cases of angina pectoris of coronary heart disease have been studied, in which the effective rate for angina pectoris was 84.62 percent; the rate of improvement of the ECG was 55.08 percent; and good results for palpitation, the depressed feeling of the chest, and short breath, etc.

The application of the above-mentioned chief and secondary points also produced definite effects on certain arrythmia. Dr. Li once treated a patient in Sapporo City of Japan who had suffered from "paroxysmal supraventricular tachycardia" due to myocarditis. The patient had one attack every week although he had received all sorts of long term treatments. He had to go to the hospital during the attack for intravenous injection. Differentiation: Deficiency of qi. The points were selected accordingly. His attack stopped after a two-week treatment. Except that there was a relapse induced by common cold one and a half months later, no more attacks occurred. No relapse occurred since the follow-up visit five months later. The Japanese doctors were so surprised that the patient was invited to the Hokkaido TV center to publicize the acupuncture treatment.

As for selecting points on bronchial asthma patients, the chief and secondary points could also be selected with the same method as mentioned above. Most of the patients asking for acupuncture treatment were those with chronic diseases and there were very few acute cases. The acute patients, if any, were mostly due to the acute attack of a chronic disease. No matter which type they belonged to the disease is located in the lungs, so the treatment must focus on the lungs. The chief points selected were Tanzhong (Ren 17), Zhongfu (L 1), Chize (L 5), Taiyuan (L 9), Dingchuan (Extra 17) and Feishu (B 13), and the secondary points, Fengchi (B 20) and Fengmen (B 12) were added for cases complicated with wind and cold; Tiantu (Ren 22), Hegu (LI 4), and Fenglong (S 40) for cases complicated with phlegm heat; Pishu (B 20) and Zusanli (S 36) for those complicated with spleen deficiency; and Shenshu (B 23) and Taixi (K 3) for those complicated with deficiency of kidney. Generally, an effective rate of 60 to 70 percent could be obtained when bronchial asthma patients were treated with the above method.

Dr. Li holds that although we have to follow the principle of syndrome differentiation in clinical acupuncture treatment, the key point is to localize the lesion. The other factors can be solved by the secondary points.

2. With the modern scientific knowledge to enrich the method of selecting the local acupoints

Lesions on cervical or lumbar vertebrae are frequently encountered diseases in clinic. Patients with the diseases are often seen in the acupuncture department. Jiaji points are very important in treating the diseases besides the points selected with the traditional syndrome differentiation. Good effects will be obtained if the points at both sides of the spinal column and around the lesion can be selected correctly. There are two methods for correctly taking local Jiaji points. One is to choose the bilateral Jiaji points at both sides of the spine which have positive findings according to the X-ray examination. Once Dr. Li treated a cervical spondylotic patient who had neck and shoulder pain and paresthesia, and weakness of the upper limb. X-ray showed a narrowing change in the space between C5-C6. Better results were obtained after he selected the Jiaji points at C5 in addition to Jianzhongshu (SI 15), Jianwaishu (SI 14), Jianjing (G 21), Jugu (LI 16), Tianzong (SI 11), Quchi (LI 11), Waiguan (SJ 5) and Hegu (LI 4) points. The other method is to select Jiaji points according to the innervation of the spinal nerves. For example, to treat the radiating pain of femoral and obturator nerves due to lumbar spondylosis, the Jiaji points at L1-L3 can be selected and L4-L5 Jiaji points for the radiating pain of sciatic nerve.

Dr. Li once treated a middle aged woman at Hokkaido who suffered from hereps zoster. The disease was located at the travelling range of the T6-T7 intercostal nerve. The patient had white tongue coating and string-taut pulse. He used the Jiaji points of T6 to T7 and supplemented them with the bilateral Zhigou (SJ 6) and Yanglingquan (G 34) points. The patient was cured only after five treatments.

When he was in Yugoslavia, he cured a hiccup patient who had received many kinds of modern treatment. Dr. Li believed that hiccup was caused by the intermittent spasm of the diaphragm which was controlled by the diaphragm nerve at C3-C5, and chiefly at C4. So he needled bilateral Futu (LI 18), and the hiccup stopped several minutes after the needling. As Futu (LI 18) is situated near the diaphram nerve, it also falls within the category of local selection of points. The etiology of hiccup is ascending stomach qi. The stomach belongs to Foot Yangming, while Futu (LI 18) to Hand Yangming. These two Yangming communicate with each other, so needling them has the effect of harmonizing the stomach and descending the stomach qi.

II. Case Analysis

Case 1: Chest pain (coronary heart disease)

Name, Guan x x; sex, male; age, 47.

Complaints The patient suffered from precordial pain for three years, which attacked him two or three times a day. The pain radiated towards the left axillary and the interior of the upper limb, complicated by a compressive sensation on the chest. Each time the pain would last two minutes. The attack often occurred after emotional excitement and overeating, but could be relieved by rest. When the attack came, it was often complicated with oppressive sensation of the chest, short breath, and palpitation, etc. On examination, it was found that the patient's tongue proper was red, with white coating, the pulse was thready and rapid. ECG: S-T segment: Low horizontal position 0.1 mv at II, III and avF. He was diagnosed as having coronary heart disease, angina pectoris.

Differentiation Yin deficiency of the heart. The treatment is directed to nourish the heart yin.

Prescription Juque (Ren 14), Xinping (Extra), Sanyinjiao (Sp 6) and Taixi (K 3).

Treatment procedure The ECG was normal after twenty treatments. All the symptoms diminished after twenty-seven treatments. Altogether the patient had thirty treatments before he was cured.

Case 2: Chest pain (anginal pectoris of coronary heart disease)

Name, Liu x x; sex, female; age, 36.

Complaints The patient was a doctor who had suffered from intermittent precordial pain for half a year, accompanied with an oppressive sensation of the chest, palpitation, short breath, loose stool, pale tongue proper, thin white coating, deep and thready pulse. ECG: S-T segment: Descending 0.05 to 0.1 mv in II, III, avF, V_3 and V_5. The diagnosis was coronary heart disease, angina pectoris.

Differentiation Qi deficiency. The treatment is directed to reinforce qi and help to restore the cardiac function.

Prescription Jueyinshu (using the interior Jiaji points instead), Tanzhong (Ren 17), Neiguan (P 6), Qihai (Ren 6) and Zusanli (S 36).

Treatment procedure All the symptoms disappeared after twenty treatments with the above-mentioned method. ECG restored to normal after thirty treatments.

Case 3: Chest pain (angina pectoris of coronary heart disease)

Name, Zhao x x; sex, male; age, 52.

Complaints The patient had a history of hypertension. He had precordial pain for six months with one or two attacks every week. He was obese with profuse phlegm, white greasy tongue coating, string-taut and slippery pulse. ECG: S-T segments: Lowering in II, III, avF. The diagnosis was coronary heart disease, angina pectoris.

Differentiation Obstruction of phlegm. The treatment is directed to resolve the phlegm and dredge the meridians.

Prescription Juque (Ren 14), Xinping (Extra), Feishu (B 13) and Fenglong (S 40).

Treatment procedure After the first treatment with the above-mentioned method, no relapse was found. After thirty treatments, ECG showed that the lowering of II, III, avF in S-T segment improved.

Case 4: Chest pain (angina pectoris)

Name, Yang x x; sex, Male.

Complaints The patient had hypertension in general, and suffered from precordial pain for half a year. The pinching-like pain attacked two or three times a day and lasted about four to ten minutes. It usually happened during excitement or exertion, sometimes at night. It could only be relieved after taking nitroglycerine. His tongue proper was dark with thin coating, and the pulse was string-taut. Normal ECG was often found between attacks. The diagnosis was doubtful coronary heart disease, angina pectoris.

Differentiation Blood stagnation. The treatment is directed to remove the stagnation and dredge the meridians.

Prescription Jueyinshu (B 14) (substituted by Jiaji points), Tanzhong (Ren 17), Neiguan (P 6), Geshu (B 17) and Xuehai (Sp 10).

Treatment procedure The attack of precordial pain was reduced from three or four times a day to once in several days after three treatments.

STANDARDIZATION OF REINFORCING AND REDUCING METHOD, IMPROVEMENT OF MOXIBUSTION

—Li Zhiming's Clinical Experience

Li Zhiming (1927-1987) was born in Tangxian County of Hebei Province in 1927. During his adolescence, he followed his uncle Li Xiugang to learn medicine. He served as a medical worker in the Bethune International Peace Hospital in 1946. He graduated from the Qahar Medical School in 1952. Since 1954, he had followed Dr. Zheng Yulin and studied acupuncture for twelve years. In 1959, he attended the third course of traditional Chinese medicine for Western medical doctors held by the Ministry of Public Health, and studied TCM for two years. Since 1964, he had been working in the Institute of Acupuncture and Moxibustion, the China Academy of Traditional Chinese Medicine and the Acupuncture Department of Guang'anmen Hospital until 1987. In the last several decades, Dr. Li has been absorbed in writing and collecting acupuncture literature and in his clinical practice. He concluded that the four methods of promoting the arrival of qi, regulating qi, retaining qi and leading qi could be regarded as the basic maneuvers of heat reinforcing and cold reducing. He contributed to the standardization of the reinforcing and reducing method. He was good at selecting points from the meridians of the same name and the related meridians. The number of points he selected was less but the quality of his selection was good.

He developed the strong points of moxibustion therapy, and he used more than twenty methods of moxibustion. Several dozens of his articles and papers had been published. He was the professor of the Guang'anmen Hospital, China Academy of Traditional Chinese Medicine, and the executive member of the China Association of Acupuncture and Moxibustion.

I. Academic Characteristics and Medical Specialities

1. Studying elaborately the reinforcing and reducing methods, and standardizing heat-reinforcing and cold-reducing methods

Dr. Li summerized the promoting the arrival of qi, regulating qi, retaining qi and leading qi as the basic manipulations for the reinforcing and reducing methods.

1) *Promoting the arrival of qi* According to *The Classic on Medical Problems*, he was fully aware that "the specialist of acupuncture regards the left hand as the chief side, while the layman only believes the right hand," indicating the importance of the coordination of the both hands. He uses his left hand for palpation, grasping, pressing, following and holding the acupoint and the place, where the meridians pass through, and his right hand to hold the needle for rapid insertion or for twisting and rotating the needle

into the points. The needle tip is directed to the diseased area with continuous lifting and thrusting, or twirling and rotating in order to obtain the arrival of qi immediately and keep the qi reaching the affected area. For example, with the promoting technique while needling Guangming (B 37), Hegu (LI 4) and Ligou (Liv 5) points, he pressed his left hand at the inferior border of the point tightly, and directed the needle tip upward. With continuous lifting, thrusting or twirling and rotating, the qi will transmit along the meridians to the ophthalmic area.

2) *Regulating qi* As stated in *Miraculous Pivot* that "regulating qi should be performed from the beginning to the end," Dr. Li realized that the key of regulating qi is to harmonize the interior and exterior in the whole process from the beginning to the end. After the promoting qi technique is performed, slow lifting and thrusting and left-right and forward-backward twirling and rotating should be appropriate to make the patient comfortable and have a sore and distended sensation. For example, needling the Shenshu (B 23) point to treat knee joint pain promotes the arrival of qi to the affected area, then follow the method of regulating qi, that is to lift and thrust the needle slowly or twirl and rotate the needle evenly to make the patient feel comfortable, a foundation for further application of the reinforcing and reducing method.

3) *Retaining qi* It is used in the heat-reinforcing method. Dr. Li followed the principle recorded in *Plain Questions*: "Once qi reaches the meridian, do not lose it. The hand should hold the needle as tightly as if it held a tiger" during the manipulation. The method is as follows: Following the regulating qi method, insert the needle 0.1 to 0.2 cun deep and thrust it deeper with the thumb rotating forward for three to five or nine times. Most of the patients will have heat and distension sensations.

4) *Leading qi* Leading qi means to lead the pathogenic factors out of the body when it is used in the cold-reducing method. The procedure is as follows: Following the regulating qi method, lift the needle upward 0.1 to 0.2 cun and scrape the handle of the needle upward with the thumb six to eighteen times, then most of the patients will have a cold feeling.

Promoting the arrival of qi, regulating qi, retaining qi and leading qi are a series of actions of the reinforcing and reducing methods, which may be applied integratedly in the heat-reinforcing and cold-reducing method. Different waveforms and amplitudes can be measured by means of the modern scientific instruments.

5) *The heat-reinforcing and cold-reducing method* This is a compound reinforcing and reducing technique, which may produce either local or general warm or cold sensation in the patient if it is applied properly. The procedures of the heat-reinforcing and cold-reducing are as follows: For the reinforcing method, insert the needle superficially first and then deeply, and vice versa for the reducing method; for the reinforcing method, press the needle tightly and lift it slowly, and vice versa for the reducing method; for the former, twist the needle with the thumb forwards more than backwards, and vice versa for the latter; for the former, scrape the needle handle downwards and vice versa for the latter; for the former, press and knead the acupoint after withdrawing the needle, and vice versa for the latter. The reinforcing effect is a warm sensation, while the reducing effect is a cold feeling. Promoting the arrival of qi, regulating qi and retaining qi are adopted in reinforcing, and promoting the arrival of qi, regulating qi and leading

qi are applied in reducing.

a. The heat-reinforcing method: Press the acupoint tightly with the left index finger, and twist or insert the needle quickly into the point 0.5 cun deep, in combination with slow lifting and tight pressing in order to get qi first. Insert the needle 0.1 to 0.2 cun downward based on the arrival of the soreness and distension. The warm distension will appear after rotating the thumb forward for three to five or nine times. In case of failure, proceed as above-mentioned method for two to three times and most of the patients will have the heat distention. The acupoint should be kneaded and pressed after withdrawing the needle. For the patient whose sensation is dull, let him exhale three to five or nine times or scrape the needle handle with the thumb downwards for thirty seconds. This method can be used in any kind of deficiency-cold syndromes, such as seminal emission, menopause, hypotension, dysmenorrhea, abnormal menstruation, insomnia, epigastric pain, optic atrophy, fundus bleeding, flaccid type of wind stroke and arthritis. Dilatation of blood vessels and elevation of the skin temperature have been observed by taking the capacity of the blood vessels and skin temperature as an index. The difference is significant statistically. Since 1980, fourteen cases of familial optic atrophy had been treated, seventeen years old on the average, the course of the disease varying from several months to three years, and twenty-eight diseased eyes in all. Fengchi (G 20), Taiyang (Extra 2), Tongziliao (G 1), Neijingming (Extra), Qiuhou (Extra 4), Shenmen (H 7), Hegu (LI 4), Guangming (G 37) and Ligou (Liv 5) were selected as the main points according to the differentiation, and the heat-reinforcing method was used. The results are shown in the following table.

Item	**Diseased eyes**	**Cured**	**Markedly effective**	**Improved**	**Total effective**	**Failed**
Number of eyes	28	5	6	10	21	7
%	100	17.86	21.43	35.71	75.00	25.00

In this group, all of the fourteen patients had been treated with Chinese herbs or Western medicine with no effect. When treated with the heat-reinforcing method, the effective rate was 75 percent, which shows that the reasonable application of the technique could obtain good therapeutic effects.

b. The cold-reducing method: Press the acupoint tightly with the left index finger, and insert the needle into the acupoint 1 cun deep by rapid twisting and rotating. Then lift the needle tightly and press it slowly to get qi. Lift the needle 0.1 to 0.2 cun upward based on the arrival of numbness and distension. Cold numbness will result after rotating the thumb backward three to five or six times. Repeat the procedure two to three times if nothing happens. Most of the patients will have cold-numbness. Neither kneading nor pressing of the points is necessary after withdrawal of the needle. Let those patients with dull sensation inhale for five to six times or scrape the needle handle upwards with the thumb for thirty seconds. This method is effective to all kinds of excess-heat syndromes, such as Yangming fu heat, high fever, hypertension, menopause, conjunctivitis, and tense type of windstroke. Construction of the blood vessels and drop of skin temperature have been observed by taking the capacity of blood vessels and skin temperature as the index. The difference is significant statistically. For example, a male patient, twenty-three years old, complained of pain of the right eye, photophobia, lacrimation for half a month, distension of the eyes, and blurred vision. His tongue coating was thin and white and his pulse was string-taut. The diagnosis was punctate keratitis. Differentiation: Wind-heat in the Liver Meridian. The principle of treatment was to clear and dredge the liver and gallbladder, dispel the wind and brighten the eyes. Fengchi (G 20) and Guangming (G 37) points were selected with cold-reducing method. During the treatment, the cold distension was transferred to the eye area. The eye pain disappeared after two treatments.

2. The advantage of moxibustion in treating diseases

"If acupuncture fails in treatment, moxibustion may be used instead." Moxibustion can not only supplement the inadequacy of acupuncture, but also possess the specific therapeutic action. Better effects can be obtained if it is used in combination with acupuncture. In treating diseases, Dr. Li used the best of both ancient or modern moxibustion methods, and applied them in the clinic. He invented moxibustion with walnut shell spectacles in treating ophthalmic diseases (Fig. 1.), and improved moxibustion with the external auditory meatus through the reed tube in treating facial paralysis (Fig 2.). He developed scarring moxibustion and riding bamboo horse moxibustion, and ear point moxibustion. He had applied moxibustion in the treatment of chronic and deficiency-cold syndromes as well as the acute and excess-heat syndromes. He was also proficient in using moxibustion at Zusanli (S 36) point to keep fit and prolong longevity.

1) *Moxibustion with walnut shell spectacles* The frame of spectacles is made of iron wire, provided with a wire hook in the front used for fixing the moxa stick. During moxibustion, rest the walnut shell which has been previously immersed in chrysanthemum water for three to five minutes on the frame of the spectacles and then put a 1.5

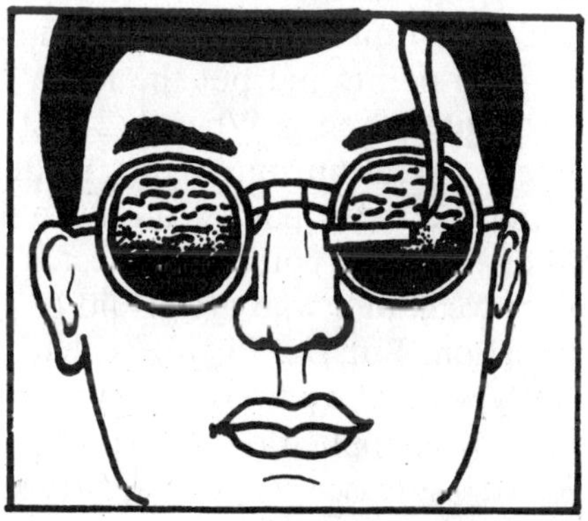

Fig. 1 Moxibustion with walnut-made glasses

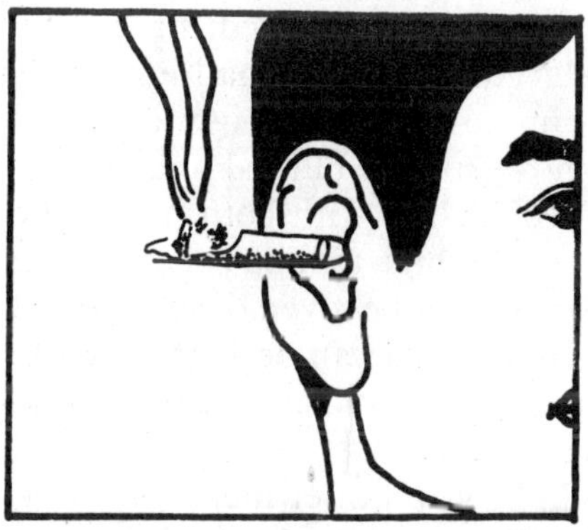

Fig. 2 Moxibustion with a reed tube

cm-long moxa stick into the iron wire hook. Ignite the external end of the moxa stick and apply moxibustion on the affected eye for one to three cones. The clinical practice has proved effective for conjunctivitis, styl, keratitis, myopia, senile cataract and optic atrophy. Ten cases of conjunctivitis were treated and all of them were cured after one to three treatments in average. For myopia with 43 eyes, the vision of 3 eyes was restored to 1.0 after five treatments, that of 24 eyes restored to 0.3, that of 15 eyes restored to 0.1 and only one eye failed. The walnut, relating to the Kidney Meridian, has the function to nourish the kidney and improve the vision; chrysanthemum, relating to the liver, has the function to nourish the liver and kidney, and dispel the wind and brighten the eyes; the moxa, relating to the Liver, Spleen, and Kidney Meridians, may activate qi and blood circulation, dredge the meridian and remove the stagnation, dispel the wind and improve the vision. Therefore, this method has a therapeutic effect on eye diseases. This technique is easily performed.

2) *Improving the reed tube moxibustion* Making and manipulation The reed tube moxa instrument consists of two segments of the reed stem. The segment on one end is about 4 cm long, the mouth of the tube is 0.8 to 1 cm in diameter. Cut the end into the shape of the lower duck beak. The other end is 3 cm long and 0.6 to 0.8 cm in diameter. This part is used to be inserted into the external auditory meatus, and can be fixed in place with adhesive tape. Put a little bit of fine dry moxa, about half a peanut in size, into the duck-beak-shaped reed tube instrument, and then ignite it, three to nine cones each time. Ten times constitute one course. Care should be taken not to burn the patient's clothes. Seventy-four cases of peripheral facial paralysis were treated, in which the curative rate was 56.76 percent; and the effective rate, 98.65 percent. The method is easy to be performed and has definite therapeutic effects. It is also effective for deficiency-cold syndrome, infants, pregnant women, patients with a weak constitution and serious visceral disease, or those who are afraid of needles.

3) *Scarring moxibustion and riding bamboo horse moxibustion* Scarring moxibustion, also called purulent moxibustion, is effective for some chronic diseases such as asthma, tuberculosis, epigastric pain, masses in the abdomen, underdevelopment, epilepsy, impotence, gangrene of the finger or toe, irregular menstruation, dysmenorrhea, and prevention of hypertension. He advocated that this method should be further explored, elevated and popularized. Procedure: After a suitable position is chosen and acupoints are selected, apply a small amount of garlic juice on the point, and put the moxa stick on it immdiately. Then ignite it (standard moxa stick) with incense. When 1/2 or 2/3 of the moxa stick is burned and the patient begins to feel a local burning pain, the doctor can beat lightly with both hands the area surrounding the moxa points to reduce pain. Generally, three to nine cones should be burned and one to three points are selected. The treatment can be given once a year. For those who are weak and who are afraid of pain, local anesthesia can be performed before the moxibustion. But Dr. Li thinks that local anesthesia can not help the therapeutic effect, especially when the pain is in fact bearable. After the moxibustion, a "clear liquid paste (self-made)" is applied on the wound. Care should be given after moxibustion. Dr. Li had observed 182 cases of asthma, fifty-seven cases of late-staged schistosomiasis complicated with enlargement of liver and spleen, and twenty-three cases of pulmonary tuberculosis. In the treatment, Dazhui (Du 14) was

always selected as the chief point, and different Shu points were chosen as the auxiliary points symptomatically. Satisfactory therapeutic effects were obtained. Experimental studies on scarring moxibustion were also carried out at Dazhui (Du 14) of rabbits. The result revealed that the twenty rabbits in the moxibustion group were more active and with better appetite compared with the ten rabbits in the control group. Also the prominent increasing of the sheep hemodilution dissolution, and proliferation of the lymphocytes among the interstitial tissues of the viscera of the rabbits were found in the moxibustion group, and there were no such changes in the control group. This indicates that the scarring moxibustion offers beneficial influence on the human body. The reasons may be that the local inflammation of the tissue produced by the moxibustion will give a long-term sustained stimulation of different degrees to the body and a protective inhibition within the cerebral cortex. Meanwhile, the decomposed products by the local inflammation can produce local stimulation action, which, through the reflection of the central nervous system and changes of the body fluid, can strengthen the immunological function and reach the aim of treatment. Riding bamboo horse moxibustion is one kind of the scarring moxibustion which had been recorded early in the Song Dynasty in the *Main Rules in Medical and Health Service.* Based on the observation data and clinical treatment of a hundred patients, Dr. Li determined that the points for riding bamboo horse moxibustion is 1.5 cun lateral to the T7, i.e. the location of Geshu (B 17) point. This method was used chiefly to treat thirteen cases of "gangrene of hands and feet," among them, four cases were cured; three, markedly effective; and six, improved.

4) *Auricular moxibustion* Since the ear is closely related to the meridians and zang-fu organs, moxibustion can warm and dredge the meridians, activate qi and blood circulation, reduce the swelling, check the pain, and regulate the functions of the zang-fu organs. Syndrome differentiation must be used in selection of the points for auricular moxibustion with either moxa stick fumigation, burning rush moxibustion or reed tube moxibustion. Auricular moxibustion offers better therapeutic effect in treating facial paralysis, ophthalmic pain, mumps, painful Bi-syndromes, herpes zoster, aphthae, and auricle chondritis.

5) *Moxibustion on Zusanli (S 36) for keeping fit and prolonging life* The moxibustion on Zusanli (S 36) is called longevity moxibustion. Dr. Li thought that Zusanli (S 36) is the He-Sea point of the Stomach Meridian and relates to the earth. The spleen and stomach are the origin of acquired substance. Frequent moxibustion over it can prevent diseases and prolong life. When combined with Zhongwan (Ren 12) and Sanyinjiao (Sp 6), it has the function to reinforce the middle jiao and regulate the spleen and stomach; if combined with Guanyuan (Ren 4) and Juegu (G 39), it functions to reinforce the source of the inherited and acquired constitution, regulate yin and yang, and prolong life. It also has a preventive and therapeutic action on cough and asthma, pulmonary tuberculosis, hypertension, coronary heart disease, and windstroke. In the mid 1950s Dr. Li had blood pressure of 170/100 mmHg. Since 1958 when he received the scarring moxibustion over his Zusanli (S 36) point, his blood pressure dropped to normal for more than twenty years. Fourteen out of fifteen hypertension patients were treated with the scarring moxibustion over Zusanli (S 36) and Juegu (G 39) points. Satisfactory long-term effects were achieved.

3. Skill in selecting acupoints on the connecting meridians, and leading qi to the diseased area

There are two commonly used methods:

1) *Selecting the points from the affected meridians, and directing qi to reach the affected area* For example, in treating toothache, Hegu (LI 4) may be needled with the needling sensation reaching to Quchi (LI 11); which is needled again with the needling sensation reaching to Jianyu (LI 15), which is needled with the needling sensation reaching the affected tooth.

2) *The method recorded of Main Rules in Medical and Health Service* "In the treatment of paraplegia, needle the related meridians from yang to yin, Zhiyin (B 67) and Yongquan (K 1), Zhongchong (P 9) and Guanchong (SJ 1), Qiaoyin (G 44) and Dadun (Liv 1), Shaoshang (L 11) and Shangyang (LI 1), Lidui (S 45) and Yinbai (Sp 1), Shaochong (H 9) and Shaoze (SI 1) can be selected; or needle the related meridian from yin to yang, Shaochong (L 11) and Shangyang (LI 1), Lidui (S 45) and Yinbai (Sp 1), Shaochong (H 9) and Shaoze (SJ 1), Zhiyin (B 67) and Yongquan (K 1), Zhongchong (P 9) and Guanchong (SJ 1), Qiaoyin (G 44) and Dadun (Liv 1) may be selected." Take the treatment of sciatica with acupuncture as an example. When Dr. Li treated the disease, he combined the differentiation with the selection of points according to the meridians. Reinforcing was used for deficiency syndrome, and reducing used for excess syndrome. The differentiation according to the etiology can be divided into the cold-damp type, the kidney deficiency type, and the blood stagnation type; while the differentiation according to the meridians divided into the Bladder Meridian of Foot-Taiyang type, the Gallbladder Meridian of Foot-Shaoyang type, and the mixed type. The Shu points from the involved meridians and Shu points from the meridians with the same name were selected respectively in combination with suitable Shu points according to the different causative factors. For example, a male worker, fifty-four years old, had left dry sciatica, which was differentiated in traditional Chinese medicine as the Gallbladder Meridian type. Sizhukong (SJ 23) was needled alone with heat-reinforcing method. The left Laseque's sign restored to 90° after the treatment, and the pain disappeared after another four treatments. Sizhukong (SJ 23) is a point of the Sanjiao Meridian of the Hand-Shaoyang, the meridian with the same name. This point can promote qi circulation of the Hand and Foot-Shaoyang Meridians.

4. Application of Fengchi (G 20) point in treating various diseases

Fengchi (G 20) is a point of the Gallbladder Meridian of Foot-Shaoyang, and a crossing point of the Hand, Foot-Shaoyang and the Yangwei Meridians, and the point externally-internally related to the Liver Meridian. It has the function of expelling the wind and dispelling the exogenous pathogenic factors from the body surface, activating the blood circulation to check pain, and benefit the eyes and inducing resuscitation. Dr. Li was good at using this point in the treatment of ophthalmic diseases. Procedure: Press Futu (LI 18) with the left thumb, and Fengchi (G 20), Yifeng (SJ 17), Qubin (G 7) and Taiyang (Extra 2) points respectively with the index, middle, ring and small fingers.

When a 1.5-cun-long filiform needle (No. 30) is quickly inserted 1 to 1.2 cun deep into the point with the right hand, its tip should point toward the unilateral eyeball. The heat-reinforcing or cold-reducing method can be adopted according to deficiency or excess, cold or heat syndrome. Following is an example for prescription:

Taiyang (Extra 2), Sizhukong (SJ 23) and Hegu (LI 4) are often combined to treat the redness, swelling and pain of the eyes; Sibai (S 2), Hegu (LI 4) and Sanyinjiao (Sp 6) combined to treat stye; Renzhong (Du 26) and Yongquan (K 1) to treat hysteric blindness; Neiguan (P 6), Shenmen (H 7), Guangming (G 37), Ligou (Liv 5) or Taichong (Liv 3) to treat glaucoma; Taichong (Liv 3), Yanglao (SI 6), Hegu (LI 4), Zusanli (S 36) and Guangming (G 37) to treat cataract; Jingming (B 1), Taiyang (Extra 2), Zanzhu (B 2), Hegu (LI 4), Shenmen (H 7), Guangming (G 37), Ligou (Liv 5), Zusanli (S 36) and Sanyinjiao (Sp 6) to treat blurring of vision and optic atrophy; Qiuhou (Extra 4), Jingming (B 1), Taichong (Liv 3), Hegu (LI 4), Shenmen (H 7), Guangming (G 37), Ligou (Liv 5) and Erbai (Extra 24) to treat vitreous opacity; Feiyang (B 58), Ganshu (B 18), Taichong (Liv 3) and Pishu (B 20) to treat night blindness; Yangbai (G 14), Sibai (S 2), Taiyang (Extra 2), Neiguan (P 6) and Hegu (LI 4) to treat myopia; Dazhui (Du 14), Waiguan (SJ 5) and Lieque (L 7) to treat common cold, headache and neck rigidity; Quchi (LI 11) and Hegu (LI 4) added in case of wind-heat; Shuaigu (G 8), Sizhukong (SJ 23), Hegu (LI 4) and Qiuxu (G 40) to treat migraine; Quchi (LI 11), Yangchi (SJ 4), Xuehai (Sp 10), Yanglingquan (G 34), Zusanli (S 36) and Sanyinjiao (Sp 6) to treat urticaria; Baihui (Du 20), Neiguan (P 6), Taichong (Liv 3), Zusanli (S 36) and Fenglong (S 40) to treat dizziness; Luozhen (Extra 26) and Juegu (G 39) to treat stiff neck; Lieque (L 7), Tanzhong (Ren 17) and Hegu (LI 4) to treat asthma; moxibustion with moxa stick to treat cold and congestion; and massage on the points for the prevention of cold, windstroke and myopia.

5. Using intention to lead the qi and applying fingers to replace the needle

Dr. Li practised qigong in combination with acupuncture. In practice, he combined qigong with needling to let the patient get qi quickly, and make the qi reach the affected area, so that the effect of the treatment was greatly elevated. On the other hand, he devoted himself to the study of health massage. He put forward the point massage exercise on the head and face, and the self-health massage exercise on the body. Long-term sustained practice of qigong (in combination with respiration and intention) and massage on certain acupoints on the head, face and trunk, that is, applying the finger instead of a needle, and using "qi" instead of needle, and using "qi" instead of a drug, can prolong the life and prevent illness.

6. Qi reaching the affected area is the key point in raising the therapeutic effect

"Qi reaching the affected area" is recorded in many medical literatures in the past dynasties. According to Dr. Li's clinical experience, the application of "promoting the arrival of qi" with the coordination of the left and right hands, can make the qi quickly reach the affected area. Whether qi has reached the affected area or not can be confirmed by the inspection, palpation and inquiry. In July of 1968, a 40-year-old man who had suffered from blindness bilaterally for more than one month was treated. The diagnosis in Western medicine was optic atrophy. The differentiation of TCM was deficiency of the essence and blood in the liver and kidney. Fengchi (G 20), Hegu (LI 4), Neiguan (P 6), Guangming (G 37) and Ligou (Liv 5) were selected with heat-reinforcing method to lead the heat distension transmit along the meridian to the eye region. The vision was recovered evidently after seventy-two treatments, the vision of the right eye was 0.6 and that of the left eye, 0.4. The therapeutic effect was so consolidated that no relapse was found in a follow-up visit eighteen years later. Another example was a French patient who suffered from herpes zoster at his lumbar region for three days. He could not sleep due to the pain, which was diagnosed as herpes zoster in Western medicine and as damp-heat in the liver and gallbladder in TCM. Taichong (Liv 3) and Zhigou (SJ 6) points were selected with the cold-reducing method. The cold distension was transmitted to the lumbar region. Shenmen (H 7) and Lieque (L 7) were needled with the even reinforcing and even reducing method, and the heat distension was transmitted to the affected area. The pain was greatly reduced, and he could fall asleep the same night. He was cured only after four treatments. A 60-year-old patient from West Germany had suffered from asthma for thirty years. This time the attack was so serious that he had dyspnea, insomnia, and a wheezing sound in both lungs. The diagnosis was asthma (deficiency of both lung and kidney). Dingchuan (Extra 17), Lieque (L 7), Shenmen (H 7) and Taixi (K 3) points were selected. During the needling, the patient had experienced an electric-current-like sensation propagating along the meridian and reaching the affected area. The asthma stopped immediately. A hundred and twenty-four cases (213 eyes) of optic atrophy were also treated with the heat-reinforcing method at Fengchi (G 20) point, in which the needling sensation in 84 eyes was radiated to the eye region, and 71 eyes (84.52 percent) were effective; the needling sensation in 68 eyes reached the vertex, and 42 eyes (61.76 percent) were effective; the needling sensation in 61 eyes was restricted at the local area, and 26 eyes (42.62 percent) were effective. If the needling sensation reached the eye region, the best therapeutic effect can be obtained. On the contrary, the result is poor. The difference is significant statistically ($P<0.001$), indicating that qi reaching the affected area is the key point to raise the therapeutic effect.

II. Case Analysis

Case 1: Optic atrophy

Name, Liu x x; sex, male; age, 21; date of the first visit, March 24, 1982.

Complaints The patient suffered from gradually blurred vision for one year without any evident cause. It was diagnosed as "familial optic atrophy" in another hospital. He had no response after taking various kinds of Chinese herbs and Western drugs, so he was transferred to our hospital. Examination: Blurred vision, headache, blood pressure 120/80 mmHg, the vision of right eye 0.05 and that of the left eye 0.07, thin white tongue coating, deep and thready pulse. Funduscopy: pale bilateral optic papillae, clear margin, the slightly curved blood vessels, the visible macular reflex. Central visual field examination showed that dark spot existed on the papilla and the center area. There were dark spots on the central peripheral visual field. According to the differentiation combined with the pulse and symptoms observed, the disease was yin deficiency of the liver and kidney, and loss of nutrition of the eyes. The treatment should be directed to nourish the kidney and liver, and clear the eyes.

Prescription Fengchi (G 20), Taiyang (Extra 5), Zanzhu (B 2), Hegu (LI 4), Shenmen (H 7), Guangming (G 37), Ligou (Liv 5) and Jingming (B 1).

Treatment procedure Fengchi (G 20) was needled with the heat-reinforcing method and the heat distension was directed to the eye area. He was treated for ten and a half months, eighty-one treatments in all. The vision of the right eye was restored to 1.2; and that of the left eye to 1.0. He was clinically recovered and could undertake his work again.

Explanation Needling Fengchi (G 20) point with the heat-reinforcing method can promote the meridian, benefit the liver and improve the eyesight. When the Luo-Connecting point Guangming (G 37) of the Gallbladder Meridian and the Luo-Connecting point Ligou (Liv 5) of the Liver Meridian are added, it can help nourish the liver and improve the eyesight. Jingming (B 1) is a crossing point of the Foot-Taiyang, Foot-Yangming, Yangqiao and Yinqiao Meridians. Needling of this point has the function of promoting meridians and activating blood circulation, benefiting the kidney and improving eyesight. Shenmen (H 7) is the Yuan-Source point of the Heart Meridian. When it is needled, it can nourish the blood and tranquilize the mind. Taiyang (Extra) is used locally in clearing the brain and improving the eyesight. Hegu (LI 11) is an experience point. Better results can be obtained if all the points are used in combination. Sixty-four cases (118 eyes) had been treated with this method, among them, 15 eyes were cured; 20 eyes markedly effective; 48 eyes improved; and the total effective rate was 75.45 percent.

Case 2: Hemiplegia (cerebral thrombosis)

Name, Li x x; sex, male; age, 43; date of the first visit, March 27, 1980.

Complaints The patient fell down suddenly four days before, and his mind was still clear. Shortly after that he suffered from right hemiplegia and aphasia. He was sent to a hospital in Beijing, where cerebral thrombosis and motor aphasia were diagnosed. No response was found after he was treated with Chinese herbs and Western drugs, so he was transferred to our hospital. When he was admitted he had right hemiplegia complicated with aphasia, poor appetite and constipation. He had had a history of hypertension. Ordinarily he had a nervous in character and was a heavy smoker and drinker. His mother had died of wind stroke. Examination: Clear mind, blood pressure 140/80 mmHg, the heart rate 70 times/minute, the heart rhythm regular, the bilateral biceps reflex (++), triceps reflex (++), bilateral knee jerk (++), Achilles reflex (++), right Babinski's sign (+), and the muscle strength of the right upper and lower extremities grade III, yellow greasy tongue coating, fine and string-taut pulse. Differentiation: Wind attacking the meridian, kidney deficiency and hyperactivity of the liver-fire, qi deficiency and stagnation of blood. The principle of the treatment should nourish the kidney and regulate the liver, promote the meridian and activate the collaterals, and dispel the wind and induce resusctation.

Prescription Yinbai (Sp 1), Dadun (Liv 1), Fengchi (G 20), Sizhukong (SJ 23), Quchi (LI 11), Hegu (LI 4), Yanglingquan (G 34), Sanyinjiao (Sp 6) and Shanglianquan (Extra 12).

Treatment procedure The muscle strength increased to grade IV and he could walk with help after Yinbai (Sp 1) and Dadun (Liv 1) were needled. His symptoms were greatly alleviated and he could speak after seven treatments when the rest points were needled and the "Buyang Huanwu Decoctions" was administered. He was recovered as a normal person after he received fifty-three treatments. No relapse was found after a follow-up visit for five years. He could undertake his original job again.

Explanation This is a hemiplegia due to windstroke which is caused by the kidney deficiency and the liver hyperactivity, deficiency of qi and stagnation of blood. According to the experience by Dr. Luo Tianyi in treating apoplectic hemiplegia, Yinbai (Sp 1) and Dadun (Liv 1) were selected as the chief points. Yinbai is the Jing-Well point of the Spleen Meridian, and is the outlet of the Spleen Meridian. Needling it can strengthen the spleen and benefit qi, dissipate phlegm and induce resuscitation. Dadun (Liv 1) is a Jing-Well point of Liver Meridian, and is the origin of qi of the Liver Meridian. Needling it can dredge the meridian qi, restore from syncope and wake up from coma, nourish the blood and promote the growth of new tissue. When these points are used together with other points, they will have the functions of toning the kidney and regulating the liver, dredging the meridians and inducing resuscitation. Among 57 cases treated with this method, 14 cases were cured; 18 markedly effective; 24 improved; and the total effective rate was 98.25 percent.

Case 3: Frozen shoulder (periarthritis humeroxcapularis)

Name, Liu x x; sex, female; age, 50; date of the first visit, March 28, 1979.

Complaints She suffered from right shoulder pain due to wind and damp, and the pain gradually got worse, especially at night. The movement of her shoulder was limited. No response was reached after various kind of treatments and she was transferred to our hospital. Examination: Her right arm could only lift to 100°; the left, 170°; abduction was 65° at the right side; 90° at the left; when the right hand turned backward and rotated internally, it could only touch her L1; left side to T5. There were tenderness points on her right acromion and interscapularis. The tongue coating was thin and yellow and the pulse was thready. In light of the differentiation and the pulse and symptoms observed, the syndrome was frozen shoulder, which was caused by the stagnation of cold and damp, and obstruction of qi and blood circulation of the Lung Meridian. The treatment was to dispel the cold and expel the dampness, promote the meridian and stop the pain.

Prescription Yinlingquan (Sp 9), Tiaokou (S 38) towards Chengshan (B 57), Jianyu (LI 15), Jianliao (SJ 14), Jianzhen (SI 9) and Quchi (LI 11).

Treatment procedure The heat-reinforcing method was used in needling Yinlingquan (Sp 9), Tiaokou (S 38) towards Chengshan (B 57) first. No retaining of the needle was needed; then Jianyu (LI 15), Jianliao (SJ 14), Jianzhen (SI 9) were needled (warm needling with one cone of moxa). After Quchi (LI 11) was needled five times, her shoulder pain was markedly alleviated. The pain disappeared and the patient recovered after fifteen treatments.

Explanation Periarthritis humeroscapularis falls within the range of Bi-syndrome in TCM. It is also called the frozen shoulder. Dr. Li realized that good effects can be obtained if the acupoints were selected according to differentiation on the meridians. When the points of the lower limbs were needled, the patient was ordered to move her upper limbs to elevate the therapeutic effects. Yinlingquan (Sp 9) is the He-Sea point of the Spleen Meridian, and has the function of dissipating the dampness and expelling the cold, promoting the movement of joints and articulations, strengthening the spleen and nourishing the muscle; Tiaokou (S 38) penetrating towards Chengshan (B 57) can dredge the meridian qi, dispel the frozen joints and stop the pain. These two points were selected from the meridian with the same name and they are also the experienced points for taking the points on the lower limbs to treat the illness on the upper limbs. In the early stage of frozen shoulder, if these two points are needled and the patient is ordered to lift the arm after the arrival of qi quicker results can be gained; Jianyu (LI 15), Jianliao (SJ 14) and Jianzhen (SI 9) (three famous points on the shoulder) are locally-selected points. Needling them can relax the tendon and muscle, activate the collaterals and stop the pain. If moxibustion is performed, it can warm and promote the meridian. Quchi (LI 11) is the point of the Large Intestine Meridian of Hand-Yangming where there is plenty of qi and blood in this meridian, so needling it can activate qi and promote blood circulation, dissipate the stasis and expel stagnation. When all these points are used together, it can expel dampness and cold, and promote the meridian. Of forty-two cases of frozen shoulder treated by acupuncture and moxibustion, 42 were cured; 34 markedly effective; 68 improved and the total effective rate was 94 percent. The therapeutic effect in the acupuncture-moxibustion group was better than that in the heat-reinforcing group, and the even-reinforcing and even-reducing group.

Case 4: Asthma (bronchial asthma)

Name, Chen x x; sex, male; age, 34; date of the first visit, November 9, 1963.

Complaints The patient had had asthma since September of 1954 following a cold. During the attack, he had dyspnea, with mouth opened and shoulder elevated, and he couldn't lie down. The attacks were more frequent and serious in autumn and winter. The asthma could be temporarily relieved after injection of aminophylline and epinephrine but couldn't be cured, so he was referred to our hospital to take the scarring moxibustion treatment. The patient was found to have cough and asthma, and inability to lie down, especially at night. He felt dry in the mouth, and was afraid of cold. He preferred hot drinks. He had three bowel movements a day. The physical examination revealed that his face was sallow. He had a pale tongue without any coating. His pulse was thready and rapid. His heart rate was 105/min., and his heart rhythm was regular. Moist rales was detectable in his right lung. Coarse lung markings were found on fluoroscopy. In the light of both pulse and symptoms observed, the syndrome was deficiency asthma, and deficiency of both lung and kidney. The patient should be treated to support the body resistance, benefit the lung and soothe asthma.

Prescription 1) Dazhui (Du 14), left Fengmen (B 12), right Feishu (B 13) and Tanzhong (Ren 17); 2) Right Fengmen (B 12), left Feishu (B 13) and Huagai (Ren 20).

Treatment procedure Scarring moxibustion was performed over the above-mentioned points. In the first treatment, Dazhui (Du 14), left Fengmen (B 12), right Feishu (B 13) and Tanzhong (Ren 17) were selected for moxibustion and good inflammatory reaction was obtained after the moxibustion. The moxa wound healed forty-five days later. After moxibustion, no attack was found for four months. In June, 1964 he suffered from asthma again due to a sudden change of weather. The symptoms were the same as mentioned above. So the second scarring moxibustion treatment was performed on July 16, 1964, and five cones were burned over the right Fengmen (B 12), left Feishu (B 13) and Huagai (Ren 20). No relapse was found in the follow-up visit for twenty years.

Explanation Dr. Li thought that the scarring moxibustion was better than any other method in the treatment of asthma. Since Dazhui (Du 14) is the crossing point of the yang qi of the whole body, and connects with the meridian qi of all the yang meridians, needling it can support the body resistance and eliminate the pathogenic factors; Feishu (B 13) is the place where the lung qi assembles, so needling it with moxibustion can open the inhibited lung qi and calm the breathing; Tanzhong (Ren 17) is the influentical point of qi, and it regulates qi of the whole body. So needling all these points with moxibustion can obtain good effects for asthma of the lung, spleen and kidney. Three hundred cases of asthma have been treated with scarring moxibustion with good short-term and long-term effects.

Case 5: Twisting of the eye and mouth (peripheral facial paralysis)

Name, Sun x x; sex, female; age, 56; date of the first visit, February 5, 1984.

Complaints The patient began to suffer from deviation of the mouth and eye nine days before and she thought that the disease might be caused by invasion of the wind and cold. As no response was found at the local hospital, she was referred to our department. She failed to close the right eye and had lacrimation, accompanied with chest distress and short breath. She had a history of coronary heart disease. Examination: Inability to raise the eyebrow and to close the eye, the palpebral fissure 0.2 cm, narrowing of the nasolabial groove, inability to show the teeth, thin yellow tongue coating, deep and thready pulse. In the light of both the pulse and symptoms observed, the syndrome is due to wind and cold invading the collaterals, and resulting in twisting of the mouth and eye. The principle of treatment was to warm the meridians and dispel the cold, expel the wind and activate the circulation of qi and blood.

Prescription External auricular meatus.

Treatment procedure Five moxa cones with the reed tube moxibustion were applied to the external auricular meatus once a day. The symptoms were alleviated after three treatments. When ten treatments in all were completed within twenty-one days, she could elevate her eyebrow, wrinkle her frontalis muscle, blow her cheeks, show her teeth and shrug her nose, and she could close her eyes completely.

Explanation The disease is mainly caused by weakness of body resistance, and invasion of the external wind and cold. The lesion lies in the crossing place of meridians. The reed tube moxibustion over the auditory meatus can offer the function of warming the meridians, dissipating the cold, expelling the wind and activating the circulation of qi and blood. This method is easy to carry out and the effect is reliable. The patient can treat the disease by himself.

Case 6: Herpes zoster

Name, Li x x; sex, female; age, 55; date of the first visit, March 16, 1985.

Complaints The patient had pain in the right lower limb and three pieces of red rashes appeared four days before. Because no response was found after numerous treatments, the patient was referred to our hospital. She complained of burning pain on the right lower extremity, which became aggravated at night, accompanied by restlessness, easily angered, dryness of the throat, and poor appetite. She had a history of diabetes, hypertension and nasopharyngeal carcinoma. Examination: Three pieces of red herpes at the right buttock, and external aspect of the thigh, and the largest being 3 x 2 cm^2, blood pressure 140/90 mmHg, thin yellow tongue coating, fine and rapid pulse. In the light of the pulse and symptoms observed, the diagnosis was herpes zoster due to damp-heat of the liver and gallbladder. The principle of treatment was to expel the damp-heat of the liver and gallbladder, and tranquilize the mind and check pain.

Prescription Auricle points for Liver, Kidney, Shenmen and Sciatic Nerve.

Treatment procedure Moxa sticks were applied over the above-mentioned points, five minutes for each point, twice daily. The pain disappeared after the first treatment and ten treatments in all were given. The patient was completely cured after fourteen days of treatment.

Explanation This illness occurs chiefly at the lumbar region, the head and face, and then the four extremities. The red and dry herpes were caused by the blood heat of the heart and liver; while the light and transparent, herpes resulted from the damp-heat of the spleen and lung. There were very few reports about the treatment with moxa stick on the auricle points. Three cases were treated by Dr. Li with rapid satisfactory results.

BLOODLETTING THERAPY AND SELECTING POINTS
—Yang Jiebin's Clinical Experience

Yang Jiebin was born on November 9, 1929, in Jintang County, Sichuan Province. He began to learn traditional Chinese medicine in his father's clinic when he was still a child, and then hung out his own shingle after graduation from the middle school. After the founding of the People's Republic of China, he was assigned to work in the Integrated Clinic, and then the People's Hospital in the county. Later, he was sent to study in the Teacher's Course of Chengdu College of Traditional Chinese Medicine, where he became a teacher after graduation in 1959. He was fortunate to learn from two famous doctors of traditional Chinese medicine, Wu Zhaoxian in Chongqing, and Pu Xiangcheng in northern Sichuan Province. He learned systematically from them the classics of traditional Chinese medicine, the knowledge of acupuncture and internal medicine, "Zi Wu Liu Zhu" (selection of points in terms of heavenly stems and earthly branches), and "Lin Gui Ba Fa" (selection of eight points from the eight extra meridians). Dr. Yang is good at acupuncture, and especially proficient at bloodletting therapy and selection of points. He has written more than thirty books and articles including *Theory of Meridians and Collaterals*, *Explanation to the Questions in Studying Acupuncture* and *A Brief Introduction to Zi Wu Liu Zhu*. At present, he is the director of the Acupuncture Clinic Teaching and Research Section of Chengdu College of Traditional Chinese Medicine.

I. Academic Characteristics and Medical Specialities

1. Bloodletting therapy

Dr. Yang is adept at bloodletting therapy, and considers it to be effective in eliminating exogenous pathogenic factors, inducing perspiration, draining heat and poison, expelling stagnation, removing obstruction from meridians, harmonizing qi and blood and activating blood. For some emergency, critical, or intractable cases, this method is extremely good. Dr. Yang often applies bloodletting therapy in treating more than thirty diseases including apoplexy, hypertension, epidemic influenza, ictero hepatitis, acute gastroenteritis, food poisoning, epilepsy, malaria, tonsillitis, abscesses, canker sore, leprosy and asthma. The methods are as follows:

1) *Pricking method* Using a three-edged needle or a thick filiform needle on the chosen area, prick the skin with a quick, deft motion, about 0.05 to 0.1 inch, allowing 0.5 to 1.0 ml of blood or 2.0 to 3.0 ml of blood in severe cases to be released.

2) *Piercing method* Insert a three-edged needle or a thick filiform needle perpendicularly about 0.5 inch, allowing 0.1 ml of blood to be released. The method is mainly used for a disease with deep location or for an area of thick musculature.

A male patient aged fourteen suffering from acute conjunctivitis had pain and swelling of the eyes for four days. Both eyes were swollen and had the appearance of two small peaches, accompanied by photophobia, profuse discharge from the eyes, visible blood capillaries in the white of the eyes, severe distending pain in the eye sockets and forehead, chills and fever. For treatment, Jingming (B 1), Apex (ear point) and Taiyang (Extra) were selected. Deep insertion was applied to Jingming (B 1), allowing the needling sensation to cover the entire eye. Bloodletting therapy, using a thick filiform needle, was applied to Taiyang (Extra) and Apex (ear point), 0.5 ml of blood was released from each point. Pain was greatly relieved after the treatment and the boy was cured after the second treatment. (Notes: Deep insertion and bloodletting therapy must be carefully applied at Jingming (B 1) point.)

Accurate selection of points is emphasized when Dr. Yang applies bloodletting therapy. The following examples are given to show his applications:

1) *Tense syndrome of windstroke* The principle of treatment is to soothe the liver, eliminate wind, and clear the mind. Prescription: The Wu Xin points (five-center points) are used. These include Baihui (Du 20) (center of vertex), Laogong (P 8) (centers of palms), and Yongquan (K 1) (centers of soles). For severe cases, Renzhong (Du 26), twelve Jing-Well points, Shixuan (Extra), Hegu (LI 4) and Taichong (Liv 3) are added. For rashes on the body, Quze (P 3) and Weizhong (B 40) could be pricked to cause bleeding so as to drain heat.

2) *Acute vomiting and diarrhoea* The principle of treatment is to eliminate heat and damp, regulate the middle jiao, and pacify qi going in the wrong direction. Shixuan (Extra), Weizhong (B 40), Quze (P 3), Neiting (S 44), Jinjin (Extra) and Yuye (Extra) are pricked to cause bleeding. Zusanli (S 36), Zhongwan (Ren 12), Neiguan (P 6) and Chengshan (B 57) are punctured with a thick needle.

3) *High fever due to disorders of qi and nutrients* The principle of treatment is to drain heat and fire, cool the blood and clear the mind. Baihui (Du 20), Zanzhu (B 2), Taiyang (Extra), Apex (ear point), Renzhong (Du 26), and the twelve Jing-Well points are pricked; Chize (L 5) and Weizhong (B 40) are punctured with a three-edged needle or a thick needle to cause bleeding. For quick effect, it is also good to needle between the spinous processes from Dazhui (Du 14) to Changqiang (Du 1).

4) *Numbness in the distal extremities* The principle of treatment is to eliminate wind and damp, activate blood and remove obstruction from the meridians. Hegu (LI 4), Taichong (Liv 3), Sifeng (Extra), Bafeng (Extra), Baxie (Extra), Waiguan (SJ 5), Yanglingquan (D 34) and the twelve Jing-Well points are needled. Points are also selected from the corresponding meridians, and local points are used according to symptoms. For local numbness, the diseased area may be tapped with a seven-star needle to cause bleeding. This will then be followed by cupping.

5) *Intractable itching of tinea* The principle of treatment is to disperse wind, tone blood and relieve dryness to stop itching. Quchi (LI 11), Xuehai (Sp 10), Hegu (LI 4), Shenmen (H 7), Sanyinjiao (Sp 6) and Neiguan (P 6) are pricked to cause bleeding. Scattered pricking with a seven-star needle over the diseased area may be combined with moxibustion, or else with cupping. For itching in the elbow or popliteal fossa, Chize (L 5) and Weizhong (B 40) may be pricked to cause bleeding in order to drain heat and

relieve itching. For itching in the palms, Shaofu (H 8) and Laogong (P 8) may be added to eliminate heat and relieve dryness.

6) *Asthma of the excess type* The principle of the treatment is to eliminate heat, induce perspiration and stop asthma. Shixuan (Extra), Weizhong (B 40), Chize (L 5), Tanzhong (Ren 17), Tiantu (Ren 22), Renzhong (Du 26), Shaoshang (L 11) and Shangyang (LI 1) are pricked to cause bleeding. Dazhui (Du 14), Dingchuan (Extra) and Taiyuan (L 9) are cupped after needling to release 1.0 to 1.5 ml of blood from each point.

7) *Acute and subacute hepatic necrosis* The principle of treatment is to eliminate heat, relieve jaundice, cool the blood and expel poisons. Dazhui (Du 14), Zhiyang (Du 9), Ganshu (B 18), Danshu (B 19), Zhongchong (P 9), Shixuan (Extra), Taichong (Liv 3) and Wangu (SI 4) are pricked quickly, releasing more than 0.5 ml of blood from each point.

2. Selection of specific points according to principles

1) *Adept in selecting specific points* Dr. Yang often selects specific points according to symptoms. For example, his method of pricking the Jing-Well points of each meridian for acute febrile diseases or intractable itching and numbness is effective in clearing the mind, draining heat and removing obstruction from the meridians. For disorders of the stomach and intestines, the Lower He-Sea Points, Front-Mu points and the influential point of the Fu organs are often punctured to maintain a free flow of qi and a normal function of ascending and descending. For disorders of the five zang organs, the Yuan-Source points, Back-Shu points and Luo-Connecting points of the corresponding meridian may be selected, and combined with the Xi-(Cleft) points for prolonged diseases. This method will tone the essential qi of zang-fu organs and remove obstruction from the meridians. Following the theory that a disease usually occurs along the course of a meridian, points are selected from the affected meridian. Dr. Yang believes that selection of points from corresponding meridians, combined with local and distal points, is an important principle in orthodox acupuncture treatment.

It should also be mentioned that Dr. Yang is able to intelligently select the proper points among Zusanli (S 36), Neiting (S 44), Quchi (LI 11), Hegu (LI 4), Weizhong (B 40), Chengshan (B 57), Taichong (Liv 3), Kunlun (B 60), Huantiao (G 30), Yanglingquan (G 34), Tongli (H 5), Neiguan (P 6), Gongsun (Sp 4), Waiguan (SJ 5), Houxi (SI 3), Shenmai (B 62), Zhaohai (K 6) and Linqi (G 41), which are also included in the eight Confluent points and twelve Heaven Star points. These points are considered as important points in treating various diseases. The twelve Heaven Star points are located on the Seven-Heaven Meridians of the human body, which relate to the twelve regular meridians. It is said that the functions of the 365 regular points are generalized by the twelve Heaven Star Points, and that therefore they are the key points in regulating the functions of zang-fu organs. The eight Confluent points, located on the regular meridians and connecting with the extra meridians, are effective in regulating the balance of yin and yang, strengthening the functions of the zang-fu organs and harmonizing qi and blood. The experience of the acupuncturists through the ages has shown that these points are highly effective and to be recommended.

2) *Combination of points by applying the dan method and the jie method* Ma Danyang, a well-known acupuncturist of the Jin Dynasty, once said: "The *dan* method or *jie* method may be used when appropriate." Later, in the Ming Dynasty, this was further explained by Wang Ji that: "The jie method implies that one point is selected; whereas the dan method denotes two points, one selected from the hand, and the other from the foot, which may be used bilaterally." Dr. Yang agrees with this explanation and believes the dan and jie methods are just combinations of points selected from the upper or lower portions of the body, used either unilaterally or bilaterally. These methods are applied clinically in three ways:

a. In combination with the twelve Heaven Star points: For toothache, the selection of Hegu (LI 4) bilaterally is considered as the dan method, and the selection of Hegu (LI 4) unilaterally is the jie method. For infantile convulsion, the selection of Hegu (LI 4) bilaterally, combined with Taichong (Liv 3), unilaterally is referred to as a combination of points with the method of upper dan and lower jie.

b. In combination with the eight Confluent points: For disorders of the heart, chest and stomach, Neiguan bilaterally, combined with Gongsun (Sp 4) unilaterally, is regarded as a combination of upper dan and lower jie. For rigidity and pain of the neck, Shenmai (B 62) bilaterally, combined with Houxi (SI 3) unilaterally, is recognized as a combination of upper jie and lower dan.

c. Combination of points from the same meridian: Selecting points from the ends of a meridian is considered the dan method, while selecting one point from the middle of a meridian is the jie method. For example, in the case of arm pain, the selection of Jianyu (LI 15) and Hegu (LI 4) is referred to as the dan method, whereas selection of Quchi (LI 11) is considered as the jie method. For leg pain, the selection of Huantiao (G 30) and Qiuxu (G 40) is taken as the dan method, whereas the selection of Yanglingquan (G 34) is recognized as the jie method. For asthma, selecting Tiantu (Ren 22) and Qihai (Ren 6) is dan, while selecting Tanzhong (Ren 17) is jie. For migraine, selecting Tongziliao (G 1) and Zuqiaoyin (G 44) is dan, and selecting Fengchi (G 20) is jie. Dr. Yang points out that the changes of the number of points in dan and jie methods seem to be significant. For instance, when the methods are used in combination with the eight Confluent points or the twelve Heaven Star points, the therapeutic effect of these points is especially good, particularly if the proper reinforcing and reducing methods are applied. As written by Yang Jizhou: "The stubborn disease may be cured if the dan or jie methods are used in treatment."

3) *Combination of points for the paired meridians* The paired meridians with the same name are generalizations of the twelve regular meridians. These include Taiyin Meridians of Hand and Foot, Jueyin Meridians of Hand and Foot, Shaoyin Meridians of Hand and Foot, Yangming Meridians of Hand and Foot, Shaoyang Meridians of Hand and Foot, and Taiyang Meridians of Hand and Foot. These six pairs of meridians connect and communicate with each other on the head and face or on the upper part of the body. Selecting one point from each of two paired meridians and using them as paired points in the clinic are considered a combination of points from the paired meridians with the same name. In theory, the function of the paired meridians is relatively similar. Modern research has shown that the needling sensation will usually propagate between the paired

meridians. It is said that the paired meridians with the same name connect with each other. Dr. Yang often pairs one of the eight Confluent points with one of twelve Heaven Star points on the basis of the principle of combining points from the paired meridians with the same name. For example, Neiguan (P 6) Taichong (Liv 3) from the Jueyin meridians of Hand and Foot are selected to treat hypertension, dizziness and vertigo. Hegu (LI 4) and Neiting (S 44) from the Yangming Meridians of Hand and Foot are selected to treat toothache due to stomach fire. Houxi (LI 3) and Weizhong (B 40) from the Taiyang Meridians of Hand and Foot are selected to treat shoulder and back pain. These above paired points have an excellent therapeutic effect. In addition, Shaoshang (L 11) and Yinbai (Sp 1) from the Taiyin Meridians of Hand and Foot are used to treat mania. Shenmen (H 7) and Taixi (K 3) from the Shaoyin Meridians of Hand and Foot are used to treat insomnia due to disharmony between the heart and kidney. Zhigou (SJ 6) and Yanglingquan (G 34) from the Shaoyang Meridians of Hand and Foot are selected to treat chest and hypochondriac pain. All of these points are selected according to the principle of combining points from the paired meridians with the same name. These prescriptions are effective and have been tested over many treatments.

II. Case Analysis

Case 1: Sunstroke

Name, Xia x x; sex, female; age, 24; date of the first visit, July 15, 1965.

Complaints Earlier that morning, she fainted suddenly on the way home after a hurried shopping trip under a hot sun. Clinical manifestations included disturbance of the mind, severe headache, restlessness, rough breathing, capillaries visible in the white of the eye, extreme thirst, profuse sweating, nausea, scanty dark-red urine, yellow sticky tongue coating, and soft, rapid pulse. Body temperature was 41°C. The diagnosis was injury of the heart and mind by heat. The principle of treatment is to clear the mind and drain summer heat.

Prescription Shaoshang (L 11), Shangyang (LI 1), Zhongchong (P 9), Taiyang (Extra), Zanzhu (B 2), Hegu (LI 4), Weizhong (B 40), Quze (P 3).

Treatment procedure Hegu (LI 4) was punctured forcefully with a filiform needle, and all other points were pricked with a three-edged needle, with 0.5 to 0.1 ml of dark purple blood was squeezed out. The patient was also advised to drink as much water as possible. Ten minutes after needling, the patient improved. One hour later, the fever subsided, the pulse became normal and sweating ceased. All the symptoms were alleviated and the patient went home alone.

Explanation Sunstroke should be treated first with the principle of clearing the mind and eliminating summer heat. Dr. Yang prefers to use the bloodletting method in the first treatment. For a severe case of sunstroke, Dr. Yang often pricks the Wuxin (Five Centers) points (Baihui (Du 20), bilateral Laogong (P 8) and bilateral Yongquan (K 1)), Renzhong (Du 26), and Shixuan (Extra) may also be combined.

Case 2: Hiccup

Name, Yang x x; sex, male; age, 30; date of the first visit; March 29, 1986.

Complaints Eleven days before, hiccups appeared immediately after eating noodles for lunch, which became worse and worse, even disturbing his sleep at night. He could not control the hiccuping, even though he was taking pills and injections of ritalin and diazepam. He was admitted into the hospital on March 26. Clinical examination showed a healthy body build, suffering expression, frequent strong hiccups which never stopped even at night, short and rapid breathing, stomach distension, sour regurgitation, stretching pain in the head, chest and hypochondriac regions, thin, white tongue coating, and a string-taut and slippery pulse. The diagnosis was upward attack of stomach qi. The principle of treatment is to strengthen the stomach and pacify the qi going in the wrong direction.

Prescription Zhongwan (Ren 12), Neiguan (P 6), Zusanli (S 36), Tanzhong (Ren 17), Geshu (B 17).

Treatment procedure All of the above points were forcefully punctured, using a gauge 28 filiform needle and the reducing method. The needles were retained for half an hour, and manipulated once every three minutes during that time. After withdrawing the needles from Tanzhong (Ren 17), Geshu (B 17) and Zhongwan (Ren 12), the cupping method was applied until the skin colour turned purplish. Ten minutes after treatments, the hiccup improved markedly, and stopped completely half an hour later. The patient slept soundly for ten hours that night. There was no recurrence of the condition during one week's observation, and the patient was subsequently discharged from the hospital.

Explanation Hiccup is usually caused by irregular food intake which injures the spleen and stomach, resulting in the upward movement of the rebellious qi. It is often spontaneously relieved, or may be cured by some folk methods. This particular case, however, involved hiccup for eleven days which had not improved by taking drugs and herbal medicine. It was a rare case. In ancient medical books, descriptions of treatment for hiccup include: "Moxibustion on Zhongwan (Ren 12) and Guanyuan (Ren 4) with a hundred moxa cones," and "For hiccup, drugs are not effective, while moxibustion on Zhongwan (Ren 12), Tanzhong (Ren 17) and Qimen (Liv 14) is definitely effective." Dr. Yang synthesizes these two methods into his own method. He selects Zhongwan (Ren 12), the Front-Mu Point of the stomach, Zusanli (S 36) and Neiguan (P 6) to ease the middle jiao, pacify the qi going in the wrong direction and stop the hiccuping. Tanzhong (Ren 17) is considered as the sea of qi and Geshu (B 17) is the influential point of blood. Puncturing these two points will regulate the balance of yin and yang, smooth qi and activate the blood. This prescription, which aims at regulating and is directed to the cause of the disease, is usually effective.

Case 3: Hypochondriac pain

Name, Chen x x; sex, female; age, 63; date of the first visit, June 26, 1980.

Complaints She reported that at midnight on June 6, she suddenly had a severe hypochondriac pain on the right side. This pain, which radiated to the back and lumbar region, was aggravated by breathing, coughing and turning the body. She went to the hospital as an emergency case, where she was treated as a case of chest pain, since the

X-ray examination was normal. Sedative drugs and gentamycin were given, and herbal medicine was also added the next day. However, the disease improved only slightly during the past twenty days, so the patient had come to visit Dr. Yang. On examination, she had a rosy face with a suffering expression, restlessness, dizziness, tinnitus, marked tenderness between the third through the seventh ribs on the right side of the chest, slightly red tongue with little coating, and string-taut, tense pulse. Diagnosis: Stagnation of liver qi. Principle of treatment: Regulate qi and stop pain.

Prescription Zhigou (SJ 6), Yanglingquan (G 34), Rugen (S 18), Tianchi (P 1).

Treatment procedure Zhigou (SJ 6) and Yanglingquan (G 34) were punctured with a filiform needle with the reducing method. The needles were then manipulated once every five minutes, and retained for thirty minutes. The cupping method was then applied to Rugen (S 18) and Tianchi (P 1) for fifteen minutes. The condition was improved after the first treatment.

Explanation Dr. Yang is particularly good at selecting the paired points which are highly effective. The selection of Zhigou (SJ 6) and Yanglingquan (G 34) for hypochondriac pain has proved effective even in ancient times. However, Dr. Yang understands the selection of these two points is the combination of points from the paired meridians with the same name, since both of the points are from the Shaoyang Meridians.

STUDIES OF SELECTION OF POINTS, COMBINATION OF POINTS AND THE MANIPULATIONS

—Yang Jiasan's Clinical Experience

Dr. Yang Jiasan was born in Wujin County, Jiangsu Province on January 2, 1919. He was very interested in medicine in his childhood and learned from Dr. Wu Bingsen. After his apprentice he followed a famous acupuncturist Cheng Dan'an to learn acupuncture. In 1936, he graduated from the China Wuxi Acupuncture Training Course, and since then has been practising medicine in Wujin County, Jiangsu Province. For more than fifty years, Dr. Yang has contributed a great deal to the study of the location of the Shu points, the clinical indicating features, the combination of acupoints and manipulations of acupuncture and moxibustion. He adopted and brought forth a lot of new ideas. He was the editor-in-chief of the book *The Shu Points*. Based on the book *Yang Jiasan's Experience in Selection of Acupoints* the film *Methodology in Selection of Acupoints* won the second class award of the Ministry of Public Health in 1985. In 1962, working together with Mr. Yue Meizhong, he cured the former President of Indonesia Sukarno's disease with traditional Chinese herbs and acupuncture. Now he is standing member of Beijing College of Traditional Chinese Medicine, deputy chairman of the Academic Committee, member of the Standing Committee of the All-China Acupuncture Association, member of the Medical Science Association of the Ministry of Public Health. He was a representative of the Third National People's Conference and member of the fifth and sixth Chinese People's Political Consultative Conference.

I. Academic Characteristics and Medical Specialities

1. Exploring and summerizing the rules for selecting the points

In the 1950s according to the acupuncture literature of past dynasties, and after a careful examination and research on the distribution of the acupoints on the fourteen meridians, Dr. Yang edited and published *A Hanging Chart of the Acupoints*. It is one of the earliest hanging charts published in China after liberation. It is not only a vivid diagrammatic material for acupuncture teaching and clinical practice, but also a valuable academic literature for location of the Shu points. In the 1960s, Dr. Yang combined the experiences of all the famous acupuncturists in selecting the points with what he had learned in clinic and teaching for several decades, and wrote a book *Atlas for Clinical Location of Acupoints*, in which the methods for locating 189 commonly used points, especially the methods for locating some important acupoints were introduced. His characteristics in locating the points are based on the surface anatomical landmarks and the simple methods are used as much as possible. In 1979, the book *Yang Jiasan's*

Experience in Locating Points was published. It was a systematic conclusion of Dr. Yang's method of selecting points. In the book the surface anatomical landmarks are regarded as the key points. In combination with the bone-length measurement, the adjacent points are classified according to the meridians and regions, and then comparison and location are done. On the basis of analysing and defining the distribution and characteristics of the acupoints of the fourteen meridians, he summarized the various rules for locating the acupoints. The method is easy to learn and remember, so it is useful both in clinical practice and teaching. Following is the explanation of the location of different points on the three Yin meridians of the Hand.

1) *The finger tip portion* Points can be located at the finger tip and the root of the nail. At the finger tip: Locate Zhongchong (P 9) at the finger tip of the middle finger. At the root of the nail: Locate Shaoshang (L 11) at the radial aspect of the root of the thumb nail (i.e. the internal side, pertaining to yin); and Shaochong (H 9) at the root of the nail of the radial aspect of the small finger.

2) *The metacarpophalangeal joint portion* Locate the points at the posterior aspect of the metacarpophalangeal joint. For example, Yuji (L 10) is located at the posterior aspect of the first metacarpophalangeal joint and at the radial side of the first metacarpal bone; Laogong (P 8) is located at the posterior aspect of the third metacarpophalangeal joint and at the radial aspect of the third metacarpal bone; and Shaofu (H 8) is located at the posterior aspect of the fifth metacarpophalangeal joint and at the radial side of the fifth metacarpal bone.

3) *The wrist portion* Two bones, two tendons and one transverse crease. Two bones refer to the os triguetrum and os pisiforme, two tendons refer to the palmaris longus and flexor carpi radialis, and one transverse crease refers to the first transverse crease behind the palm. Taiyuan (L 9) is located at the lower border of the radial aspect of os triguetrum, Shenmen (H 7) at the radial aspect of os pisiforme, and Daling (P 7) is located between the two tendons. These three points are all at the first transverse crease behind the palm.

4) *The forearm portion* Points can be located beside the bone, beside the tendon and between the tendons. "Beside the bone" refers to the border of the radial bone and the styloid process of the radius; "beside the tendon" refers to the radial side of the tendon flexor carpi ulnaris; and "between the two tendons" means between the tendon palmaris longus and the flexor carpi radialis. Beside the bone: Jingqu (B 64) is located beside the palmar aspect of the highest point of the styloid process of the radius; Kongzui (L 6) is located at the ulnar side of the radius, and 7 cun superior to the first crease of the posterior aspect of the palm. Beside the tendon: Lingdao (H 4), Tongli (H 5), Yinxi (H 6) and Shenmen (H 7) points are located at the radial side of the tendon flexor carpi ulnaris, and 0.5 cun apart from each other. Between the tendons: Ximen (P 4), Jianshi (P 5), Neiguan (P 6) and Daling (P 7) points are located between the tendon palmaris longus and flexor carpi radialis. Daling (P 7) is situated at the transverse crease of the wrist, Neiguan (P 6) is located 2 cun above the transverse crease of the wrist, and Jianshi (P 5) and Ximen (P 4) are located 3 and 5 cun above this crease respectively.

5) *The elbow joint portion* The points should be located at the transverse crease, at the end of the crease and on both sides of the tendon. For example, Chize (L 5) is located

at the radial side of the tendon biceps on the transverse crease of the elbow, Quze (P 3) is located beside the ulnar aspect, and Shaohai (H 3) is located at the end of the transverse crease of the ulnar aspect of the elbow when the elbow is flexed.

6) *Upper arm portion* Points are located at one muscle and between the two sulci. One muscle refers to the biceps and two sulci to the sulci at the radial side and ulnar side of biceps. Tianquan (P 2) is located 2 cun below the end of anterior axiliary crease and between the biceps, Tianfu (L 3) and Xiabai (L 4) are located at the radial aspect of the biceps, and 3 and 4 cun respectively below the end of anterior axiliary crease; and Qingling (H 2) located at the ulnar sulcus of the biceps, and 3 cun above the medial condyle of the humerus.

2. The characteristics, indications and application of the Five Shu Points

Dr. Yang holds that there are not only rules for the distribution of the five Shu points and the infusing depth of the meridian qi, but there are also the different characteristics of the needling sensations. In general, the Jing-Well point has sharp pain; the Ying-Spring point has sensitive pain; the Shu-Stream point has pain distension and soreness; the Jing-River point has distension and soreness; and the He-Sea point has soreness, distension, numbness and referring pain. Therefore, common regulations in the indications may be followed. Dr. Yang advocates that the indicating function of the five Shu points should be combined with the pathogenesis of the five zang organs and be utilized according to the differentiation: The indicating action of the five Shu points: The Jing-Well points are related to the liver, and able to disperse the depressed liver qi and eliminate the wind, regulate qi and dissipate the depression, dredge the meridians and connect qi, and induce resuscitation. The Ying-Spring points are related to the heart, and able to clear and tranquilize the mind, reduce the heat and cool the blood; the Shu-Stream points are related to the spleen, and able to strengthen the spleen and stomach, and transport the water and eliminate the dampness; the Jing-River points are related to the lung, and able to strengthen the dispersing function of the lung and dispel the exogenous pathogenic factors from the body surface, stop coughing and descend the perverted qi; and the He-Sea points are related to the kidney and able to regulate the kidney and nourish yin, and treat the stomach. The application of the five Shu Points is chiefly based on the disorders of the twelve meridians. Through the four diagnostic methods, the involved meridian should be determined and then the disorders of the meridians or disorders of zang-fu organs should be understood. In the light of the chief indications of the five Shu points and the pathogenesis, the points are selected and the auxiliary points are added according to the conditions of the disease. Here is the example for the Lung Meridian of Hand-Taiyin:

1) *Manifestations* a. Diseases of the meridians: Chest pain, cough due to cold, swelling pain of the supraclavicular fossa, sore throat, cold and pain of the shoulder and back, or fever with sweating, pain at the radial side of the arm, cold arm, and burning sensation in the palms. b. Visceral disease: Cough due to internal injury, asthma, hemoptysis, distension of the lung, irritability, difficulty in urination, edema, or frequent urination, changes of the urine color, loose stools.

2) *Selection of points according to differentiation* a. For the excess syndrome of the meridian, the Ying-Spring point Yuji (L 10) is selected; while for the deficiency syndrome, the Shu-Stream point Taiyuan (L 9) is selected; for syndromes of the viscera, the Jing-River point Jingqu (L 8) is selected. If the disease is complicated with fullness of the upper abdomen or without fullness of the upper abdomen, but with liver disease, the Jing-Well point Shaoshang (L 11) is added; if complicated with body heat or without body heat, but with heart disease, the Ying-Spring point Yuji (L 10) is added; if complicated with joint pain or without joint pain but with spleen symptoms, the Shu-Stream point Taiyuan (L 9) is added; and if with adverse flowing of qi or without adverse flowing of qi, but with kidney symptoms, the He-Sea point Chize (L 5) is added.

As to the treatment of the external meridian diseases, according to "Ying-Spring and Shu-Stream points for external meridian diseases" stated in *Miraculous Pivot*, the Ying-Spring point Yuji (L 10) which is related to the heart should be selected with the reducing method (bleeding) for such Hand-Taiyin external meridian excess syndromes as cough due to cold, sore throat, red swelling, and pain along the meridian, while for such deficiency syndromes as cold and numbness on the areas where the meridian passes, the Shu-Stream point Taiyuan (L 9) which is related to the spleen and connected with the primary qi should be selected with the reinforcing method (moxibustion is advisable). In case of the excess syndromes of the Hand-Yangming external meridian such as fever, aversion to cold, nasal disorders, toothache, deviation of the mouth and nose, skin disease and red swelling on the area where the meridian passes, the Ying-Spring point Erjian (LI 2) should be used with the reducing method; while for deficiency syndromes such as the dysfunction of the index finger, numbness and cold on the area where the meridian passes, the Shu-Stream point Sanjian (LI 3) is preferable with moxibustion.

For zang-fu syndromes, the corresponding five Shu points should be selected. For the disease of Hand-Taiyin Lung, the corresponding Jing-River point Jingqu (L 8) is selected to disperse the lung and descend qi. If the both internal and external meridians are affected, the disease should be treated both internally and externally, so that the Jing-River point Jingqu (L 8) and Shu-Stream point Taiyuan (L 9) or Ying-Spring point Yuji (L 10) should be selected. Shaoshang (L 11) will be added for those complicated with liver syndromes, because Shaoshang (L 11) is not only related to the Lung Meridian, but also is the Jing-Well point of the five Shu Points which is related to the liver. When this point is needled, it can not only soothe the liver and regulate qi, but also treat the lung and liver simultaneously, Yuji (L 10) is added if complicated with heart syndrome because Yuji (L 10) is the Ying-Spring point of the Lung Meridian, and is related to the heart. It is able to reduce heat and cool blood, and to treat lung and heart simultaneously. Taiyuan (L 9) is added if complicated with spleen diseases, because it is the Shu-Stream point of the Lung Meridian, and related to the spleen. As its function is to strengthen the spleen and resolve the dampness, it can regulate both the lung and spleen. Chize (L 5) is added if kidney disease is involved, because it is the He-Sea point of the Lung Meridian and related to the kidney. Its function is to descend the perverted qi and nourish the kidney, both the lung and kidney are considered.

As with the other twelve meridians, the involved meridian should be first determined, followed by point selection and then the reinforcing or reducing method. The characteristics of this diagnostic method are to combine the treating principle of the place where the meridian passes for indication with the therapeutic function of the five Shu points so as to define the longitudinally diseased meridian and locate transversely the position with the indication of the five Shu points, thus the range of indications is expanded.

3. Inserting the filiform needle with one hand

The method of one-handed insertion is a new technique which was put forward by Dr. Yang in his clinical and teaching practice. Taking the advantages from the method of inserting the needle with both hands, he uses one hand instead of the penetrating hand and pressing hand. During the treatment the operation is performed completely with the right hand, and the left hand holds the needles for use. There are four ways of inserting the needle: a. the hanging and pressing way (or pressing way), b. the pressing with inclined angles (or inclined pressing way), c. the twisting and pressing way, and d. the continuous pressing way. The details are as follows:

1) *The hanging and pressing way* a. Holding the needle: Hold the handle of the needle with the right thumb and index finger, and the middle finger supporting the needle body, and the ring and small fingers holding the lower part of the needle, leaving the tip 0.05 cun exposed. In case a long needle is used, hold the needle body with the thumb and index fingers of the right hand moving downward. b. inserting the needle: Hang the hand which holds the needle, and keep the tip of the needle 2 cun away from the skin. The angle between the needle and the skin is about 90°. Point exactly to the acupoint and insert the needle quickly into the skin with a downward pressure. This method is applicable to most points and all kinds of filiform needles of various lengths. This method is suitable to those points such as Hegu (LI 4), Quchi (LI 11), Shousanli (LI 10), Waiguan (SJ 5), Zusanli (S 36), Sanyinjiao (Sp 6) on the four extremities and abdomen where the muscles are thick and flat in case the perpendicular or deep insertion is required. c. Chief points for manipulation: The distance between the tip of the needle and the skin should be suitable, generally about 2 cun. If the distance is too large, the point will not be easily punctured and the downward pressing will be heavy to cause pain. If it is too short, the insertion of the needle will be blocked because of the insufficient pressing force, and this may also cause pain. In addition, the exposed needle tip must not be too long, but should be at the same line with the lower border of the finger, about 0.05 cun. If it is too long, the tip of needle will directly reach the deep muscular layer, resulting in difficulty in regulating qi and in manipulating the needle because the needle body can easily bend. Due to the pressing force of the thumb and index finger, the depth of needling can reach 0.2 to 0.3 cun which can penetrate completely through the skin or the superficial layer of the muscle, although the needle is only 0.05 cun exposed.

2) *The inclined pressing way* a. Holding the needle: There are two methods: When perpendicular insertion is performed, the method is the same as the pressing method; and when the oblique insertion is needed, hold the handle of the needle with the thumb and index fingers of the right hand, support the needle body with the other three fingers, keeping the needle tip at the same level with the lower border of the small finger. b.

Inserting the needle: For perpendicular insertion, a 75° angle is needed between the needle body and the skin surface. The ring and small fingers can be used to press lightly the both sides of the point to make the skin taut. Then point the needle tip to the acupoint, and internally rotate the wrist, rapidly turn the angle from 75° to 90°, and penetrate the needle into subcutaneous tissue with a downward pressure. For oblique insertion, the angle between the needle and the skin is 90°. The small finger is used to press the skin lightly to make it taut, the tip of needle should be directed to the acupoint. Then internally rotate the wrist, at an angle from 90° to 110°, and insert the needle quickly into the subcutaneous tissue. This method is suitable for all points of the body, especially for the points on the abdomen (where the skin is loose and wrinkles are available). One cun to 1.5 cun filiform needle is suitable for the perpendicular, oblique or superficial insertion. c. Main points for the manipulation: For perpendicular insertions, the angle between the needle body and the skin surface should be around 75°. If the angle is too small, the longer distance of the needle tip to the acupoint will cause difficult insertion and the pressure produced by the angle change may be too big and cause pain. If the angle is too large, the downward pressure produced by the angle turning will be not enough to insert the needle to the required depth. In addition, during the oblique insertion, the angle is quickly turned from 90° to 110°, so when the needle tip penetrates the skin, the gesture and angle will be suitable for oblique insertion. The turning of the angles should be quick rather than slow. The internal rotation of the wrist should be flexible and natural. Quick insertion of the needle will produce less pain. But for certain important acupoints, such as Jingming (B 1) point, the insertion should not be too quick, because it is situated very close to the eyeball, where there are abundant blood vessels. The method of holding the needle with the inclined pressing method is different from that of the hanging and pressing method. For oblique insertion, the lower end of needle body is not held by the ring and small fingers. If the small finger is held inside, it will hinder the needle body turning from 90° to 110° in the oblique insertion. During the perpendicular insertion, the ring and small fingers should press both sides of the point slightly, while in the case of oblique insertion, the small finger should press the skin to make it taut, in order to facilitate the insertion.

3) *Twisting and pressing method*, a. Holding the needle: Make the thumb about 0.4 cun anterior to the index finger, and hold the needle handle together with the index finger and the other three fingers. The needling technique is the same as that for the hanging and pressing method. b. Inserting the needle: The angle will be 90° in case of perpendicular insertion, and 45° or 135° in case of oblique insertion. In perpendicular insertion, the ring and small fingers should be used to press slightly the skin near the point. In 45° oblique insertion, press the skin around the acupoint slightly with the ring finger (the small finger not touching the skin) and in 135° oblique insertion, the tip of the small and ring fingers can be used to press the skin near the point lightly. Then, put the needle tip on the point, and quickly insert the needle by twisting the needle handle backward and downward with the thumb, and the needle tip will penetrate the skin. b. Chief points for manipulation: The needle is inserted into the skin chiefly by the force produced by the thumb and index finger when they are used to twist the needle handle backward and downward. The insertion will be quick and cause less pain if the force of the fingers big

enough. So more exercises should be done to train the finger strength. This method depends chiefly on the twisting, i.e. twisting with downward pressing, however, repeated twisting should be avoided. The angle of twisting is quite large when this method is performed, so that thumb should be placed 0.4 cun perpendicular on the index finger in holding the needle handle. After the twisting, the thumb tip should withdraw backward to 0.2 cun on the index finger. The twisting angle should be increased as much as possible. This method is suitable for the 1.5 cun filiform needle, and is applicable to the points on the thin subcutaneous region or points at the tendon or the bone, such as Lieque (L 7), Kunlun (B 60), Dubi (S 35), Neiguan (P 6), Zhongzhu (K 15). It can also be applied to the points on the chest or on the back where the important viscerae are located.

4) *The continuous pressing method* a. Holding the needle: Hold the needle handle with the right thumb and index finger with the middle, ring and small fingers, supporting the needle body. The needle tip is at the same level with the lower border of the small finger. b. Inserting the needle: There are subcutaneous insertion and intradermal insertion: In case of subcutaneous insertion, the angle between the needle body and the skin surface should be 165°, with the ring and small fingers pressing the skin of the point tightly. Touch the needle tip lightly on the point, and quickly insert the needle into the skin subcutaneously with the finger force and wrist force. Then press the needle downward several times until the needle reaches the affected area. In case of intradermal insertion, the small, ring and middle fingers should all press the skin surface tightly and the angle between the needle body and the skin surface is about 170°. The needle is inserted into the skin by using the same method. c. Chief points for manipulation: Since this is subcutaneous insertion and intradermal insertion, the angle between the needle body and the skin should be quite large (165° and 170° respectively). During the manipulation, when the wrist which holds the needle rotates internally, the posture and angle required will be in position. During insertion the local pain is very sensitive, and the insertion is rather difficult. Therefore, the pressing force on the skin by the middle, ring and small fingers should be increased. These three fingers, which play the role of the pressing hand, can prevent the skin from sliding on the bone surface and help fix the points. After the needle is inserted into the skin, continuous and even force should be applied to press the needle two to three times to the expected depth. Neither interrupted pressing nor one pressure is applied. Otherwise, the manipulation will be stiff and too heavy. The method is usually applicable to the points on the head, or face where the skin and muscle are thin and superficial, such as Sishencong (Extra 6), Shangxing (Du 23), Baihui (Du 20), Touwei (S 8), Shuaigu (G 8), and Sizhukong (SJ 23) and is used for various syndromes which can be treated with subcutaneous or intradermal insertion.

4. Manipulation of the needle and flexible application of reinforcing and reducing method

The manipulation of the needling includes promoting qi, waiting for qi, manipulating qi and retaining qi. Different manipulations may be applied to stimulate qi and promote the arrival of qi in case of failure to get the needling sensation after inserting the needle. This process is called promoting qi. Qi still fails to arrive after promoting, retains the needle to wait for the arrival of qi, and five minutes later perform the promoting method again. This is called the waiting for qi method. After the arrival of qi, in order to radiate qi to the remote region or to the affected area, the different manipulations are performed, this is called manipulating qi. Once the qi arrives, the needle is retained in the required depth and angle to keep the qi gathering in the meridian. This is called retaining qi. After that, regulating qi (the reinforcing or reducing method) should be carried out on the basis of the retaining qi method.

Inspired by the saying recorded in *Miraculous Pivot* that, "slow insertion and slow withdrawal of the needle is the method of leading qi. Both the reinforcing and reducing methods are to prevent the essential qi," Dr. Yang put forward the idea of the manipulation values for the essential qi. He said that in a sense, acupuncture therapy is a therapy for the treatment of trauma. Rough needling shall in no case be applied not only on the head, neck and trunk, but also on the extremities. There had been a case where numbness lasted for a lifetime when Neiguan (P 6) was needled. Therefore, the needling sensation is by no means the bigger, the better. The stimulating amount should be suitable. In a word, prevent the essential qi from being damaged, and the meridian qi should be stimulated as much as possible. In addition, the depth for manipulation should be taken into consideration, which will depend on the arrival of qi. If qi fails to arrive, lift the needle and manipulate it from superficial to deep again. Dr. Yang uses four words to explain the basic manipulations as "short and small, quick and slow." "Short" means that the distance between the lifting and thrusting is short; "small" means that the twisting angle is small; "quick" means that the frequency for lifting, thrusting, twisting and rotating is quick, lifting, thrusting, twisting and rotating are applied simultaneously, forming a compound method, and "slow" means that the insertion of the needle is slow when applying short, small, quick maneuvres for lifting, thrusting, twisting and rotating. According to the clinical experience, the injury of the tissues can be avoided and the quick arrival of qi is ensured by using Dr. Yang's method. It also facilitates the performance of retaining qi and manipulating qi. Dr. Yang holds that the reinforcing and reducing should attach importance to the selection of points and the necessary needling apparatus in addition to the general needling techniques. The theory, method, acupoints, needle apparatus and technique are closely related and should be considered as a whole. Each is correlated with the reinforcing and reducing, but the "technique" lies in the last. Therefore, reinforcing and reducing should be applied dialectically. For example, the spleen deficiency should be treated differently. For the patient with spleen yang deficiency, the method should be to tone the Hand-Jueyin Neiguan (P 6), selected in combination with Xinshu (B 15). The reinforcing method should be used in combination with moxibustion. In case of qi deficiency complicated with dampness, the method should be to reinforce qi and eliminate dampness. The Yuan-Source point of Foot-Taiyin, Taibai (Sp 3) in combination with Qihai (Ren 6) is needled with the reinforcing method. In case of spleen deficiency and liver hyperactivity, the method used should be to support the earth and restrain the wood. The Front-Mu point of the spleen and the Confluent point of zang Zhangmen (Liv 13) should be selected in combination with Yiny-Spring point of the Liver Meridian, Xingjian (Liv 2) with the reducing method; in case of spleen deficiency complicated with qi stagnation, the method should be to regulate the stomach and remove the stagnation from fu organs. Zhongwan (Ren 12) the Front-Mu and the Influential point of fu is selected in combination with Tianshu (S 25), the Front-Mu point of the large intestine and Zusanli (S 36), the Lower-He point of the Stomach Meridian with reducing method. Although these cases all belong to the spleen deficiency, the cause and mechanism of the disease are different, the method and prescription of acupoints are different, as are the reinforcing and reducing methods. Among the five Shu points, the Jing-Well and Ying-Spring points incline to reducing and the Yuan-Source and Front-Mu points incline to reinforcing. The Lower He-Sea points are used chiefly to treat the fu syndrome and it inclines to reducing. The Shu points in the chest, abdomen, back and lower back tend to treat the Yang syndromes (the fu, heat, and excess syndromes); the Back-Shu points tend to treat the Yin syndromes (zang, cold and deficiency syndromes). The Shu points below the chest, abdomen and the umbilicus tend to tonify the deficiency. As to the methods of acupuncture and moxibustion, the former inclines to the reducing and the latter inclines to the reinforcing; as to the needle instruments, the three-edged needle for bleeding has a function of reducing, the plum-blossom needle inclines to reinforcing, and the filiform needle can be served for the purpose of both. The ancient nine needles have different functions and their reinforcing and reducing features are clear. As to the quantity of the stimulation (it depends upon the density of the points selected, the strength of the manipulation, times of needling, duration of retaining the needles), the heavy stimulation inclines to reducing, and the light stimulation inclines to reinforcing; as to the selection and prescription of points, the combination of the shu points can evidently influence the therapeutic effect of the prescription. For example, Hegu (LI 4), the Yuan-Source point of the Hand-Yangming of the Large Intestine, is the chief point in regulating qi. If it is combined with Quchi (LI 11), it can reduce the heat, dispel the wind, activate the blood and release the muscle spasm. This is an important method to regulate the upper jiao. If it is combined with Sanyinjiao (Sp 6), it can regulate qi, nourish the blood, regulate menstruation and stimulate lactation. This is an important prescription for gynecological disorders. If it is combined with Neiting (S 44), it can reduce heat, stop nausea and vomiting and regulate the stomach. If it is combined with Taichong (Liv 3), it can soothe the liver and dispel wind, dredge the meridians and stop the pain. The techniques of reinforcing and reducing in acupuncture are various, and different actions can result from different methods. For example, Hegu (LI 4) and Fuliu (K 7) can either induce the sweat or stop it if a different kind of maneuvre is performed; Hegu (LI 4) and Sanyinjiao (Sp 6) can be used either to induce abortion or to protect the fetus according to different manipulations. In conclusion, the application of the reinforcing and reducing methods in acupuncture is determined by different factors. If any aspect is neglected, it will influence the effect of regulating qi. Of course, correct differentiation and definite character (excess or deficiency) of the disease are the premise of the reinforcing and reducing, because it is a fundamental rule not only for acupuncture, but also for all fields of traditional Chinese medicine.

5. Use of the head points, and flexible combination of the Yuan-Source points

1) *Application of the Shu points on the head and neck* Dr. Yang uses the Shu points

on the head and neck in a very broad range. According to our incomplete statistics, he can treat more than forty kinds of diseases which are involved in internal medicine, surgery, gynecology, pediatrics, and ENT. He once treated an old woman who had suffered from hyperactive liver-fire, lassitude and anxiety. She fell suddenly into a coma with stiffness of the tongue and aphasia, salivation, incontinence of urine, and dystrophy of the right hand. Dr. Yang took such points on the head as Fengchi (G 20), Fengfu (Du 16), Yamen (Du 15), Baihui (Du 20), Qianding (Du 21), Houding (Du 19), Tongtian (B 7) and Shenting (Du 24). She improved markedly within ten days. In treating windstroke, Dr. Yang always follows a general principle, that is, to soothe the liver and diminish the wind. According to the pathological conditions, and the principle of "in emergency case treat the acute symptoms first, when these being relieved treat its root cause." The two prescriptions took the points on the head, Baihui (Du 20), Tongtian (B 7), Qianding (Du 21), Houding (Du 19) or Fengchi (G 20), Fengfu (Du 16), Tianzhu (B 10) were taken as the chief points. In case of aphasia, Yamen (Du 15) and Fengfu (Du 16) are selected; for loss of consciousness, Shenting (Du 24) and Benshen (G 13) selected; for dysphagia, Fengfu (Du 16) and Lianquan (Ren 23) selected; for dizziness, Tianzhu (B 10) and Yifeng (SJ 17) selected; for tremor, Naokong (G 19) and Naohu (Du 17) selected; for hemianopsia, Shuaigu (G 8) penetrating Luxi (SJ 19) selected. Besides the above-mentioned windstroke, the most commonly seen internal wind are epilepsy, convulsion, liver wind, migraine, thunder-headache, alopecia areata, internal oculopathy depression and mania. The diseases caused by the external wind include wind-cold, rheumatics, wind heat, sun stroke, infantile convulsion, urticaria and acute epidemic febrile diseases. In treating all these diseases, Dr. Yang always chooses Fengchi (G 20), Fengfu (Du 16) and Baihui (Du 20) as the chief points; if it is combined with mental problems, Shenting (Du 24) and Benshen (G 13) are added, because he thinks Fengchi (G 20) and Fengfu (Du 16) are the general points in treating wind; and Shenting (Du 24) and Benshen (G 13) are important points in treating mental disorder. These four points are all named according to their specialities. Baihui (Du 20) can elevate the clear qi and soothe the liver and dispel the wind, and is the first important point on the head. For example, Dr. Yang once treated a young girl who was introverted. She could not concentrate, and suffered from insomnia, dizziness and anorexia with acoustic and visual hallucinations because of too much stress from her studies. No response was revealed after she had taken Western drugs for two months. Examination: Yellow complexion, sluggish eyesight, distension of the upper abdomen, constipation, red tip of the tongue, yellow greasy tongue coating, string-taut, thready and slippery pulse. Differentiation: Epilepsy. Prescription: Baihui (Du 20), Fengchi (G 20), Shenting (Du 24), Benshen (G 13), Sishencong (Extra 6), in combination with Neiguan (P 6), Gongsun (Sp 4), Zhongwan (Ren 12) and Zusanli (S 36). She was recovered and returned to school after over twenty treatments. Another case was an old man who was suffering from a bad cold. Examination: Aversion to cold, fever, anhidrosis, headache, absence of thirst, nasal obstruction, itching of the throat, coughing, and lassitude, thin white tongue coating, deep pulse. Differentiation: Yang deficiency and attack by the exogeneous pathogenic cold. Shangxing (Du 23), Baihui (Du 20), Fengfu (Du 16), Fengchi (G 20), Fengmen (G 12), Dazhui (Du 14) (with moxibustion) were selected to restore the Yang and expel the pathogenic factors, eliminate the wind and remove the cold. He was cured after the second treatment.

2) *The combination of the Yuan-Source points* Dr. Yang thinks that the Yuan-Source points are the places where the primary qi of the Sanjiao passes and is retained. Therefore, the Yuan-Source point can not only expel the pathogenic factors, but also tonify the deficiency and support the body resistance. Needling the Yuan-Source points can promote the flow of the primary qi of Sanjiao so as to irritate the primary qi to maintain the body resistance and defend against the pathogenic factors. They are often used coordinately with some specific points. a. Combination with the Yuan-Source point of zang-fu organs: This is a point combination of the Yuan-Source points of five zang organs and six fu organs, yin and yang, upper and lower. It is suitable for the diseases of the internal organs which are mainly reflected on the superficial organs. The points of the Yin Meridians are chiefly for the internal organ diseases and the points of the Yang Meridian are chiefly for the disease of the superficial organs. Under the condition when the internal organ diseases are mainly reflected on the superficial organs, the Yuan-Source points of the Yin Meridians should be selected in combination with the Yuan-Source points of the Yang Meridian to strengthen the effects. The principle of the combination: Shaoyin combined with Shaoyang, Taiyin with Taiyang, and Jueyin with Yangming, that is, the points on the upper extremities should correspond with those on the lower extremities, and the Yin Meridian should correspond with the Yang Meridian. For example, for dizziness and vertigo caused by yin deficiency leading to liver hyperactivity, or the spasm of hands and feet due to the injury of the liver by depression and anger, although the disease is chiefly in the liver, the symptoms are mostly reflected on the head, eyes and the four extremities. Therefore the Yuan-Source point Taichong (Liv 3) of the Liver Meridian of Foot-Jueyin should be selected in combination with the Yuan-Source point Hegu (LI 4) of the Large Intestine Meridian. The combination of these two points is called the "Four Passes," which nourish the blood, regulate the qi, pacify the liver, diminish the wind, promote the meridian and expel the dampness. b. Combination of the Yuan-Source points and the Back-Shu points: This is to combine the Yuan-Source points of the zang-fu organs with the corresponding Back-Shu points, therefore, the common characteristics of the Yuan-Source points and the Back-Shu points could work in coordination to strengthen the therapeutic effects. It is suitable for various yin syndromes (including interior, deficiency and cold syndromes). As to the indication properties, the Yuan-Source points can support the body resistance and expel pathogenic factors, and the Back-Shu points are inclined to be used to treat yin diseases. The combined use of these two points can treat various deficiency syndromes of the zang-fu organs. c. Combination of the Yuan-Source points and the Luo-Connecting points: It can be divided into combination of the Yuan-Source points and the Luo-Connecting points of exteriorly-interiorly related meridians and combination of the Yuan-Source points and the Luo-Connecting points of the same meridian, that is to select the Yuan-Source points and the Luo-Connecting points from the same upper or lower extremities. The combination of the Yuan-Source and Luo-Connecting points of the externally and internally related meridians is suitable for diseases of certain meridians or those complicated with externally related meridians or internally related meridians. The

method of combination of points is as follows: If a meridian is affected, the Yuan-Source point of the involved meridian should be taken as the main point in combination with the Luo-Connecting point of the related internal and external meridians. Because we take the Yuan-Source point as the main point and the Luo-Connecting point as the secondary point, it is also called the combination of chief Yuan-Source and secondary Luo-Connecting point. For example, if cough, asthma, and dyspnea appear in the Lung Meridian of Hand-Taiyin, accompanied with toothache and incontinence of stool of the Large Intestine Meridian of Hand-Yangming, Yaiyuan (L 9), the Yuan Source point of the Lung Meridian should be selected as the main point in combination with Pianli (LI 6), the Luo-Connecting point of the Large Intestine Meridian. Based on the principle; disease at the early stage will affect the meridian and prolonged disease usually affects the collaterals and persistent disease results in deficiency. Dr. Yang thinks that in treating chronic diseases caused by internal injury or exogeneous pathogenic factors, the Yuan-Source point is selected, and simultaneously combined with the Luo-Connecting point of the meridian. For example the persistent cough is treated by penetrating the Yuan Source point Taiyuan (L 9) towards the Luo-Connecting point Lieque (L 7) of the Lung Meridian; palpitation and chest pain are treated by penetrating the Yuan-Source point Daling (P 7) towards the Luo-Connecting point Neiguan (P 6) of the Pericardium Meridian. Usually the therapeutic effect is satisfactory. d. Combination of the Yuan-Source point with the He-Sea points: It can be divided into the combination of the Yuan-Source point with He-Sea point of the external and internally-related meridians and combination of these points of the same meridians or the different collaterals. For the combination of the Yuan-Source point with the He-Sea point of the external and internally-related meridians, the Yuan-Source point of yin meridian (interior) and the He-Sea or Lower He-Sea point of the yang meridian (exterior) are usually selected. For example, nausea, vomiting, abdominal distension and diarrhoea caused by the dysfunction of the spleen and the stomach can be treated by selecting the Yuan-Source point Taibai (Sp 3) of the Spleen Meridian in combination with the He-Sea point Zusanli (S 36) of the Stomach Meridian to strengthen the spleen and stomach, elevate the clearance and descend the turbidity. For combination of the Yuan-Source point with He-Sea point of the same meridian, the Yuan-Source point Hegu (LI 4) of the Large Intestine Meridian of Hand-Yangming in combination with He-Sea point Quchi (LI 11), can treat such diseases caused by the wind-heat as headache and ophthalmic pain, toothache and swelling of the gum, dryness of the throat and epistaxis. It is a wonderful method in regulating both the qi and blood, and clearing the upper jiao, also, the Yuan-Source point Taichong (Liv 3) of the Liver Meridian of Foot-Jueyin in combination with the He-Sea point Ququan (Liv 8) can treat hernia and swelling pain of the penis. Its function is to regulate the deficiency of yin, relax the tendons and stop pain. For combination of the Yuan-Source point with the He-Sea point of different meridians, the Yuan-Source point Hegu (LI 4) of the Large Intestine Meridian of Hand-Yangming in combination with the He-Sea point Zusanli (S 36) of the Stomach Meridian of Foot-Yangming can regulate the gastro-intestinal tract, dissipate stagnation and promote defecation; also, the Yuan-Source point Taichong (Liv 3) of the

Liver Meridian of Foot-Jueyin in combination with the He-Sea point Zusanli (S 36) of the Stomach Meridian of Foot-Yangming is an experienced prescription in treating gastric pain, chest pain, and irritability by soothing the liver and harmanizing the stomach.

II. Case Analysis

Case 1: Pharyngitis

Name, Hou x x; sex, female; age, 31; date of the first visit, December 25, 1984.

Complaints She had suffered from chronic pharyngitis for many years, and the symptoms were sometimes mild and sometimes serious for two years. Recently it became worse because of a cold, and she suffered from pain and swelling of the throat, dryness of the mouth, and had a sensation of a foreign body in the throat when she came to the hospital. She had a fever, aversion to cold, nasal obstruction, flushed face, headache, sore throat, thirst, preference for cold drinks, cough, yellow and sticky sputum, constipation, normal appetite, thin and white coating, red tongue, superficial and rapid pulse. Examination: Temperature 37.8°C, congestion of the pharyngeal mucus, the lymph follicle of the posterior wall of the pharynx was red with slight congestion of the uvula. In this case, the symptoms such as swelling and pain of the pharynx and larynx, complicated with fever and aversion to cold, and the superficial and rapid pulse were due to wind-heat invading the lung. Differentiation: Excess syndrome of the Hand-Taiyin. Treatment should be given to disperse the lung qi and dispel the exogeneous pathogenic factors.

Prescription Yuji (L 10), Shaoshang (L 11) and Fengchi (G 20).

Treatment procedure The reducing method was carried out on these three points. A three-edged needle was used to bleed at Yuji (L 10) and Shaoshang (L 11) points. Fengchi (G 20) was needled with moderate stimulation without retaining the needle once a day. The pain stopped after the first treatment, and the swelling subsided after the second treatment. She was cured after three treatments.

Explanation In this case, as the wind and heat invaded the lung, sore throat appeared, pertaining to excess syndrome of Hang-Taiyin. According to the differentiation of the five Shu points, the Ying-Spring point Yuji (L 10) was selected to reduce the heat and facilitate the pharynx, the Jing-Well point Shaoshang (L 11) was selected to expel the wind and dissipate the nodule; Fengchi (G 20) was added to expel the wind and promote sweating, eliminate the swelling and stop the pain.

Case 2: Wandering Bi-syndrome

Name, Lin x x; sex, female; age, 58; date of the first visit, September 25, 1985.

Complaints She was attacked by wind-cold last autumn, then she had pain in the small joints, but the pain was not fixed, and the pain gradually affected the elbow, knee and hip joints. It was diagnosed as rheumatoid arthritis in one hospital. When she visited Dr. Yang, the finger joints were slightly swollen, deformed and contracted and movement of the knee joints was slightly limited. She couldn't walk long distances due to the joint pain. She got tired easily and was weak. Sallow complexion, abdominal distension, loose stool, spontaneous coating, pale tongue, greasy and slight yellow tongue coating, string-taut and thready pulse. Differentiation: Wandering Bi-syndrome. The treatment was directed to expel wind and nourish the blood, to dissipate cold and resolve the dampness and dredge the meridians.

Prescription Fengchi (G 20), Fengfu (Du 16), Geshu (B 17), Hegu (LI 4), Taichong (Liv 3), Ashi (moxibustion), Dazhui (Du 14) and Taibai (Sp 3).

Treatment procedure The reducing method was used at Fengchi (G 20), Fengfu (Du 16) and Huge (LI 4) with slightly strong stimulation, and the reinforcing method used at Geshu (B 17), Taibai (Sp 3), Dazhui (Du 14) and Taichong (Liv 3) with retention of the needle for twenty minutes. Treat once a day. After three treatments, the joint pain was alleviated and the spontaneous sweating disappeared. After more than thirty treatments, the complexion became rosy, the spirit was good, and she could walk faster than before and the joint pain disappeared. She was advised to take some medicinal herbs to consolidate the effect.

Explanation Both Fengchi (G 20) and Fengfu (Du 16) points are good in treating the wind. When they are used together with Geshu (B 17), a point of blood, it follows the principle: If you want to treat the wind, you must treat the blood first because when the blood circulation is promoted, the wind will be diminished. Taichong (Liv 3) is the Yuan-Source point of the Liver Meridian and is also a Shu point of the spleen. It is able to regulate the liver, strengthen the spleen and expel dampness. When it is combined with the Yuan-Source point Hegu (LI 4) of the Large Intestine Meridian of Hand-Yangming, it is the combination of Yuan-Source point of zang-fu organs, which has the function of expelling the wind and dissipating dampness, dredging the meridians and stopping the pain. As the patient had complications of spleen deficiency and weak external yang, Dazhui (Du 14) of the Du Meridian was added to facilitate yang, expel the cold and consolidate the exterior; the Yuan-Source point Taibai (Sp 3) of the Spleen Meridian was added to strengthen the spleen and expel the dampness. Good effects were obtained through the combination of the above points.

Case 3: Hiccup

Name, Li x x; sex, male; age, 65; date of the first visit, April 13, 1985.

Complaints Because the patient suffered from headache, fever, aversion to cold and coughing, he was diagnosed as having a common cold. He took some tetracycline to treat the disease by himself. Before long, he had hiccups. It was diagnosed as spasm of the diaphragm in another hospital. There was no response after he took Western drugs. Then he had insomnia and anorexia because of the uncontrollable hiccup. He vomited what he had eaten with purplish mucus, accompanied by lassitude, discontinuous breathing, epigastric palpitation, which was relieved on pressure, clear urine, loose stool, thin white tongue coating, pale tongue and weak pulse. Differentiation: Deficiency of the primary qi and disharmony of the lung and stomach. The treatment was to reinforce the primary qi, harmonize the stomach and the lung.

Prescription Jingqu (L 8) penetrating Taiyuan (L 9), Daling (P 7) penetrating Neiguan (P 6), Gongsun (Sp 4) penetrating Taibai (Sp 3), Zusanli (S 36) penetrating

Shangjuxu (S 37).

Treatment procedure Every point was penetrated along the skin with the reinforcing method and the needle was retained for twenty minutes. Treat once a day. The hiccup stopped at the same night and he began to have a good appetite as well as sleep. After the second treatment, the hiccup improved a great deal and he was cured after the third treatment.

Explanation Taiyuan (L 9) and Jingqu (L 8) are the Yuan-Source point and Jing-River point of the Lung Meridian respectively; Daling (P 7) and Neiguan (P 6) are the combination of the Yuan-Source and Luo-Connecting points of the Jueyin Meridian. They can reinforce the primary qi, calm the lung and tranquilize the mind. When the Yuan-Source point Taibai (Sp 3) is penetrated towards Gongsun (Sp 4) of the Spleen Meridian and the He-Sea point Zusanli (S 36) of the Stomach Meridian penetrated towards the Lower He-Sea point Shangjuxu (S 37) of the large intestine, they can strengthen the spleen and regulate the stomach, elevate the clearance and descend the turbidity. This prescription emphasizes the function of the primary qi of sanjiao. The Yuan-Source point of the kidney in combination with the Luo-Connecting point and Jing-River point can treat lung and stomach simultaneously, and regulate the spleen and kidney at the same time.

Case 4: Enuresis

Name, Wang x x; sex, male; age, 9; date of the first visit, August 14, 1986.

Complaints He had suffered from enuresis since childhood, one to three times per night. He couldn't wake up after being called. Examination: Listlessness, sallow complexion, delicate constitution, scanty yellow urine, pale tongue proper, flabby tongue body, thready and weak pulse. Differentiation: Deficiency of the kidney qi and imbalance of yin and yang. The treatment was directed to reinforce the kidney qi and regulate yin and yang.

Prescription Lieque (L 7), Zhaohai (K 6), Shenting (Du 24) and Benshen (G 13).

Treatment procedure The reinforcing method was used on the above four points. Shenting (Du 24) and Benshen (G 13) were needled subcutaneously. Light stimulation was given and the needles were retained for twenty minutes. Treat once a day. He had no more enuresis after two treatments. After needling for two weeks, he was ordered to take "Jingui Shenqi Pills" to consolidate the therapeutic effects.

Explanation Lieque (L 7) communicates with the Ren Meridian and Zhaohai (K 6) communicates with the Yinqiao Meridian. These two points are the Confluent Points of the eight meridians. Lieque (L 7) is also the Luo-Connecting point of the lung. Water can be generated, so it can reinforce the kidney qi. When Zhaohai (K 6) of Yinqiao is selected in combination with Shenting (Du 24) of the Du Meridian, and Benshen (G 13) of the Shaoyang Meridian, it can support yang and inhibit yin, refresh the mind and strengthen the brain.

Case 5: Abdominal distension after operation

Name, Zhang x x; sex, male; date of the first visit, June 8, 1960.

Complaints He suffered from slight abdominal distension and pain around the operative wound with difficult respiration after his left nephedectomy due to kidny stone one day before. Then the abdominal distension was aggravated with dyspnea and anorexia. His tongue coating was white and greasy. The pulse was string-taut. Differentiation: Damage of the kidney qi after operation, and water failing to nourish wood, and wood attacking the earth reversely. The abdominal distension was caused by the dysfunction of the spleen and the stomach. The principle of treatment should be to strengthen the water and to nourish the wood, and to strengthen the spleen.

Prescription Taixi (K 3), Zusanli (S 36), Zhigou (SJ 6), Yanglingquan (G 34) and Tianshu (S 25).

Treatment procedure The reinforcing method was used at Taixi (K 3) and Zusanli (S 36), and reducing was applied at Zhigou (SJ 6), Yanglingquan (G 34) and Tianshu (S 25) with moderate stimulation. Retain the needles for fifteen minutes. The intestine flatus could be discharged from the anus one hour after the needling. The abdominal distension was basically relieved and the respiration was restored to normal after two treatments. The symptoms vanished after three treatments.

Explanation Taixi (K 3) is the Yuan-Source point of the Kidney Meridian and functions to reinforce the kidney qi, and nourish the water to irrigate the wood. Yanglingquan (G 34) is the He-Sea point of the Gallbladder Meridian. Zhigou (SJ 6) is the Jing-River point of the Sanjiao. The combination of these two points can pacify the liver and regulate qi and remove the stagnation. When the He-Sea point Zusanli (S 36) of the Stomach Meridian and the Front-Mu point Tianshu (S 25) of the large intestine were added, they can regulate the stomach and the intestine, and strengthen the spleen. When the kidney qi is sufficient, the earth and wood are harmonized, the turbid qi descends and the clear qi ascends. Then the abdominal distension is eliminated.

Case 6: Pain after operation

Name, Zhai x x; sex, male; age, 26; date of the first visit, May 11, 1960.

Complaints The patient had suffered from osteomyelitis of his left leg since 1954. The attack occurred every year and there were ulcer and pus at his interior and exterior aspect of the thigh. The attack in 1958 resulted in a high fever and limitation of the movement of the left lower limb. He was restrained in bed for eight months with rigidity of the knee. The sinus over the wound refused to heal. The X-ray film taken on May 16, 1960 showed numerous cavities and plenty of dead bone fragments. After debridement, he felt severe pain which was hard to tolerate. When Dr. Yang saw him on June 8, the patient cried due to severe pain. The pulse was string-taut and strong.

Differentiation Deficiency of kidney water, wood fire burning inside, and excess of the toxic heat. The principle of treatment was to nourish the kidney and to replenish the marrow, and remove the toxic heat.

Prescription Taixi (K 3), Juegu (G 39), Xingjian (Liv 2) and Futu (LI 18).

Treatment procedure Reinforcing was applied on Taixi (K 3) and Juegu (G 39), and the reducing method was used at Xingjian (Liv 2) and Futu (LI 18) with strong stimulation. The needles were retained for fifteen minutes. The pain was stopped immediately after the needling.

Explanation Taixi (K 3) is the Yuan-Source point of Kidney Meridian, and Juegu

(G 39) is the point of thc Gallbladder Meridian, and is also the point of marrow. The kidney controls the bone and produces marrow, and Shaoyang dominates the bone disease. When these two points are used together, it can nourish the kidney and replenish the marrow to treat its root cause. Xingjian (Liv 2) is the Ying-Spring point of the Liver Meridian and belongs to fire. When used with the local Futu (LI 18), it can remove the toxic heat and treat the symptoms.

FIVE STEPS IN DIFFERENTIATION AND MULTIPLE SHALLOW NEEDLING

—He Shuhuai's Clinical Experience

He Shuhuai was born in a famous TCM family at Zhengding County, Hebei Province, in 1937. In 1957, he enrolled at Beijing College of Traditional Chinese Medicine, and was assigned to work in the Acupuncture Department of the affiliated hospital after graduation. He has experience in the application of the syndrome differentiation, especially proficient in treating windstroke, headache, Bi-syndrome, asthma and facial paralysis. He advocates needling superficially with more points. Thus widening the indications of Huatuojiaji and Ashi points. He wrote dozens of papers and compiled *Acupuncture and Moxibustion in Clinical Practice*, and *Acupuncture*. He is now the director of the Acupuncture and Tuina Department and the Teaching room of the Acupuncture Therapy of Beijing College of Traditional Chinese Medicine, and associate professor, and standing member of the China Association of Acupuncture-Moxibustion.

I. Academic Characteristics and Medical Specialities

1. Five steps in differentiation in acupuncture and moxibustion

Dr. He holds that differentiation in acupuncture and moxibustion should proceed in five steps.

1) *Locating according to zang-fu and meridian* This is to determine the location of the disease according to TCM theory of zang-fu organs and meridians in combination with the signs and symptoms of the patient. Diagnosis is very important in acupuncture treatment, as treating methods vary according to the location of the illness. It is the first step in differentiation.

a. Location according to the position of the lesion: For this method, the location chiefly accords to the running course of the meridian and zang-fu organ to which it pertains. Since the twelve meridians pertain to zang-fu organs internally, and communicate with the extremities and organs externally, they all have fixed running courses and communicating relations. So the locating diagnosis can be made according to the combination of the position of the disease. For example, headache may be differentiated into Shaoyang, Yangming, Taiyang and Jueyin syndrome according to different locations of the disease and the running course of the meridians. Another example is head and neck pain. Shaoyang and Taiyang are clinically differentiated according to the motor disturbance and the location of pain. If the Taiyang meridian is involved, the pain should be located at the nape and back because it runs from the vertex to the brain, diverting from the neck, and running along the medial aspect of the shoulder and arm. Since the Shaoyang meridian is distributed at both sides of the neck, the Hand-Shaoyang turns round to the neck behind the auricle, and Foot-Shaoyang travels along the neck in front of the Hand-Shaoyang meridian. The neck pain should be located at the lateral aspect of the neck and if the patient fails to turn the head, this is largely due to the disorder of the Shaoyang Meridian. In addition, the ear problems are mostly related to the diseases on the Foot-Shaoyin and Shaoyang meridians, because the Foot-Shaoyin pertains to the kidney interiorly and opens to the ear. The collateral of Hand-Shaoyang goes around the ear and enters the ear, and so does the collateral of Foot-Shaoyang. Gingivitis is usually related to Yangming and Foot-Taiyin Meridians. This is because the Hand-Yangming Meridian enters the lower teeth and the Foot-Yangming Meridian enters the upper teeth. The Foot-Taiyang Meridian pertains to the spleen internally, and dominates the muscles, so the disorder of the tooth and gum is related to them. Ophthalmic diseases are chiefly related to the Foot-Jueyin, Taiyang and Shaoyang Meridians. Bilateral hypochondriac pain is usually related to the Foot-Jueyin and Foot-Shaoyang Meridians, because the Foot-Shaoyang Meridian pertains to the gallbladder and is connected with the liver, passing along the hypochondriac region, and the Foot-Jueyin Meridian pertains to the liver and connects with the gallbladder, running upward to the diaphragm and distributing to the hypochondriac and costal region.

b. Location according to the characteristics of the symptoms. This means that if the same symptoms or sign occurs at a different part of the body, the location can be made according to the running course of the meridians. But if similar symptoms occur at the same position, the location should be found together with other symptoms. For example, a sore throat may be located either at the Lung Meridian of Hand-Taiyin or the Kidney Meridian of Foot-Shaoyin, because these two meridians both pass through the larynx. Whether the disease pertains to the lung or kidney, the location should also refer to the type of pain. Severe pain mainly pertains to the Lung Meridian of Hand-Taiyin, while mild pain chiefly pertains to the Kidney Meridian of Foot-Shaoyin. Sore throat with swelling mainly belongs to the lung and that without swelling refers to the kidney; the pain with a short course of illness is mainly due to the lung, and that with a long duration chiefly pertains to the kidney; sore throat accompanied with cough is usually due to the lung and sore throat combined with soreness of the lower back, and seminal emission is mainly due to the kidney. For this we can see that if the same symptoms occur at the same position, and at the same time two or more organs are involved, the location will have to be done in combination with the characteristics of the syndrome and zang-fu organs.

c. Location based on the physiological function of zang-fu organs. According to TCM theory, zang-fu organs and the meridians have their own functional characteristics. Clinically the location can be carried out according to the functional characteristics of the zang-fu organs.

d. Location in combination with the etiology: In clinical practice, location can also be carried out based on the etiology. For example, wind can be divided into external wind and internal wind. External wind is usually the cause of the illness resulting from the exogenous pathogenic factors and is mostly related to the Lung Meridian of Hand-

Taiyin, while the internal wind is chiefly caused by the hyperactivity of the liver yang and is mainly related to the Liver Meridian of Foot-Jueyin. Cold can be divided into external cold and internal cold. If the external cold invades the body surface, the location may be at the lung. The external cold can also directly invade zang-fu organs such as the middle jiao, where vomiting and diarrhoea will result. In this case, the location is in the intestine and stomach. Internal cold is mainly due to deficiency of yang, and the cold is produced from inside. This can be located according to the characteristics of the zang-fu organs. In case of aversion to cold, chest and back pain, cough, asthma and dyspnea, the location should be at the heart and lung. For abdominal distension and loose stool, cold extremities, vomiting of clear water, the location should be at the kidney. Summer-heat is caused by the qi of the fire heat, so it is very easy to invade the pericardium; besides, summer-heat is easily associated with dampness which is mainly related to the spleen and stomach, so location for summer-heat is usually in the pericardium, spleen and stomach. Dampness can be divided into internal dampness and external dampness. No matter what kind of dampness it is, the location can be considered to be in the spleen. External factors can influence the internal factors. For Example, overexcitment may lead to disorder of the heart, anger may harm the liver, too much thinking may injure the spleen, grief may damage the lung, fear may hurt the kidney.

2) *Determination of the nature* Determination of the nature means to determine the nature of the illness according to the various manifestations of the patient. Great attention has been paid to this problem for many dynasties. It is stated in *Miraculous Pivot* that "in acupuncture treatment, it is necessary to examine the excess and deficiency of meridians first, and then touch along the meridians and press them, and snap them in order to elicit their responses, and then apply the appropriate method of treatment." It is said again in the *Miraculous Pivot* that "in order to find out the location of the pain, one should examine the cold and heat sensation and determine the affected meridian." The method is performed according to the eight principles, based on the symptoms and signs as well as the causes of the illness, to make a comprehensive analysis and classification to determine whether the disease belongs to yin or yang, heat or cold, deficiency or excess.

3) *Combination of the location and determination of the nature* After determining the location of the disease and the nature of the syndrome, these two aspects should be combined. The aim is based on TCM theory to find out the causes of the disease, differentiate the nature of the disease, and observe the position and its changes, so as to differentiate and recognize the disease accurately. For example, with palpitation, short breath, spontaneous sweating, which became worse after exertion, pallor, pale tongue proper, white coating and weak pulse, the location should be at the heart, and deficiency syndrome (deficiency of either yang or yin) should be differentiated because all these are manifested in hypofunction. In combination of the location with determination of the nature, it may be deficiency of the heart qi or deficiency of the heart yang. Diseases of the meridian are the same to those of the viscera. For example, if the pain of the knee joint often occurs at the lateral side, and becomes worse after fatigue, disliking wind but liking warmth, the location will be at Shaoyang and the nature belongs to deficiency-cold. In combination of these two, weakness of qi and blood of the Shaoyang Meridian and

short nourishment of the tendons and vessels are differentiated.

4) *Differentiation of the root cause and the symptoms* According to the record in *Plain Questions*, "Each disease has its symptoms and root cause." The symptoms and the root causes reflect the relation between the primary and secondary pathological changes of a disease, excess or deficiency of the body resistance and the pathogenic factors, and the interrelationship between the etiology and the symptoms. They are regarded as the basis of acupuncture treatment in clinical practice. Therefore it is very important to distinguish the root cause from the symptoms of an illness. The manifestations and changes of the disease are complicated. So only after we know the essence of the illness from the complicated changes and find out which pathological changes in the zang-fu organ and meridian plays a main role, can we determine a suitable therapeutic method. First of all, we have to analyse whether the illness is due to the affection of its original meridian or zang-fu organ. If only the involved meridian is affected, the treatment should be directed to treat the qi of the involved meridian. The disease of a zang may be influenced by the involved zang or by other zang organs. For example, gastric pain and vomiting can be caused by dysfunction of the stomach or by the liver. The root cause is at the liver, but the symptoms appear in the stomach.

5) *Treatment method* From the above analysis, after the location and the nature of the illness are determined, the key point of the disease is grasped through pathological analysis, and the root cause and the symptoms of the disease are determined, the next step will be to selecte a suitable method of treatment. The disease may be treated either by acupuncture or moxibustion, either with reinforcing or reducing to dredge the meridians, regulate qi and blood, balance the yin and yang, and recover the function of zang-fu organs. Then the disease will be cured.

The following is an example: A female, thirty-one years old, paid her first visit to the doctor on December 21, 1981. She complained of toothache on the left side for three days. The patient had received acupuncture treatment on Hegu (LI 4) and Xiaguan (S 7) in a local hospital, but the result was not good, even the pain-killers had no effect. Examination: Severe pain of the left upper and lower teeth which affected the head of the same side, accompanied by dry and bitter mouth, distension pain on both hypochondriac regions, oppressed chest, fullness in the epigastrium, yellow tongue coating, and string-taut and rapid pulse. According to the analysis in five steps, the main manifestations were at the gum, gastric region and hypochondrium. Based on the theory that Yangming meridian enters the upper and lower teeth, and Jueyin meridian is distributed at the hypochondrium region, the disease was located in the liver and stomach. According to the analysis with the Eight Principles, severe toothache, dry and bitter mouth, yellow tongue coating and rapid pulse were the heat-excess syndrome. In combination with the location and the nature of the illness, the disease was heat-excess in the liver and stomach, which was caused by anger and anxiety attacking the liver, which produced heat attacking transversely the middle jiao and disturbing upward along the meridian. So, the root cause of this disease was in the liver, but its symptoms were in the stomach. The treatment should be to reduce the liver-fire and stomach-fire, treating the root cause and the symptoms simultaneously. The Foot-Jueyin was selected as chief meridian and the Yangming meridian as the secondary. Taichong (Liv 3), Hegu (LI 4), Jiache (S 6) and

Taiyang (Extra 2) were needled by the reducing method, retaining the needle for thirty minutes. Toothache and other symptoms were relieved after treatment. No relapse was found in the follow-up visit three days later.

2. Application of Ashi point in differentiation of syndrome

Ashi point is also called Tianying point. It has been widely used in clinic. Good threapeutic effect can be obtained if the treatment is based on differentiation. The points are selected accurately and proper manipulations are applied.

1) *Manifestation and examination method of Ashi point* Dr. He found out that the clinical manifestations of Ashi point include the positive reaction substance and the positive sensation. The positive reaction substances are the nodules and cords which can be palpated, while the positive sensations are the local subject pain, soreness, distension and numbness. The examination method of Ashi point can be divided into the superficial palpation method and the meridian measuring method:

a. The superficial palpation: Press the abdomen with the thumb along a certain definite direction and slide or knead in order to detect the positive reaction substance or the positive sensation. Strength should be applied evenly during the examination, and attention paid to compare the sensation bilaterally. Generally the back and lumbo-sacral region should be examined first, then the chest, abdomen and the four limbs. Of course, some important regions may be examined according to the symptoms. For example, the back or abdomen is examined in case of gastric pain; the back or chest examined for asthma; the neck, scapula and the upper limbs for the pain of the upper extremities; the spinal column, lumbo-sacrum and lower limbs for lower leg pain.

b. Meridian-measuring method: When the diseased point is not apparent or the Ashi point can't be determined by the palpation method, the meridian-measuring method is often adopted to detect the volume of electric conduction with a meridian-measuring instrument. The point with the highest electric conduction is regarded as the Ashi point. This method is mostly used in internal diseases and meridian diseases.

2) *Clinical application of Ashi point*

a. Examining the diseases: When a disease occurs in the internal organs, it can be reflected on the body surface through the meridians, showing the spontaneous pain, tenderness, hyperesthesia, and some special changes, such as subcutaneous nodules, rashes and changes of skin colour. Respiratory diseases often have tenderness around Feishu (B 13), Zhongfu (L 1) and Kongzui (L 6) points, and the heart and chest diseases have tenderness at Ximen (P 4) point, indicating the close relations between the internal organs and the body surface. Clinically this specific correlation can be applied in diagnosing the disease.

b. Treating diseases: Ashi points have a very wide range of indications, which include not only the diseases of the internal organs, but also the meridian diseases. For example, gastric pain may be treated by needling the tenderness of hypersensitive points at the gastric region and on the back, and appendicitis treated by needling the tenderness appeared on the abdomen or Lanwei (Extra 33) point. Ashi points can be used independently or in combination. When used in combination, the location and nature of the disease should be determined according to the Four Diagnostic Methods and differentiation of zang-fu organs and meridians, then the suitable Shu points will be selected. For example, distension and pain at the gastric region, distension and fullness of the chest and hypochondrium, anorexia, belching, depression, and string-taut pulse may be differentiated as stagnation of liver qi, failure in dispersing depressed liver qi and attacking of the stomach. Therefore, Zusanli (S 36) of the Stomach Meridian of Foot-Yangming and Taichong (Liv 3) of Liver Meridian of Foot Jueyin are added in addition to Ashi points. Another example is the shoulder and arm pain, with difficulty in lifting the arm. The prominent tenderness was found at Jianneiling (Extra) point. Differentiation was wind-cold and damp blocking the Hand-Taiyin Meridian. Good result was obtained when the Ashi points were needled in combination with the point Chize (L 5) of Hand-Taiyin Meridian.

c. Selection of the needling method: When Ashi points are needled, the acupuncture principle must be followed and suitable manipulations should be adopted according to the pathological conditions and location of the disease, whether it is an excess or deficiency, cold or heat. Either deep insertion or superficial insertion, either single needling or multiple needling, either reinforcing or reducing method, moxibustion or fire needling method, or bleeding method is used. Deep and shallow insertion: Ashi points should be needled according to the location of the disease. The needling depth will vary, because the disease is either at the interior or exterior, at the zang or fu organ, at the flesh or tendon. It is said in *Plain Questions* that "since the disease is located superficially and deeply, needling will be applied accordingly." According to Dr. He's experience, the following five kinds of manipulations are applied: First, shallow needling should be used for superficial illness, the commonly used are skin needling and shallow needling. Shallow needling refers to the subcutaneous needling which is mainly used to treat common cold or cold and numbness of the skin. Good therapeutic results can be obtained with this method. Second, if the disease is situated in the meridian, shallow puncture to bleeding, also called collateral puncture method, is often used. The three-edged needle, the cutaneous needle and cupping with bleeding fall within this aspect. In general, it is used to treat the blockade of the collaterals, or stagnation of the heat in the blood, such as sprain, acute superficial lymphangitis, erysipelas. Third, if the disease is situated at the tendon, puncture the tendon, that is the joint needling or relaxing needling. The former is to insert the needle perpendicularly to the attachment of the tendon, and to prevent bleeding during treatment, while the latter is to insert the needle at the side of the tendon towards the tendon with various directions. Clinically, it is mainly used to treat tendon diseases, such as external humeral epicondylitis, tendinitis, of supraspinatus muscle, inflammation of patella ligment, paraligmentous injury of knee joint. Fourth, when the illness affects the muscle, puncture the muscle with the superficial needling and intermuscular needling methods. The superficial needling is to insert the needle obliquely penetrating the muscle. Clinically, it is often used to treat the pain syndromes caused by muscle spasms, such as acute lumbago. After Ashi point is selected, a 2 to 3 cun long filiform needle is punctured obliquely towards the spine. Good results can be obtained when the needle penetrates through the spasmodic muscle transversely. Intermuscular needling is to insert the needle in several directions like a chicken's claw, so it is also called the chicken claw puncture, and is often used to treat rheumatism of the muscle, such as periarthritis humeroscapularis, tendinitis of infraspinatus tendon and lumbar muscle strain. Fifth, if the illness lies in the bone, puncture deeply with Shu needling and short thrust needling. Shu needling is to insert and withdraw the needle directly to the bones. It is often used to treat rheumatism of the bones. Short needling is to insert the needle with a little vibration until it reaches the bone. It is a method of lifting and thrusting the needle at the skeleton, and it is often used to treat bone diseases such as hyperplasia. For example, Ashi points at the side of the spine are selected in the treatment of cervical spondylosis and hypertrophic spondylitis. The Ashi points surrounding the patella are selected in treating chondromalacia of the patella. The needle should be inserted deeply to the bone, and lifted and thrusted several times after the arrival of qi. Single or multiple needling: According to the size of the positive reaction substance, and the range of pain, single or multiple needling may be applied. The single needling means a single puncture on the Ashi point, which is effective for smaller positive reaction substance and small sensation, while the multiple needling refers to the method of giving more than two needles on the affected area and tender points. The most commonly used methods are triple needling, adjacent needling, quintuple needling, repeated shallow puncture, and leopard-spot needling. The triple needling is a method in which the needles are inserted at three spots. With one in the center and two on both sides; the adjacent needling is a method in which the needling is applied vertically and laterally with one needle each to treat large areas of pain, such as injury of nervi clunium superiores, or injury of piriformis; the quintuple needling is a method in which the needles are inserted at the five spots with one in the center of Ashi point and the four scattered around it. It is also named as the surrounding puncture, and used to treat the superficial and large area disorders, such as external humeral epicondylitis and tensoynovitis; the repeatedly shallow insertion is also one of the twelve punctures. The leopard-spot puncture is one of the five punctures, a technique in which the needles are used to pierce small blood vessels around the affected area to treat erysiples and carbuncle. Contralateral needling and resistant needling; The contralateral needling refers to needling applied to the points on the right side when the affected region is on the left and vice versa. For example, Ashi point which should be needled on the left side of the human body, but puncture on the right corresponding area. Resistant needling is to puncture the painful point when the patient is asked to move the limb to the extent he can tolerate. This is often used to treat the sprain or pain syndrome caused by the exogeneous pathogenic factors obstructing the meridians. Satisfactory results can also be obtained by applying the bird-pecking method. In addition to the above-mentioned methods, moxibustion, point injection, point blocking, intradermal imbedding, cupping and magnetic therapy can also be applied.

3. "Shallow needling with multiple needles"

1) *Characteristics* Shallow puncture is often used in treating superficial disorders. There are many records about its manipulation and indications in *Internal Classic*, such as shallow needling, extreme shallow needling, superficial needling, quintuple needling

and straight needling, etc. The indications are the meridian disease where the pathogenic factors lie at the surface or at the shallow place of the body. This method is a kind of reinforcing method, and is suitable for deficiency syndrome and weak patients.

2) *Clinical application*

a. For the treatment of late-stage facial paralysis or long-term facial paralysis: The facial paralysis is due to the invasion or the wind of the wind-cold leading to flaccid paralysis of muscles. At the early stage of the disease, when the pathogenic factors are prosperous, the reducing method should be used to expel them. At the late stage, when the pathogenic factors become weak, and the body resistance is still deficient, the reinforcing method must be used in combination with the method of dredging the collaterals and dispelling the pathogenic factors to support the body resistance. Old facial paralysis refers to a disease with a course of more than half a year. Because of long-term retention of pathogenic factors in the meridians, the local muscles and blood vessels are short of nourishment of qi and blood. This is regarded as a deficiency syndrome. Therefore, shallow insertion with multiple acupoints is used to support body resistance and expel the pathogenic factors. Commonly used points are Zanzhu (B 2), Jujiao (S 3), Yingxiang (LI 20), Heliao (LI 19), Renzhong (Du 26), Quanliao (SI 18), Dicang (S 4), Jiachengjiang (Extra 5), Xiaguan (S 7), Jiache (S 6), Fengchi (G 20), Hegu (LI 4) and Zusanli (S 36). Needling method: The points on the face should be needled 0.1 to 0.2 cun deep by a 1 cun filiform needle with tight pressing and slow lifting. Twenty-seven cases of old facial paralysis with a course of disease of more than half a year were treated with the above-mentioned method. Among which, twelve were basically cured; fourteen were effective; and one failed.

b. For the treatment of late-stage sciatica: Primary sciatica falls within the Bi-Syndrome in TCM, and it is due to the invasion of wind, cold, and dampness attacking the meridians and obstructing qi and blood. The treatment should focus on warming the meridians, dispersing cold, and dredging the meridians. Huantiao (B 30) and Yanglingquan (G 34) are often needled with a reducing method to remove the obstructions from the meridians and expel the pathogenic factors. Severe pain may be controlled very quickly but not radically. At the late stage of the disease, patients often suffer from soreness and pain on the lumbar region, weakness of the affected limbs, numbness on the lateral aspect of the leg, and distending pain on the calf, which may become aggravated on exertion and can be improved after rest. At that time although the pathogenic factors are weak, the body resistance is still deficient. The treatment should be to reinforce qi and nourish the blood, in combination with the method of dredging collaterals and expelling the pathogenic factors. "Shallow needling with multiple points" can be applied to consolidate the results.

For example, a male cadre of fifty-six years old paid his first visit on December 5, 1969. He complained of left lumbar and hip pain for about one month. The pain radiated downward along the posterior aspect of the thigh and lateral aspect of the leg. The pain was continuous and deteriorated paroxysmally, especially during coughing and sneezing. He had difficulty in turning his body, cold lower extremities, aggravated at night, and insomnia. He was first treated with the points of the Taiyang and Shaoyang Meridians namely, Shenshu (B 23), Huantiao (G 30), Yinmen (B 37) and Yanglingquan (G 34) with the reducing method. The needling sensation was propagated along the meridian. Moxibustion was combined. The pain was alleviated after ten treatments, but he still felt soreness and weakness over the lower back and the lower extremities, and distending pain on the leg. Ten more treatments with the above method were given, but without effect. Because of the deficiency of essence and blood of the kidney, insufficient qi and blood failed to nourish the meridian and blood vessel and to fill in the bone marrow. Thus soreness and weakness of the lower back and the knee, numbness of the leg and easy fatigue resulted. All this belonged to deficient qi and blood. So the treatment was changed to reinforce kidney qi and regulate qi and blood in combination with expulsion of the pathogenic factors. Geshu (B 17), Ganshu (B 18), Danshu (B 19), Pishu (B 20), Weishu (B 21), Shenshu (B 23), Dachangshu (B 25), Guangyuanshu (B 26), Yaoyangguan (Du 3), Weizhong (B 40), Feiyang (B 58), Yanglingquan (G 34), Waiqiu (G 36), Yangjiao (G 25), Xuanzhong (G 39), Taixi (K 3), Zusanli (S 36), Shangjuxu (S 37), Xiajuxu (S 39) and Taichong (Liv 3) were selected and punctured shallowly. Treat once every other day. The patient was cured after eight treatments.

c. For the treatment of old or late-stage sprain: This disease usually has a long duration with the main symptoms of soreness and pain of the muscle and joints, swelling which become aggravated after fatigue, or attacks on cloudy or rainy days. The symptoms may be relieved after treatment, but the soreness and pain of the muscle was still left. Treatment of this case should remove the blood stasis. Most cases can be cured with the method of "shallow needling with multiple points." For example, a man, thirty-eight, first visited the doctor on March 16, 1981. His right shoulder was dislocated after a fall from a bicycle one month before. He suffered from shoulder pain after the shoulder joint was put back manually. Soreness and pain of the upper arm appeared whenever he placed his arm in a fixed position. The examination showed that the muscles of his shoulders had slight atrophy and limited mobility. "Shallow needling with multiple points" was applied to remove the long-term blood stasis and the obstruction from the meridians, and to nourish qi and blood. Therefore, Xiabai (L 4), Tianfu (L 3), Chize (L 5), Jianyu (LI 15), Jianliao (SJ 14), Jugu (LI 16), Binao (LI 14), Naoshu (SI 10), Naohui (SJ 13), and Quchi (LI 11) were needled 0.2 to 0.3 cun deep with the filiform needles and sparrow-pecking used at Jianneiling (Extra) and Jianyu (LI 15). He was greatly improved after two treatments and recovered after four treatments.

d. For the treatment of superficial and localized disorders: It refers to Bi-syndrome of the superficial muscles, numbness and soft tissue lesions, such as external humeral epicondylitis and neuritis of lateral cutaneous nerve of thigh. A hundred and ten cases of the above-mentioned diseases were treated with this method, among which, ninty-five were cured, and the curative rate was 84.6 percent.

e. For the treatment of neurasthenia: Good therapeutic effects were obtained in treating deficiency of the heart and spleen and difficulty between the heart and kidney.

4. Selecting Jiaji points

Huatuojiaji (Jiaji) is first described in *Prescriptions for Emergencies* and it has been used to treat chronic diseases. Jiaji points are distributed at both sides of the spine on the back and the lumbar region, and located 0.5 cun lateral to the lower border of the spinous process of T1 to L5, and there are altogether thirty-four points bilaterally. They are very close to the Back-Shu points and have similar functions, and are often used alternately. Clinical practice has proved that different reactions may appear on the back in case of zang-fu diseases, which are usually called the positive reaction substance or positive sensation. For example, respiratory diseases can be reflected at both sides of T3-T5, digestive diseases at T5-T12, and urinary disease at both sides of lumbosacral vertebra. Needling Jiaji points can treat visceral diseases effectively.

Dr. He believes that Jiaji points can be needled to treat not only internal organ diseases, but also some diseases related to the internal organs through the regulation of the visceral functions.

1) *Vascular migraine* Migraine is an intractable disease, in which the location of pain pertains to Shaoyang Meridian and relates to the heart, liver, spleen and kidney. Seventy cases have been treated by Dr. He since 1973. Most of them had received acupuncture, moxibustion or other therapies, but the effect was not satisfactory. Jiaji points Nos. 5, 7, 9, 11, 14 were needled in combination with Fengchi (G 20). Thirty-four cases were cured; 20 markedly improved, 13 improved, the total effective rate being 95.7 percent.

2) *Acroparesthesia* The chief manifestation of this disease is paroxysmal numbness of both hands, especially during sleeping or upon waking up for a short time. For the serious cases, the numbness may involve the tongue, lips and lower limbs, causing motor disturbance of the hands. It is commonly seen in women of fifty years old. The disease is due to overwork, deficiency of qi and blood or stagnation of qi and blood in the meridians, and loss of nourishment of the muscles. Thirty-one cases were treated by needling Jiaji points Nos. 5, 7, 9, 11 and 14, among which 22 (71 percent) were cured; 3 cases (9.7 percent) were markedly improved, and 6 cases (19.3 percent) relieved.

3) *Impairment of the vegetative nerves* The manifestations of this illness are very complicated. Here we only deal with dizziness, cold limbs, hemiparesthesia, profuse sweating or scanty sweating caused by dysfunction of the vegetatve nervous system. Traditional Chinese medicine ascribes this disease to insufficiency of ying (nutrient) and Wei (defensive qi) and weakness of qi and blood. Among the 18 cases who were treated with Jiaji points, 13 cases were cured, and 5 improved.

4) *Cerebrovascular disease* Here refers to windstroke of the collaterals being attacked due to cerebral ischemia attack. Traditional Chinese medicine regards this case to be deficiency of qi and blood, sudden hyperactivity of liver yang, excess of heart-fire, stirring of wind-fire, the reverse circulation of qi and blood associated with phlegm attacking the meridians. The location of the disease is mainly in the heart, liver, spleen and kidney. Forty cases were treated with Jiaji points, and 33 were basically cured; 5 markedly improved, and 4 relieved.

Besides, better therapeutic results have also been obtained when Jiaji points were needled to treat the Raynaud's disease and erythromelalgia which are related to qi and blood.

Needling Jiaji points can cure zang-fu disorders and diseases related to the qi and blood of zang-fu organs, because these points regulate the qi and blood. Jiaji points 3, 5,

7, 9, 11 and 14 have a similar function with those of Feishu (B 13), Xinshu (B 15), Geshu (B 17), Ganshu (B 18), Pishu (B 20) and Shenshu (B 23). All these Back-Shu points can regulate the functions of their corresponding zang-fu organs. Acroparesthesia and dysfunction of the vegetative nerves are both due to insufficiency of the Ying (nutrient) and Wei (defensive qi) and weakness of qi and blood. The defensive qi is originated from the lower jiao, nourished in the middle jiao and developed in the upper jiao. Qi is the substance which maintains the life activities and the external reaction of the physiological functions of zang-fu organs. Yin qi is the essence of water and cereal which regulates the five zang organs and spreads over the six fu organs. The blood is promoted from the spleen, governed by the heart, stored in the liver, distributed in the lungs and excreted from the kidney. So needling Jiaji points can regulate qi and blood, dredge the meridians. Such symptoms as numbness of the limbs, cold and weakness can be relieved when qi and blood are regulated, and the meridian is dredged and then the muscles are nourished. Though the location of migraine is at Shaoyang Meridian, the cause is mainly due to upward disturbance of the wind-fire of the Liver Meridian. It is either complicated by deficiency of the spleen producing phlegm, or by insufficiency of the kidney water, or long-term illness affecting the collaterals. Needling Jiaji points 5, 7, 9, 11 and 14 can calm the liver to eliminate the wind, support the kidney to nourish the liver, strengthen the spleen to expel phlegm, and regulate qi and blood to promote the collaterals, thus headache is relieved. In case of windstroke caused by deficiency of qi and blood, imbalance of yin and yang and hyperactivity of liver yang associated with fire and phlegm, Jiaji points 5, 7, 9, 11 and 14 are often needled to calm the liver and eliminate wind, nourish the water to restrain wood, strengthen the spleen to resolve the phlegm, regulate the blood to activate the circulation of blood in the collaterals.

5. Treating different types of facial paralysis

Facial paralysis is a common disease caused by wind-cold invading the Yangming Meridians. Dr. He classified this case into four types:

1) *Obstruction of wind-cold* The symptoms for this type include paralysis of the facial muscles at the affected side, deviation of the mouth and eye, lacrimation, superficial, tense or string-taut pulse, and thin white tongue coating. It is again divided into two types in clinic: The first is due to wind-cold invading the Yangming Meridian, and its chief manifestations are paralysis of the facial muscles; the other one is due to wind-cold invading the Yangming and Shaoyang Meridians, where there is pain at the posterior part of the ears and below the ears with prominent tenderness at the mastoid process besides the facial paralysis.

2) *Wind-cold invading the stomach* The wind-cold invades the meridian externally, and injures the spleen and stomach internally. Besides the facial paralysis, it is also complicated with tastelessness of the mouth, anorexia, thin white tongue coating and string-taut pulse.

3) *Damp-heat of the liver and kidney* The wind-cold in the meridians is not eliminated, but enters the meridian and affects zang-fu organs, and turns into heat, or the internal damp-heat associated with the external pathogenic factors. Besides the facial

paralysis, there appear hyperacousia, pain at the posterior part of the ears, or herpes at the ear, severe pain inside the ear, bitter mouth and dry throat, or tastelessness, anorexia and yellow greasy tongue coating and string-taut pulse.

4) *Deficiency of the liver and kidney* General insufficiency of the liver and kidney is associated with the attack by the external pathogenic factors and heat burns the body fluids. In addition to the facial paralysis, the accompanied symptoms are intra-ocular dryness, less or absent tears, or squint, facial spasm, and thready and string-taut pulse.

The treatment varies according to the different syndrome types and different points and manipulations are selected accordingly, Zanzhu (B 2), Yangbai (B 14), Sizhukong (SJ 23), Sibai (S 2), Dicang (S 4), Yingxiang (LI 20), Jiache (S 6), Fengchi (G 20) and Hegu (LI 4) are often selected (as the basic points). Secondary points: For example Waiguan (SJ 5) is added in case Shaoyang is involved; Zhongwan (Ren 12) and Zusanli (S 36) are added in case of the wind-cold invading the stomach; Yanglingquan (G 34), Xingjian (Liv 2) and Jiexi (S 41) are added in the case of damp-heat in the liver and gallbladder; Taixi (K 3), Shenshu (B 23) and Taichong (Liv 3) are added in case of deficiency of the liver and kidney. Method of needling and moxibustion: The reducing method will be applied first. However, for those with deficiency of the liver and kidney, the reinforcing method must be used, while for those with severe cold, moxibustion should be added. Treat once a day. Ten treatments constitute a course. The treatment can be divided into two steps: At the onset of the disease when the pathogenic factors are abundant, and body resistance is sufficient, the disease, pertaining to excess syndrome, should be treated with the reducing method to expel the external pathogenic factors. At the later stage, reinforcing is chiefly used because the external pathogenic factors were expelled, but body resistance was also impaired. The method of "shallow needling with multiple points" in combination with Zusanli (S 36) is therefore selected to support the body resistance and expel the pathogenic factors. The therapeutic effects are promoted after being treated with the above-mentioned method. The effects were observed in 75 cases, among which, 46 belonged to the obstruction of wind-cold; 9, wind-cold invading the stomach; 17, damp-heat of the liver and gallbladder; and 3, deficiency of the liver and kidney. The curative rate was raised from 62 percent to 82.7 percent, and the therapeutic effects increased. Dr. He also summed up the following factors which influenced the therapeutic results on facial paralysis: a. Among the 75 cases, 46 cases whose disease lies in the meridian, and 35 cases were cured; 29 cases with zang-fu organs affected, and 12 cases were cured. The statistical difference is very significant ($P < 0.05$). Among the 75 cases, 3 cases with the liver and kidney disorder were affected, and no case was cured after 6 months' treatment. This indicates that it is easy to cure the disease when the meridians are affected, but difficult to treat cases in which the zang-fu organs are affected. b. Mild cases are easy to cure while severe cases are difficult to treat. The degree of the facial paralysis is closely related to the strength of the body resistance and the condition of the pathogenic factors. If the body resistance is strong and the pathogenic factors are not so vigorous, the illness may be mild. Therefore the incomplete paralysis can be cured more easily. On the contrary, complete paralysis is difficult to be cured. For example, among the 75 cases, there were 33 cases who suffered from complete paralysis. However only 10 cases (13.3 percent) were cured; for the 42 cases of incomplete paralysis, 37 (49.3 percent) cases were cured. The statistical difference is significant ($P < 0.005$). c. Among the 75 cases, 34 cases which had a course within 3 days, 26 cases were cured; of 18 cases which had a course within 7 days, 12 cases were cured; of 23 cases which had a course more than 8 days, only 9 cases were cured. This also indicates that the difference is significant ($P < 0.01$).

6. Treating asthma by dispelling and eliminating the wind

An attack of asthma is usually related to the mental factors. Anger injures the liver, wind, after being transformed from yang, disturbs the lung upward, then resulting in asthma. Dr. He thinks that branchial asthma is related to "wind." In the treatment, Dr. He often added the points Fengchi (B 20), Fengfu (Du 16), Fengmen (B 12), Neiguan (P 6), and Taichong (Liv 3) to the commonly used points in order to expel the wind, soothe the liver and stop the wind. Thus good therapeutic results are usually obtained. For example, in April, 1977, a patient who had been suffering from asthma for more than ten years came to see Dr. He. Before that he had had many kinds of treatment with no effect. As the attack occurred two to three times a month, he suffered a great deal. The time when he came to the clinic, his asthma was bothering him. Immediately Fengchi (G 20) and Fengfu (Du 16) were needled and the asthma began to be relieved five minutes after the treatment. The asthma stopped after needling the points Neiguan (P 6), Tanzhong (Ren 17), Zusanli (S 36), and Lieque (L 7). He was cured after another twenty treatments. No relapse was found after a follow-up visit for two years. In the last several years, Dr. He has treated 62 cases of asthma. The curative rate was 29 percent and a markedly effective rate was 38.7 percent.

II. Case Analysis

Case 1: Dizziness

Name, Li x x; sex, male; age, 60; date of the first visit, December 10, 1981.

Complaints He had suffered from dizziness for half a year and the disease had worsened for one month. The patient had had gastric pain for more than ten years, and the pain attacked him very frequently. In the last half a year, dizziness and dull sensation, which was mild in the morning, and severe in the afternoon, especially after fatigue appeared, accompanied with sallow complexion, weakness of the four extremities, loss of appetite, loose stool, pale tongue, deep and thready pulse, blood pressure 180/100 mmHg. Differentiation: Weakness of the spleen and stomach. The principle of treatment should be to regulate the spleen and stomach, reinforce qi of the middle jiao. The points of the Foot-Yangming Meridian were selected as the main points.

Prescription Baihui (Du 20), Zhongwan (Ren 12), and Zusanli (S 36).

Treatment procedure Reinforcing with heavy pressing and light lifting was used. The patient improved remarkably after five treatments with the above-mentioned points needled. He was cured after ten treatments. His face turned pink, and his general health recovered. He could ride a bike two hours a day without feeling tired, and he had no more gastric pain.

Explanation In this case, the heavy pressing and light lifting method was adopted with good results. The patient was needled at Zusanli (S 36) with a 1.5 filiform needle, and after the arrival of qi, the heavy pressing and light lifting method was performed five to ten times. The patient felt distension going upward along the Stomach Meridian of Foot-Yangming. The distension as broad as a thumb was felt with indistinct borderline. He felt a tight sensation in the stomach and borborygmus, then it reached the face through the chest, and finally arrived at his vertex. The propagation route of the sensation at the head and the face was not clear. When the treatment was continued, the tight sensation turned into heat stream going upward with a faster speed. After it reached the head and the face, he felt hot at the head and the face, then the face became flushed. Almost in every treatment he could feel the hot sensation. The patient was very comfortable after withdrawing the needle. His mind was clear and his spirit was high. From these, we can see that the five key links, that is, theory, methodology, prescription, acupoints and technique are extremely important in acupuncture. Through this case, we can also see the importance of the manipulation in the acupuncture treatment.

Case 2: Facial paralysis

Name, Shi x x; sex, female; age, 13: date of the first visit, February 6, 1979.

Complaints She had left facial paralysis one year ago when she was in a bus and invaded by the wind. She received many kinds of treatment with no response. Examination: Incomplete closing of the left eyelid, loss of the frontal wrinkles on the forehead, lacrimation, shallowing of the left naso-labial fissure, deviation of mouth corner to the right side, difficulty in whistle, malposition of teeth showing, tightness of the face, thin white coating, and deep and thready pulse. Differentiation: Retention of pathogenic factors, deficiency of qi and blood, loss of nourishment of the muscle and blood vessels, and disuse of the facial muscle. Principle of the treatment should be to support the body resistance and expel the pathogenic factors. The "shallow needling with multiple points method" should be selected.

Prescription Yangbai (B 14) , Zanzhu (B 2), Sibai (S 2), Juliao (S 3), Dicang (S 4), Sizhukong (SJ 23), Quanliao (SI 18), Shangyingxiang (Extra), Yingxiang (LI 20), Heliao (LI 19), Jiache (S 6), Jiachengjiang (Extra 5), Xiaguan (S 7) and Fengchi (G 20) were needled at the left side, and Hegu (LI 4) and Zusanli (S 36) bilaterally.

Treatment procedure The needles were retained for thirty minutes. The symptoms were alleviated after the treatment, and he was greatly improved after fifteen treatments, and basically recovered after twenty-five treatments.

Explanation The long duration of the facial paralysis often occurs when the pathogenic factors remain in the meridians, resulting in the consumption of qi and blood, short nourishment of the local muscles, tendons and blood vessels. In addition to the paralysis of the facial mimetic muscle, the disease is usually complicated with muscular spasm, tic or atrophy of the small muscles on the affected side. Since the disease belongs to deficiency, the reinforcing method should be adopted. Owing to the pathogenic factors still remaining, and the meridians still obstructed, the supplemented treatment should be considered to expel the pathogenic factors and promote the collaterals. The "shallow needling with multiple points method" has proven effective in treating deficiency syndrome, and it also has the functions, to dredge the meridians and expel the pathogenic factors. Therefore, it is suitable to treat long-term facial paralysis.

Case 3: Migraine

Name, Yin x x; sex, female; age 45; date of the first visit, September 21, 1973.

Complaints The patient complained of migraine headaches for twenty years which was aggravated in recent two years. The pain attacked repeatedly. After various treatments, instead of being alleviated the disease deteriorated. Even ergotamine drugs could not control it. Usually an attack occurred every two or three days with rebounding pain which first started from the frontal region, either the left or right side, and then spread to the opposite side and gradually to the whole head. The peak of the pain often appeared after three hours of the attack, and would gradually be relieved after twenty-four hours. The accompanying symptoms were nausea, vomiting and irritability.

Prescription Huatuojiaji points 5, 7, 9, 11 14, and Fengchi (G 20).

Treatment procedure Treat once every other day, and the headache became alleviated remarkably after ten treatments. Only a mild attack took place for about two hours. No more attacks occurred after another fifteen treatments, and no relapse was found in the follow-up visit for one year.

SELECTING POINTS AND IMPROVING ACUPUNCTURE IMPLEMENTS

—Yu Zhongquan's Clinical Experience

Yu Zhongquan was born in 1912 in Wanxian County, Sichuan Province. As a young boy, he was influenced by his grandfather and father in the field of traditional Chinese medicine. In 1941 he graduated from Sichuan National University of Medicine. Upon the invitation of Chengdu College of TCM, he lectured there on acupuncture and did research and clinical work.

Dr. Yu had thorough knowledge of Chinese medical classics and the achievements of modern research in addition to extensive clinical experience. He realized that we should learn from the ancients, but not simply imitate them. He also stresses careful differentiation of symptoms and signs and proper selection of points. Dr. Yu is for needling according to time, but simplified the needling technique of Mid-night Ebb-flow Method. He developed new methods of treatment, especially new acupuncture implements, such as retaining small pills on the ear points, applying a rolling needle on the skin and using a spring needle device in puncturing. These implements are effective for the treatment of windstroke, pain, laryngospasm and stranguria.

Now Yu Zhongquan is a professor and academic committee member of Chengdu College of Traditional Chinese Medicine. He is also the advisor of Sichuan Acupuncture Society and editor of TCM teaching material for national colleges.

I. Academic Characteristics and Medical Specialities

1. Taking the meridians as the key link and the symptoms as the principle to summarize the indications of the points

Facing many scattered point indications, Dr. Yu thought of using meridians and collaterals as the key links for generalizing these indications. In this way we can modernize the experience of the ancients.

Taking the present textbook *Acupuncture* published in 1985 as an example, the 361 points of the fourteen meridians indicate more than one hundred different cases, which repeat the fourteen meridians more than nine hundred times. For instance, there are 11 points for the Lung Meridian of Hand-Taiyin, indicating in more than 30 cases, and there are 67 points for Bladder Meridian, indicating in more than 140 kinds of conditions. If the indications are not summarized, it is difficult to use them. Thus Dr. Yu has categorized the point with the same functions. For example, the main indications of the points from the Lung Meridian are to promote the function of the lung, eliminate exterior syndromes, check coughing, ease asthma, promote the descending and dispersing function, regulate lung qi, and promote the free flow of qi of the meridians and collaterals.

The indications of the points from the Bladder Meridian are to promote the function of the lung in descending and dispersing, to regulate the functions of the spleen and stomach, warm up the kidney yang, reduce the fire from liver and gallbladder, regulate menstruation, check leukorrhea, reduce heat, calm the mind, eliminate toxins, brighten the eyes and activate the qi and blood flow of the meridians and collaterals. Dr. Yu classified the points from all the meridians according to the similar indications. From this, he concludes that one disease can be treated by different points from different meridians. Then, based on the differentiation according to the meridians, the proper points can be selected quickly.

1) *Headache* a. Yangming headache (frontal headache), points from the Large Intestine Meridian are Hegu (LI 4), Yangxi (LI 5), Wenliu (LI 7), Xialian (LI 8), and Shanglian (LI 9) and points from the Stomach Meridian are Sibai (S 2), Touwei (S 8), Fenglong (S 40) and Jiexi (S 41). b. Taiyang headache (occipital headache), points from the Small Intestine Meridian are Wangu (SI 4), Houxi (SI 3), Qiangu (SI 2), Zhizheng (SI 7) and Xiaohai (SI 8) and points from the Bladder Meridian are Zanzhu (B 2), Meichong (B 3), Kunlun (B 60). c. Shaoyang headache (temporal headache), points from the Sanjiao Meridian are Guanchong (SJ 1), Yemen (SJ 2), Zhongzhu (SJ 3), Waiguan (SJ 5) and points from the Gallbladder Meridian are Tongziliao (G 1), Yangbai (G 14), Yangfu (G 38), Zulinqi (G 41) as well as Lieque (L 7) from the Lung Meridian. d. Jüeyin headache (vertex headache), points from the Liver Meridian are Xingjian (Liv 2), Taichong (Liv 3). e. Headache due to deficiency of kidney, point from the Kidney Meridian is Yongquan (K 1). If the pathogenic factors predominate, points from the Du Meridian are Baihui (Du 20), Shangxing (Du 23), Shenting (Du 24), Xinhui (Du 22), Qianding (Du 21), Qiangjian (Du 18), Fengfu (Du 16), Dazhui (Du 14).

2) *Sore throat* All the meridians have certain points which treat sore throat, except the Spleen Meridian. Therefore, we cannot treat sore throat by simply bleeding on the points Shaoshang (L 11) and Yuji (L 10). We must select points based on differentiation. a. Invasion by the exogenous pathogenic factors: The points from the Lung Meridian are Shaoshang (L 11), Yuji (L 10), Jingqu (L 8), Lieque (L 7), Kongzhui (L 6), Chize (L 5) and Yunmen (L 2) and those from the Du Meridian are Baihui (Du 20), Dazhui (Du 14) and Fengfu (Du 16). b. Excessive heat of the Yangming Meridian: The points from the Large Intestine Meridian are Shangyang (LI 1), Erjian (LI 2), Sanjian (LI 3), Hegu (LI 4), Yangxi (LI 5), Pianli (L 6), Wenliu (LI 7), Quchi (LI 11) and Tianding (LI 17) and those from the Stomach Meridian, Lidui (S 45), Neiting (S 44), Fenglong (S 40), Xiajuxu (S 39), Zusanli (S 36), Biguan (S 31), Quepen (S 12), Qishe (S 11), Shuitu (S 10) and Renying (S 9). c. Flare-up of heart-fire: The points from the Heart Meridian are Tongli (H 5) and Shenmen (H 7), points from the Pericardium Meridian are Laogong (P 8), and Daling (P 7) and those from the Small Intestine Meridian are Shaoze (SI 1), Qiangu (SJ 2), Tianchuang (SI 16), Tianrong (SI 17) and Xiaohai (SI 8). d. Liver and Gallbladder fire: The points from the Gallbladder Meridian are Zuqiaoyin (G 44), Yangjiao (G 35) and Wangu (G 12), and those from the Liver Meridian are Taichong (Liv 3), Xiyangguan (G 33) and Xingjian (Liv 2), and those from the Sanjiao Meridian are Yemen (SJ 2), Zhongzhu (SJ 3), and Guanchong (SJ 1). e. Sore throat due to deficiency of yin: The points from the Kidney Meridian are Yongquan (K 1), Rangu (K

2), Taixi (K 3), Zhaohai (K 6) and Dazhong (K 4), those from the Bladder Meridian are Dazhu (B 11), Tianzhu (B 10), Feishu (B 13), Geshu (B 17), Danshu (B 19), Pishu (B 20) and Chengshan (B 57) and those from the Ren Meridian are Jiuwei (Ren 15), Huagai (Ren 20), Yutang (Ren 13), Xuanji (Ren 21), Tiantu (Ren 22), and Zigong (Ren 19).

2. Combination of meridian differentiation and the point properties to select a few but effective points

1) *Qihai (Ren 6) and Dazhui (Du 14)* In the spring of 1974, Dr. Yu met a male patient suffering from thin body build, pallor, feeble speech and trembling of the larynx for the past sixteen years. Sixteen years ago he fell into a snow-filled hold. When he was rescued he was frozen stiff. After the snow melted, he had general trembling. After the treatment by acupuncture and Chinese herbs, trembling stopped, except for the spasm in the larynx. Since then, he has had spasm and trembling of the larynx. During these sixteen years, he was treated by many doctors without success. The pulse was slightly thready and slow, the tongue proper was pale with a white coating. Differentiation: Excessive yin with the chief problem being located along the Ren Meridian. Therefore, points from the Ren Meridian were used. Qihai (Ren 6) is the point where the general qi is converged.

Deep insertion with a 3 cun needle was applied. Immediately after insertion, the patient's throat felt better. The needle was retained for thirty minutes, then the trembling and spasm of the larynx disappeared.

2) *Dazhui (Du 14)* A male adult had motor impairment for years. Since the case was mild, he ignored it. One year before, the patient had general choreic movements and was treated by both electro-acupuncture and Chinese herbs but without improvement. The disease became more severe until he could not control his right arm and he had hypsokinesis of his head every few minutes. It was worse at day than at night. The patient also complained of insomnia. This symptoms indicated that the yang meridians were involved. Thus, the point Dazhui (Du 14), the meeting point of all the yang meridians was needled once a day. After forty-five treatments, the illness was cured.

3. Herbal pills on ear points

In the fifties, Dr. Yu began to use auricular therapy to stimulate the sensitive points of the appropriate area of the ear. He used a small bamboo probe instead of a needle, which may relieve the pain and achieve good therapeutic results. Later he improved this method during his clinical practice by applying herbal pills sticking to the desired ear point covered with adhesive tape. In addition to the physical pressing function, herbal pills may provide a medicinal effect which relates to the disorder.

1) *The use of tranquilizing herbal pills for mental disease*

a. Ingredients: Magnetite poria with hostwood, rhizoma ligustici chuanxion, radiz angelicae dahuricae and moschus. The pills are coated with Cinnabaris and kept in a sealed bottle.

b. Indications: Insomnia, mental disorder, emotional depression, mania, tinnitus and chorea.

c. Ear points: Endocrine, Subcortex, Ear Shenmen.

Here are several cases for explanation:

Case 1: A female aged fifty suffered from insomnia for more than thirty years. Chinese herbs, Western medicine and injection of Flecceflower failed to respond to the treatment. Dr. Yu applied tranquilizing herbal pills on the ear points Shenmen and Subcortex. The pills were changed every three days. The patient was asked to press the pills three or four times a day. Within one month treatment, insomnia was gone.

Case 2: A male aged twenty-four complained of insomnia, because he was troubled with depression after failing to enter university two years ago. The diagnosis of Western medicine was depressive schizophrenia. The patient tried sedatives for a long period to help him sleep. Dr. Yu applied tranquilizing herbal pills on ear points Shenmen and Subcortex. Since the patient's body constitution was weak, Dr. Yu used the cutanenous rolling needle described later in this article in combination with the tranquilizing herbal pills. The rolling needle was applied from Xinshu (B 15) to Shenshu (B 23). Dr. Yu also asked the patient to press the herbal pills on the ear three or four times a day, and try to reduce the intake of Western medicines gradually. The tranquilizing herbal pills were changed once every three days. After a month treatment, the patient could fall asleep without the help of the Western drugs.

Case 3: A male, aged forty was troubled for three years with a distending feeling in the ear and tinnitus (worse on the left). The diagnosis from Sichuan Medical College was vestibulitis. He was hospitalized for more than one year without relief. His body build was thin and he was weak. The tongue proper was pale, and the pulse was weak. Differentiation: Tinnitus due to deficiency of the kidney. He applied tranquilizing pills on the ear points Endocrine and Subcortex. After one month of treatment, the condition was cured.

Case 4: A girl aged twelve, who generally had an excellent academic record, suddenly became hyperactive and she had a poor memory. She had to stop her schooling because of her bad results. Dr. Yu used herbal pills on the ear points Kidney and Subcortex. After three months of treatment, the condition was improved and she resumed her schooling.

2) *The use of sedative herbal pills for relief of pain*

a. Ingredients: Rhizoma cyperi, Radix clematidis, lignum sappan plus some other herbs which promote the flow of qi and blood and relieve pain.

b. Indications: Different kinds of muscular skeletal pain.

Although the therapeutic result of treating pain by acupuncture is good, some patients can not return for treatment every day or every other day, because of their work, traffic problems, or living far away. Thus Dr. Yu applies tranquilizing herbal pills on the ear after needling. With this method, they need to return for acupuncture only once every two weeks. It is convenient for the patients and good results can still be obtained. Body needling can stimulate and regulate the qi flow of the meridians to stop pain. Dr. Yu thought that the use of tranquilizing herbal pills on the corresponding ear points can prolong this stimulation of qi and strengthen the sedation of pain. This creative method is simple, useful and convenient.

The following are the treating methods for several kinds of pain:

a. Headache: The points should be selected based on the differentiation. Then tranquilizing herbal pills are used on the ear Shenmen and Subcortex after needling.

b. Low back pain: Kidney, Bladder and Lumbar Vertebra.

c. Abdominal pain: Appendix, Small Intestinc and Large Intestine.

d. Stomach pain: Stomach, Liver and Gallbladder.

e. Toothache: Toothache area.

f. Dysmenorrhea: Uterus, Endocrine and Subcortex.

g. Painful joints: Antihelix and the area corresponding to the lower limbs.

h. Sore throat: Throat and Large Intestine.

Remarks: The ingredients of the tranquilizing herbal pills can be added, reduced or changed according to the different symptoms and signs. For instance, Liushenwan can be used for acute sore throat. Here are some cases of headache:

Case 1: A male, twenty-six, had headache for more than one year. He felt numb in the scalp, which became worse when reading. He also complained of insomnia. The pulse was thready and rapid and the tongue slightly red. Because the patient lived in the suburbs, it was difficult to come to the hospital daily. After doing acupuncture on Sishenchong (Extra) and Dazhui (Du 14), Dr. Yu applied herbal pills on the ear points Shenmen and Subcortex, once a week. After two months of treatment, the problems were gone.

Case 2: A woman, thirty-four, had had a left side headache since she was a child. Four years before, tinnitus appeared and the headache continually became more severe. The pulse was thready and the tongue proper was red. Because of her busy work, she could not come for treatment every day. Dr. Yu decided to use herbal pills in combination with body acupuncture. After needling Sishenchong (Extra), Fengchi (G 20) and Taichong (Liv 3), he applied the pills on the ear points Shenmen and Subcortex. Treated once a week for two months, her symptoms were gone.

4. Simplifying and enlarging the application of Ziwuliuzhu (Midnight-noon Ebb-flow Method)

Dr. Yu thinks that it is very important to select an acupuncture point according to the time of day when the point is most effective. This optimal time can be determined by several methods. Dr. Yu describes the circulation of the qi in the body as being like the tides of the ocean-flourishing and declining at certain hours of a day in the various meridian. The Midnight-noon Ebb-flow Method is more complicated. The "Na Zhi" method (although this method is more simple than "Na Gan") is used according to the flourishing and declining of qi during the day (Horary Clock). When we consider the interpromoting, interacting, overacting and counteracting relationships of the Five Elements, the points are limited to sixty-six.

Since the flourishing and declining rule of qi says that the qi of the meridian swells and diminishes, Dr. Yu believes that all the points of the meridians may be used not just the Five Shu points. For instance, qi of the Lung Meridian flourishes on the third of the twelve Earthly Branches. Dr. Yu thinks the qi of all the eleven points of this meridian (not only the Five Shu points) is more active at this time of a day. Thus, any point of the Lung Meridian will be more effective on the third of the twelve Earthly Branches. Likewise, since the qi of the Large Intestine Meridian reaches its optimum during the fourth of the twelve Earthly Branches, any of the twenty points will be more active during that time. The qi of the Stomach Meridian peaks during the fifth of the twelve Earthly Branches and any point of the meridian will be more effective during this time. Points from other meridians can be selected in the same way.

Dr. Yu has simplified the Mid-night Ebb-flow Method and has developed the theory of flourishing and declining qi of the meridians. With these improvements, the doctor has a larger number of points available for selection. The new method is simple and useful for enhancing the therapeutic results.

Case 1: A male, fifty-nine years old, suffered from hemiplegia for seven months. He had received acupuncture for several months without any improvement. When he went to Dr. Yu, the myodynamia of his left upper extremity was "O" and that of his left lower extremity was "III." Differentiation: Deficiency of qi and blood with wind-phlegm obstructing the meridians and collaterals. Principle of treatment: Eliminate wind, remove the obstruction from the meridians and resolve phlegm. Points were selected from the three yang meridians with even movement. Dr. Yu gave the acupuncture treatments according to the specific time of the twelve Earthly Branches. For instance, Chengqi (S 1), Dicang (S 4), Liangmen (S 21), Biguan (S 31), Zusanli (S 36), Jiexi (S 41) from the Stomach Meridian were punctured during the time of the fifth of the twelve Earthly Branches. Two to four points were selected each time. After insertion, the patient felt a strong sensation which propagated quickly along the meridian. After being treated for fifteen days, the myodynamia of both left extremities reached "IV."

Case 2: A female aged thirty-two had chief complaints of a spasmatic pain on the epigastic region for six years, accompanied by restlessness, insomnia, quick temper and scanty menstruation. Diagnosis: Gastroptosis. Differentiation: Sinking of qi due to deficiency of the spleen and stagnation and depression of liver qi. The principle of treatment was to tonify the qi of the middle jiao and raise the yang qi. Dr. Yu decided to use points from the Stomach Meridian on the fifth of the twelve Earthly Branches and points from the Spleen Meridian on the sixth of the twelve Earthly Branches. For instance, he punctured Tianshu (S 25), Zusanli (S 36), Neiting (S 44), Weishu (B 21) and Zhongwan (Ren 12) on the fifth of the twelve Earthly Branches. The patient felt a strong needling sensation which spread quickly along the meridians. The patient felt a spasm-like sensation extending upward in the epigastric region. After two weeks of treatment, all the symptoms were gone. Then the patient took an upper GI X-ray with barium which showed that the gastroptosis had lessened. Compared to before, the distance between the notch of the ventriculi minor curvatura and the iliac bone went from 7.5 cm to 4.8 cm. The distance between the notch of the ventriculi major curvatura and the iliac bone changed from 14 cm to 12 cm.

From the above, we can see that this simplified method can not only enlarge the choice of points, but also improve the therapeutic effect. The new method is useful and easy to learn.

5. Invention of the Cutaneous Rolling Needle

In 1954, Dr. Yu and Xiong Xiuwu created a new cutaneous needle with a rolling device, because the tapping with the old cutaneous needle was uneven.

1) *Making of the cutaneous rolling needle* Take a rubber spigot 1.5 to 2.5 cm in diameter and 2 to 3 cm in height as the roller. Secure fifty to ninty short stainless steel needles in it with the tips lining even.

2) *Objects* Patients with weak body condition and children.

3) *Manipulation* Repeatedly roll the needle along the course of the meridian with even force and smooth rolling. The rolling pressure may be either light or heavy according to the patient's constitution, age and tolerance. Generally, the needle is rolled five to nine times along the involved meridian until a pink skin appears.

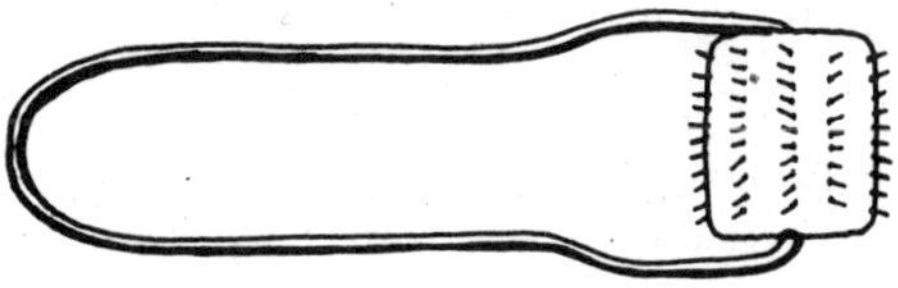

Fig. 1 Cutaneous Rolling Needle

4) *Commonly used meridians* a. The first line of the Bladder Meridian on the back: This is the most basic and frequently used line for the cutaneous rolling needle. Generally, it is rolled from above to below. For the patient with general weakness, deficiency of kidney and lung, or the elderly patient, the rolling needle can be applied from Feishu (B 13) to Shenshu (B 23) up and down; for those with weakness of the spleen and kidney, and insufficiency of the liver and kidney, the device should be applied from Ganshu (B 18) to Shenshu (B 23); for those with problems with the liver and spleen, the rolling needle is performed from Ganshu (B 18) to Weishu (B 21). b. The meridians on the four extremities: If the yin meridians of the upper extremities are involved, roll the needle from the heart to the end of the extremity, and vice versa if the yang meridians are involved. If the yin meridians of the lower extremity are involved, the needle should be applied from the foot to the heart, and vice versa if the yang meridians of the lower extremity are involved. c. The meridians on the abdomen: Roll the needle from below to above along the Liver, Spleen, Kidney and Ren Meridians. d. Principle: As said in *Miraculous Pivot* that "shallow insertion should be used when Bi-syndrome occurs on the superficial position of the body." Therefore, the cutaneous rolling needle can be applied for any indications which can be treated by cutaneous needle. In comparison with the seven star needle, the rolling needle stimulates the skin smoothly with an even force. And said again in *Miraculous Pivot* that: "The thin person has less muscle, colourless skin and speaks softly. In this case, the blood is dilute and the qi flows freely. Therefore, the qi and blood are easily disrupted. For the treatment, quick and shallow insertion are required. Babies are weak with less blood and qi and delicate skin. Therefore the filiform needle with shallow insertion is required." So the cutaneous rolling needle can be applied on patients with a weak body condition, elderly patients and infants because it only pricks the skin at a shallow depth.

The action of the rolling needle along the running course of the meridians is to induce the meridian qi and restore the function of the zang-fu organs. In light of the patient's condition, either light or heavy force is used. In any case, the manipulation should be stopped when redness of the skin appears, which indicates the free flow of qi and blood in the meridians.

6. The Spring-Loaded Acupuncture Implement

Considering infants and patients who are afraid of needles and pain, Dr. Yu has created a spring-loaded acupuncture implement. The following is an introduction of this new implement.

1) *Structure* a. Needle. b. Spiral regulator. c. Draw handle. d. Spring piece. (Fig. 2)

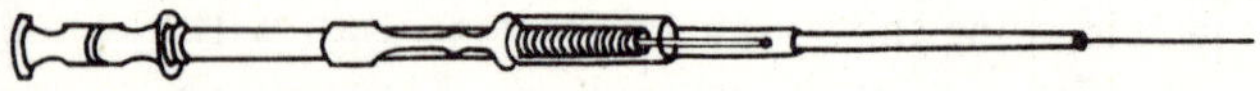

Fig. 2 Spring Needle Helper

2) *Operation* a. installation: Put the selected filiform needle in the tube with the tip facing outward and the handle inward, leaving the tip 0.2 to 0.3 cm exposed. b. Regulate the length of the tip of the needle with the spiral regulator according to different diseases. c. Pull the draw handle 0.5 cm backward after adjustment to keep the whole needle inside the tube. d. Place the mouth of the tube (needle is inside) on the point and apply the proper pressure. e. Fix the mouth of the tube and press the spring piece. Insert the needle into the point with the spring pressure.

3) *Advantages* The patient will not be afraid of needling because he cannot see the tip. The pain of insertion can be reduced with this implement because the needle can be inserted quickly under the pressure of the spring.

II. Case Analysis

Case 1: Prostatitis

Name, Ma x x; sex, male; date of the first visit, June 20, 1979.

Complaints Frequent urination suddenly occurred in May, 1979. The patient complained of urinating more than ten times during the day, and worse at night. Incontinence, scanty and painful urination developed later. There was an uncomfortable electric sensation on the penis whenever he urinated. He was treated with acupuncture in the local area without results. On June 12, he went to the Department of Urology in the People's Hospital of the province. The diagnosis was prostatitis. He received injections of antibiotics and antiphlogistics, but with no response. Then he went to Dr. Yu, at the time the tongue coating was dark grey with cracks and the pulse was thready and rapid. Differentiation: Descent of dampness and heat into the lower jiao, resulting in dysfunction of the bladder.

Prescription 1) Zhongji (Ren 3), Sanyinjiao (Sp 6), Jiaji (L 2) 2) Guanyuan (Ren 4), Yinlingquan (Sp 9), Shenshu (B 23), 3) Shimen (Ren 5), Xuehai (Sp 10), Zhishi (B

52).

Treatment procedure The above three groups of points can be used alternately. The needles were retained for twenty minutes after the arrival of qi. Then the cutaneous rolling needle was applied along the first line of the Bladder Meridian on the back from Ganshu (B 18) to Shenshu (B 23) until the skin appeared red. On June 29, when he came for the second treatment, urination was normal, three or four times a day, with clear urine. The uncomfortable feeling while urinating disappeared.

Explanation As said in *Miraculous Pivot* that "kidney is internally and externally-related to the bladder, which is the organ where urine is stored.... Sanjiao is the passage where the water passes through and enters the bladder...." So, urination syndrome is often due to dysfunction of the kidney, bladder, sanjiao and small intestine. The Back-Shu points in combination with the Front-Mu points are good for the diseases of the zang-fu organs. Therefore, Shimen (Ren 5), Zhongji (Ren 3), Guanyuan (Du 1) and Shenshu (B 23) are used as the main points. With the correct differentiation, the therapeutic result was obtained quickly.

Case 2: Facial muscular twitching (facial spasm)

Name, Fan x x; sex, female; age, 35; date of the first visit, May 30, 1979.

Complaints The patient complained of intermittent episodes of muscular spasms on the left side of the face since 1972. The patient sometimes did not feel the twitching. After overexertion, she would feel a tight sensation of the muscle on the left side of the face, accompanied by poor appetite and scanty menstrual flow. In 1972, she received acupuncture treatment in the hospital in a local clinic, but with no improvement. When she went to Dr. Yu, she had uncontrollable muscle spasms on the left side of the face. The tongue proper was pale, the pulse was thready and weak. Differentiation: Blood deficiency producing the endogenous wind.

Prescription Zusanli (S 36), Yanglingquan (G 34) and Hegu (LI 4) (right side).

Treatment procedure The needles were retained for twenty minutes after the arrival of qi. Meanwhile, the cutaneous rolling needle was applied from Xinshu (B 15) to Shenshu (B 23) until the proper redness of the skin appeared. Then the rolling needle was applied on the left side of the face until the redness appeared. By June 7, after six treatments, the frequency of the spasms was reduced. Later the spasm disappeared and her appetite returned to normal.

Explanation Based on two principles, treat disease on the upper part of the body with the points on the lower part of the body, and treat the disease on the left side of the body with points on the right side of the body, and the point Hegu (LI 4) on the right side was used to regulate the qi of the Yangming Meridians on the left side. Also, the cutaneous rolling needle was applied from Xinshu (B 15) to Shenshu (B 23) to adjust the function of zang-fu organs through the Back-Shu points. Here, point Zusanli (S 36), the He-Sea Point of the Yangming Meridian of Foot, is used to strengthen the function of producing qi and blood. Yanglingquan (G 34) is the influential point of the tendons to stop twitching. The purpose of applying the rolling needle on the face is to promote the free flow of qi and blood of the meridians on the diseased area.

Case 3: Mydriasis

Name, Chen x x; sex, female; age, 26; date of the first visit, April 23, 1980.

Complaints The patient suddenly developed headache, vertigo, dizziness, nausea, vomiting, blurred vision and enlargement of the pupils. When she went to the hospital, the tests of EEG, CSF, B-ultra sonic wave of the brain, ESR and tuberculin check were all normal. The hospital diagnosis was "tonic mydriasis." When she went to the department of ophthalmology and neurology in our hospital, her left pupil was 0.5 cm, there was slight cornea of the right eye, and her light reflex was dull. The diagnosis from our hospital was the same as that of the other hospitals. Medical doctors thought the disease could not be cured. Thus, the patient came to acupuncture treatment. Examination: Thin body, general lassitude, emotional depression, poor appetite, dryness of the eyes and fear of light, which was alleviated at night, string-taut and rapid pulse, red tongue tip, and thin yellow coating. Differentiation: Deficiency of the five zang organs resulting in failure of the essence going upward to nourish the eyes.

Prescription Body Needling: 1) Chengqi (S 1), Sibai (S 2), Qiuhou (Extra), Fengchi (G 20), Baihui (Du 20), Taixi (R 3), and Rangu (K 2).

2) Zusanli (S 36), Shenshu (B 23), Mingmen (Du 4), Yaoyangguan (Du 3) and Yongquan (K 1).

3) Cutaneous rolling needle: Roll the needle on the Bladder Meridian from Xinshu (B 15) to Shenshu (B 23).

4) Apply herbal pills on the ear points: Liver, Eye 1, Eye 2, Shenmen, Sanjiao, Endocrine and Subcortex.

Treatment procedure Select three or four points from the first group for one treatment. Withdraw the needles after the arrival of qi without retaining. Select two or three points from the second group for another treatment and apply the moxa stick for ten to twenty minutes. Use the cutaneous rolling needle on the third group in the manner described earlier. Select two to four ear points for each treatment. The pills are changed once every week.

Combination with herbal pills First she took "Fuzi Lizhongwan" for nine doses, followed by fifteen doses of "Shiquandabuwan." The last visit was on August 6, 1980. The duration of treatment was three months. During the course of treatment, Dr. Yu maintained certain principle mentioned above and the patient cooperated well. Thus, the pupil contracted gradually until it was normal, and headache, insomnia, poor appetite and general lassitude relieved.

Explanation The liver opens into the eyes, and the eyes are nourished by the essential qi of all the five zang and six fu organs. According to the theory of Five-Circles and Eight-Regions, the pupil refers to the kidney. So this disease is related to the liver, gallbladder and kidney. The patient also had some symptoms of heart and spleen deficiency, manifesting in poor appetite, general lassitude, insomnia and thin body. Thus, this disease is not caused by only one zang or one fu organ dysfunction, but by all of the five zang organs. We should treat all the involved zang-fu organs, especially the liver, gallbladder, spleen and kidney.

According to Dr. Yu's clinical experience, he prefers to select fewer and effective points, but for some chronic and intractable diseases, which involve several zang or fu organs, the new methods of treatment should be followed based on correct differentiation. In this way, successful therapeutic results can be obtained.

THREE STEPS IN NEEDLING, THREE PRESCRIPTIONS IN TREATING PARALYSIS

—Song Zhenglian's Clinical Experience

Dr. Song Zhenglian was born in Wuxian County, Sichuan Province, in December, 1926. He worked as a physician and a surgeon after he graduated from Hubei Medical College in 1951. In October, 1955, he attended the first training course of Traditional Chinese Medicine for the Western-trained doctors, which was run by the Academy of Traditional Chinese Medicine, and the Ministry of Public Health. He was awarded a silver prize after studying for two and a half years. After graduation, he was assigned to work in the Acupuncture Department, Affiliated Hospital of the Academy of Traditional Chinese Medicine, where he learnt from Dr. Huang Zhuzai. At the end of 1962, he was promoted as the deputy chief of the first research room of the Acupuncture Institute. He has been engaged in clinical and laboratory researches on cerebral vascular disease, syringomyelia, sequlae of encephalitis, sciatica, and cervical syndrome. He has had more than twenty papers published, and he is one of the editors of the book, *Essentials of Chinese Acupuncture and Moxibustion.* Now he is the professor and chief of the Department of Neurology of the Acupuncture Institute of China Academy of Traditional Chinese Medicine.

I. Academic Characteristics and Medical Specialities

1. Three steps of needling

1) *Avoiding pain in needling* Many patients are afraid of pain during needling. Pain, however, can be avoided if the operator is proficient in manipulation, that is, the needling should be performed lightly, skillfully and gently. The three techniques are as follows: a. Inserting the needle with twirling and rotating: Put the needle slightly with the right hand on the disinfected point, perpendicular with the skin, and twist the needle within a range of 90°. While twisting the needle, the doctor must concentrate with gentle and even manipulation. b. Finger nail pressing and swift needling method: The acupoint should be pressed heavily with the nail of the left thumb or the index finger, and a 1 to 1.5 cun needle should be penetrated quickly into the skin with the right hand. c. Inserting the needle with the help of fingers: Hold the needle tightly with the left thumb and index finger, the needle tip is wrapped with wet disinfected cotton ball. The needle tip lightly touches the disinfected acupoint. The disinfected right thumb and index finger should hold tightly the needle at the place 0.5 cm away from the left thumb and index finger, and penetrate the needle quickly into the skin with the right hand. Needles of 1.5 cun or longer, either coarse or fine, are used. Similarly, the needle tip with disinfected cotton ball can be held with the right thumb and index finger, leaving the needle tip 0.5 to 1

cm exposed, and then is inserted swiftly into the skin.

2) *Arrival of qi* a. Such maneuvers as twirling and rotating, lifting and thrusting, flicking and scrapping are used to wait for the arrival of qi. Dr. Song often uses twirling and rotating combined with lifting and thrusting to wait for the arrival of qi. This method is gentle and mild, and the patient feels comfortable. b. In addition to the above-mentioned maneuver, a definite needling depth is required especially on the place with thick muscles such as the buttock and the thigh. c. In case of failure to obtain the needling sensation on the head, face and fingers and places with thin muscles, needling should reach the periosteum, thus qi arrives. d. If the abdomen is needled without arrival of qi, the needling sensation may appear when the needle is inserted to the peritoneum or penetrated through the peritoneum. e. For the superficial diseases, such as abscess, style and blepharitis with red swelling, and burning pain, the ancient acupuncturists said: "Use shallow puncture for superficial illness." The needle should be inserted shallowly by twirling and rotating into the point subcutaneously to ensure the needle sensation.

3) *Reinforcing and reducing* This is related to the needling stimulation. The difference between the reinforcing and reducing method in ancient times depends mainly on the frequency, amplitude, strength and duration of lifting, thrusting, twirling and rotating. For twirling and rotating the needle, small amplitude, slow speed and short duration are applied; and vice versa. For lifting and thrusting, when the needle is inserted to a certain depth and qi arrives, the light lifting with slow speed and heavy thrusting with quick speed in short duration is the reinforcing, and vice versa. The even strength used during lifting and thrusting with moderate speed is considered as the even reinforcing and even reducing. Clinically, Dr. Song takes the stimulation strength as a criteria and often achieves good effects. Besides the twirling, rotating, lifting, and thrusting in reinforcing and reducing, he also combines these techniques and applies the vibrating method for reinforcing and reducing as well as even reinforcing and even reducing in the treatment of excess and deficiency syndrome.

2. Three prescriptions for paraplegia

There are three chief prescriptions in treating apoplexy, paraplegia or other paralysis:

1) *Points on the head* Baihui (Du 20), Fengchi (G 20), Tongtian (B 7) and Chengguang (B 6), Baihui (Du 20), a point of the Du Meridian, is the crossing point of all the yang meridians. It has the function of calming the liver and suppressing yang hyperactivity, tranquilizing and easing the mind, dredging the meridians, regulating qi and blood, and elevating yang and benefiting the qi. Chengguang (B 6) and Tongtian (B 7), Shu points of the Bladder Meridian, are situated on the vertex of the head and pertaining to the Liver Meridian of Foot-Jueyin. The ancient acupuncturists used these two points to treat headache, dizziness, and vertigo, so they have the functions of nourishing yin, calming the liver to dispel wind, activating the blood, dredging the meridians and collaterals and stopping pain. These three points in combination with Fengchi (G 20) are effective to expel wind, dredge the meridians, promote blood circulation, stop pain, and nourish yin and calm the liver.

2) *Points on the four extremities* Quchi (LI 11), Waiguan (SJ 5), Hegu (LI 4), Huantiao (G 30), Yanglingquan (G 34), Zusanli (S 36), Sanyinjiao (Sp 6) and Taichong (Liv 3). Hegu (LI 4), Waiguan (SJ 5), Huantiao (G 30), Yanglingquan (G 34) and Taichong (Liv 3) can dredge the meridians and activate the blood circulation and regulate the qi and blood; while Quchi (LI 11), Zusanli (S 36), and Sanyinjiao (Sp 6) can regulate the spleen and stomach.

3) *Huatuojiaji points* a. For paralysis of the upper limbs: C5, 6; and T1, 2. b. For paralysis of the lower limbs: T11, 12; and L 1, 2, 3, 4. All the points have the functions of regulating the spleen and stomach, expelling the wind and activating the blood circulation, and dredging the meridians and collaterals.

The above prescriptions for treating paralysis can be used either independently or in combination in case of chronic and difficult cases.

II. Case Analysis

Case 1: Hemiplegia (cerebral hemorrhage)

Name, Zhang x x; sex, female; age, 59; date of the first visit, July 10, 1983.

Complaints She began to feel uncomfortable in her head five days ago, accompanied with irritability, hot temper, and numbness of the fingers. The headache got worse in the afternoon after she got angery with her child. On the following day she felt heaviness of the left side, inability to lift the left arm, numbness aggravated and she still had headache. Though she could lift her left leg slightly, she couldn't stand. After she was examined in the hospital, the blood pressure was 170/110 mmHg. The Western-trained doctor diagnosed it as "hypertension and cerebral thrombosis." The headache was alleviated, but hemiplegia became worse after taking anti-hypertensive and sedative drugs. On the ninth day, the left upper arm was completely paralysed, and the left lower leg could only move slightly. She could not speak clearly and when she extended her tongue, it was deviated to the left. She was referred to the acupuncture department due to her deteriorated condition. Examination: Clear mind, emaciation, flushed face, dark red tongue proper, yellow thin coating, string-taut, slippery and forceful pulse, but weak at "chi" region, the blood pressure 160/100 mmHg, completely paralysed left upper limb, and the left lower limb could move slightly, inability to extend or flex all the joints, weak pharyngeal reflex, left deviation of the tongue, pain of the left limbs relieved, the left physiological reflex hyperactive, Hoffmann's sign (+), Babinski's sign (±).

Differentiation Deficiency of the liver and kidney yin leading to stirring of the liver wind which attacks the meridians causing stagnation of qi and blood. The principle of treatment was to nourish the yin, pacify the liver and activate the blood circulation.

Prescription Baihui (Du 20), Tongtian (B 7), Quchi (LI 11), Yanglingquan (G 34) and Taichong (Liv 3).

Treatment procedure Electro-acupuncture was performed on the head points with even reinforcing and even reducing. Reduce Quchi (LI 11) and Yanglingquan (G 34), retaining the needle for thirty minutes. Treat once every other day. The patient felt comfortable in the head and headache vanished after one treatment. The blood pressure elevated 10 mmHg at the beginning of the treatment, but lowered during the retaining period. The left leg could move better, and the upper arm could move slightly after the third treatment. She could flex her knees and elevate the left upper limb a little at the sixth treatment. As she had throbbing pain sometimes in the head, she had a CT scan on the brain, and a small hematoma was found at the right parietal area, which falls into the aspect of "hemorrhagic hemiplegia." With her condition and blood pressure under close observation, the needling was continued to the fifteenth treatment, then the left extremities could extend except for the fingers and toes. The treatment was continued for another two months, twice a week. After that movement was basically recovered. During the treatment, Tianshu (S 25) and Zusanli (S 36) were supplemented due to fluctuation of the blood pressure, dry stool and yellow thick tongue coating in order to regulate the qi of the middle jiao and to promote bowel movement.

Explanation At the early stage of cerebral hemorrhage, the changes of blood pressure must be closely observed. The fluctuation of blood pressure under 10 mmHg during the acupuncture treatment is advisable.

Case 2: Wei syndrome (sequela of encephalitis)

Name, Yu Zi; age, 32; sex, female; date of the first visit, July 20, 1986.

Complaints She had suffered from the tetraplegia for thirteen years. When she was a child, she had injury of the head, and then she suddenly couldn't hold objects stably. On December 8, 1969, she had a craniotomy in a university hospital in Tokyo and left hemiparesis on the left side after the operation. She had a high fever up to 40°C three days later and the fever remained for three weeks, during which she was in a state of coma. The dianosis was encephalomyelitis. Though the fever subsided after the treatment, she became tetraplegia with incontinence of both urine and stool, and downward deviation of the eyes. A few days later, she had complications with pneumonia and was hospitalized again. In 1975, she suffered from another high fever and coma for five days. In 1976, she had a high fever again with a longer duration. She was hospitalized for several months fed with a nasal tube. Because of incontinence of urine, a catheter was used for more than three years. The catheter was removed in 1978, but there was still retention of urine and enuresis. Since February, 1984, she had been treated with passive physical therapy for three months. But there was still severe muscular atrophy, bilateral strephenopodia and deformity, frequent epilepsy and enuresis, sore joints, insomnia and loss of appetite. Examination: Pallor, listlessness, pale red tongue proper, thick coating, and white greasy on the root, thready and weak pulse, bed-ridden and unable to move, tetraplegia except the right hand, severe muscular atrophy, bilateral strephenopodia and deformity, dark and lustreless small legs and toes, hypoalgesia, pain of head, neck, shoulder, low back, ankle and toes, medication of antiepileptic and analgesic drugs, frequent convulsions, the reflex of knees and Achilles disappeared, the tendon reflex of the left upper extremity diminished, while that on the right upper extremity active blurred vision, high fever for several times, and coma for several weeks. Differentiation: Attacking of the pericardium, heart, spleen, liver, kidney and lung leading to deficiency of qi and blood, and loss of nourishment of the meridians which resulted in the obstruction of the meridians and disturbance of qi and blood. The dark and lustreless skin indicates the dysfunction of the spleen in transportation and transformation and failure of the stomach in receiving. Long standing muscle atrophy brings about Wei syndrome. The principle of treatment was to strengthen the spleen and stomach, to regulate qi and blood, and to dredge the meridians.

Prescription Pishu (B 20), Weishu (B 21), Zusanli (S 36), Sanyinjiao (Sp 6), Baihui (Du 20), Tongtian (B 7), Xinshu (B 15) and Geshu (B 17).

Treatment procedure Reinforcing method was used for Pishu (B 20) and Weishu (B 21). Tongtian (B 7), Baihui (Du 20) and Zusanli (S 36) were needled with electro-acupuncture for thirty minutes, and even reinforcing and even reducing applied for the other points with retaining for thirty minutes. Treat once every three or four days. No more headache was felt three days after the first treatment. She began to have a clear mind, sound sleep, good appetite, normal bowel movement, and less pain. On the third treatment, the tongue coating turned from greasy to thin and the pain in the body and headache had lessened. Because she still sometimes had pain on the neck, spine and lower back, Jiaji points of C5, 6, T1, 2 were added with quick puncture and even reinforcing and even reducing. A plum-blossom needle was applied to relieve pain on the head, both sides of the spine, and hypoalgesic area. Massage and chiropractic were also applied. After five treatments, the muscle strength of the left upper arm was increased, and the visual acuity was improved. She could control her urine for a longer duration and began to have a better appetite and sleep and she could move her right leg a little. After ten treatments, the pain of the head, neck, back, and lower back was diminished. Analgesics were no longer necessary. No convulsion occurred and the colour of the skin of the four extremities was better. The dark colour of the feet faded a great deal. She could take meals in a sitting position. Since August 20, functional exercises of the limbs were strengthened. After thirty-nine treatments within 4 months, she could move after thirteen years of paralysis and sit by the bed with support. Urination and bowel movement were normal, and she could take meals by herself. Active movements have been found at the bilateral hip, knees and ankle joints. She is expected to be able to stand and walk after correcting of her foot deformity.

Explanation The ancient doctors realized that "in treating Wei syndrome, the Yangming Meridians should be selected." So it is essential to regulate the spleen and stomach first and restore the source of qi and blood. Only when the appetite is recovered and the spleen functions improved, can the patient have sufficient qi and blood to dredge the meridians, regulate qi and blood, and balance yin and yang. This is the important point in treating paralysis. Furthermore, active exercise by the patient is also important in treating Wei syndrome.

Case 3: Neck and shoulder pain (cervial spondylotic syndrome)

Name, Shen x x; sex, male; age, 36; date of the first visit, November 27, 1986.

Complaints On September 14, 1986, the patient suffered from right neck and shoulder pain due to fatigue. He had limitation of the neck movement and numbness of his thumb. He was treated in an Orthopaedic Hospital with traction, neck supporter and drugs, and the diagnosis was "prolapse of C5, 6 intervertebral disc." After the abovementioned treatment, the symptoms were alleviated for one week, then the neck and shoulder pain, numbness of the fingers, and limitation of the neck reappeared. Examination: Sallow complexion, normal body constitution, painful appearance, white thin tongue coating, pale red tongue proper, string-taut and slippery pulse, tenderness at the left neck and shoulder. X-ray film: Straightening of physiological curvature of the cervical vertebra, posterior vertebrae subluxation of C5 and C6. Differentiation: Injury of the neck and shoulder leading to obstruction of qi and blood and blockage of the meridians, thus pain and numbness appeared.

The principle of treatment Activate the blood circulation and dredge the meridians.

Prescription Tianzhu (B 10), Dazhui (Du 14), Quyuan (SI 13) and Quchi (LI 11).

Treatment procedure Even reinforcing and even reducing was used with elctro-acupuncture. The pain was alleviated after the needling, but there was still pain during extension of the neck and thoracic segments. After the second treatment on October 29, his neck was more comfortable. Paresthesia of the hand and the back pain during extension of the neck posteriorly was alleviated. He was treated with the above prescription supplemented with T1 and T2 Jiaji points with the reducing method. The needles were retained for thirty minutes with a small amount of electric stimulation. The patient was told to extend and flex his neck back and forth. The pain was evidently relieved. To consolidate the result, the patient was ordered to perform neck exercises three times a day. After the third treatment on November 1 the patient was found to be in good spirits, and he could have a sound sleep and normal movement of the neck, but he still had finger paresthesia. The tongue was pale red and the coating was thick and white. So Shousanli (LI 10) was used instead of Quchi (LI 11) supplemented with Waiguan (SJ 5), Yangxi (LI 5) to activate the blood circulation and dredge the meridians to release the numbness. On November 4, after the fourth treatment, the dull pain of the neck, shoulder and back was diminished, and only paresthesia of the thumb remained once in a while. His tongue coating was thin and white and his pulse was string-taut and slow. Prescription used in the third treatment was applied to consolidate the therapeutic effect.

THE CLINICAL STUDY ON THE NEEDLING SENSATION
—Zhang Jin's Clinical Experience

Zhang Jin was born in Heishan County, Liaoning Province, in September, 1930. He graduated from the China Medical University in 1951 and has been engaged in teaching, practice and research of acupuncture and moxibustion for thirty years. He has been studying needling manipulations, meridians, and literature. In cooperation with others, he invented the acoustoelectric needle, the electric blunt needle, acoustoelectric blunt needle and the thermo-electric blunt needle. He emphasized the importance of qi reaching the affected area and method to raise the rate of qi reaching the affected area. He has proven the existence of latent propagated sensation and its theoretical significance. He has published more than sixty papers and he has won eight scientific awards. Now he is a professor and president of Heilongjiang Academy of Traditional Chinese Medicine, a member of the Professional Group of Traditional Chinese Medicine, the State Scientific and Technological Committee, a member of the Medical Science Committee of the Ministry of Public Health and permanent member of the China Acupuncture Association.

I. Academic Characteristics and Medical Specialities

1. How to control the property of the needle sensation

Clinical experience has indicated that the needling sensation with different characteristics has different therapeutic effects on different diseases. For acupuncture anesthesia, heavy numbness sensation is expected, and the longer the transmission, the better the effects. This is the reason why the needling sensation should be controlled.

The clinical significance of the needling sensation is mainly manifested in cold and heat sensations. Of course there is no need to seek the needling sensation from every patient. In fact, even if the special manipulation has been adopted, it is not necessarily successful in every case. The result depends on the operator's experience, the patient's pathological condition and the reaction of the body. In general, the purpose can be achieved if the operator has sufficient finger force, the patient is suitably selected, the needling depth is well-moderated, the movement is quick enough and the different techniques such as picking-up, rubbing, flicking, pressing, twisting and twirling are well combined.

1) *Soreness* It is one of the commonly seen needling sensations, often appearing at the local area and sometimes radiated to the remote end, especially in the deep muscle layers, and at the points on the four extremities, then to the lower back, the neck, the back and the face. It is seldom seen in the chest and abdomen, and it is never seen at the peripheral sensitive points. As to its property, it is similar to the sensation produced by

the accumulation of lactic acid in the muscle. In order to promote the appearance of soreness, the application of the pressing hand is very important. In general, numbness and distension will be produced after the needling. If the numbness appears, the pressing hand should be used with more strength; if distension appears only, the pressing hand should be lightly pressed. At that time, the needle should be twisted towards one direction. If pain appears, the successful rate is small; if the distension becomes stronger, change the manipulation to quick lifting and thrusting with small amplitude. Repeat the manipulation if necessary. See the following table:

Basic Sensation	Pressing hand	Twisting	Amplitude of lifting and thrusting	Speed of lifting and thrusting	Direction of the needle tip
Distension	Light	Towards one direction	Small	Quick	No change
Numbness	Heavy				

2) *Numbness* This needling sensation is mostly seen, but it seldom occurs at the distal ends of the four extremities. The sensation is strip-like, thread-like or band-like, usually in a state of radiating. If numbness fails to appear after the needling, the manipulations may be performed in order to get numbness. Usually, the pressing hand is not used, or light pressing applied. The twisting angle and the lifting and thrusting amplitude should be large, but the lifting and thrusting speed may be either quick or slow, and the direction of the needle tip should be changeable. See the following table:

Pressing hand	Angle of twisting	Amplitude of lifting and thrusting	Speed of lifting and thrusting	Direction of the needle tip
Not used or slightly used	Larger	Larger	No limitation	Changeable

3) *Distension* This sensation is frequently felt, often at the local region around the soreness. Sometimes it radiates as a patch to the surrounding areas, similar to the compressive sensation caused by local injections. To produce this sensation, the pressing hand is essential. Pressing should be done together with twisting, sometimes with lifting and thrusting in quick speed and small amplitude. The direction of the needle tip doesn't change. See the following table:

Pressing hand	Twisting and rotating	Amplitude of lifting and thrusting	Speed of lifting and thrusting	Direction of the needle tip
Heavy pressing	To one direction	Smaller	Quicker	No change

4) *Pain* The pain of the epidermis is not included. This kind of needling sensation may limit locally or radiate. If the pain is local, the pain can be eliminated by moving the needle tip a little bit. Pain usually leads to local tension, and twisting and rotating or lifting and thrusting may increase the pain. Flick the handle or lift the needle a little bit or completely withdraw the needle to relieve the pain.

5) *Electric shock-like sensation* A kind of uncomfortable sensation which can radiate to the distal end, and is commonly felt at the four extremities. Sometimes it can induce muscle spasm and bend or break the needle, so it should be avoided. Even in order to promote qi reaching the affected area, suitable strength should be used; otherwise, an electric shock-like sensation would result. Special attention should be paid to those who are sensitive to needling, and care should be taken when the points on the four limbs are needled. The amplitude of the lifting and thrusting should be small, and blind needling should be avoided. When the points on the four limbs are needled, the pressing hand should be used to fix the points and to prevent bending the needle due to the contraction of the limbs.

6) *Water wave-like or air bubble-like sensation* It is a comfortable needling sensation which is easily produced when the manipulation of even reinforcing and even reducing is used. It appears mostly at the points on the four limbs. The basic sensation is numbness. During the time shortly after the numbness appears, the right index and middle fingers are used to hold the needle handle on one side, and the nail of the right thumb should scrape the needle handle slowly up and down on the other side. Meanwhile, based on the different basic sensations, lift and thrust the needle with small amplitude. At this time, numbness will radiate towards the distal end, and the gentle and even stimulation will exert on the point area one after another, just like the posterior wave pushing the anterior wave. The needling sensation will appear succeedingly, so it is called the water wave-like needling sensation. The distance and direction of the movement of this kind of needling sensation depends on the distance and direction of the radiated basic numbness.

See the following table:

Basic sensation	**Method of holding the needle**	**Movement of the nail of thumb**	**Index and middle fingers**	**Lifting and thrusting the needle**
A weak numb sensation radiating to a definite direction	Index and middle fingers at one side, the thumb at the other side	Scraping the needle handle upward and downward	The needle handle is attached to the index and middle fingers	Lifting and thrusting the needle upward and downward in small range during scraping the needle handle

7) *Cold and heat* Much experience about needling sensations has been accumulated since ancient times. Lifting and thrusting, twisting and rotating, inspiration and expira-

tion, forward and backward, quick and slow, nine and six manipulations are frequently used. Different accounts have been handed down from past dynasties. For the eight techniques found in the literature, each simple type of needling sensation can be divided into two groups:

Group A: Heaviness, distension, soreness and heat.

Group B: Itching, formication, wave-like sensation, numbness, electric-shock and cold.

The pain sensation seems to be in between the above two, when it combines with group A, local manifestations appear, and when it combines with group B, the conducting radiation mostly appears.

For the techniques of these two groups of needling sensation, see the following table:

Group	Location of the sensation	Amplitude of lifting	Speed of lifting and thrusting	Angle of twisting the needle	Strength exerted on the needle	Pressing hand
A	Most local	Large	Quicker	Larger	Heavy	Heavy
B	Most radiating	Smaller	Slower	Smaller	Light	Light, or not used

The process for the needling sensation to be produced has the following regularities: The numbness, soreness and distension will appear after needling. The soreness and distension are the basis of the heat sensation. In order to make the qi transmit to the affected area, usually the numbness should be induced first. After the qi reaches the affected area, the numbness should be changed into distension, then into soreness and heat according to the above method. After the appearance of numbness, the formication, wave-like sensation and electric shock-like sensation will appear gradually based on the different strength exerted.

2. How to control the direction of the propagation of the needling sensation

1) *The general propagation (without control)* Under certain conditions the needling sensation will transmit along a definite direction towards the distal end, and generally it is called the propagation of the needling sensation, or "the propagated sensation" which can be controlled by the special manipulation. For example, the ordinary needling sensation of Zusanli (S 36) usually propagates to the external malleolus, but if it is controlled by certain techniques, the sensation can be transmitted upward to the lateral aspect of the abdomen or even higher. If anyone wants to know how to control it, he must know needling sensation when it is not under special control. In general, if the operator is skillful, the appearance of the needling sensation will be faster, and the distance propagated will be longer.

2) *How to control the direction of the needling sensation propagation* a. Relation with the Shu points: The needling sensation is easily transmitted at the points of the four limbs, especially the big points. Its direction of propagation is also easily controlled.

Selection of the needle and technique of insertion—the angle for twisting and rotating should be large. The techniques such as rubbing, flicking, thrusting, lifting and pressing should be applied. The needle is neither too long nor too fine, and the elasticity of the needle must be good with a smooth needle body. No pain should be produced during the insertion, and the patient's cooperation is important. Careless lifting and thrusting is prohibited after the needling. Attention should be paid to the needling sensation, and avoid missing the needling sensation under the needle tip. b. The basic sensation—finding out the basic sensation is the prerequisite of controlling the needling sensation. It is easy to propagate if the numbness appears first, and vice versa if the soreness appears first. So try to find the numbness first, let it transmit to its natural position, then change the manipulation to let it propagate to the expected direction. If the basic sensation is not good, it will be difficult to reach the purpose, and needling should be stopped to avoid causing more suffering to the patient. c. The direction of twisting the needle—it is one of the key manipulations. The operator must be skillful and careful to catch every possible change in a moment. He must be steady and patient, and quick to adjust the twisting and rotating direction. In general, find the numbness first, then try to twist the needle towards one direction. If the results are satisfactory, proceed to the original technique in order to let the needling sensation transmit to the remote area. If the direction is reversed, the direction of twisting and rotating should be changed with the needle tip remaining in the same position, and pay attention to maintaining the original basic sensation. d. The direction of the needle tip—in general, the direction of the needling sensation is the same as that of the needle tip. The following two methods can be used when there is no need to change its direction: The first one is to keep the needle tip in its original position, and turn the needle handle to the opposite direction. This method is suitable for the shallow puncture with thick needles. Only when the patient is sensitive can it be used. The other one is to change the position of the needle tip. It is suitable for deep puncture. If failed in transmitting the needling sensation with the above method, lift the needle a bit, and change the direction and press the needle downward trying to find out a new basic sensation. The direction of the needle tip should point towards the required propagation direction. With lifting and thrusting, twisting and rotating, the needling sensation can be propagated towards the expected area. The amplitude of lifting and thrusting should be small, and strong strength should be used to press downward. With the cooperation of the pressing hand, try to avoid the soreness. e. Application of the left hand—the left hand is essential both for pressing and holding the needle. In controlling the direction of the needling sensation, the function of the left hand is to block one end of the meridian, and let the needling sensation radiate to another end. The next step is to press along the meridian to induce the appearance of the needling sensation. The left hand can also be used to block one end of the meridian and move forward slowly to exert strength on the needle tip. In practice, the procedures of closing, inducing and moving the needle tip should be applied simultaneously. f. The closing method: In general, close one side of the meridian with the left thumb, which is close to the area to be punctured, and the strength exerted should be towards the open side of the meridian. If the strength is too much, the needle sensation will transmit to the opposite direction, causing pain. The closing can be applied by the finger tip instead of the nail.

g. The inducing method: The left index, middle, ring and small fingers are placed on the skin perpendicularly in a shape of "-" on the meridian to be transmitted. Of course, if two or three fingers are placed on the centre of the Shu point, it is better. Knead the meridian with strength or gradually increase the strength during needling. Sometimes, the fingers can be put on certain parts of the meridian (such as the big point region or the area where the dispersion is blocked) and apply the pressing method. The former is mainly used at the head and face and the condition where the lesion is close to the needling spot, while the latter is applicable to the condition where the lesion is far from the needling spot.

3) *How to make the needling sensation pass through the joints* Usually the needling sensation passes through the joints with difficulty unless certain manipulations are adopted. Just as recorded in *Compendium of Acupuncture and Moxibustion*: "If the qi is blocked by the joint, the technique of 'dragon fighting against the tiger' can be applied to dredge the meridians and promote the flow of qi." It is also recorded that: "First apply the method of 'dragon rolling its tail,' then 'red phoenix shaking its head,' followed by the method of 'eight finger methods upward and downward,' thus the qi will flow eloquently in the joint." What is mentioned here is a method to make the needling sensation pass through the joints and cross at the meridian. a. "Dragon rolling the tail" is a method in which the needle tip is directed to the affected area and gradually moved from left to right after finding out the basic sensation. b. "Red phoenix shaking its head" is a method in which the needle is generally inserted to the earth region (deep region), then to the heaven region (shallow region), and further more lifting to all the directions. After the suitable needling sensation is found, shake the needle left and right like ringing a bell.

4) *Relationship between the needling sensation and the radiation* The numbness can radiate a long distance, but its radiating route is narrow and the duration is short. The soreness and distension transmit a shorter distance, but the route is broader, and the duration is longer. If you want a prolonged duration of the numbness, you must twist the needle diligently.

5) *Retention of the needling sensation* After the needling, there usually exists a period for needle retention, which is related to the strength of stimulation. It usually disappears automatically after twenty to thirty minutes. For some senstive patients or when the stimulation is too strong, the duration of the needle retention may last a few hours or a few days. The uncomfortable retaining sensation can radiate to the distal region, which appears as a soreness, distension, heaviness, or pain. It can be removed by massage and moxibustion, gentle kneading at the local area or heavy pressing on the big points of the affected meridian, or repeated pressing of the skin on the affected meridian. Sometimes the needling sensation is retained on purpose, but the patient should be informed beforehand. This method is commonly used in treating pain syndrome. The method to retain the needling sensation is to lift and thrust the needle heavily before withdrawing the needle.

6) *Distinguishing between good and poor needling sensation* The empty sensation in the tissue after needling indicates that the "qi" has not arrived, and the manipulation can only be performed after arrival of qi. Sometimes the needle body in the tissue is

abnormally tight, and it is caused by the "pathogenic qi." This phenomenon should be checked by certain manipulations; otherwise, sticking the needle or retention of uncomfortable sensation will occur. How to distinguish the "pathogenic qi" from the "normal qi"? The ancients have accumulated an explanation: "The normal qi comes slowly and gently; while the pathogenic qi comes quickly and urgently." Therefore we are asked to manipulate various techniques on the basis of "cereal qi."

7) *How to observe the propagation of the needling sensation* The objective manifestations of the needling sensation which are detectable are the patient's facial expression, local tics or tremor. The operator must pay attention to them in order to trace the direction of the needling sensation, the patient's perception, the nature of the needling sensation and the relative strength of the stimulation. Of course, these should be determined together with the patient's chief complaints. It is ideal if we can find a pure objective parameter, but we can't undervalue the importance of the chief complaints. According to the present conditions, we can observe from the following aspects: a. First of all, careful inquiries should be made in order to get full cooperation from the patient. Care should be taken to the rapid changes of the needling sensation, otherwise, something will be lost. In inquiries, the age, sex, cultural background and the impression of the acupuncture treatment should be asked. The needling sensation should be controlled properly. The inquiry should include the basic sensation, strength, direction and the area reached, duration, nature of the needling sensation, existence of pain, and radiating condition. b. Next is the local examination by the operator. This is a careful work which needs the patient's cooperation. In general, local spasm, tremor, vibrating, convulsion and jumping of the limbs may appear after the needling. As these phenomena disappear quickly, it is hard to differentiate them. Here experience is needed. When "deqi" appears locally, the expression is in tension, but the strength is not very strong. Tremor or vibration will appear in case of stronger stimulation. The appearance of convulsion and jumping movement indicates that the stimulation is even stronger. See the following table:

Manifestation	**Strength of stimulation**	**Condition of deqi**	**Details of the manifestation**
Local tension	Light	Deqi, distension and numbness	Deep and tight sensation around the needle, locally slight solid sensation
Local tremor	Relatively light	Mostly numbness, not radiating or nearby, comfortable	Slight tremor locally, which can only felt by touch of the hand, especially along the meridian
Nearby tics	Rather heavy	Mostly numbness, accompanied by propagation	More evident than above, appears during twisting of the needle, interruptedly
Convulsion	Heavy	A complex numbness, radiating towards a definite direction	It can be seen obviously, locally or remotely
Tics	Heavier	Numbness, rapid transmission, Like electric shock	It can be seen clearly and the patient is hard to tolerate. The needle may be bent due to tics

Jumping of the limbs	Heaviest	Electric shock feeling	Large movement of the limb. Sometimes the limb can leave the bed very high. This can be seen when needling the large points, such as Huantiao, Hegu, Weizhong, etc.

3. Application of "setting the mountain on fire" and "penetrating-heaven coolness"

Dr. Zhang holds that the manipulations of "setting the mountain on fire " and "penetrating-heaven coolness" were formed from the *Ode to the Gold Needle* (1439), and were completed 160 years later when the *Compendium of Acupuncture and Moxibustion* was published. These two kinds of manipulations are described by the motions of lifting and pressing, forward and backward, shallow and deep, the direction of turning the needle with the thumb, whether in combination with respiration or not, whether the number of nine yang and six yin are performed or not, and whether the points are pressed or not after withdrawing the needle. The clinical effect of these two maneuvers is hot and cold. The manipulations used are entirely different and have been developed since the 1950s. This is chiefly manifested in "scraping" (scraping the needle handle with the nails), "flying needle," needling directly to the bottom without considering the layers and emphasizing the basic needling sensation.

As to the relations between slow and quick, and shallow and deep, or forward withdrawing, Dr. Zhang agrees the opinion mentioned in *Miraculous Pivot,* that is, "Slow insertion and rapid withdrawal of the needle is the reinforcing, while rapid insertion and slow withdrawal of the needle is the reducing."

"Shallow and deep" is based on the trinity of heaven, man and earth. Only when needling is divided into layers can we say shallow and deep, otherwise we can't differentiate deep or shallow if the needle is inserted directly to the bottom. Shallow first is a manipulation from shallow to deep through the three layers, i.e. from the heaven region through the human being region to the earth region, a manipulation of needling layer by layer. Then deep indicates a method of withdrawing the needle from deep to shallow. It is the opposite action of shallow first. Shallow first is performed in three layers, one by one. Therefore, it is slower than one withdrawing of the needle. Shallow first is in fact one of the manifestations of slow insertion, or it is derived from slow insertion. On the contrary, deep first then shallow means inserting the needle directly once to the bottom, then withdrawing gradually through the earth, human and heavenly regions. The core of the deep first then shallow is then shallow. In other words, slow insertion and quick withdrawing is shallow first then deep, and quick insertion and slow withdrawing is deep first then withdrawing to the superficial layer.

Three insertion or three withdrawing indicates the insertion to the heavenly, human and earth layers. As to one insertion or withdrawing, it indicates inserting or withdrawing the needle. The three steps of insertion and one step of withdrawing means slow insertion and rapid withdrawing, which is a method of reinforcing with the heat effect, while the one insertion and three steps of withdrawing means rapid insertion and slow withdrawing, which is considered as the reducing with cold effect. Dr. Zhang thinks that if an acupuncturist

Group	Famous acupuncturist	Manipulation	Lifting and thrusting	Forward and backward	Deep and shallow	Twisting and rotation	Respiration	Nine, six	Books
Ancient acupuncturists	Yang Jizhou	Setting the mountain on fire	Lifting slowly, thrusting tightly	Three forward, 1backward	Shallow first then deep		Inhale via nose once, exhale via mouth fifth	Insert 9 times, yang number	*Compendium of Acupuncture and Moxibustion*
		Penetrating heaven coolness	Lifting tightly, thrusting slowly	Three backward, 1 forward	Deep first then shallow		Inhale via mouth once, exhale via mouth fifth	Lifting 6 times, yin number	
	Nan Fengli	Setting the mountain on fire	Lifting slowly, thrusting tightly		Shallow first then deep		Inhale 5	Old yang number	*Compendium of Acupuncture and Moxibustion*
		Penetrating heaven coolness	Lifting tightly, thrusting slowly		Deep first then shallow		Exhale 5	Young yin number	
	Dou Hanqing	Heat-reinforcing	Pushing inward	Inserting slowly		Turning anticlockwise			*Ode to the Standard of Mystery*
		Cold-reducing	Withdrawing with vibrating	Withdrawing slightly		Twisting clockwisely			
	Xu Feng	Setting the mountain on fire	Lifting slowly, thrusting tightly	Three inserting, 3 withdrawing	Shallow first then deep			Nine yang in number	*Ode to the Gold Needle*
		Penetrating heaven coolness	Lifting tightly, thrusting slowly	Three withdrawing, 3 inserting	Deep first then shallow			Six yin in number	
	Wu Zhaoxian	Setting the Mountain on fire	Thrusting 3 times and lifting once				Exhale during lifting, inhale during thrusting	Even number of yang day	*Discussion on Ziwuliuzhu*
		Penetrating heaven coolness	Lifting 3 times and thrusting once				Exhale during thrusting, inhale during lifting	Odd number for yin day	
Modern acupuncturists	Jiao Mianzhai	Setting the mountain on fire	Lifting slowly, thrusting tightly	Three inserting, 1 withdrawing	Shallow first	Twisting clockwise	Operator exhales with strength		*Maneuvres of Acupuncture*
		Penetrating heaven coolness	Lifting tightly, thrusting slowly	Three withdrawing, 1 inserting	Deep first	Anticlockwise	Inhale during lifting exhale in thrusting		
	Zheng Yulin	Setting the Mountain on fire	Lifting slowly, thrusting tightly	Three inserting, 1 withdrawing	Half cun deep, exhale during insertion	Twisting 9 times towards one direction	Inhale via the nose	Nine for yang	*Journal of TCM*
		Penetrating heaven coolness	Reversely (three steps)	Three withdrawing, 1 inserting	One cun inhale during insertion	Twisting 6 times (3 steps)	Reversely	Six for yin	
	Lu Shouyan	Setting the mountain on fire	Lifting slowly, thrusting tightly	Three inserting, 1 withdrawing	Shallow first		Insert during exhalation	Thrusting 9 times	*Compendium of Acupuncture and Moxibustion*
		Penetrating heaven coolness	Reversely	Three withdrawing, 1 inserting	Deep first		Insert during inhalation	Lifting 6 times	

can't understand these problems, they could not master these two manipulations.

II. Case Analysis

Case 1: Headache

Name, Wang x x; sex, male; age, 21; date of the first visit, March 18, 1955.

Complaints He had suffered from headache for one year, which had gradually become aggravated. The pain was chiefly located on both sides of the temples. The pain became severe when he studied hard. The symptoms were distension of the head, excessive dreaming, anorexia and weakness of the four limbs, pallor, pale purple tongue proper, thin white moist coating, rapid and thready pulse. Differentiation: Deficiency of the kidney yin, and upward attacking of the mind by the liver fire. The principle of treatment was to calm the liver and nourish the kidney, regulate the stomach and ease the mind.

Prescription Taichong (Liv 3), Taixi (K 3), Zusanli (S 36), Shenmen (H 7) and Fengchi (G 20) (spot puncture without retaining of the needle).

Treatment procedure He was needled every other day. His headache was greatly alleviated and his appetite and sleep improved after four treatments. Each time his headache was alleviated when the needle sensation at Fengchi (G 20) propagated upward. At the fifth treatment, the right Zusanli (S 36) was needled first in the lying position until the qi arrived, then the left thumb was used to press the distal end of the Zusanli (S 36) point of the Stomach Meridian to let the needling sensation propagate upward. The needling sensation was blocked at the knee area, and the "green dragon rolling its tail" method was adopted (shallow with big rolling) to promote the meridian and connect the qi, assisted by kneading along the Stomach Meridian above the knee to let the qi cross the point and transmit upward to the head. When the right Zusanli (S 36) was needled with the same way, the same effect was obtained. The needle was retained for twenty minutes. A sitting position was adopted after withdrawing the needles. Then Fengchi (G 20) was needled bilaterally, and the lower end of Fengchi (G 20) was blocked with the fingers to send the needling sensation from the lateral side towards the temporal region. Then retain the needle for ten minutes. His headache was basically cured after the fifth treatment, and completely cured after another treatment three days later. No relapse was found since the last treatment.

Case 2: Fixed Bi-syndrome

Name, Wu x x; sex, male; age, 48; date of the first visit, December 15, 1955.

Complaints He had suffered from left shoulder pain after catching cold three years ago. The pain was worse in winter or on rainy days, but alleviated with heat. He had numbness on his left elbow, and his skin was cold. He had difficulty in lifting his arm. There was no muscle atrophy. The patient had anorexia, loose stool and insomnia. The tongue proper was pale, the tongue coating was slippery and the pulse was deep and weak. No response was received after five treatments by needling in other hospitals. The diagnosis was fixed bi-syndrome caused by cold.

Prescription Quchi (LI 11), Jianyu (LI 15) (with the technique of setting the mountain on fire), Zusanli (S 36) and Sanyinjiao (Sp 6).

Treatment procedure Quick insertion was used on the left Quchi (LI 11) point, and the needling sensation was propagated to the shoulder. The arrival of qi was enhanced with the rubbing method. Then the left thumb was used to press the point, and the right thumb and index finger were used to lift and thrust the needle (small amplitude and quick movement). Then the patient first had a soreness. After the needle handle was scraped with the right thumb twenty times, the patient felt a hot sensation locally going upward to the shoulder and the hot sensation lasted for five minutes. A hot sensation was also produced when Jugu (LI 16) was needled with the above method. After the needles were withdrawn, the patient was asked to lie down when his bilateral Zusanli (S 36) were needled to strengthen the spleen, improve the appetite, and invigorate the flow of qi. Sanyinjiao (Sp 6) was also needled to nourish the liver and kidney.

The patient had half of his pain relieved before his second treatment, and was cured after another treatment five days later.

Case 3: Heat syncope

Name, Liu x x; sex, male; age, 34; date of the first visit, October 20, 1965.

Complaints He suffered from cold, headache, soreness of the four limbs and fever for two days, and the symptoms became worse gradually though he had taken drugs for a common cold. His temperature was 40.8°C, and his face was flushed. His neck was stiff and both hands were cold. His mind was not clear and he had carphology. His eyes were upward staring. His pulse was superficial, tight and slippery. As his jaw was tightly clenched, it was impossible for the doctor to see his tongue. He was diagnosed as having convulsions due to high fever.

Prescription Pricking Shixuan (Extra 30) to bleeding to recover his consciousness, and needling Neiguan (P 6) to tranquilize the mind.

Treatment procedure He gradually became quiet for ten minutes after the treatment, but the fever refused to subside. Then a round sharp needle with quick puncture method was applied on the Back-Shu points [from Fengmen (B 12) to Shenshu (B 23)], and the moving cupping method was also applied at both sides of the Shu points from upward to downward, from left to right, and repeated three times. His temperature dropped to 38.5°C after twenty minutes. He was then conscious, with a normal facial colour, and his neck was soft. He recovered two days later.

POINT INJECTION AND EAR ACUPUNCTURE THERAPY

—Zhang Heyuan's Clinical Experience

Dr. Zhang Heyuan was born in Guiyang in 1934. She graduated from Guiyang Medical College in September 1957. From 1959, she studied traditional Chinese medicine at the first course of the Traditional Chinese Medicine for the Western Medical Doctors in Guizhou province for three years. In 1965, she studied with the famous acupuncturist Professor Xia Senbo in Guizhou. She is good at using strychnine for point injection to treat various diseases with good results. Guided by Dr. Li Dongyuan's "spleen and stomach theory," she has accumulated a great deal of experience in acupuncture treatment. She is also good at treating gynecological diseases with auricular acupuncture and emphasizes the selection of points based on differentiation. She has published several papers, such as the *Therapeutic Effects on Fifty-one Cases of Dilatation of Cervix with Auricular Acupuncture.* Now, she is an associate professor and Director of the Acupuncture Research Office of Guiyang College of Traditional Chinese Medicine and a council member of Guizhou Association of Traditional Chinese Medicine.

I. Academic Characteristics and Medical Specialities

1. New investigation on strychnine point injection

Clinically, Dr. Zhang, in addition to the use of traditional acupuncture, has widely applied vitamin B12 and strychnine for point injection to treat various diseases. Strychnine is a stimulant of the central nervous system, and an alkaloid extracted from Semen Strychni, and is often used in the treatment of paraplegia and hemiplegia. Dr. Zhang first achieved good results in treating sequela of poliomelitis with strychnine. During the process of treatment, she found that when the function of the diseased limbs was gradually restored, such symptoms as lassitude, general weakness, anorexia and nocturia also improved and some even disappeared, indicating that this drug effectively dredges the meridians, strengthens resistance, supports primary qi, and strengthens the body. Based on clinical reports and observations, she concluded that the long-term use of strychnine nitrate injection has positive effects. Half to 2 mg (smaller dosage for children) on one or two points once daily or every other day had a good tonic action rather than the accumulated toxic reaction. It is beneficial to the treatment of many diseases of the nervous, circulatory and motor systems. Modern pharmacological studies have also proved that strychnine is able to excite the cerebral cortex and medulla oblongata. When used in a small dosage, it excites certain spinal nerves. Through the elevated spinal excitement, it can strengthen the tone and the nutrition of the skeletal muscle, and the visceral smooth muscle, and can stimulate the optic nerve, olfactory nerve and auditory nerve and promote the regulation of insulin secretion. It has also been proved by clinical observations that the drug dredges the meridians, promotes the circulation of qi and blood, and warms the kidney and strengthen the spleen. Therefore, it is suitable for the patients with chronic diseases, a delicate constitution, hypofunction or serious functional damage to show such symptoms as lassitude, weakness, abdominal distention, poor appetite, lustreless complexion, low voice, soreness and weakness of the lower back and knee, nocturia, loose stool, cold limbs, weak pulse, painful and flaccid limbs, and obstruction of the meridians by blood stasis. Since 1964, it has been broadly used in the treatment of peripheral facial paralysis, poliomyelitis sequelae, amyotrophic lateral sclerosis, traumatic paraplegia, gastro-duodenal ulcer, gastroptosis, gastritis, diabetes, impotence, vertigo, swelling pain after fracture, traumatic muscular atrophy, alopecia areata, facial acne nervous deafness, and optic atrophy. Good results have been achieved.

For example, an army man had pain and numbness on the right lower limb, which became aggravated during walking, for nine years. He had two bullet wounds in 1946 and 1948, and the metal fragments remained in his body. Since 1968, the pain had gradually become exaggerated. He had received many treatments both in army and civilian hospitals, but without any effect. Examination: Numbness and stabbing pain on the right leg, aggravated by walking, the fixed location of the disease, dark red skin on the affected area, thermoanesthesia below the knees on the affected side, pale tongue with ecchymosis, thready and hesitant pulse. After a careful investigation, Dr. Zhang held that his disease was caused by long-term stagnation of blood, leading to insufficiency of yang qi. One mg of strychnine was injected into Zusanli (S 36), Fenglong (S 40), Jugu (LI 16) and Ashi points, two points for each treatment. Treat once every other day. The pain and numbness were alleviated after five treatments, and diminished after fifteen treatments. The temperature sense and motor activity were restored to normal. No recurrence was found in the follow-up visit for two years.

2. Treating gynecological and dermatological diseases with auricular acupuncture

1) *To dilate the cervix with auricular acupuncture* In light of the theory of zang-fu and meridians, which are related to the ear, Dr. Zhang selected the subject of dilating the cervix with auricular acupuncture. The method is as follows: The points of the Uterus, Ovary and Endocrine are first sterilized with cotton balls containing 75 percent alcohol and then needled with the filiform needles, gauge No. 28 to 30 into the auricular cartilage until the heat and distending pain appear and the ear is congested. Altogether 56 cases were observed, among which 47 cases with normal cervix were found to have dilatation and relaxation of the opening of the cervix only 30 seconds after the needling; 8 cases with mild adhesion of the opening of the cervix were found to have dilatation of the opening after twirling and rotating and retaining the needle one to three minutes; and no change was found only in one case with deformity and a severe adhesion. For the fifty-five cases whose cervical openings were successfully dilated, the uterine probe failed to enter the uterine cavity before the acupuncture, but uterus dilators No. 4 to 8 could enter after the auricular needling for one second to three minutes. Meanwhile the embryo

sucking time was one to one and a half minutes shorter than that under the normal conditions. The embryonic sac was intact, and the bleeding during the operation was only 1 to 3 ml. The success rate was 98 percent.

2) *Treating leukorrhea with auricular acupuncture* Leukorrhea is divided into three types according to the differentiation. a. Deficiency of the spleen: The treatment is directed to strengthen the middle jiao and reinforce qi. The points such as Spleen, Lung and Uterus are used. b. Damp-heat: Treatment is given to clear the heat and eliminate the dampness. The points such as Spleen, Adrenal, Uterus, Pelvic Cavity and Sanjiao are selected. c. Deficiency of the kidney: The treatment is directed to reinforce the kidney and strengthen the primary qi. The points such as Kidney, Endocrine, Uterus and Ovary are used. Through clinical observation on 21 cases (the criteria for treatment: Restore to normal amount of leukorrhea, check the lower abdominal and low back pain, and negative findings in the gynecological examination), 2 cases were cured after one treatment; 16 cases were cured after 2 to 5 treatments; 2 cases were cured after more than 5 treatments; and 1 case was not reexamined. All twenty cases had satisfactory results.

3) *Treating nodules of the breast with auricular acupuncture* This disease is diagnosed as hyperplasia of the mammary gland in Western medicine. According to the theory of "the breast pertaining to the Stomach Meridian of Yangming and the nipple pertaining to the Liver Meridian of Jueyin" recorded in the ancient medical book *Dan Xi's Experiential Therapy,* Dr. Zhang holds that this disease is chiefly due to phlegm obstructing the Stomach Meridian of the breast, so the principle of treatment is to regulate the liver qi, promote the flow of qi of the Stomach Meridian, and regulate qi to resolve the phlegm. Points of Liver and Stomach should be selected as the chief points in combination with Mammary Gland and Endocrine. Needling with filiform needle or the pill-pressing method is used. Clinical observation showed that the masses of breasts in ten cases were completely diminished after the treatment.

4) *Treating dermatological disease with auricular acupuncture* According to the records of "sores and pruritus all due to disturbance of the five zang organs" in *Revelation of the Mystery of Surgery* and "the lung being connected with the skin, and nourishing the hair" in *Plain Questions,* Dr. Zhang holds that a close relationship is present between the skin diseases and the lung. The chief etiology is the insufficiency or stagnation of the lung qi. If the lung qi fails to distribute the essence of water and food, the skin and hair will become short of nutrition and the defence ability of the body will become weak. Therefore, the root cause of skin disease is the failure of the lung qi in dispersion, while the symptom is the exogeneous pathogenic factors. The treatment is to disperse the lung qi by needling the auricular points such as Lung and Large Intestine, in combination with Small Intestine and Heart in case of heat in blood; in combination with Adrenal Gland in case of excess of dampness; with Shenmen in case of excess of wind; and in combination with Endocrine and Stomach in case of deficiency of qi. In each treatment three to five points are embedded with needles. Altogether 29 cases were observed, among them 14 cases were urticaria; 5 flat wart; 4 arthroncus; 3 acne; 2, itching; and 1 allergic dermatitis complicated with infection. All the cases were cured except for one case with improvement.

II. Case Analysis

Case 1: Optic atrophy

Name, Guo x x; sex, female; date of the first visit; March 15, 1982.

Complaints The patient often suffered from dizziness, tinnitus and fatigue. Her visual acuity began to decrease half a year before. She was diagnosed as having bilateral optic atrophy at the department of ophthalmology, the affiliated hospital of Guiyang Medical College. There was no response to treatment with Chinese herbs. Examination: Gradual diminution of vision, left visual acuity 0.1; right, 0.2; accompanied with dizziness, tinnitus, soreness of the lower back, weakness of the knees, emaciation, pale tongue, white coating, and deep and thready pulse.

Differentiation Deficiency of the liver and kidney leading to failure of the blood in nourishing the eyes. The principle of the treatment was to nourish the liver and kidney.

Prescription Shenshu (B 23), Geshu (B 17), Fengchi (G 20), Taiyang (Extra 2), Guangming (G 37), Sanyinjiao (Sp 6), Jingming (B 1), Qiuhou (Extra 4), Sibai (S 2) and Yangbai (G 14).

Treatment procedure A mixture of Vitamin B12 (0.1 mg.) and Strychnine nitrate (1 mg.) was injected into the points, one point each time, in combination with needling of two points by the filiform needles. Shenshu (B 23), Geshu (B 17), Fengchi (G 20) and Sanyinjiao (Sp 6) were injected respectively, and the other points were needled. The right visual acuity increased from 0.2 to 0.5 after 5 treatments; and after 10 treatments, the right increased to 0.9, and the left increased from 0.1 to 0.3; and after 20 treatments, the right increased to 1.2, and the left to 0.9.

Explanation This case was due to chronic deficiency of the liver and kidney, and insufficiency of the essence and blood. Dr. Zhang, in the light of the differentiation according to the theory of the Liver, Kidney and Spleen Meridians, selected Shenshu (B 23), Geshu (B 17) and Sanyinjiao (Sp 6) and used strychnine to regulate the zang-fu and the general functions with satisfactory therapeutic effects.

Case 2: Chorea minor

Name, Huang x x; sex, female; age, 16; date of the first visit, October 14, 1978.

Complaints She had "acute rheumatic arthritis" in early March, 1978. She was admitted to the Affiliated Hospital of Guiyang College of Traditional Chinese Medicine, and was discharged two months later. She continued the treatment with anti-rheumatic therapy. At the end of September 1978, she began to suffer from coldness of both knee joints, weakness of the four extremities, slow reaction and involuntary muscle spasm. She was diagnosed as having chorea minor in the affiliated hospital of Guiyang Medical College on October 6. No response was found after she took Chinese herbs and Western medicine. Examination: Frequent involuntary movement of the four limbs, twinkling of the eyes and pouting of the lips, twitching of the muscles of the four limbs, inability to physically control herself until she went to sleep, coldness of both knees, weakness of the four extremities, sluggish reactions, dizziness, anorexia, insomnia, flabby tongue with pale and slight purplish proper, thin white coating, string-taut and thready pulse.

Differentiation Deficiency of the liver blood leading to stirring of the deficiency wind. The principle of treatment was to strengthen the spleen and reinforce qi and to nourish the blood and eliminate the wind.

Prescription a. Geshu (B 17), Ganshu (B 18), Jinsuo (Du 8), Yanglingquan (G 34) and Zusanli (S 36) b. Zhongwan (Ren 12), Xiaguan (S 7), Yanglingquan (G 34), Zusanli (S 36) and Geshu (B 17).

Treatment procedure The reinforcing method with the filiform needles was performed. Treat once a day. Mild moxibustion was given until the colour of the skin changed to pink. The muscles of the whole body were relaxed and tics of the face, eyes and the mouth corner decreased after ten treatments on the first group of points, and the tics of the face all vanished after ten more treatments on the second group of points. She was cured after another ten treatments.

Explanation Dr. Zhang took Zusanli (S 36) and Zhongwan (Ren 12) as the chief points to regulate the spleen and stomach. Zhongwan (Ren 12) is a fu point, Front-Mu point of the stomach and the crossing point of Hand-Taiyang, Shaoyang, Foot-Yangming and Ren Meridians. It is situated in the middle jiao, close to the liver, gallbladder, stomach, large intestine, and small intestine. It has the function of regulating the middle jiao, strengthening the spleen to eliminate the dampness, reinforcing qi, and regulating the stomach to descend the perverted qi. Zusanli (S 36) is the He-sea point of the Stomach Meridian of Foot-Yangming, which has the function of strengthening the spleen and stomach, regulating the intestine and removing the stagnation, reinforcing qi and nourishing blood, eliminating the dampness and dredging the collaterals. The effects are better when these two points are used in combination. Good results have been obtained in treating various difficult diseases with these two points.

Case 3: Depressive psychosis (schizophrenia)

Name, Hu x x; sex, male; age, 16; date of the first visit, September 22, 1979.

Complaints He suffered from insomnia, restlessness, mental distress, dullness, and anorexia after his failure in passing the college entrance examination. He was diagnosed as schizophrenic at an early stage and treated with Western drugs, but with no response. He was transferred to the acupuncture department due to aggravation of the symptoms in the last week. Examination: Mental distress, dullness, insomnia, nightmares, speechlessness, anorexia, and abdominal distension after meals, pale tongue, white coating, string-taut and thready pulse.

Differentiation Deficiency of the spleen, depression of the liver and obstruction by the phlegm. The principle of treatment was to strengthen the spleen and harmonize the stomach, resolve the phlegm and remove the depression.

Prescription Zhongwan (Ren 12), Zusanli (S 36) and Neiguan (P 6).

Treatment procedure Moxibustion was used in combination with the reducing method with filiform needles. He felt the oppression of the chest and abdomen alleviated after one treatment. He recovered after the continuous moxibustion at Zhongwan (Ren 12) and Zusanli (S 36) with moxa sticks for one month.

Explanation Dr. Zhang cured the patient successfully with moxibustion at Zusanli (S 36) and Zhongwan (Ren 12) which indicates the effects of these two points.

Case 4: Alopecia areata (alopecia neurotica)

Name, Wan x x; sex, male; date of the first visit, June 29, 1979.

Complaints He had sudden occipital alopecia areata one day due to overwork. Examination: A 2 x 3 cm alopecia area at the occopital region, accompanied with insomnia and excessive dreams, pale red tongue, thready and rapid pulse.

Differentiation Deficiency of the liver and kidney. The principle of the treatment was to reinforce the liver and kidney.

Prescription Geshu (B 17), Shenshu (B 23) and Ganshu (B 18).

Treatment procedure Vitamin B12 (0.1 mg) and strychnine nitrate (1 mg) were injected to one point, once daily. White villus appeared after seven treatments, and then turned to black. New hair grew up after seventeen treatments.

Case 5: Infertility (underdevelopment of the uterus)

Name, Wu x x; sex, female; date of the first visit, May 4, 1982.

Complaints She was thin and weak, born when her mother was forty years old. Her menstruation was delayed until seventeen years old, small in amount and dark in colour. The period lasted only for two or three days with lower abdominal pain. The vulva was usually dry. Gynecological examination: Poor development of the vulva, dryness, underdeveloped uterus, and the appendix negative. The diagnosis was underdevelopment of the uterus. Her family was told that she was unable to get pregnant. No response was found after all sorts of treatments, then she came for acupuncture treatment. Examination: Emaciation, lassitude, anorexia, flabby tongue with pale proper, deep, thready and forceless pulse.

Differentiation Deficiency of qi and blood, and disturbance of Chong and Ren Meridians. The principle of treatment was to regulate the Chong and Ren Meridians.

Prescription Shenshu (B 23), Ganshu (B 18), Pishu (B 20), Zusanli (S 36), Ciliao (B 32) and Guanyuan (Ren 4).

Treatment procedure One ml of Radix Angelicae Sinenses injection was given to two points each time with moxibustion at Guanyuan (Ren 4). The dryness of the vulva improved and the appetite increased after five treatments. She was pregnant after twenty treatments, and delivered a girl after nine months.

Explanation Dr. Zhang holds that the regulation of the Chong and Ren Meridians is for nourishing the liver and kidney, especially for reinforcing the spleen and stomach to promote the hemogenesis. The injection of Radix Angelicae Sinensis is able to nourish the blood, and the results will be strengthened through the point injection.

Case 6: Nodules of the breast (hyperplasia of the mammary gland)

Name, Xu x x; sex, female; age, 31; date of the first visit, July 9, 1985.

Complaints She had distending pain of the breasts, and four masses in different sizes could be palpatable, which was diagnosed as hyperplasia of the mammary gland in a Western hospital. She complained of a distending pain of both breasts, fullness of the chest, irritability, insomnia, loss of appetite, thin yellow tongue coating, and string-taut pulse. Examination: Four hard masses of 3 x 2 cm^2 of the breasts with clear margin and prominent tenderness.

Differentiation Depression of the liver and condensation of the phlegm leading to obstruction of the Stomach Meridian. The principle of treatment was to remove the depression of the liver qi and dredge the Stomach Meridian.

Prescription Auricular points: Liver, Stomach, Mammary gland and Endocrine.

Treatment procedure Semen Vaceariae were pressed on the points, and changed every other day. The patient was told to press them with the hands three or four times a day until the auricle became hot. The distending pain disappeared after the first treatment, and the four masses were eliminated after four treatments.

Case 7: Leukorrhea (parametritis)

Name, Zhang x x; sex, female; age, 34; date of the first visit, October 11, 1974.

Complaints She had profuse leukorrhea, bearing distention of the lower abdomen, and soreness of the lower back after a cesarean section and ligation of the oviduct in 1962. The gynecological examination two months ago showed normal vulva, smooth cervix, enlarged uterus, with evident tenderness, thickened bilateral appendix and profuse and white vaginal secretion. Blood routine examination: The total number of the white blood cell, $12000/mm^3$, neutrophile, 82 percent, and lymphocytes, 18 percent. Parametritis was diagnosed. No response was found after an injection of penicillin. The symptoms worsened in the last three days due to overstraining so she came for acupuncture treatment. The tongue was pale with white coating, and the pulse was deep and thready.

Differentiation Weakness of the kidney yang, and descending of cold-dampness. The principle of treatment was to warm the kidney and reinforce the primary qi, and to stop leukorrhea.

Prescription Auricular point: Kidney, Endocrine and Ovary.

Treatment procedure Warm needling was applied with the needles retained for thirty minutes. Treat once every other day. The leukorrhea was reduced and the cold pain of the lower abdomen alleviated after one treatment. All the symptoms disappeared after three treatments. Two more treatments were given to consolidate the effects. No relapse was found in the follow-up visit for a year.

Explanation Though the disease was serious with a long course, the patient was cured very soon after auricular acupuncture was performed on the basis of differentiation. The long-term effects are also good.

CONGENITAL AND ACQUIRED SITUATIONS IN PULSE DIAGNOSIS, WARMING TONIFICATION AND COLD REDUCING IN ACUPUNCTURE TECHNIQUES

—Lu Shouyan's Clinical Experience

Lu Shouyan (1909-1969), a native of Kunshan County, Jiangsu Province, learned medicine from his family at an early age. In 1927, he started practising medicine and published *Medical Words from Lu's House* recommending acupuncture therapy. In 1948, he and his wife, Dr. Zhu Rugong, jointly established the New China Acupuncture and Moxibustion Research Society, the Acupuncture and Moxibustion Correspondence Class and the Acupuncture and Moxibustion Training Class. In 1958, he created the first electric glass manikin of meridians and acupoints in China coordinated by the former Shanghai Teaching Model Factory, which was rewarded with the second prize of national industrial product. His major works are *Orthodox School of Acupuncture and Moxibustion, Pictorial Book of Meridians, Acupoint Concept, Collection of Techniques in Acupuncture and Moxibustion, Acupuncture Atlas,* etc. During his lifetime, he had successively held the posts of TCM advisor in the Second Military Medical University, director of the Acupuncture and Moxibustion Department in Shanghai College of Traditional Chinese Medicine, director of the Acupuncture and Moxibustion Clinic of the Affiliated Longhua Hospital, president of the Shanghai Acupuncture and Moxibustion Research Institute, member of the National Scientific Committee, vice-chairman of the Shanghai Association of Traditional Chinese Medicine, and Chairman of the Shanghai Association of Acupuncture and Moxibustion.

I. Academic Characteristics and Medical Specialities

Dr. Lu devoted his life to acupuncture theory and clinical research and gradually formed his individual academic thought and medical style. He especially emphasized meridian theory in clinical work. He pointed out that it was necessary to identify the diseased area and the meridian. The correct prescription could only be obtained by understanding the relationship between the disease and relative meridian.

1. Pulse diagnosis and the influence of kidney and stomach qi

He considered that in acupuncture clinic, pulse diagnosis was one of the important bases for deciding needling techniques, depth of insertion as well as the choice between acupuncture and moxibustion, and whether therapy was correctly used or not, as it determined the results. He put forward that besides Cunkou pulse (radial artery), one must diagnose Shen-qi pulse (inferior epigastric artery), Xuli pulse (apical pulse),

Chongyang pulse (dorsal artery of foot), Taixi pulse (tibial artery), Hanyan pulse (temporal artery) and Taichong pulse (dorsal metatarsal artery). At the same time one must carefully palpate the skin of the meridian and relative acupoints. This overall pulse diagnosis in syndrome differentiation fully reflects his academic thought—"with the theory of meridians as the principal part for syndrome-differentiation and treatment."

1) *Dr. Lu considered that the Shen-qi pulse referred to the primary force of human life and could not be neglected* In harmonizing yin and yang, the Yuan (source) qi must be even and well, its pulse regular and not too rapid, four or five beats one breath, equivalent to Cunkou pulse. If the Yuan (source) yin is insufficient, the yang qi will be restless and uneasy and its pulse will be palpated on hand as string-taut quality. The treatment should be applied to strengthen the qi of the Yuan (source) yin with Taixi (K 3), Fuliu (K 7), Shenshu (B 23) and Guanyuan (Ren 4). If the qi of Yuan (source) yang declines, its pulse will be felt in a knotted quality. If the disease is indicated to turn for the worse, then moxibustion on Guanyuan (Ren 4) and Qihai (Ren 6) should be applied to warm and consolidate the Yuan (source) yang in the prevention of sudden prostration.

2) *Xuli pulse could help diagnose the condition of stomach qi and the Zong (essential) qi* Dr. Lu considered that this pulse should be felt on the hand neither too slowly nor too rapidly. If this pulse is felt as a slight beat on the hand, it indicates the interior deficiency of the Zong (essential) qi and no stomach qi in the pulse. If this pulse can be visualized on the surface, it indicates the discharge of the Zong (essential) qi and is a dangerous stage of the disease. Therefore, Feishu (B 13), Pishu (B 20) and Weishu (B 21) must be strengthened immediately to support and nourish the earth as well as to regulate the lung qi. Simultaneously Tanzhong (Ren 17) should be strengthened in order to regulate the qi action of the whole body. In this way, the disease can be cured.

3) *Taixi pulse and Chongyang pulse could help to tell the prognosis of the disease* Dr. Lu specially emphasized the deficiency and excess in stomach qi as well as kidney qi. Therefore he paid much attention to the diagnosis on Taixi pulse and Chongyang pulse, which are respectively attributed to the Kidney Meridian of the Foot-Shaoyin and the Stomach Meridian of Foot-Yangming, corresponding to the right Guan pulse and both Chi pulses. Dr. Lu relied upon these two pulses for estimating the prognosis of the disease. If the Chong pulse does not decline, it tells that stomach qi still exists, that the disease is severe, but vital functions do not cease. If Chongyang pulse disappear, it means the exhaustion of stomach qi and it is a dangerous condition. If Chongyang pulse disappears occasionally while Taixi pulse is still vigorous, it indicates that kidney qi does not vanish and the congenital root has not been broken off, and the disease can still be relieved though it is serious. If Taixi pulse vanishes, it indicates the illness is very critical.

Besides, Dr. Lu also noticed that Cunkou pulse was often bigger than Chongyang and Taixi pulses in the patient with upper hyperactivity and lower deficiency; that Cunkou pulse was smaller than Chongyang and Taixi pulses in the patient with lower excess and upper deficiency. The hyperactivity in Chongyang pulse indicates the surplus of the stomach fire; the preponderance of Taixi pulse shows the excess in the ministerial fire.

4) *Dr. Lu thought that Hanyan pulse could diagnose the condition in clear orifices, and Taichong pulse could tell the situation of liver qi* In the patient with hyperactivity

of liver yang, Hanyan pulse always throbs strongly, while Cunkou pulse and Taichong pulse are often string-taut and thready. In the patient with deficiency in spleen and kidney as well as with descent of qi in the middle jiao, the Hanyan pulse throbs weakly and is felt with difficulty. Correspondingly, Cunkou pulse and Taichong pulse also show a thready and weak quality. For the former, Dr. Lu advocated to strengthen (or with moxibustion) Yongquan (K 1) in order to guide the circulation of qi and blood downward, simultaneously to reduce Xingjian (Liv 2) for balancing liver and extinguishing wind, to strengthen Taixi (K 3) for nourishing water and supporting wood; for the latter, moxibustion on Baihui (Du 20) should be applied to guide qi ascension of clear yang. Besides, Pishu (B 20), Shenshu (B 23) and Zusanli (S 36) should be punctured to strengthen the spleen and kidney fundamentally.

5) *Dr. Lu pointed out that in the palpation of Cunkou pulse, one should notice if it was predominant either in the left or in the right hand* Although there was the expression, "left pulse in male and right pulse in female," he thought that the predominant pulse in either the left or right hand was not a good sign. The predominance of qi and blood in either the left or right hand is often the indication of apoplexy. Therefore it cannot be neglected, it must be dealt with properly for the prevention of possible trouble.

The overall pulse palpation enables the doctor to get the patient's general condition and to do the correct syndrome differentiation, which gives rise to better therapeutic result. The following examples are able to confirm this expression. For instance, one young female patient had muscular and joint soreness for more than ten years, accompanied by palpitation (her heart rhythm: 120-130 times/minute), aversion to cold, poor appetite, facial puffiness, blue nails, shortness of breath, stuffy chest, insomnia, pale facial complexion, deficient body constitution with hyperactive appearance, which had not been relieved by long-term treatment. The examinations showed that the Cunkou pulse was string-taut, thready and rapid, and the spiritless quality in the two Chi portions, as well as the motive force of qi below the umbilicus and Xuli pulse were rapid, accompanied by dark-red tongue proper and thin tongue coating. These symptoms were identified as insufficiency of kidney qi and discharge of the Zong (essential) qi which gave rise to ascension of fire and dysfunction of meridian qi. Treatments were applied to soothe heart and calm the spirit to remove obstruction, clear the meridians and nourish the kidney qi. Prescription: Reducing Hunmen (B 47), Shenmen (H 7), Neiguan (P 6), Hegu (LI 4), Taichong (Liv 3), reinforcing Guanyuan (Ren 4), Zusanli (S 36). Technique: Twisting-rotating and lifting-thrusting methods. After three treatments, palpitation and insomnia decreased. With twenty continuous treatments, all the symptoms disappeared gradually, and all the pulses came slowly again. In another example, a young male patient had exhaustion of kidney yang due to too much sexual activity, which gave rise to disability of essence in qi transformation, manifested by shortness of breath and complicated asthma, accompanied by dizziness, blurring of vision, frequent nocturnal emission, palpitation, poor memory, lassitude and weak limbs, soreness in the back and lumbar region, thin tongue coating and dark-red tongue proper. The problems lasted for ten years and were not relieved by long-term treatments. In the acupuncture clinic, the pulse was identified as having a deep, thready and rapid quality, in deficient and big quality on Chi portion. Taixi pulse was much more hyperactive than Chongyang pulse. Caused by deficiency of the lung and kidney as well as yin deficiency and yang hyperactivity, the disease was treated by the principle of nourishing yin, descending qi, soothing mind and astringing essence. Prescription: Reinforcing on Feishu (B 13), Guanyuan (Ren 4), Shenshu (B 23), reducing on Taixi (K 3), Fuliu (K 7) and Shenmen (H 7). Technique: Lifting-thrusting method. After four treatments, insomnia, dizziness, blurring of vision and nocturnal emission were eliminated. Spirit and mind were strengthened. Pulse came in deep and thready quality, accompanied by calm Taixi pulse. At the time when ministerial fire was reduced, Taixi (K 3) was punctured with reinforcing method instead for enhancing the nourishment of kidney. All the symptoms disappeared with a total of twelve treatments.

2. Research on needling techniques, warm tonification and cold reduction

Dr. Lu thought the correct needling was essential. Generally speaking, in the treatment of internal diseases, the therapeutic results were much better with the reinforcing and reducing technique than those without.

In view of the numerous complicated and confusing needling techniques recorded in classical literature, Dr. Lu systematized and classified needling techniques.

1) *Two forms* By the structure and form, Dr. Lu classified techniques into three categories: Basic techniques, auxiliary techniques and compound techniques. The basic techniques could be further classified into five types: insertion and withdrawal method, lifting-thrusting method, twisting-rotating method, needle direction and needle retention. He summarized auxiliary techniques into sixteen methods, while compound techniques referred to combined use of various single techniques.

2) *Three Functions* In terms of functions, Dr. Lu classified needling techniques into three types: Waiting for qi, circulating qi and the reinforcing-reducing method. Waiting for qi refers to the method of inducing qi in acupuncture. Circulating qi means to circulate qi and blood to the diseased area. And the reinforcing-reducing method is designed to deal with excess and deficiency of the disease.

3) *Two reinforcing-reducing methods* Dr. Lu summarized the reinforcing-reducing method into two types: to regulate yin and yang, and to harmonize the ying (nutrient) qi and wei (defensive) qi. The former is especially for the surplus and insufficiency of qi of yin and yang in the meridians and zang-fu organs. Inducing yang into the interior tones, while guiding yin outwards is reduction. With the reinforcing-reducing method lifting and thrusting the needle to regulate yin and yang can be used for various cold, heat, deficient and excessive syndromes in the meridians and zang-fu organs. The latter is designed for hyperactivity and weakness in the circulation of the ying (nutrient) qi and wei (defensive) qi, to puncture along the course of meridian is reinforcing while to puncture against the course of meridian is reduction. With the reinforcing-reducing methods by puncturing the needle along or against the course of the meridian and by twirling and twisting the needle, the technique can be applied to various syndromes due to problems with ying (nturient) qi and wei (defensive) qi and due to obstructions in the meridians. The reinforcing-reducing methods of opening and closing the acupoint hole and following the phases of respiration

are also attributed to the category of regulating yin and yang. The two methods, needle retaining and the nine-six manipulation, can be applied randomly in accordance with combined techniques. Dr. Lu analysed the laws of the compound techniques combination and their functions. As well he classified them into three categories and eighteen methods. a. The simple combination of toning and reduction: Composed of the techniques in similar functions, it strengthens the therapy. Among these, the techniques of "setting the mountain on fire" and "cool like a clear-sky night" are considered representative. b. Cross combination of toning and reduction: The reinforcing method and the reducing method are used alternately, techniques such as "yin hiding in yang" and "yang hiding in yin." c. The mutual combination of the reinforcing-reducing method and the circulating-qi method: The combination of method of reinforcing the deficiency and reducing the excess with the method of circulating the meridian qi is able to promote the circulation of qi and blood, and to remove stagnation, with techniques such as the "blue dragon wagging its tail" and the "white tiger shaking its head." As such, the techniques used clinically have their selective foundations and basis.

4) *Five techniques of circulating qi* The techniques of circulating qi have the special ability to transmit needling sensation and are able to enhance results. In his *Collections of Techniques in Acupuncture and Moxibustion*, Dr. Lu listed and summarized the following five types: Circulating qi by twisting the needle, circulating qi by lifting and thrusting the needle, circulating qi by following the phases of respiration, circulating qi by pressure and the circulating qi with the needle tip. In order to study the transmission of qi and substantive phenomena of meridians, Dr. Lu performed experiments with the needling sensation, the direction of transmission of the electric situation in relative acupoints, in which the technique of circulating qi was applied and an electromyogram (EMG) of multiple positions was used. He did his work in coordination with the Zhongshan Hospital affiliated with the Shanghai Medical University. The results showed: a. The relation between puncturing direction and the transmission of needling sensation in subjects: It was found that in ninety-nine punctures using the technique of circulating qi, the direction of the needling sensation in the subjects followed the puncture direction in seventy cases, accounting for 71 percent, and it was higher in the downward puncture direction than upwards, 93 percent and 66 percent respectively. b. The relation between the needling technique and electric response in the relative acupoint: In the downward puncture on Zusanli (S 36) using the technique of circulating qi, the acupoints below Zusanli (S 36) on the Stomach Meridian of Foot-Yangming had an electric response, accounting for 69 percent; while in the upward puncture, the acupoints of the Stomach Meridian of Foot-Yangming in the above reached 62 percent with an electric response. The electric response in acupoints on other meridians was not obvious. c. The conformation among the puncture direction, the transmitting direction of the needling sensation and the electric response in acupoints: In 99 punctures, the total response following the puncture direction appeared in 52 punctures, accounting for 53 percent; partial response following the puncture appeared in 38 punctures, reaching 37 percent. No response following the puncture appeared in only 9 punctures, accounting for 10 percent. It indicated the relationship among the above three aspects. d. The relation between the technique of circulating qi and ordinary

needling techniques in the direction of the needling sensation: It was found that the direction of the needling sensation accounted for 71 percent of the technique of circulating qi, while it accounted for only 43 percent in ordinary techniques. There was a significant difference between them. It was confirmed at first that there was a significant difference in the direction of the needling sensation created by different techniques.

5) *"Setting the mountain on fire" and "Cool like a clear-sky night"* These are the two types of compound techniques respectively belonging to pure toning and reduction. Dr. Lu described the origin, development, theory and practice of these two compound techniques: a. The sequence of needle insertion and withdrawal as well as the amplitude of lift and thrust must be manipulated distinctively and evenly. b. The intensity of stimulation must be moderate. c. The techniques must be manipulated on the basis of qi arrival (needling sensation). The heat sensation often develops from a sore and distending sensation which starts from a heavy sensation. d. The patient should concentrate on feeling the needling sensation, otherwise slight needling sensation would be neglected. e. If the technique is repeated three times without result, the needle should be retained 10 to 13 minutes in coordination, the therapeutic result often would be enhanced. In clinical application of the techniques of "setting the mountain on fire" and "cool like a clear-sky night," Dr. Lu treated 32 cases of 11 diseases, such as painful syndromes, postpartum wind-, damp- and cold-syndromes, gastroptosis, nail cyanosis, common cold, fever, spleen yang deficiency, kidney yang deficiency, deficient heat, chyluia and muscular paralysis. Effectiveness appeared in 21 cases, while 11 cases failed to obtain the needling sensation which indicated that two techniques are significant in clinical work. It was also noticed during the treatment that in 136 punctures, there was heat sensation if 73 of 82 punctures treated by the techniques of "setting the mountain on fire," accounting for 89 percent; and there was cold sensation in 43 of 54 punctures using the technique of "cold like a clear-sky night," accounting for 79 percent. The positive reaction between the two was 84 percent. The body temperature increased in 58 punctures after the technique of "setting the mountain on fire," accounting for 71 percent, and the body temperature decreased in 32 punctures after the technique of "cool like a clear-sky night," accounting for 60 percent. The positive rate between the two was 66 percent.

Expecting to explain further their functions and principles, Dr. Lu made experiments on the influence of these two techniques on body temperature and composition of some body fluid in cooperation with a biochemical teaching group in the Shanghai College of Traditional Chinese Medicine. All the procedures of the experiments were designed by the principle of double blindness. The experiment results showed that the technique of "setting the mountain on fire" increased body temperature generally and the content of blood sugar and plasma citric acid obviously; that the technique of "cool like a clear-sky night" decreased body temperature and the content of blood sugar and plasma citric acid, and that the technique of "even movement" produced no difference in the above three aspects.

Dr. Lu treated a middle-aged male patient who had a history of asthma, sudden dizziness and blurring of vision, inability to move for more than ten hours and he couldn't lie flat. When he looked at objects they spinned around. He also had low voice, stuffy chest, pale facial complexion. The symptoms were identified as deficiency of yang qi, insufficiency of the Yuan (source) qi and the ascension of the Jue qi. The treatment was given to check the liver and harmonize the stomach. Prescription: Tonification on Zusanli (S 36), reduction on Taichong (Liv 3). Technique: Toning or reduction with the needle along or against the direction of the meridians as well as effecting method were applied in order to lower qi; toning or reduction by lifting or thrusting the needle was used to regulate yin and yang. The needles were retained for twenty minutes. At the beginning of puncturing Zusanli (S 36), only an empty and hollow sensation was felt on the needle tip. Afterwards using the waiting-for-qi method for four minutes, a tight sensation appeared on the needle tip. But the patient still had no obvious reaction. Then the needle was lifted gently to a superficial sequence and was thrusted obliquely downwards about one inch. At once the patient started to have a sore and distending sensation radiating along the tibia to Fuyang (B 59) on the dorsum of foot, as well as having some slight improvement in chest and epigastric region. Again the needle was lifted about one inch and then was thrusted forcefully. The needle was held still for about one minute. The patient promptly had a needling sensation radiating to the toes with a slight throbbing. The patient said the tight symptoms in the chest and epigastric region disappeared. Afterwards the second point, Taichong (Liv 3), was punctured and rotated for about three minutes. After qi arrived, the needle was manipulated with rapid lift and slow thrust twenty times in order to discharge hyperactive liver yang, then the patient promptly felt the blurring of vision disappear and the head relax. He was able to lie on the bed in any position. On the visit the second day, the illness was nearly cured except for the poor spirits and weakness of the limbs, thus Zusanli (S 36), the He-Sea point of the Stomach Meridian of Foot-Yangming, was toned with the lifting-thrusting method, and the needle was retained for five minutes to harmonize stomach qi. With needle withdrawal, the patient felt better and became slightly vigorous. In the follow-up the next day, all the symptoms disappeared and physical power was restored.

3. Recommending warm-needle technique, summer acupuncture, summer moxibustion

Dr. Lu realized that warming the needle not only warmed and circulated meridian qi, but also strengthened the technique. Therefore he highly recommended it. He thought the moxa-warming and heat-burning the needle handle, could transmit and penetrate through needle body to the interior of muscles. When meridian qi is deficient and feeble, toning in coordination with the warm-needle technique can promote the circulation of meridian qi and can warm and enrich yang; when meridian qi is obstructed by exterior pathogenic factors, the reducing technique is used to expel exterior pathogenic factors and reopen the meridian and collaterals, then the warm-needle technique is used to increase the circulation of qi and blood to remove stagnation, therefore the warm-needle technique can be used either in the toning method or the reducing method. But it is not suitable to be used in the treatment of high fever, local congestion and swelling, convulsion and tremor which cannot be treated by retaining the needle. The warm-needling method and moxibustion are two different therapeutic approaches. The warm-needling method works to assist inadequacy of the needling power with its warmness, while moxibustion works with heat to invigorate yang and warm the meridians. Therefore in the practice of the warm-needle method, moxa cones cannot be too big and too many, generally one moxa cone is enough.

There is no way of verifying the summer acupuncture and summer moxibustion in the classic literature. But in clinical practice with his father and from his own experience for many years, Dr. Lu realized that the striations of the body opened and yang qi became vigorous in hot summer weather when either acupuncture or moxibustion could easily expel the retained exterior pathogenic factors in the deep muscles and bones by perspiration; twice the result could be got with half an effort in either toning deficiency or reducing excess. For example, asthma often reoccurs in autumn and winter. If moxibustion is done on Dazhui (Du 14), Shenzhu (Du 12), Fengmen (B 12), Feishu (B 13), Jueyinshu (B 14), Tiantu (Ren 22) and Shanzhong (Ren 17) in summer months, serious attacks would be prevented. Cure can be expected with moxibustion for three summer seasons. This is the effective approach for the treatment of winter disease in summer season.

4. The technique of reducing south and toning north as an expedient measure

The technique of reducing south and toning north is put forward according to the pathological change of "excess in east" and "deficiency in west." Excess in east means wood excess, while deficiency in west equals metal deficiency. Reducing south is to reduce fire and toning north means to tone water. Pathologically in wood excess and metal deficiency, wood excess produces fire and attacks metal. As a result the treatment should be guided to check fire and save metal for controlling liver wood. This is the method of reducing excess. Why water is toned instead of toning earth, in metal deficiency? Dr. Lu thought that this was the expedient measure put forward by the ancients. Under the normal condition of earth, toning on earth would make it excessive, and excess in earth overstimulates water, and the deficiency of water is unable to restrain fire. Consequently hyperactive fire could attack metal further; therefore, a therapeutic effect is unobtainable, but a vicious circle results instead. Anyhow toning water is suggested. When water is not deficient, it is able to restrain fire. The restrained fire would not attack metal. As a result metal deficiency could be cured. In other words, strong metal can restrain wood, and wood becomes even and normal. In view of the above, for fire excess and water deficiency, it is advisable to tone wood and reduce earth when metal is normal and even; for earth excess and wood deficiency, it is advisable to tone fire and reduce metal when water is normal; for metal excess and fire deficiency, it is suitable to tone earth and reduce water when wood is even and good; for water excess and earth deficiency, it is good to tone metal and reduce wood when fire is normal.

5. Slight or strong stimulation only being taken as dosage

At present someone says that the toning and reducing techniques can be replaced by slight or strong stimulation. Slight stimulation is able to excite nerves, which tones and strong stimulation can inhibit nerves, which is a reducing method. Recently practice shows that this viewpoint does not conform to facts. Excitement by slight stimulation and inhibition by strong stimulation are only the response of nerves, while the toning and reducing method is created from the theories of meridians, qi and blood. The bases of both are different and cannot be considered equally. Dr. Lu thought that the complete replacement of the toning or reducing method with slight or strong stimulation needs further discussion and study.

Slight-strong stimulation and toning-reducing method are not absolutely irrelevant. Any motion in the needling techniques includes the different degrees of stimulation. For example, in the reducing and toning method by lifting and thrusting the needle, the manipulation of rapid thrust and slow lift means toning, while the manipulation of slow thrust and rapid lift means reducing the techniques. The rapid and slow manipulation is made standard according to the degree of stimulation. Rapid implies heavy, and slow equals slight over here. Therefore, in the toning-reducing method with lifting and thrusting the needle, whether the toning method or reducing method, every manipulation includes slight or strong stimulation. For another example, in the tonifying and reducing method by twisting the needle, the clockwise twist and the counter-clockwise twist are also related to the degree of stimulation. Respectively, the counter-clockwise twist implies that the needle is twisted first counter-clockwise with heavy force and then clockwise with slight force; the clockwise twist shows that the needle is twisted first clockwise with heavy force and then counter-clockwise with slight force. As a result, slight and strong stimulation can only be taken as a dosage and cannot be lumped together with the toning and reducing techniques.

6. The toning and reducing function of needle retention created by the techniques

Generally, it is believed that short-term needle retention tones while long-term needle retention is a reducing function. At present almost all diseases are treated by retaining the needle and better therapeutic results are obtained. Therefore the toning and reducing functions by retaining needle are questioned. Dr. Lu thought that the duration of needle retention was relative and not absolute. At the same time the toning and reducing functions in needle retention are believed to be created by the techniques. For example, that the needle is retained after performing the toning method is able to strengthen the toning function, while the needle retained after the reducing method is able to increase reducing ability. Needle retention is able to strengthen and deepen the stimulation of the techniques to give the greatest effect. During needle retaining, the needle also can be manipulated repeatedly with either the toning method or the reducing method, which enables several slight stimulations to work together for the strengthening, toning or reducing functions. Therefore needle retention is an important step in the procedure of the toning and reducing methods.

II. Case Analysis

Case 1: Vomiting

Name, Cheng x x; sex, male; age, 68.

Complaints Epigastric pain, tasteless, vomiting, acid regurgitation, pain with food intake and vomiting with severe pain for one year. The treatments with Chinese and Western medicines didn't bring any obvious result. Vomiting aggravated and low spirit, lassitude ensued. Afterwards the patient was hospitalized for further treatment. Seven days later his general condition improved and he was discharged from the hospital. Two months later the patient was able to go to work. But twenty days later illness reoccurred with lassitude, aversion to cold, aggravated vomiting and anorexia. Further treatment with Chinese and Western medicine was ineffective. The patient was dispirited and his family started to prepare his funeral. In the afternoon that day, Dr. Lu was invited to deal with the patient. The illness was identified as weakness and deficiency in spleen yang which failed to decompose and process water and grain. The treatment was designed to warm and tone the spleen and stomach by moxibustion.

Prescription Zhongkui (Extra), Zusanli (S 36).

Treatment procedure Each acupoint was applied with eleven cones of ricegrain size moxa, moxibustion was done alternately on the two acupoints. Vomiting was eliminated immediately after moxibustion. The next day moxibustion was repeated on Zusanli (S 36), and the patient began to have a wrm and comfortable sensation in the epigastrium and was able to take porridge. Epigastric pain decreased swiftly. Afterwards treated and cared with herbal medicine, the patient's appetite increased gradually. In ten days he was able to get up and about. In one month he was able to work.

Explanation This critical illness, caused by long-term regurgitation which resulted in weakness and deficiency of spleen yang, could not be cured without moxibustion. Zhongkui (Extra) is an acupoint for relieving hiccup and regurgitation. Dr. Lu applied moxibustion on it repeatedly to obtain cure.

Case 2: Cerebellopontileatrophy

Name, He x x; sex, male; age, 34; date of the first visit, September 29, 1964.

Complaints Over four years, the patient had unstable steps in walking, constant headache and vertigo, blurring of vision, occasional tremor, double vision, inclination to right in walking, choking while eating, lassitude and restlessness. He was diagnosed as having cerebellopontileatrophy in one hospital. Flabby, thin and yellow tongue coating, deficient, thready and rapid Cunkou pulse (radial artery) were noticed in acupuncture diagnosis. The patient was identified as having deficiency in liver and kidney, ascension of wind-yang and a long-term weak body which resulted in deficiency of qi and yin. The treatment proposed to tone the kidney, soften the liver, to raise the clear and descend the turbid.

Prescription 1) Fengchi (G 20), Fengfu (Du 16), Sizhukong (SJ 23), Xingjian (Liv 2), Kunlun (B 60), Weizhong (B 40). 2) Ganshu (B 18), Shenshu (B 23), Fuliu (K 7), Taixi (K 3), Zusanli (S 36).

Treatment procedures The first group of acupoints were punctured with the reducing method and the second group of acupoints, with the toning method. The needles were punctured using the techniques of lifting, thrusting, twisting and rotating movements, without retaining needles. In the fifth treatment on October 20, 1964, the patient was better. The patient didn't need to be supported in walking. The tongue and pulse were still the same as before. The same treatment was repeated. In the eighth treatment, on November 11, 1964, the illness improved, the lower legs became more powerful in walking, especially the left leg. In two to three days after each treatment, symptoms improved prominently. But visual ability was still poor, accompanied by double vision. There were thready rapid pulse, pale tongue body with cracks in the centre, thin and sticky tongue coating. Treatment was given again for toning the liver and kidney, raising the clear and descending the turbid. Prescription: Reducing method with needles on Fengchi (G 20), Fengfu (Du 16), Sizhukong (SJ 23) and Xingjian (Liv 2); toning method with needles on Ganshu (B 18), Shenshu (B 23), Zusanli (S 36), Taixi (K 3), Guangming (G 37) and Taichong (Liv 3). The needles were still manipulated with lifting, thrusting, twisting and rotating movement without retaining needles (in puncturing Sizhukong (SJ 23), a warm sensation was felt in the foot sole). One course of treatments on the above acupoints brought a satisfactory effect.

Explanation This case was diagnosed as cerebellopontileatrophy in Western medicine and no improvement was obtained by various therapies. The effective result in acupuncture therapy was mainly due to simultaneous application of toning and reducing methods for dealing with both symptoms and causes of the disease, which is the key for treating chronic and intractable diseases. Dizziness, blurring of vision, restlessness, double vision, unstable steps in walking, thready and rapid pulse, flabby tongue body and yellow tongue coating in the patient were the manifestations of deficiency in liver and kidney, and ascension of wind-yang. Therefore, Dr. Lu chose Fengchi (G 20), Fengfu (Du 16) and Xingjian (Liv 2) in order to decrease hyperactive yang in the liver and gallbladder for relieving blurred vision and dizziness, and chose Sizhukong (SJ 23) to clarify accumulated heat in the liver and gallbladder to improve the eyes, which was the method of treating symptoms. Besides, Ganshu (B 18), Shenshu (B 23), Taixi (K 3) and Fuliu (K 7) were toned to regulate qi in the liver and kidney, which was the method for dealing with the cause. Zusanli (S 36) was chosen to adjust the spleen and stomach in the application of treating Wei-atrophy syndromes only by the Yangming Meridians. Here Weizhong (B 40) and Kunlun (B 60) were chosen to regulate qi and blood in the Bladder Meridian of Foot-Taiyang, because this meridian dominates tendons and its branch, the Yangqiao Meridian which starts from Shenmai (B 62). When qi and blood are harmonized, they strengthen tendons to improve walking.

Case 3: Tinea

Name: Zhang x x; sex, male; age, 32; date of the first visit, October 14, 1963.

Complaints The patient had tinea on the nape and back, intolerable pruritus, and dry and hard skin with flakes. Since 1954, the disease was treated with acupuncture and herbal medicine. Recurrence appeared three times in ten years. The disease was identified as the accumulation of wind and dampness in the superficial muscles. The treatment was designed to expel wind and dampness, to regulate and open meridians.

Prescription Fengchi (G 20), Fengmen (B 12), Sanyinjiao (Sp 6), Yinlingquan (Sp 9), Weizhong (B 40), Tianjing (SJ 10).

Treatment procedure The acupoints were punctured by the reducing method with lifting, thrusting, twisting and rotating movements. A seven-star needle was used to tap the local tinea for fifteen minutes. In the fourth treatment on October 21, 1963, pruritis decreased but intractable tinea still scattered on the nape and back, accompanied by dry skin, which were due to wind produced by blood heat, due to accumulation of dampness in the superficial muscles. Therefore, treatment was repeated to dispel dampness and improve muscle. Prescription: Puncture with the reducing method on Fengchi (G 20), Fengmen (B 12), Weizhong (B 40), Xuehai (Sp 10) and Tianjing (SJ 10), puncture with the toning method on Shaohai (H 3). A seven-star needle was used to tap the tinea for fifteen minutes. In the sixth treatment on November 1, 1963, the pruritus decreased a lot, but there was still the tendency of recurrence. The skin was dry, thick and coarse. This condition was due to accumulation of wind and heat, and stagnation of turbid dampness. The same treatment was given and supplemented with external application of herbal medicine. Prescription: Reducing method on Fengchi (G 20), Xuehai (Sp 10), Tianjing (SJ 10), Dazhu (B 11) and Tainzhu (B 10), tonifying method on Shaohai (H 3). The reducing and toning methods were practiced with twisting movements. As well a seven-star needle was used to tap the tinea for fifteen minutes. Prescription for external use: Rhizoma atreactylodis 12 g, cortex phellodendri 9 g, radix paeoniae alba 9 g, radix scutellariae 9 g, radix sophorae flavescentis 9 g, sulfur 6 g, cortex hibiscus syriacus 9 g, fructus kochiae 12 g, caulis peperis dadsurae 30 g, and ginseng leaves 15 g. The decoction of the above prescription, with 15 g of vinegar, was applied to the local tinea three to four times per day, and then the skin was wiped and applied with vaseline. With the application of acupuncture and herbal medicine, the disease started to disappear after six treatments, and the tinea was cured in two months.

Explanation In classic literature, tinea was classified into five types: damp tinea, intractable tinea, windy tinea, horse tinea and ox tinea. Although the conditions differ variously, the causative factors are heat and dryness in the blood, which results in accumulation of wind-toxin and dampness in the skin. Therefore the treatment must be designed to expel wind and remove dampness, and clean blood and get rid of dryness. In Dr. Lu's experience, Fengchi (G 20) and Fengmen (B 12) were punctured with the reducing method to expel wind; Sanyinjiao (Sp 6) and Yinlingquan (Sp 9) were reduced for removing water and dampness; Weizhong (B 40) was used to cool blood; Tianjing (SJ 10), the earth point and the He-Sea point of the fire meridian, was chosen to clarify heat in excessive syndromes, and tapping with the seven-star needle on tinea, the unusual use of "shallow puncture," described in *Internal Classics* was supposed to expel wind-toxin in the superficial skin and muscle. Therefore when pruritus decreased after four treatments, the acupoints for removing dampness were taken out, and Xuehai (Sp 10) was added to clarify heat in blood. All the pruritus and pain of ulcers are attributed to the heart, and Shaohai (H 3), the He-Sea point and water point of the Heart Meridian of Hand-Shaoyin, was toned to nourish water to check heart fire. When the condition started to disappear after six treatments, it was advisable to deduct points for expelling wind and cooling blood, such as Fengmen (B 12) and Weizhong (B 40). The problem was still on the nape and back; therefore, besides the shallow puncture on the local area with a seven-star needle, Dazhu (B 11) and Tianzhu (B 10) were reduced to promote qi flow in the meridians, supplemented by external herbal medications. The condition was cured in two months.

Case 4: Epigastric pain

Name, Xie x x; sex, male; age, 44.

Complaints The patient had an acute stomach ache for one day. The pain didn't decrease after treatment, and therefore the patient was sent for emergency treatment that night when he had hidden pulse on both hands, pale and delicate tongue, pale facial complexion, cold sensation on four limbs, lassitude, watery vomiting, dizziness and vertigo. The syndromes were identified as deficiency and cold in the spleen and stomach, which resulted in dysfunction of yang qi. The treatment was designed to warm up the middle jiao and dispel cold, dilate the middle jiao and regulate qi.

Prescription Reducing method on Neiguan (P 6), the toning method on Zusanli (S 36).

Treatment procedure The reducing and toning methods by puncturing the needle along and against the pathway of the meridian were performed together with the efforting method. Both sides of Neiguan (P 6) were twisted simultaneously. After qi arrived the needles were punctured obliquely upwards about one inch, and then the needle was pressed to wait for the arrival of qi. The patient felt a sore and distending sensation which radiated to the chest and epigastrium. Afterwards epigastric pain and distension were relieved. The pulse then appeared. Zusanli (S 36) was punctured further. Ten minutes after the needle withdrawal, the patient was able to go home, accompanied by his wife. The follow-up next day showed recovery.

Explanation Dr. Lu emphasized the reducing and toning methods. He thought that the onset of disease was due to deficiency and excess. Pathogenic factors were able to be expelled and body constitution supported, qi and blood, regulated only by applying reducing and toning methods in acupuncture therapy. The present stomach ache was due to insufficiency of middle yang and dysfunction of qi. Both reducing and toning methods should be considered for use in treatment. Here Neiguan (P 6) was reduced to guide meridian qi to reach the diseased area to relieve pain, and then Zusanli (S 36) was toned to support the stomach qi. When the stomach became normal and well, middle yang can be smooth and even and all the symptoms can be eliminated.

Case 5: Edema

Name, Xu x x; sex, female; age, 54.

Complaints The patient had edema on the lower limbs, poor appetite, paste stool, scanty and yellowish urine, progressive edema on abdomen and puffy face, lassitude, cold limbs, a stuffy and distending sensation in the epigastric and abdominal region, pale and flabby tongue, white and sticky tongue coating, deep and thready pulse. The syndrome was identified as yang deficiency in spleen and kidney, which failed to transform water, resulting in the accumulation of water. The treatment was designed to warm up yang and strengthen the spleen for flowing qi and removing water.

Prescription Feishu (B 13), Pishu (B 20), Shenshu (B 23), Qihai (Ren 6), Shuifen (Ren 9).

Treatment procedure Puncture with toning methods of lifting, thrusting and twisting movements. Pishu (B 20) and Shenshu (B 23) were applied with the warming-needle method. Qihai (Ren 6) was punctured with the lifting and thrusting method, without retaining the needle. Shuifen (Ren 9) was applied with moxibustion for five to ten minutes. In the second treatment, urine increased and general edema decreased by half; the stuffy and distending sensation in the epigastric and abdominal region also decreased. But still there were paste stool, pale tongue with a white coating and deep and thready pulse. The treatment brought effectiveness, and therefore the prescription was still composed of Feishu (B 13), Pishu (B 20), Shenshu (B 23), Qihai (Ren 6), Yinlingquan (Sp 9) and Shuifen (Ren 9). The toning method by lifting, thrusting and twisting was applied. Yinlingquan (SP 9) was punctured with the warming-needle method. The other acupoints were given without retaining the needles. Shuifen (Ren 9) was applied with moxibustion. In the third treatment, urine was free and normal, general edema nearly disappeared, and the patient had a good appetite, normal urine and stool, vigorous spirit, harmonized abdomen, slight pale tongue and thin and white tongue coating. The treatment was given again to warm yang and harmonize earth. Prescription: Toning puncture on Pishu (B 20), Shenshu (B 23), Qihai (Ren 6) and Zusanli (S 36). Zusanli (S 36) was applied with the warming-needle method, Qihai (Ren 6) was punctured with warming-needle method by lifting and thrusting movements. Pishu (B 20) and Shenshu (B 23) were punctured without retaining the needles. Three treatments brought complete recovery.

Explanation In this case, poor appetite, scanty urine, paste stool, deep and thready pulse, pale and flabby tongue body were the the manifestations of yang deficiency of spleen and kidney. Pulse diagnosis showed yin edema. In Dr. Lu's experience, Feishu (B 13) was punctured to tonify lung and circulate qi, Pishu (B 20) was used to support earth to control water, Shenshu (B 23) to nourish kidney for warming yang, Qihai (Ren 6) here was applied to tone the Yuan (source) qi, and the acupoint Shuifen (Ren 9) was added with moxibustion to remove water for cleaning the fu organs. Therefore after treatments, urine increased and edema disappeared. In the second treatment, Yinlingquan (Sp 9), the water point of the earth meridian, was added to support earth by the toning method, and to remove water by the reducing method. The simultaneous application of the reducing and toning methods was the secret of Dr. Lu's success. Therefore in the third treatment, the method of supporting earth was supplemented to consolidate the therapeutic effect.

Case 6: Acute convulsion (cerebrospinal meningitis)

Name, Chen x x; sex, male; age, 7.

Complaints The symptoms were opisthotonos, delirium, high fever, loss of consciousness, red and dry tongue tip. The syndrome was identified as consumption of fluid due to high fever and stirring-up of liver wind. The treatment was designed to clarify heat to resuscitate yang, and to extinguish wind to soothe the mind.

Prescription 1) Acupoints: Reducing method on Fenglong (S 40), Fengchi (G 20),

Fengfu (Du 16), Dazhui (Du 14), Shendao (Du 11), Zhongshu (Du 7), Jizhong (Du 6). 2) Herbal medications: a. One pill of divine rhinoceros elixir; b. radix isatidis 9 g, radix scrophulariae 9 g, flos lonicerae 9 g, fructurs forsythiae 9 g, folium bambusae 90 g for decoction.

Treatment procedure In the treatment the next day, convulsion stopped and consciousness was restored after relieving excessive black stool. The disease was cured with four treatments.

Explanation Cerebrospinal meningitis in TCM is classified in the category of spasm syndrome and belongs to critical condition. In Dr. Lu's experience, Fenglong (S 40) was used to release phlegm-heat for soothing the mind and spirit, Fengchi (G 20), Fengfu (Du 16) and Dazhui (Du 14) were used to clarify heat and extinguish wind, Shendao (Du 11), Zhongshu (Du 7) and Jizhong (Du 6) were used to remove stagnant pathogenic factors in the Du Meridian. The above method, together with herbal medicine, soothed the mind, eliminated spasm and brought swift results.

CLASSIFICATION IN TONING AND REDUCTION, BENEFITS FROM ACUPUNCTURE AND MOXIBUSTION

—Chen Dazhong's Clinical Experience

Chen Dazhong, a native of Wuxi, Jiangsu Province, was born in June, 1909. After graduation from senior high school in 1927, he was apprenticed to Zhang Jilu and Chen Dingxue in the study of acupuncture-moxibustion and internal medicine for eight years. From 1935-1954, he served successively as director in the Chinese Medical Department in the Wuxi Hospital of Chinese and Western Medicine and as deputy director in the No. 4 United Clinic, Songshan District, Shanghai. Since September of 1954, he has been working as an acupuncturist in Ruijin Hospital affiliated with the No. 2 Shanghai Medical University. Dr. Chen has special experience in the treatment of cervical cancer, malignant oxyhhil cellular tumour, hypertension, insomnia, vertigo, intractable constipation, and various painful syndromes. He wrote and compiled three volumes of acupuncture teaching materials, as well as two volumes of textbooks and one volume of an acupuncture atlas in cooperation with colleagues. He designed and manufactured acupuncture substitute pills, acupuncture-needle forceps, electric auricular apparatus, and non-traumatic qi-guiding therapy which has been approved by the Shanghai municipal government. Dr. Chen has published more than forty academic papers and works. At present he is a TCM professor in the Shanghai Second Medical University, chief doctor of the acupuncture department in the affiliated Ruijin Hospital, deputy director of the Shanghai Acupuncture and Moxibustion Association, member of the First Committee of China Acupuncture and Moxibustion Association, and deputy director of the editorial board of the Shanghai Journal of Acupuncture and Moxibustion.

I. Academic Characteristics and Medical Specialities

Dr. Chen thinks it is necessary to use moxibustion by toning and reduction, manipulate needles with techniques, choose precise acupoints and to emphasize extraordinary points.

1. On toning and reducing techniques in moxibustion

The disease is differentiated as cold, heat, deficient and excessive syndromes and the treatment is classified as toning, reducing, warming and cooling techniques.

There were descriptions about toning and reducing techniques in moxibustion among classic literature. For example, it was said in *Miraculous Pivot* that only by moxibustion can the stagnant blood in blood vessels be dealt with and removed. It was said in *Plain*

Questions that moxibustion was used to treat patients living in northern areas where it was cold and windy. These above descriptions indicate that moxibustion disperses cold and circulates blood, which belongs to reducing techniques. Now it is necessary to explain further with some examples.

Theoretically in Chinese medicine, hypertension is differentiated as the result of preponderance of liver yang, upward disturbance of liver wind and fire hyperactivity in the heart and liver. Accordingly, it should be treated with the principle of balancing liver and reducing yang, and clarifying heat and expelling wind. Dr. Chen has got satisfactory therapeutic effects from treating this disease with moxibustion.

See the following description.

a. Prescription: Baihui (Du 20), Zusanli (S 36), Xuanzhong (G 39).

b. Method: Direct moxibustion is done on each point with seven cones of pure moxa wool wheat-grain size (with the reducing method of quick-burning technique). Zusanli (S 36) and Xuanzhong (G 39) are stuck with plaster after moxibustion for suppuration.

c. Explanation: Baihui (Du 20), situated in vertex, and the gathering site of all the yang meridians, is able to raise yang and awake brain with the toning method, and to reduce yang and calm the mind with the reducing method. Zusanli (S 36), one of the four tonic points and the He-sea point of the Stomach Meridian of Foot-Yangming, is able to regulate the blood pressure. Xuanzhong (G 39), one of the eight Confluent points, is able to awake the brain and calm the mind with reducing method, and strengthen the brain and benefit marrow with the toning method. The combination of these three points is able to balance yang and yin and regulate and adjust qi and blood.

2. Toning and reducing techniques guided by differentiation of syndromes

Dr. Chen emphasizes the toning and reducing techniques in acupoint selection along meridians and differentiation of syndromes. Now for some examples.

Vertigo: This is a spontaneous symptom and can be caused by several factors. In accordance with clinical experience the treatment is given by differentiation of syndromes and puncturing points along the meridian.

1) *Upward disturbance of liver yang*

a. Treatment principles: To balance liver and reduce yang, as well as to nourish yin and calm the mind.

b. Prescription: Taichong (Liv 3) is punctured with reduction first and then toning (slow-rapid movement); Neiguan (P 6) and Sanyinjiao (Sp 6) are punctured with toning (slow-rapid movement).

c. Explanation: Taichong (Liv 3) is the Yuan-source and Shu-stream point of the Liver Meridian of Foot-Jueyin, one of the four-gate points, and belongs to earth in five elements; therefore, it is able to balance, soften and smooth liver. Neiguan (P 6), the Luo-connecting point of the Pericardium Meridian of Hand-Jueyin and belonging to the Yinwei Meridian, is able to dilate chest and smooth qi circulation with reducing technique and able to calm the mind and soothe the heart with toning techniques. Sanyinjiao (Sp 6), the major point in the Spleen Meridian of Foot-Taiyin and the gathering point of the Liver, Spleen and Kidney Meridians, is able to nourish blood and prevent miscarriage with the toning technique and able to activate and circulate blood with the reducing technique. This point must be used carefully in pregnant women.

2) *Qi and blood deficiency*

a. Treatment principle: To strengthen spleen and stomach, to tone and nourish qi and blood.

b. Prescription: Shaofu (H 8) and Laogong (P 8) are punctured with the toning technique (slow-rapid movement); Taibai (Sp 3) and Chongyang (S 42) are punctured with the reducing technique first and then the toning technique (slow-rapid movement).

c. Explanation: Shaofu (H 8) and Laogong (P 8) are the Ying-spring points respectively in the Heart Meridian of Hand-Shaoyin and the Pericardium Meridian of Hand-Jueyin, which belong to the fire in the five elements. Fire points in the fire meridians, are able to regulate the functions of heart and pericardium, as well as able to strengthen spleen and stomach with the toning technique and to remove stagnation in the liver with the reducing technique. Taibai (Sp 3), the Yuan-source point and the Shu-stream point in the Spleen Meridian of Foot-Taiyin, belonging to earth in the five elements and the earth point in the earth meridian is able to adjust the function of the Spleen Meridian of Foot-Taiyin. It is able to tone the lung and benefit qi with the toning technique and able to clean the heart and nourish the blood with the reducing technique. Chongyang (S 42), the Yuan-source point of the Stomach Meridian of Foot-Yangming, serves to harmonize and strengthen the spleen and stomach.

3) *Type of insufficiency in kidney essence*

a. Treatment principles: To tone the kidney and assist yang in prominence of yang deficiency, to tone the kidney and benefit yin in prominence of deficiency.

b. Prescription: Main points: Jingqu (L 8). Additional points: Taixi (K 3) for yang deficiency, Fuliu (K 7) for yin deficiency.

c. Explanation: Jingqu (L 8) is the Jing-river point of the Lung Meridian of Hand-Taiyin and belongs to metal in the five elements. This point, the metal point of the metal meridian, is able to regulate the function of the Lung Meridian of Hand-Taiyin. Theoretically, metal produces water; therefore, it is able to clean the heart and benefit the Kidney. Here the combination of Jingqu (L 8) and Taixi (K 3), the Yuan-source and Shu-stream point of the Kidney Meridian of Foot-Shaoyin, is able to strengthen kidney yang. Fuliu (K 7) is the Jing-river point of the Kidney Meridian of Foot-Shaoyin and belongs to metal in the five elements. Metal produces water, so that the combination of Jingqu (L 8) and Fuliu (K 7) benefits kidney yin.

4) *Accumulation of turbid phlegm*

a. Treatment principles: To disperse dampness and expel phlegm, to strengthen spleen and harmonize stomach.

b. Prescription: Yinlingquan (Sp 9) is punctured with reducing technique (slow-rapid movement) and Fenglong (S 40), with the toning technique (slow-rapid movement), Gongsun (Sp 4) is punctured with the reducing technique first and then the toning technique (slow-rapid movement).

c. Explanation: Reducing technique on Yinlingquan (Sp 9), the He-sea point of the Spleen Meridian of Foot-Taiyin and belonging to water in the five elements, proposes to remove dampness. Fenglong (S 40), the Luo-connecting point of the Stomach Meridian of Foot-Yangming, is the main point for dispersing phlegm. Gongsun (Sp 4), the Luo-connecting point of the Spleen Meridian of Foot-Taiyin, serves to remove dampness, strengthen the spleen and harmonize the stomach.

3. Precise selection of acupoints

Dr. Chen is specialized in the precise selection of acupoints and often eliminates severe and intractable illness only by one acupoint.

Insomnia: It can be caused by several factors. The illness was generalized by Zhang Jingyue as pathogen-involved type and nonpathogen types, that pathogen-involved insomnia was an excessive pattern. Clinically, there are many cases of insomnia which cannot be improved by taking Western and Chinese medication for years. Dr. Chen only punctures one acupoint, Sanjian (LI 3), for various types of insomnia, using the toning technique on a deficient pattern and a reducing technique on an excessive pattern. He analysed the therapeutical effects of 102 cases. The effective rate reached 95.09 percent. Sanjian (LI 3) is the Shu-stream point of the Large Intestine Meridian of Hand-Yangming and is classified as wood in the five elements. It is able to strengthen the spleen for dispersing phlegm with the reducing technique and able to soothe the heart and calm the mind with the toning tcchnique.

4. Extraordinary points

Extraordinary points were discovered from clinical practice by successive practitioners. Extraordinary points are able to relieve severe illness immediately if used correctly.

Acute lumbar sprain: This is a commonly encountered disease and even be aggravated by breathing in severe cases. Dr. Chen can often get results in the treatment of this illness by only one point, Yintang (Extra).

Yintang (Extra) is situated between the eyebrows and where the Du Meridian goes through. Therefore it is closely related to the back, lumbar region and vertebral column. This point is punctured with pinching-up technique downwards subcutaneously about 1.0 inch. And then the needle is manipulated with the reducing technique first and afterwards with the toning technique (slow-rapid movement). During manipulation, the patient should be asked to move the lumbar region with progressive amplitude. Usually within one or two minutes, pain would gradually decrease and disappear. Clinical observation on sixty-six cases showed that the effective rate reached 90.9 percent. This belongs to selection of acupoints along meridian and the method of upward points for downward illness.

II. Case Analysis

Case 1: Chronic diarrhoea

Name, Huang x x; sex, female; age, 59; case No, 73-12632.

Complaints Over ten years of intermittent paste stool aggravated as diarrhoea about times per day without abdominal pain after taking a little greasy food or raw and cold fruits. There was no improvement in treatment by Western and Chinese medicine. At present, she had poor appetite, distending and full sensation in the abdominal region, aversion to cold, puffiness in the face, lassitude, emaciation, soft and thready pulse, pale tongue and white tongue coating. This was differentiated as accumulation of dampness due to spleen deficiency, which resulted in dysfunctions of spleen in transportation and transformation. This case was treated with the principle of warming up the stomach and strengthening the spleen for eliminating dampness.

Prescription Zhangmen (Liv 13), Guanyuan (Ren 4), Gongsun (Sp 4), Yinlingquan (S 9).

Treatment procedure Zhangmen (Liv 13) and Guanyuan (Ren 4) were inserted slowly by the warming-needle technique with three moxa cones and then taken out swiftly. It served to warm up qi in the lower abdominal region for strengthening the spleen and raising yang. Gongsun (Sp 4) and Yinlingquan (Sp 9) were punctured with technique of swift insertion and slow withdrawal for eliminating dampness. The treatment was given once a day. After three treatments, bowel movement returned to normal, and other symptoms disappeared. No recurrence was found out in the follow-up examination after one year.

Case 2: Diarrhoea

Name, Jiang x x; sex, male; age, 68; case No, 74-31860.

Complaints Diarrhoea due to bromatoxism for two years, there was abdominal pain along naval and borborygmus before every dawn, which resulted in diarrhoea with undigested food, aversion to cold, cold sensation in limbs, soreness and weakness in the lumbar region and knees, poor appetite, pale tongue, white tongue coating, deep and thready pulse. It was differentiated as weakness of the constitution due to old age, involvement of kidney due to spleen deficiency and decline of fire of Mingmen (vital gate). Before dawn, yang qi has not become vigorous yet, while yin-cold is still hyperactive, causing borborygmus and diarrhoea or early morning diarrhoea. Therefore this type of illness should be treated with the principle of warming up the kidney and strengthening the spleen.

Prescription Taibai (Sp 3), Taixi (K 3), Pishu (B 20), Shenshu (B 23), Guanyuan (Ren 4).

Treatment procedure Taibai (Sp 3) and Taixi (K 3), The Yuan-sourse points respectively of the Spleen Meridian of Foot-Taiyin and the Kidney Meridian of Foot-Shaoyin, were punctured with the technique of slow insertion and swift withdrawal for regulating meridian qi of both the Spleen Meridian of Foot-Taiyin and the Kidney Meridian of Foot-Shaoyin. Pishu (B 20), Shenshu (B 23) and Guanyuan (Ren 4) were done with direct moxibustion of seven wheat grain-size moxa cones to support the spleen qi and warming up kidney yang. The treatment was given twice per week. After three treatments, symptoms improved. After twenty treatments, symptoms disappeared completely. No recurrence was found in the follow-up examination after six months.

Case 3: Diarrhoea

Name, Yang x x; sex, female; age, 57; case No, 73-23679.

Complaints The patient complained of frequent distending and stuffy sensation in the chest and hypochondriac region, belching, acid regurgitation, borborygmus and abdominal pain before bowel movements. She had a thready string-taut pulse, slight red tongue, thin and sticky tongue coating. This case was differentiated as dysfunctions in the liver, which attacked the spleen and caused dysfunctions of spleen in transportation and transformation, resulting in abdominal pain and prolonged diarrhoea. This case should be treated with the principle of compressing the liver and supporting the spleen.

Prescription Xingjian (Liv 2), Daling (P 7), Gongsun (Sp 4), Yinlingquan (Sp 9).

Treatment procedure Xingjian (Liv 2) and Daling (P 7), the Ying-spring point of the Liver Meridian of Foot-Jueyin and the Yuan-source point of the Pericardium Meridian of Hand-Jueyin respectively, were punctured with the reducing technique of lifting-thrusting movements for smoothing circulation of the liver. Gongsun (Sp 4) and Yinlingquan (Sp 9), the Luo-connecting point and the He-sea point of the Spleen Meridian of Foot-Taiyin, were punctured with the toning technique of lifting-thrusting movements for adjusting and supporting spleen qi. After treatments, abdominal pain decreased and stool formed. Diarrhoea was eliminated with 7 treatments.

Explanation The basic reason for chronic diarrhoea is due to deficiency and weakness in the spleen and stomach, which result in abnormal transportation and transformation. As well the kidney is often involved in prolonged diarrhoea. Therefore in clinical treatment, the basic therapy is to tone the spleen and promote the stomach. But the treatment must be given with differentiation of syndromes in different types of diarrhoea caused by problems between the liver and spleen or by kidney involvement due to spleen illness. The causative factors and symptoms were different in the above three cases of chronic diarrhoea. In accordance with the differentiations, different acupoints and techniques were used. Consequently, satisfactory effects were obtained.

Case 4: Night sweating

Name, Chen x x; sex, female; age, 45; case No, 82-1426; date of the first visit, November 9, 1982.

Complaints The patient complained of profuse sweating during the night for five months since a cold and febrile illness in autumn. Examination: Yellowish facial complexion, low spirits, red tongue, yellow tongue coating. Inquiring: distending and full sensation in epigastric region, slight fever, dream-disturbed sleep. Auscultation and olfaction: Low voice. Palpation: String-taut and slippery pulse, pain by pressure in epigastric region. By analysis of four diagnostic methods, the case was differentiated as accumulation of turbid dampness in middle jiao and dysfunction of spleen in transportation due to unrelieved summer pathogen. This case was treated to eliminate summer pathogen, to disperse and expel dampness and to promote functions of Sanjiao.

Prescription Quchi (LI 11), Zhigou (SJ 6), Yinlingquan (Sp 9), Yanglingquan (G 34), Zusanli (S 36), Fuliu (K 7).

Treatment procedure The reducing technique by slow-swift movement was applied on Quchi (LI 11) and Yinlingquan (Sp 9). The toning technique by slow-swift movement was applied on Zhigou (SJ 6) and Fuliu (K 7). Yanglingquan (G 34) was punctured towards Zusanli (S 36) with the reducing technique first and then with the toning technique by slow-swift movement. Afterwards the needles were retained. On the second visit on September 11, the patient said that she slept quite well without sweating on the day she was treated with acupuncture. The patient felt the full sensation in the epigastric region decreased and bowel movement became relaxed and appetite increased. The sticky tongue coating was removed and pulse became feeble and string-taut. In order to consolidate the therapeutical effect, the treatment was given once again with the previous prescription in which Fuliu (K 7) was replaced with Sanyinjiao (Sp 6).

Explanation Night sweating can be caused by either exterior pathogenic factors or interior injury, and therefore the principles of treatment can be quite different. Night sweating of interior injury is mostly caused by yin deficiency and interior heat, by hyperactivity of yang-heat. Accordingly, it must be treated to nourish yin and clarify heat, to tone blood and eliminate profuse night sweating. Night sweating of exterior factor is mostly due to invasion of factors in Shaoyang Meridian and unrelieved summer factor. Therefore it must be treated to smooth qi circulation in the Shaoyang Meridians to expel exterior pathogenic factor and clarify heat. The above case was due to unrelieved summer pathogenic factor and accumulation of dampness. The previous practitioner used toning herbs improperly, so that summer dampness remained in the body. In acupuncture treatment, Zhigou (SJ 6), the Jing-river point of the Sanjiao Meridian of Hand-Shaoyang, and Yanglingquan (G 34), the He-sea point of the Gallbladder Meridian of Foot-Shaoyang, were punctured together with the He-sea points of the Yangming Meridians of Hand and Foot in order to clarify heat and expel pathogenic factor, as well as together with the He-sea point of the Spleen Meridian of Foot-Taiyin in order to promote the flow of water and disperse dampness. Only one treatment can eliminate the problem.

PALPATION OF THE MERIDIAN AND TIME PHASE OF THE MERIDIAN

—Chen Zifu's Clinical Experience

Chen Zifu was born in Tangshan, Hebei Province in October 1935. He entered the Beijing College of Traditional Chinese Medicine in 1956. Since his graduation in 1962, he worked at Tonghua, Jilin Province. From 1979 he worked at the Tangshan Municipal Hospital of Traditional Chinese Medicine and was transferred to Beijing in 1982. Through twenty year's clinical and teaching work, he has accumulated a lot of experience in the study of the meridian Shu points. His main works included *Teaching Materials on Meridian* and *Reference on Meridian* (in progress), and more than ten papers were published. Now, he is an associate professor and chief of the Teaching Division of the Meridians of the Department of Acupuncture, Moxibustion and Tuina of the Beijing College of Traditional Chinese Medicine. He is also a standing member of the Beijing Acupuncture Association.

I. Academic Characteristics and Medical Specialities

1. Palpation of the meridian

The method of the meridian palpation was recorded early in *Internal Classic*, which included more than ten kinds such as detecting, palpating, touching, pressing, feeling, flicking, pushing, picking up, leading and dredging. As to the reaction of the palpation upon the skin, there are warm, cold, lubricating, dry, thick and thin, coarse and fine, hard and soft, etc. There are three kinds of reactions of the meridian: The first includes soreness, numbness, pain, distension, paresthesia, heaviness, hardness, tightness, warmth, cold, blood, swelling, depression, and so on; the second are tendon-like, cord-like, nodule-like, pearl-like, cereal-like, hammer-like, and wood-like sensations, etc.; and the third are electric-shock, formication, water flowing, air fleeing, warm streaming, and cold streaming, etc. Just as recorded in *Miraculous Pivot* that "acupuncturists should detect the condition of the meridian first, palpate it and follow it, press it and flick it, then select the points and needle them." So palpation of the meridian is an essential method in the diagnosis of diseases and selection of points. Dr. Chen is proficient and has much experience. For example, there was a thirty-eight-year old male worker, who suffered from sudden severe pain of his upper incisor teeth for three months. No response was found when he was treated with modern medicine including morphine. The pain could be induced by cold air, hot food, and light touching, and became worse during the night. He had received needling treatment but the pain could not be stopped. He was referred to Dr. Chen in February, 1966. From appearance, his teeth were normal and there was no swelling of the gum. His tongue was covered with thin yellow and greasy coating. Dr. Chen then needled Xiaguan (S 7) and Hegu (LI 4) with the reducing method. The patient fell asleep immediately after needling but severe pain and restlessness recurred after the needles were removed. Then Dr. Chen palpated the Five Shu points and the Yuan-Source points along the Hand and Foot-Yangming Meridians, but with no reaction. He let the patient change into a prone position and palpated the Back-Shu points. He found that there was severe pricking pain at both Jueyinshu (B 14) points when he pressed along the Back Shu points. With the pecking method, Dr. Chen punctured the point with a short needle. The toothache was stopped and the patient fell asleep. No relapse was found after retaining the needles for one hour. Dr. Chen could not understand why the Jueyinshu (B 14) point was able to kill the pain. Then he asked the patient and found out the pain was induced by a quarrel between the patient and his family, and whenever he was angry a toothache followed. Therefore, according to the theory that the heart dominates the mind and emotional activity, Dr. Chen found the cause of the disease. Another example was a female patient of thirty years old, who suffered from gastric pain for many years. The pain could be temporarily relieved by antispasmodic drugs. "Gastric spasm" was diagnosed after a barium radiography. The patient was strong, but irritable. The gastric pain would appear whenever there were emotional changes. At the time when she visited the doctor, she was having great pain of the stomach. The tongue proper was pale red with scanty coating, and the pulse was string-taut and somewhat rapid. She was diagnosed as having depression of the liver qi and affecting the spleen leading to stagnation of qi of the Foot-Yangming Meridian. The Foot-Jueyin and Foot-Yangming Meridians and the yin-yang points were palpated. Dr. Chen felt that there seemed to be a nodule at Taichong (Liv 3), and depression at Zusanli (S 36) and Yanglingquan (G 34). There was no response at the Back-Shu points of the liver, spleen and stomach, but there was a tendon-like tenderness at Geshu (B 17). Dr. Chen realized that the blood stasis at Geshu (B 17) might be due to the long-term pain invading the collateral of the stomach. So treatment should be to dredge the Jueyin Meridian and promote the Yangming Meridian and use yang to induce yin to descend the perverted qi. The pain was relieved by needling the four pass points and pricking Geshu (B 17). Yanglingquan (G 34) and Zusanli (S 36) were selected to consolidate the effect. The pain was eliminated after retaining the needle for fifteen minutes. No relapse was revealed after a follow-up visit over half a year later.

2. Penetration needling therapy to expel the wind in treating paralysis

Dr. Chen holds that the method of inducing yang from yin and inducing yin from yang is an important principle for syndrome differentiation in selection of points. Quick results could be obtained if one needle can penetrate two points, or one point can relate two meridians to induce both yin and yang. For example, a male retired worker of sixty-eight years old who suffered from left hemiplegia was sent to the Acupuncture Department in the morning. He got drunk the night before, and hemiplegia was found the next morning after he got up. The patient was tall and strong, with a pink face. His muscle was thick, his mind and speech clear, the left corner of his mouth deviated slightly to the right side. The naso-labial fissure was shallow and his left eye failed to close tightly. His left frontal wrinkle was flattened, and the limbs on the left side were paralysed. His tongue proper was light red with little coating, and his pulse was deep, string-taut and strong. The syndrome belonged to windstroke. Though the patient looked strong, his kidney yang qi was weak, due to his age. Deficiency of yang failed to lead the blood circulation and resulted in stagnation of blood in the meridians. Therefore, the principle of treatment was to reinforce qi and promote the blood circulation, warm the meridians and dispel the wind. Moxibustion was applied at Baihui (Du 20), Qihai (Ren 6) and Guanyuan (Ren 4) points, and needling applied at Xuehai (Sp 10) (bilateral) and Zusanli (S 36) (bilateral) points, and Yangbai (G 14) penetrated toward Yuyao (Extra 3), Sibai (S 2) towards Yingxiang (LI 20), Jiache (S 6) towards Dicang (S 4), Jianyu (LI 15) towards Binao (LI 14), Quchi (LI 11) towards Shaohai (H 3), Waiguan (SJ 5) towards Neiguan (P 6), Hegu (LI 4) towards Houxi (SI 3), Huantiao (G 30) towards Changqiang (Du 1), Fengshi (G 31) towards Yinmen (B 37), Yanglingquan (G 34) towards Yinlingquan (S 9), Xuanzhong (G 39) towards Sanyinjiao (Sp 6), and Kunlun (B 60) towards Taixi (K 3). Treat once a day. The patient could walk and take care of himself after one month of treatment.

3. The time phase of the meridian

Dr. Chen got the essence of the midnight-noon ebb-flow method from Dr. Shan Yutang. Under his guidance, Dr. Chen wrote a book titled *Critical Interpretation of Midnight-Noon Ebb-Flow*. After more than twenty years' work on this classic acupuncture technique, he put forward *Three Principles of Dr. Shan's Liuzhu Method:*

1) *Investigating the disease carefully and matching it with the time phase* The technique of midnight-noon ebb-flow is divided into two kinds, one is to select the points according to the routine method, and the other is to do so based on clinical differentiation. The routine method is recorded in the textbook, after calculating the day, hour, the heavenly stems and the earthly branches, points can be selected in accordance with the day to match the heavenly stems and earthly branches. The hour-prescription of acupoints is to select the points according to the method of reinforcing the mother acupoint and reducing its son acupoint. But the selection of acupoints according to the routine method can not treat all the diseases. Therefore, it is necessary to investigate the disease carefully, and match it with the time phase, that is to say, the differentiation must be integrated with the time-prescription of the points. To investigate carefully has two meanings: One refers to careful and accurate differentiation, and the second refers to the observation of the pathological condition strictly according to the principle of differentiation. There are two methods for matching it with the time phase: The first one is to wait until qi reaches the required stage, i.e. after the differentiation, do not needle the acupoints corresponding to the disease until they are open. The second is, after the differentiation, to select the acupoints which are suitable to the disease from the originally opened points, then needle them. Therefore, the midnight-noon ebb-flow method is not against the principle of treating disease based on the differentiation, but it is a very flexible method to select points according to the differentiation.

The day-prescription of acupoints is to select the yang points in clinic at yang day and yang hour and select the yin point at yin day and yin hour according to differentiation based on the diseased conditions and the meridians. Meridian produces meridian, point generates point, the five Shu points of the meridian which are on duty in the day can open one layer or several layers in the clockwise phase, or according to the rules of the motion of the five elements, A joins with F, B with G, C with H, D with J and E joins with K. Select the points from the meridians which match yin and yang, such as yang points selected at yang hour and yang day. In case of yin meridian disease, the points of yin meridian are selected. Qiaoyin (G 44) the Jing-Well point of the Gallbladder Meridian which belongs to metal is selected at time from 7 p.m. to 9 p.m. in case of spleen syndrome, Shangqiu (Sp 5), a metal point of the Spleen Meridian may be selected so that the coordination of yin and yang, and promotion of qi and blood can be achieved. And based on the relation of zang and fu which are connected with each other, the five Shu points of the meridians with the same name can be selected, such as the lung is related to the large intestine, the heart to the small intestine, the spleen to the stomach, the liver to the gallbladder, the kidney to the bladder, and the pericardium to the Sanjiao. From 7 p.m. to 9 p.m. Qiaoyin (G 44), the Jing-Well point of the Gallbladder Meridian is selected; and Dadun (Liv 1), the Jing-Well point of the Liver Meridian is used in case of the disorders of the Liver Meridian. This is called the point-selecting method from the exterior-interior related meridians. According to the principle of five elements' motion integrated with yin, yang and stems, A and F, B and G, C and H, D and J, E and K can be regarded as a combining day. The five Shu points of these combining days can be mutually selected, and it is called the mutual point-selecting method at the combining day. And it can also be supplemented with the time points according to the disease. It is named the point-selecting method of the integration between the time and the disease.

The hour-prescription of acupoints which is used in clinical differentiation for selecting points is based on the relations between yin and yang, exterior and interior of zang-fu organs, thus the Yuan-Source points and Luo-Connecting points could be applied. For example, at the time when the Yuan-Source point of the Lung Meridian is selected, the Luo-Connecting point Pianli (LI 6) of the Large Intestine Meridian can be added. This method is named as the point-selecting method of communicating zang-fu organs.

Clinically, the Linggui eight methods (selection of the Eight points in Eight Extra-Meridians related to the day and the hour in terms of heavenly stems and earthly branches) are often applied in combination with the day-prescription or hour-prescription method. According to the needs of the disease, the points can be selected with the eight methods first, then supplemented with the day-prescription method. This is called the eight method combining with day-prescription method. If the points are selected with the hour-prescription method, it is called the method of selecting points with eight methods and hour-prescription method. There are also other methods called the eight method-day-prescription Yuan-Source point selecting method, and the eight method-day-prescription-five Shu points selecting method, the eight method-day-prescription method, the eight method-day-prescription-Yin-Yang point-selecting method, eight method-day-prescription-mutual application of points at the combining day method and day-prescription-eight method combined with affected point and day-prescription hour method, etc. These methods can be used flexibly in clinic.

2) *Opening the points in the close time, and observing the ruler of the heaven* In *Cycle Diagram of Midnight-Noon Ebb-Flow,* there are twelve hours every week when no point can be selected. This is called the "close time." In ancient times, the acupuncturists called it "natural defect." Various kinds of methods had been tried to open the points at the close time by later scholars, but all were in vain. Going with the ruler of heaven, Dr. Shan invented the "1, 4, 2, 5, 3, 0" method to open the points at the close time, filling properly the twenty-four closed points, which indicated that there was no interruption for the qi and blood to irrigate the human body. The above viewpoint was agreed by modern scholars. Dr. Chen followed what is explained in *Plain Questions* "In the Heaven, there are six cycles and each cycle consists of sixty days with a total of three hundred sixty days in a year. The Heaven has ten celestial stems which make up sixty days in a cycle, and six cycles amount to a year, so that a year has three hundred sixty days which is the fixed law." He tried to find a day from the sixty cycle table. "Restriction is the origin of inborn constitution, generation is the root of the acquired constitution." After having carefully examined the midnight-noon ebb-flow cycle diagram, he found out that the order of "1, 4, 2, 5, 3, 0" is not going with the ruler of the Heaven, but is the reverse of the order of Heaven. If we follow "A is the first one," the order of A day will be "4, 1, 0, 3, 5, 2." But the points opened at the close time are similar to "1, 4, 2, 5, 3, 0." After careful investigation, he found its root: The order of "1, 4, 2, 5, 3, 0" will be the order of Yin-Yang Stems. There are "ten blankets" in this series, the lost points also have their order, so a blanket is missed for the day (of the last ten Heavenly Stems), because that day begins with the last twelve Earthly Branches). Thus, Dr. Shan filled all the close points of *Midnight-Noon Ebb-Flow Cycle Diagram.*

3) *Reinforcing and reducing* Reinforcing and reducing along or against the running course of the meridian is the essence of the midnight-noon ebb-flow method. Actually, it is the content of *Internal Classic.* The reducing method moves towards the direction of the flow of qi and blood in the meridian, while the reinforcing method is the contrary. The maneuver includes twisting and rotating, lifting and thrusting, inspiring and expirating, slow and quick, etc. In ancient times, male and female, left and right were also be considered.

The Eight Confluential Points are broadly used in clinic, and this had been recorded early in the "Directions of Acupuncture and Meridian." Therefore, the selection of points should first be based on the Linggui Eight method, then differentiation will be applied if necessary, and then open the points needed for day-prescription, for example, at Jia Xu hour of Jia Shu day, in order to treat such syndromes of the Lung Meridian as superficial pulse, asthma and cough, cold and mild fever, lower abdominal tenderness and borborygmus. Houxi (SI 3) and Shenmai (B 62) points of the eight methods are used: the Hand-Taiyin Jing-Well point Shaoshang (L 11) and Foot Taiyin Jing-Well point Yinbai (Sp 1) are supplemented in case of fullness of the upper abdomen; the Hand and Foot-Taiyin Yang-Spring points Yuji (L 10) and Dadu (Sp 2) are supplemented if the disease is complicated with heat feeling of the body; the Hand and Foot-Taiyin Shu-Stream points Taiyuan (L 9) and Taibai (Sp 3) are added if the disease is complicated with heaviness of the body and joint pain; the Hand and Foot-Taiyin Jing-River points

Jingqu (L 8) and Shangqiu (Sp 5) are added when it is complicated with asthma and cough, cold and heat; the Hand and Foot-Taiyin He-Sea points Chize (L 5) and Yinlingquan (Sp 9) are supplemented in diarrhoea. In case of the illness of the Yuan-Source point, the Yuan-Source point is added; if the close points can be used mutually in certain disease, then the close points have to be supplemented. The methods are flexible, and the key point is that differentiation according to the meridians must be accurate.

II. Case Analysis

Case 1: Facial spasm

Name, Wang x x; sex, male; age, 54; date of the first visit, July 1970.

Complaints He suffered from left facial spasm for more than ten years, accompanied with facial convulsion, inability to control the closing and opening of the left eye, and deviation of the left mouth corner. He was thin and weak. As no response was found after many kinds of treatments, he was referred to the Acupuncture Department. Differentiation: Stirring up of deficiency-wind and upward disturbing of the face.

Prescription Right Hegu (LI 4), Jiache (S 6), Sibai (S 2), Yangbai (G 14) and Yifeng (SJ 17).

Treatment procedure The opposing needling method (pucture the points opposite to the diseased side) was used for three months with no response. Dr. Chen then palpated his Hand and Foot-Yangming Meridian. He found that there was soreness at the left Shousanli (LI 10) point but there was no reaction below the elbow of the Hand-Shaoyang and Taiyang Meridians, and neither at the Back-Shu points. There was a tender or nodule-like soreness at the Tianzong (SI 11) point. After the above two points which had reaction together with Hegu (LI 4) and Waiguan (SJ 5) on the same side were needled, his attacks were gradually reduced and the patient was finally cured after two months' treatment.

Case 2: Migraine

Name, Guo x x; sex, female; age, 43; date of the first visit, October, 1965.

Complaints She suffered from left headache for two years and the pain gradually worsened. No response was found after administering of analgesic. At each attack, the pain was so severe that she even wanted to commit suicide. The face was slightly dark, and there were cupping marks at the frontal area. The tongue coating was thin yellow with red tip, the pulse was string-taut and slightly rapid. Differentiation: Long-term stagnation of the liver qi leading to transformation into fire which goes upward to disturb Shaoyang. The principle of treatment was to reduce the liver fire and facilitate the gallbladder, regulate the qi and stop the pain.

Prescription Taichong (Liv 3), Zulinqi (G 41), Yangbai (G 14), Fengchi (G 20) and Hegu (LI 4).

Treatment procedure After treatment for more than one month, the needling effect was not stable. So Dr. Chen palpated along her head and face, and found a soreness and distension at Touwei (S 8), then palpated her Back-Shu points and found tendon-like pricking burning pain at Geshu (B 17) and Danshu (B 19) points; no reaction was found below the elbow; then he palpated beneath the knee and a nodule-like sore mass was found at Zhaohai (K 6) point. Needling was given with the reducing method at the above-mentioned points and combined with points selected according to differentiation. Treat once every other day. The attacks of headache became less frequent and the headache was alleviated after three months' treatment, and the patient was cured after a longer period of treatment. No recurrence was found in a follow-up visit one year later.

Case 3: Dysuria

Name, Hu x x; sex, male; age, 82; date of the first visit, September 1972.

Complaints He was hospitalized for two months due to cirrhosis and ascites. A consultation was made by the TCM doctor for the problem of retention of urine. The face was dark yellow as if to be covered with dirt, and his chin was thin. The patient was emaciated, but his abdomen was found to be as big as a drum and soft. The urinary bladder was distended with a clear margin. The tongue was glossy and free from coating, and the tongue proper was dark purple. The pulse was deep, thready and a little hesitant. It was thought that the ascites were due to the stagnation of liver qi and blood which transformed into fire to burn the essence and fluids, leading to deficiency of the kidney water. Because the Earth (spleen) failed to transform the water, water was retained in the body. Retention of urine was due to old age and deficiency of the kidney. The principle of treatment was to treat symptoms in case of acute stage, and to use needling combined with drugs to promote the water.

Prescription Modified Composite of Zhenwuwulin should be used to promote yang and nourish the water; Taixi (K 3), Fuliu (K 7), Yinlingquan (Sp 9) (reinforcing) should be needled; and Guanyuan (Ren 4) and Zhongji (Ren 3) points should be pressed with fingers.

Treatment procedure The urine began to pass five minutes after the needling and finger pressing. Passive urination happened after the needling was given once daily. After more than ten days' treatment, he could pass water by himself. After four days' treatment with needling and herbs, the ascites disappeared and he could walk slowly. The patient was discharged after another three months' treatment with an altered prescription.

REINFORCING AND REDUCING BY SLOW AND QUICK INSERTION OF THE NEEDLE AND SCALP ACUPUNCTURE

—Chen Keyan's Clinical Experience

Dr. Chen Keyan (1930-1986), was born in Shenyang of Liaoning Province. In 1950, she graduated from the Gynecology and Pediatrics College of the China Medical Institution. In April of 1953, she was shifted to the Experimental Institute of Acupuncture and Moxibustion of the Ministry of Public Health, and in December of 1955, she attended the training course of the traditional Chinese medicine for Western-trained doctors run by the Ministry of Public Health. She was taught by the famous acupuncturist Ye Xinqing and the famous TCM doctor Zhao Xiwu. She emphasized the slow, quick, reinforcing and reducing maneuveers in her research work of acupuncture and moxibustion and successfully applied such techniques as the infrared imagine technique in the clinical studies. In clinic, she was good at using scalp acupuncture, and good therapeutic results had been obtained in treating cerebral vascular disease, hypertension, epilepsy, bulbar paralysis, polyneuritis, peptic ulcer, etc. with the reinforcing and reducing method. She published more than 30 papers in *China Acupuncture* and *Journal of Traditional Chinese Medicine*. She directed and specified the International Standard Terminology of Scalp Acupuncture which was accepted by the West Pacific Region Acupoints Working Conference, WHO, in 1984. She was an associate professor and chief of the Acupuncture Methodology Research Room of the Institute of Acupuncture and Moxibustion, the China Academy of Traditional Chinese Medicine, and Chief of the All-China Scalp Acupuncture Cooperation Group.

I. Academic Characteristics and Medical Specialities

1. Importance of reinforcing and reducing by slow and quick insertion of the needle

The reinforcing and reducing method by slow and quick insertion of the needle is the oldest simple method, which is regarded as the foundation of various reinforcing and reducing methods described in *Internal Classic*. Dr. Chen had made a systematic study on the stimulation, heat reinforcing and cold reducing and their clinical applications.

1) *Stimulation of reinforcement and reduction by slow and rapid insertion of the needle* It is stated in *Miraculous Pivot* that "the assertion that slow insertion and rapid withdrawal will contribute to a reinforcement means that to insert slowly and draw out rapidly will make qi become reinforced. The assertion that rapid insertion and slow withdrawal will contribute to a reduction means that to insert rapidly and draw out slowly will reduce the qi." According to her clinical experience, Dr. Chen realized that insertion and withdrawal couldn't simply be explained as inserting or withdrawing the

needle in and out of the skin. Insertion should include pressing to penetrate the needle to the required depth until qi arrives, and withdrawal should include lifting to lift the needle out of the skin after qi arrives. Slow and rapid indicate not only the speed of insertion and withdrawal of the needle, but also the needling strength and duration. Specifically speaking, slow insertion needs to insert the needle slowly and to press it downward heavily, and the time required for the needle to reach the expected depth will be longer; Rapid withdrawal means that the needle should be withdrawn quickly, but lifted slightly, and the time required for the needle to withdraw from the skin will be shorter. The needling strength and time for rapid insertion and slow withdrawal and for slow insertion and rapid withdrawal are opposite, i.e. the speed for rapid insertion is quicker and the force of pressing should be light, and the time required is shorter, while the speed for slow withdrawal is slow, and the strength of lifting is heavier, and the time is longer.

Dr. Chen used the needling strength and time of insertion to calculate the total amount of stimulation. The formula is: Strength x time = the total amount of stimulation. With this formula the total amount of stimulation by reinforcing and reducing with rapid and slow insertion may be calculated, i.e. the total amount of stimulation for reinforcing = slow insertion (heavy strength x longer time) + rapid withdrawal (mild strength x shorter duration). It is just opposite for the reducing method, that is, the total amount of stimulation = rapid insertion (mild strength x shorter duration) + slow withdrawal (heavy strength x longer duration). From the above calculation, it is not difficult to see that the total amount of stimulation for the reinforcing and reducing by slow and rapid insertion is the same, but different from the viewpoint that light stimulation is reinforcing and heavy stimulation is reducing. It indicates that both the reinforcing and reducing have heavy and mild stimulation.

2) *The detailed procedure of the reinforcing and reducing by slow and rapid insertion of the needle* The ancient acupuncturists believed that the manipulations included light twisting, mild twisting and no twisting. Dr. Chen advocated the method of no twisting and put forward the specific depth and needling time, that is, the reinforcing is performed by inserting the needle slowly and forcefully to the earth region (about 8 cm), then by pressing the point tightly for thirty seconds and withdrawing the needle quickly, while the reducing performed by inserting the needle quickly to the earth region (about 8 cm) and then gradually withdrawing the needle. The manipulating time is four minutes for both the methods. One must perform needling attentively so that the qi could be conveyed from the hand to the Shu points and the meridian, and then to produce heat reinforcing and cold reducing functions.

3) *Heat reinforcing and cold reducing* It is recorded in *Plain Questions* that deficiency symptoms should be treated by bringing about excess which means that the patient should feel hot sensation around the tip of the needle, because when the qi is in excess, it will generate heat. The excess symptoms should be reduced which means that the patient should feel cold sensation in the region around the tip of the needle due to qi deficiency brought about by needling. The acupuncturists of later generations would use such complicated reinforcing and reducing methods as "setting the mountain on fire" or "penetrating-heaven coolness" in clinic to produce hot or cold sensations. Based on

clinical practice, however, Dr. Chen thought that the simple method of reinforcing and reducing by rapid and slow insertion of the needle might produce heat reinforcing and cold reducing. Specifically, the key point of slow insertion and rapid withdrawal is slow insertion, which is an effective method to bring about the hot sensation, pertaining to heat reinforcing, while the key point of rapid insertion and slow withdrawal is the slow withdrawal, which is an effective method to result in the cold sensation, pertaining to cold reducing.

In order to prove this phenomenon, ten subjects with normal body temperature were subjected to reinforcing by needling the left Hegu (LI 4) point every other day. The comparison of the reducing method and self-control (without needling) showed that except the soreness and distension of the reinforcing and reducing, reinforcing brought about five times the amount of hot sensation and one pain feeling induced through the reinforcing method; and reducing resulted in twice the amount of cold sensation and five times amount of pain sensation. In a comparison of these two methods, the difference was significant ($P<0.05$).

4) *Applications of the reinforcing and reducing method* a. Reinforcing method in the treatment of the toxic reaction of the chemical anticarcinoma drug: The toxic reaction of the anticarcinoma drugs, especially the inhibition of the hemogenetic function and the gastro-intestinal reaction, has become the greatest disturbance of chemotherapy. Dr. Chen once treated with needling thirty postoperative patients of breast carcinoma who were receiving chemotherapy. Each time before the administration, acupuncture was given. On the second day after the administration, acupuncture was again applied, sixteen treatments in four weeks in all. Dazhui (Du 14), and Zusanli (S 36) (bilateral) were selected in the first and third week; and Shenzhu (Du 12) and Sanyinjiao (Sp 6) were used in the second and fourth week. The results indicated that both the reinforcing and reducing had prominent toxic-relieving action. However, the action of the reinforcing to decrease the white blood cell count and to improve the clinical symptoms was better than that of the reducing method. b. Reducing method in the treatment of post operative heat absorption: In order to further prove the clinical significance of the reinforcing method by slow and rapid insertion, 111 cases of post operative patients with heat absorption were observed. All the patients had excess-heat symptoms such as fever, string-taut, slippery and rapid pulse, red tongue proper, white greasy coating, halitosis, constipation, and red urine. The patients were divided into a reinforcing group of 37 cases; a reducing group of 34 eases; and the control group of 40 cases. No antipyretics were given for all the groups. When the reinforcing and reducing methods were applied at the bilateral Quchi (LI 11) and Zusanli (S 36) points, the results indicated that the immediate antipyretic effect of needling with the reducing method was better. Compared with the condition before the needling, $P<0.001$. No immediate antipyretic effect could be found with the reinforcing method when the reducing group was compared with the reinforcing group. $P<0.05$, the difference was significant. As to the continuous needling effect, the patients in the reducing group began to have a remarkable drop of body temperature in the first day of the treatment ($P<0.01$), but patients in the reinforcing group had decreased body temperature in the second day of the treatment ($P<0.01$). The number of the days of the drop of the body temperature treatment below 37°C was 3 days for the

reducing group; 4 days for the reinforcing group, and 5 days for the control group. c. Combined with scalp acupuncture in treating hypertension: For scalp acupuncture, some adopted quick twisting method, and some used needle retaining method after insertion. Dr. Chen applied the reinforcing and reducing method in scalp acupuncture. For the reinforcing method, she inserted the needle slowly and forcefully to the earth region (8 cm), then pressed the point tightly for half a minute, and then withdrew the needle quickly, while for the reducing method, she inserted the needle quickly to the earth region (8 cm), then lifted the needle slowly and forcefully, and let the skin around the needle hole in the hillock state. Either the reinforcing or reducing was manipulated for ten minutes. For the even reinforcing and even reducing, the needle should be inserted quickly to the earth region, then the needle handle is held by the thumb and index finger and twisted evenly forward and backward for 180° at the frequency of 150 cycles/minute for one minute and retained for nine minutes, and then withdrawn. All these three methods are performed with a 1 cun filiform needle gauge No. 26 with a single hand. The effects to drop the blood pressure varied with different methods used. Fifteen patients with hypertension out of thirty cases were divided into deficiency of yin and hyperactivity of yang, 6 cases, obstruction of the phlegm-dampness in the middle jiao, 6 cases, deficiency of the kidney, 3 cases according to differentiation. The self-control method was adopted at the same time. The immediate effect on the blood pressure was observed every other day when the parietal midline was needled with alternating reinforcing, reducing and even movement each day. The statistical results indicated that both the reinforcing and reducing methods were effective for patients with yin deficiency and yang hyperactivity, and the reducing method was effective for the obstruction of phlegm-dampness in the middle jiao. There was no statistical result for the three patients with kidney deficiency because the number of cases were too few.

2. Standardization of scalp acupuncture lines

Since 1970, scalp acupuncture has been used in clinic, and now it has become a common acupuncture method used in the treatment of illness. But for a long time there were different opinions about how to localize the points for scalp acupuncture. Some selected the points by experience, others took the scalp projection area corresponding to the function of the cerebral cortex as the therapeutic points. These different viewpoints have brought about confusion on the development of scalp acupuncture. So a standarized nomenclature of scalp points should be worked out. Dr. Chen undertook this large task, and presided over a symposium, in which the decision of localizing the meridians according to the divisions and selecting the points on the meridians in combination with the ancient point penetrating method was made. Fourteen standard lines were worked out on the four areas of the scalp (the frontal area, the parietal area, the temporal area and the occipital area), which serves as locations for acupuncture treatment.

1) *The relation between scalp acupuncture and the meridians* After analysing and comparing the scalp needling standard lines with the traditional meridians, Dr. Chen found that each line of scalp acupuncture pertained to a definite meridian. For example, the occipital midline, the parietal midline and the frontal midline pertaining to the Du

Meridian; the parafrontal line 1, and the paraparietal line 1, the upper paraoccipital line and the lower paraoccipital line pertaining to the bladder Meridian of Foot-Taiyang; the parafrontal line 2, and line 3, paraparietal line 2, anterior and posterior temporal lines pertaining to the Gallbladder Meridian of Foot-Shaoyang; anterior and posterior oblique parietotemporal lines transversly cross the above three meridians. From the mutual relationship of the meridians and the Shu points, it indicates that these scalp acupuncture lines are not isolated from one another and there are intercrossing communicative relations among them, thus laying a theoretical foundation for the treatment of systemic diseases with the scalp acupuncture standard lines.

2) *The relation between scalp acupuncture and the Shu points* The Shu points on the head are usually distributed on the area with hairs. The Shu points are the places where qi of the meridians and zang-fu organs is gathered and the qi come in and out of the body surface. They play the role of dredging the meridians, invigorating qi and blood, expelling the pathogenic factors and reinforcing the body resistance, and treating various diseases and regulating deficiency and excess. Dr. Chen found there were altogether thirty-five Shu points which were situated on the hairy part of the head, while there were seventeen starting and ending points of the standard scalp acupuncture corresponding to the location of the Shu points such as the starting point of the frontal midline, Shenting (Du 24); Meichong (B 3) for the parafrontal line 1; Toulinqi (G 15) for the parafrontal line 2; Touwei (S 8) for the parafrontal line 3; Baihui (Du 20) and Qianding (Du 21) for the parietal midline; Sishencong (Extra 6) and Xuanli (G 6) parietal-temperal oblique line; Zhengying (G 17) for the parietal-temperal posterior oblique line; Hanyan (G 4) for the temperal anterior line; Shuaigu (G 8) for the temperal posterior line; Qiangjian (Du 18) and Naohu (Du 17) for the upper occipital midline; and Yuzhen (B 9) and Tianzhu (B 10) for the lower paraocciptial line. Dr. Chen thought that the function of these above-mentioned points was in accordance with that of the standard scalp acupuncture.

In order to further prove the therapeutic action of the standard line of the scalp acupuncture, Dr. Chen once treated 27 hemiplegia patients (9 with left hemiplegia, and 18 with right hemiplegia) with the combined reinforcing and reducing methods. The left paratemporal line 1, the parieto-temporal anterio-oblique line, the parieto-temporal posterio-oblique lines were needled and the influence of the treatment on the EMG amplitude of the four extremities were observed before and after the acupuncture. The results showed that the EMG amplitude on the affected limb before needling was markedly lower than that on the healthy side, and the EMG amplitude of the four extremities after needling was markedly increased ($P<0.01$), but the increased amplitude of EMG on the right limbs was evidently higher than that on the left limbs. According to the above observation, Dr. Chen realized that the main therapeutic action of the scalp needle standard line lies on the opposite side, although the effects are available on both sides.

3. Application of scalp acupuncture

1) *Needling characteristics* a. Needling direction: As the standard line is a line not

a point, it may be either long or short, and have a starting point and an ending point. There are different opinions on whether the needle should be inserted from the starting point or from the ending point. Dr. Chen advocated that the method of reinforcing and reducing by puncturing along the meridian course and against the meridian course should be used. During the treatment, the scalp needle standard line should be combined with the running course of the meridian before the needling direction is decided. If the needle tip is directed along the running course of the meridian, it is reinforcing, while with the tip directed against the running course of the meridian, it is reducing. For example, if the frontal midline (pertaining to the Du Meridian) is needled, the reinforcing is performed by needling from Shenting (Du 24) point of the frontal area towards the anterior hairline, while the reducing performed by inserting the needle from the point 0.5 cun below the hairline and directing the needle tip to the upper hairline. Therefore, the needling direction depends on the different standard lines. b. Needling depth and angle: The thickness of the scalp is about 0.2 cun for a male adult. The needling depth may be 1 cun, 2 cun, or even 5 cun, so the oblique insertion should be adopted, but the needling angle is related to the anatomical structure of the scalp. The scalp is divided into five layers (skin, subcutaneous tissue, aponeurosis and epicranius, subaponeurotic loose connective tissue, and periosteum of cranium). The first three layers are so tightly connected, that they are not easily separated, and they are regarded as one layer in clinic, so the needle is obliquely inserted 1 or 2 cun deep. The needling depth is also closely related to the needling angle. In general, an angle of 15° to 30° between the needle body and the scalp is considered to be suitable. If the needling angle is too big, the needle will penetrate the periosteum and hurt the patient, but if the angle is too small or the needle only reaches the second or third layer, it will be hard for the needle to be inserted. Thus, the needling angle determines the needling depth. c. Subcutaneous embedding method: Subcutaneous embedding is a method in which the needles are retained in the point under the skin for a longer duration. Clinically, it is usually applied to the Shu points, the points on the back, the four extremities and the auricular points. Dr. Chen made a new trial by embedding the needle on the scalp needle standard line, and satisfactory results were obtained. After the scalp acupuncture was finished, the needles were embedded subcutaneously and the needles should be replaced after three to five days. The patients were advised to massage the points themselves for one minute, three times a day. This method has certain therapeutic effect on some intractable diseases. Dr. Chen once treated epilepsy with this method. The self-massage of the embedded needle at the epileptic aura may control or alleviate the attack of epilepsy. d. Moxibustion on the scalp needle standard line: Moxibustion functions to warm and dredge the meridians and collaterals, to elevate yang and reinforce qi. There have been records of moxibustion at Baihui (Du 20) in treating prolapse of rectum in the ancient medical book. But there are also some people who hold that the head is the crossing place of all the yang meridians, so it is not suitable to apply moxibustion on the scalp. Dr. Chen used the moxibustion on the head instead of needling in clinic. This method has the function of dredging the meridians, and promoting the circulation of qi and blood to treat general diseases. Procedure: Ignite the moxa stick and play moxibustion at the place 1 cun away from the scalp needle line for fifteen minutes on both sides. Dr. Chen achieved certain effects with this method on the treatment of sequela of windstroke and brain injury on the parieto-temporal anterio-oblique line.

2) *Clinical application* a. Treating epilepsy: Seventy cases of epilepsy were treated with the rapid twisting of the needle and subcutaneous embedding method. Most of the patients in this group had been treated in vain with various antiepileptic drugs. According to their types, different therapeutic areas were selected; for the grand mal, the Motor Area (corresponding to parieto-temporal anterio-oblique line) and the Choreal Tremor Area (corresponding to anterio-temporal line) were needled; for the petit mal, the Thoracic Cavity Area (corresponding to the parafrontal line 1) was needled; and for psychomotor attack type, Vertigo-Auditory Area (corresponding to posterio-temporal line) was needled. After three months' treatment, the epileptic attacks were lessened dramatically. Such symptoms as anxiety, insomnia, mental retardation, and hypomnesia were greatly improved. The results of the observation indicated that the marked effective rate was 46.88 percent; and the effective rate, 67.71 percent. EEG examinations for twenty-nine cases were observed before and after the treatment, and the improvement rate of EEG was 55.17 percent. b. Treating pseudobulbar paralysis: This disease is mainly manifested in speech disturbance and dysphagia, which belongs to one of the difficult cases. Certain effects were obtained in the treatment of fifteen patients. Motor Area was selected as the chief needling position (corresponding to parieto-temporal anterio-oblique line) and then the Sublingual Area was taken (underneath the maxillary, at both sides of the musculi digastricus. The needle tip was directed to the root of the tongue for 3 cm), and Glossopharyngeal Area (one finger breadth from the anterior lower part of the mandible corner, needling 3 cm towards the direction of the root of the tongue). Among the fifteen patients, there were six cases who choked on water during drinking and who had the tongue contractured in the mouth, or who failed to open the mouth wide. They could open the mouth, protrude the tongue and eat food without choking after 3 to 6 treatments; 5 cases could take semi-liquid and liquid food after the nasal feeding tube was removed after 1 to 6 treatments; and 4 cases had results after 7 treatments. Among the 15 cases, 9 were basically cured; 3, markedly effective; and 3 effective after the treatment.

II. Case Analysis

Case 1: Windstroke (bulbar parlysis)

Name, Wang x x; sex, male; age, 23; date of the first visit, April 18, 1976.

Complaints The patient used to be very healthy. He had sudden soreness and pain on the back and scapular region after physical labour on the morning of March 13, 1976. He went on working until 4 o'clock in the afternoon when he felt uncomfortable on his neck. Then he had a headache, vertigo, nausea, vomiting, numbness and weakness of the left limbs. His blood pressure was 180/120 mmHg. On the following day, his voice became hoarse, sometimes even with no sound. He suffocated while breathing, and choked during eating, and his left lower limb was completely paralysed in the afternoon. The dyspnea became aggravated on the third day. The treachcotomy was performed after he was admitted to the hospital on March 18, 1976. Examination: Clear mind, cooperative, hoarse voice, dysarthria, the left pupil larger than the right one, the light reaction (++), no left pharyngeal reflex and the right sluggish, the uvula and tongue deviated to the right, mouth opening only 4 cm, flaccid paralysis of the left upper and lower limbs, the muscle strength grade 0, and that of the right limbs grade 3 to 4, low muscular tone, decreased tendon reflex, right Babinski's sign (++), feeble pulse, pale tongue proper with thin white coating. The diagnosis by Western medicine was: 1) brainstem lesion, 2) bulbar paralysis.

Differentiation Windstroke (deficiency of qi).

Treatment procedure After admission, the patient was given 2 mg of strychnine sulfate three times daily, 200 mg of Vit. B12 for i.v. drip, once a day, and antibiotics, and TCM drug Tongmai Decoction. Scalp acupuncture was applied when nasal tube was still preserved due to the choking. Bilateral Motor Area (corresponding to the Parieto-temporal anterio-oblique line) and Sublingual and Gloss opharyngeal Areas were needled, once a day. He could drink a little water after the eighth treatment; he could take the paste of half an apple and one-third of a cake after the eleventh treatment; one ounce of gruel after the twelfth treatment, and noodles and liver after the eighteenth treatment; and he could eat and speak normally after the twenty-second treatment. The bilateral pharyngeal reflex reappeared and the muscle strength of his left upper and lower limbs was grade 4. Then the needling was stopped, and he was cured and discharged.

Case 2: Epilepsy

Name, Yang x x; sex, male; age, 10.

Complaints He had recurrent attacks of temporary loss of consciousness for six years after a convulsion with high fever at the age of four. During an attack, he spat white foam, pallor, upward staring of the eyes, and occasional convulsion of the four extremities. Each attack lasted about ten minutes. The number of attacks were not definite, varying from three times a year to once a month, influenced by fatigue and emotional factors. He had medication of antiepilepitic pills for a long duration. Examination: Cooperative, clear mind, normal gait and nothing negative in the neurological examinations. An EEG examination revealed marginal changes. He was thin and weak with anorexia and loose stool, a pale red tongue proper, thin white coating, thready and weak pulse. The Western diagnosis was epilepsy.

Differentiation Deficiency of the spleen and stomach, obstruction of phlegm.

Treatment procedure Scalp acupuncture was adopted. Points selected: Bilateral Thoracic Cavity Area (parafrontal line 1), Bilateral Vertigo Auditory Area (corresponding to the posterior temporal line). Reinforcing and reducing by slow and rapid insertion of the needle was used, three times a week. After being treated for three months, he had only one attack within three months. Medication was ceased. The duration of the attack was reduced to five minutes. Then the treatment was given twice per week. Needles were embedded at the parafrontal and posttemporal lines after needling. No abnormality was found after two months' treatment. Then the needling was stopped. No relapse was found in the follow-up visit for half a year. His physical condition gradually became stronger, and no epileptic attacks occurred.

DIFFERENTIATION OF SYNDROMES IN MERIDIANS, AND BALANCING THE LIVER AND SPLEEN

—Chen Zuolin's Clinical Experience

Chen Zuolin, a native of Wujin County, Jiangsu Province, was born in August, 1925 into the family of a Chinese medical practitioner in Shanghai. He graduated from Shanghai Chinese Medical College in 1944 and afterwards he practised Chinese internal medicine under his father's instruction for six years. In 1950, he opened an independent clinic. Mr. Chen studied acupuncture by himself at an early age and afterwards he was apprenticed to Dr. Guo Jiugao in acupuncture therapy. In 1956, he started to practise in acupuncture and moxibustion in the Central Hospital of the Shanghai Railway Administration. Mr. Chen emphasized the combination of syndrome-differentiation and meridian identification. He published about twenty academic papers, among which are: *Clinical Observation of Sixty-one Cases with Hypertension Treated with Moxibustion, Experience in Acupoint Selection with Syndrome-Differentiation by Theories of Zang-fu Organs and Meridians, The Application of Theories of Spleen and Stomach in Acupuncture Clinic.* At present he is the director and deputy chief-doctor in the acupuncture department in the Central Hospital of the Shanghai Railway Administration, councillor of the China Acupuncture-Moxibustion Association and deputy director of the Shanghai Acupuncture-Moxibustion Association.

I. Academic Characteristics and Medical Specialities

1. Meridian-identification and remote acupoints along meridian pathway

Dr. Chen holds that both differentiation of syndromes according to the theory of zang-fu organs and the theory of meridians should be used interdependently, in which the differentiation of syndromes according to the theory of meridians is more important. Because of the characteristics in acupuncture therapy, the treatment can be given in accordance with the differentiated syndromes and meridian, and acupoints can be chosen along the involved meridian.

He treated a case of functional uterine bleeding. The patient was thirty-eight years old and had a lot of bleeding with menstruation and incessant drippling of blood. The condition often lasted for more than ten days and the period restarted less than ten days after it stopped. Repeatedly, the disease troubled the patient for three years so that she had a pale facial complexion, shortness of breath, low voice, lassitude, dizziness and insomnia, which were differentiated as exhaustion and deficiency of ying (nutrient) blood. Theoretically, liver dominates storing blood and and its meridian goes along the external genitalia and reaches the lower abdomen. Therefore it is often involved in gynecological diseases. The spleen controls blood, and deficiency in the spleen usually decreases its function of controlling blood and causes extravasation. The treatment should regulate the Liver Meridian of Foot-Jueyin and the Spleen Meridian of Foot-Taiyin in this patient. Therefore Ligou (Liv 5), Sanyinjiao (Sp 6) and Xuehai (Sp 10) were punctured for one course (one treatment every other day, ten treatments as one course). In the next month the menstruation came at the regular time, but still lasted for ten days. Accordingly the patient was ordered to have sparrow-pecking moxibustion with a moxa roll on the bilateral Yinbai (Sp 1) respectively before and during the period for three to five minutes every day, until the menstruation stops. It became effective immediately in that month and menstruation lasted for one week. With continuous moxibustion for three months, the condition became normal, menstrual volume decreased and the period lasted only for five days.

The differentiation of syndromes according to the theory of meridians guides the clinical selection of acupoints. For example, one female patient was fifty-one years old and had irritability and a distending sensation in the hypochondrium for six months after menopause. Every night during six months she had contractive pain between the first and second toes, which ascended along the Liver Meridian of Foot-Jueyin to the area below the nipples (about in Qimen (Liv 14)). The pain reoccurred three to four times per night and disturbed her sleep. Upon inspection the patient was found to have a thin and yellow tongue coating, purplish spots on the tongue margin and string-taut and thready pulse, which were the manifestations of climacteric syndrome. Considering her irritability, distension in the hypochondrium, menopause and repeated attacks of pain along the Liver Meridian of Foot-Jueyin, the condition was differentiated as dysfunction of liver qi and stagnation of qi and blood in the Liver Meridian of Foot-Jueyin. The liver was involved and therefore it must be regulated. Taichong (Liv 3), Qimen (Liv 14) and Yanglingquan (G 34) were punctured accordingly. After two treatments (one treatment every other day) the contractive pain decreased and only appeared once per night. Four treatments later, all the symptoms disappeared. If the differentiation was incorrect, the clinical therapeutic effect would be influenced. For instance, there was one patient who suffered from distending pain in both hypochondriac regions, uncomfortable sensation in epigastric region, bitter taste in the mouth, poor appetite, lassitude, string-taut and slippery pulse, yellow and sticky tongue coating. The condition belonged to damp-heat in the liver and gallbladder. But misled by the saying that all the symptoms of edema and swelling due to dampness-related dysfunction in spleen, the previous acupuncturist used the technique to clean and disperse damp-heat in the spleen and stomach first by puncturing Zhongwan (Ren 12), Zusanli (S 36), Yinlingquan (Sp 9), Fenglong (S 40) and Neiguan (P 6). Unfortunately, the symptoms did not decrease even in the slightest after three treatments. Dr. Chen thought that the treatment must be done to regulate the gallbladder first, and he changed Yanglingquan (G 34) for Zusanli (S 36) in the above prescription. After one treatment 50 percent of the pain disappeared and it stopped completely with two treatments (one treatment every other day). At the same time the sticky tongue coating dispersed, appetite increased and spirits improved.

It was said in *A Supplement to the Prescriptions Worth a Thousand Gold* that all the acupoints are passed through by meridians and collaterals and able to lead qi to relieve disease. This indicated that the acupoints connect with various parts of the body through the meridian system and are able to guide qi to reach remote areas for eliminating distal diseases. Consequently in the acupuncture treatment of acute sprain, acute neck pain and lumbar pain, acute pain in the back and chest, Dr. Chen differentiates the involved meridian and then punctures the related remote acupoints to relieve the symptoms. Take acute neck pain for example, the pain will appear in either the Yangming, Shaoyang, Taiyang Meridians or the Du Meridian. Respectively, it is beneficial to puncture Renzhong (Du 26) for the pain in the Du Meridian, in the middle of the cervical vertebrae, where tenderness and motor impairment can be detected in supraspinal and interspinal ligaments. And it is effective to puncture Houxi (SI 3) or Yanglao (SI 6) for neck pain in the Taiyang Meridians in which the pain appears on the lateral side of the cervical vertebrae and radiates downwards between the spinal column and the medial side of the scapula. It is advisable to puncture Waiguan (SJ 5) or Xuanzhong (G 39) for pain in the Shaoyang Meridians in which the pain occurs in the lateral side of the Taiyang Meridians and radiates along the upper border of the scapula. It is possible to puncture Hegu (LI 4) or Lieque (L 7) for neck pain in the Yangming Meridians in which the pain appears in the anterior and posterior sides of m. sternocleidomastoideus and is often accompanied by motor impairment. During the acupuncture treatment, it is advisable to manipulate a 1.5-inch needle with twisting, lifting and thrusting techniques and then to retain the needle ten to fifteen minutes after the arrival of qi. Meanwhile, it is necessary to manipulate the needle once or twice during needle retention and to ask the patient to move the neck. The symptoms usually would decrease or disappear in most patients after treatment. If there is still a tight sensation in the neck, it is advisable to puncture by an in-and-out technique on the most painful spot and then to do cupping therapy afterwards for about three minutes. At the very beginning, neck pain only involves one meridian. If untreated or mismanaged, two meridians will be involved. In the differentiation of involved meridians, the primary affected meridian or the most painful meridian should be taken for the diseased meridian, which is to be regulated with remote acupoints. If two meridians are involved to a similar degree, the joined-puncture technique can be used. For example, the pain involves the Taiyang and Shaoyang Meridians. It is advisable to puncture Waiguan (SJ 5) all the way towards Yanglao (SI 6). The joined-puncture technique is only a difference in needle manipulation and its theoretical reason still implies "selection of remote acupoints." There is the expression: The pathway of a meridian is amenable to treatment. The key importance in selection of remote acupoints relies upon correct differentiation of the involved meridian. A puncture in the distal site is able to unblock qi, activate the circulation of qi and blood; on the other hand it is convenient for the patient to move his neck. The exercise is an important step in the treatment of acute sprain and it is helpful to unblock qi and blood. It is better to have exercise slowly and on a large scale. Dr. Chen emphasizes that the needle cannot be retained locally for an acute sprain. Because there is stagnation of qi and blood, and muscular contracture in the local area, needle retention will aggravate muscular contracture. On the contrary, the distal puncture is able to regulate meridian qi, and afterwards the in-and-out puncture and the cupping therapy are enough to eliminate slight local stagnation of qi and blood. In the treatment of acute lumbar sprain, Dr. Chen does not advise to puncture the patient in a lying position. He still punctures remote points on the hand for the convenience of motion in the lumbar region and of exercise. The cupping therapy will follow in a sitting position for improving the flow of qi and blood. In the observation of therapeutical effects in three hundred cases of acute lumbar sprain, Dr. Chen worked out three effective remote acupoints: Houxi (SI 3), Renzhong (Du 26), Yaotongxue (Extra). These acupoints are respectively effective for muscular sprain in different areas. Houxi (SI 3) is most effective for the problem in the Bladder Meridian of Foot-Taiyang, with 81.6 percent of the symptoms disappearing immediately. Renzhong (Du 26) is most effective for the problem in the Du Meridian, with 77.8 percent of the symptoms disappearing. For the problem in the Bladder Meridian of Foot-Taiyang and the Gallbladder Meridian of Foot-Shaoyang (pain in the lateral sides of spinal column radiates to hip and thigh), Yaotongxue (Extra) would be most effective and 77.8 percent symptoms would disappear rapidly after treatment. Theoretically there is the connection in qi circulation between the Foot and Hand Meridians under the same names, this is why the effect would be prominent in the use of Houxi (SI 3) for the problem in the Bladder Meridian of Foot-Taiyang. Renzhong (Du 26) is much better than other acupoints for the problem in the Du Meridian. This implies that the correct differentiation of the involved meridian is the prerequisite for effective results. (Yaotongxue (Extra) is an experienced acupoint, the mechanism of which needs further study.) Except Yaotongxue (Extra), Dr. Chen prefers to puncture remote acupoints on the opposite side of the diseased meridian. Apart from the above-mentioned information, Dr. Chen also prefers to use remote acupoints of the affected meridian for pains and motor impairment basically by differentiation of the meridian. For example, one patient had paroxysmal contractive pain on the posterior vertex, which appeared in both the retroauricular region and the vertex. But no other abnormal condition was found in the examination. In this case, the pain was differentiated in the Du Meridian and Taiyang Meridians, therefore, bilateral Kunlun (B 60) were chosen. Remote acupoints often bring about effectiveness in this kind of commonly encountered disease. In the treatment of pain in the limbs, Dr. Chen punctures corresponding acupoints. For example, in the treatment of severe heel pain, Dr. Chen likes to puncture and retain the needle on the corresponding acupoint of the palmer base on the same side. Meanwhile the patient is asked to walk. Although it is difficult to explain the therapy, it produces results. Consequently the corresponding point of the lower limbs is often chosen for pain in upper limbs on the same side; the corresponding point of upper limbs is used for pain in the lower limbs. For example, one female patient, thirty-five years old, had pain on both heels for two years. The pain started one month after childbirth and the patient had rested in bed for more than seventeen months. On the first visit, the patient was able to walk, but she had pain when touching the heels to the ground even with one inch of foam plastic in her shoes. Severe tenderness was noticed in both heels upon examination. By puncturing the corresponding points on both palms, the pain disappeared swiftly and the patient was able to walk as a healthy person. The needles were retained for ten minutes in treatment. In the return visit ten days later, the patient told us that there was slight pain at home, but she was able to walk normally. The pain disappeared again by the same technique. There had been no recurrence by the follow-up examination four months later.

2. Regulating and toning spleen and stomach

Dr. Chen thinks that in the body the congenital essence has been transformed but must be regulated and toned postnatally. For those who have weak body constitutions, emaciation and insomnia belonging to dysfunction in transformation of qi and blood and to deficiency of essence, it is advisable to regulate and tone the spleen and stomach. Especially for elderly patients, it is more necessary to tone the acquired organs for transforming qi and blood as well as for regulating yin and yang. Dr. Chen treated a patient with insomnia. The woman, forty-eight years old, had insomnia for seven to eight years and was only able to sleep for two or three hours every night. Meanwhile there were palpitation, tastelessness in the mouth and weakness in the four limbs, pale tongue proper, thin white tongue coating, thready, soft and feeble pulse. The condition was differentiated as blood deficiency in the heart and spleen. Spleen qi was deficient and failed to transport and transform water and food, resulting in deficiency of qi and blood. Heart dominates blood and stores the mind theoretically. While heart blood is deficient and unable to nourish the heart and calm the mind, insomnia is the common result. Therefore it is advisable to strengthen the spleen and stomach for producing qi and calming the mind of this patient. After two treatments (one treatment every other day) with Zusanli (S 36), Sanyinjiao (Sp 6) and Shenmen (H 7) punctured, the patient was able to sleep for about five hours. After five treatments, the patient was able to sleep for six to seven hours with other symptoms eliminated. Complete recovery came after about ten treatments. For another example, a 23 year-old patient came to the clinic because of sudden serious pain in the abdomen. The patient pressed on the lower abdomen and was unable to lie flat. Meanwhile she had pale facial complexion, lustreless lips and thready pulse. Theoretically, her dysmenorrhea was differentiated as blood deficiency which failed to nourish the uterus. Therefore it was emphasized to strengthen the spleen and stomach, benefit qi and blood, smooth the meridian and warm up the uterus. After Zusanli (S 36) (warming-needle technique), Sanyinjiao (Sp 6) and Ligou (Liv 5) were punctured on her, the pain decreased five minutes later and disappeared ten minutes later. The lips had lustre fifteen minutes later. The treatment finished after the needles were retained for another five minutes.

Both of the above two cases belonged to syndromes of qi and blood deficiency. Clinically, the regulation of spleen and stomach can be emphasized not only for digestive problems but also can be used for those who have a weak constitution due to prolonged illness. When the spleen and stomach have normal physiological functions, transportation and transformation can be guaranteed and qi and blood would be vigorous and sufficient. Therefore all the ailments could be cured expectantly. In prescription, Zusanli (S 36) is often of common choice. The warming-needle technique is resorted to this point if there are deficient and cold manifestations. Besides, Guanyuan (Ren 4) and Dazhui (Du 14) are the other choice. Guanyuan (Ren 4) is situated in the region 3 cun below the umbilicus. It was expressed in *Classics on Medical Problems* that qi starting below umbilicus and between the kidneys was the foundation for human life activities and was the root of the twelve meridians. As a result, Guanyuan (Ren 4) is mostly selected for qi deficiency and weakness and the deficiency in kidneys, such as in infantile enuresis and diarrhoea due to kidney deficiency. Guanyuan (Ren 4) is situated in the Ren Meridian and connects with three yin meridians. The Ren Meridian is described as the sea of the yin meridians. To tone qi of Guanyuan (Ren 4) leads yang from yin. When yin is well and even, yang will be vigorous. Dazhui (Du 14) is located in the Du Meridian and described as the gathering site of all the yang meridians. Dazhui (Du 14) is helpful for yang and qi deficient syndromes in the expectation of toning qi and yang. For example, moxibustion on Dazhui (Du 14) is usually prescribed for thrombocy topenic purpura and rheumatoid arthritis.

Dr. Chen thinks that in the relationship between acupoints and syndromes, it is very important to apply proper stimulation for regulating and adjusting qi in meridians and collaterals. Usually the surplus can be deducted and the insufficiency can be toned. Therefore Zusanli (S 36) and Guanyuan (Ren 4) can be prescribed for both deficient and excessive syndromes. For example, there was a 61-year-old male patient who had pain on the dorsum of right foot, accompanied by tumefaction, rigidity as well as difficulty in walking. In the consideration of congestion, tumefaction and pain in the Yangming Meridian, the problem was differentiated as invasion of wind-heat into the Yangming Collaterals and obstruction of qi and blood. The doctor punctured Zusanli (S 36) and Neiting (S 44) to expel hyperactive qi in the Yangming Meridian. In theory, the flow of qi promotes blood circulation. As a result, this patient was able to walk slowly and the pain decreased after the needles were retained for twenty minutes.

Dr. Chen emphasizes that in acupuncture one shouldn't emphasize experienced and effective acupoints, while one should pay much attention to syndrome differentiation guided by the theory of meridians.

Joy and anger are the commonly noticed emotional manifestations in daily life, but on the contrary abnormal joy and anger serve as the most common causative factors of illness. Stagnation of liver qi is the typical result. Both liver and heart are classified into Jueyin and their meridian qi is mutually connected. Therefore Dr. Chen often relies upon the Jueyin Meridians for dealing with emotional ailments and syndromes in heart and liver. And Taichong (Liv 3) and Neiguan (P 6) are surely resorted to in combination for smoothing and regulating liver. Taichong (Liv 3), the Yuan-source point of the Liver Meridian of Foot-Jueyin, is advised for zang diseases. Here Taichong (Liv 3) is purposed to adjust qi in the Liver Meridian of Foot-Jueyin for its stagnation. While for stagnation of liver blood, Taichong (Liv 3) serves to remove stagnation. Neiguan (P 6) is the Luo-connecting point of the Pericardium Meridian of Hand-Jueyin and communicates with the Sanjiao Meridian of Hand-Shaoyang. The Sanjiao Meridian of Hand-Shaoyang dominates qi and the Pericardium Meridian of Hand-Jueyin governs blood; therefore, Neiguan (P 6) can be used for both qi and blood disorders. Neiguan (P 6) also connects with the Yinwei Meridian and is able to dilate chest and benefit qi. Both of the acupoints are situated on the Jueyin Meridians and communicate with each other in qi flow, and the simultaneous used is able to increase their properties of removing qi stagnation in liver. Dr. Chen treated a 60-year-old patient who had abdominal distension for six months, accompanied by irritability, nightmare-disturbed sleep, poor appetite, nausea, constipation, loss of weight, string-taut and thready pulse and thin and yellow tongue coating. The syndromes were related to emotional depression and dysfunctions in liver which attacked transversely the spleen. Therefore it was advisable to puncture Zusanli (S 36), Sanyinjiao (Sp 6) and Taichong (Liv 3) to remove liver qi stagnation and strengthen the spleen. After acupuncture therapy, abdominal distension was reduced but the nightmares continued. Added with Neiguan (P 6) and Yinlingquan (Sp 9) in the second treatment, abdominal distension decreased and appetite increased. After the third treatment with the above acupoints, abdominal distension basically disappeared, and so did the nightmares and poor appetite. In the fourth treatment, Neiguan (P 6) and Taichong (Liv 3) were omitted. With the above acupoints, most symptoms disappeared after ten treatments. But the patient still required moxibustion with moxa rolls in the mornings and afternoons on bilateral Yinbai (Sp 1) respectively for five minutes. Afterwards abdominal distension disappeared completely and appetite returned to normal.

Dr. Chen is also skilled in regulating the Jueyin Meridians for various gynecological diseases under the similar reason of adjusting emotional activities. For instance, there was a 24-year-old patient who had amenorrhea for more than ten months, which had not improved with repeated decoctions of warming up the meridian and activating blood for removing stagnation. Upon inquiry, the patient complained of breast distension every month, morbid leukorrhea mixed with scanty stagnant blood, and epistaxis five months ago. The patient was plump and had edema in the lower limbs, a puffy face, dry mouth, preference for cold drinks, a string-taut and thready pulse, and thin tongue coating. All these symptoms were differentiated as stagnation of liver qi and dysfunctions in the Chong and Ren Meridians. Therefore Ligou (Liv 5), Taichong (Liv 3), Xuehai (Sp 10), Yinlingquan (Sp 9) were punctured for removing qi stagnation in liver and adjusting the Chong and Ren Meridians. After two treatments, menstruation came in scanty volume. The same prescription was reused the next month before the expected period. As a result, her menstruation came on schedule.

II. Case Analysis

Case 1: Dermal rash (thrombocytopenic purpura)

Name, Zhang x x; sex, female; age, 42; case No, 12148.

Complaints The patient had purplish rashes and bleeding spots in the lower limbs for two years, and with increasing menstruation in the last three months, which lasted for more than ten days, and with tastelessness and general weakness in the limbs. The examination showed soft and rapid pulse, thin and clear tongue coating, and the platelets count was 41,000/mm^3. The syndrome was differentiated as spleen qi deficiency which was unable to perform controlling function. And it was treated to strengthen spleen for controlling blood.

Prescription Xuehai (Sp 10), Sanyinjiao (Sp 6), Dazhui (Du 14) (warming-needle technique, three cones).

Treatment procedure After four treatments, purplish rashes and bleeding spots gradually decreased and diminished without the occurrence of new rashes. Menstruation decreased in volume. After eight treatments with the above prescription, no new bleeding spots were noticed and menstruation lasted only five to six days. Upon examination the platelets count showed 86,000/mm^3. No recurrence was shown in the follow-up examination three months later.

Explanation Moxibustion on Dazhui (Du 14), the gathering site of all the yang meridians, is able to warm up yang and benefit qi. Qi is described as the master of blood, when qi is sufficient, it is able to have powerful control. Xuehai (Sp 10) and Sanyinjiao (Sp 6) are used to strengthen spleen for controlling blood in avoidance of extravasation.

Case 2: Cavernous hemangioma on tongue tip

Name, Huang x x; sex, female; age, 66.

Complaints The patient had a purplish painless and peanut-size tumour on tongue body. After it was diagnosed as cavernous hemangioma in a hospital, the patient was transferred to an acupuncture clinic for further treatment. Examination showed that there was a purplish tumour which was hard and adhesive to the tongue mucosa, and it was painless and unmovable. The syndrome was differentiated as stagnation of heart blood and dysfunctions of the tongue.

Prescription Shenmen (H 7), Neiguan (P 6).

Treatment procedure One treatment per day, the needles were punctured bilaterally and retained for fifteen to twenty minutes. Taichong (Liv 3) was added in the third treatment. The tumour disappeared completely after eleven treatments. No recurrence was shown in the follow-up examination after six months.

Explanation Theoretically the tongue is described as the mirror of heart which dominates blood circulation. Therefore, the symptoms would manifest on the tongue tip if the Heart Meridian of Hand-Shaoyin is diseased. In the patient with stagnation of heart blood, usually there would be a purplish spot on the tongue tip or the tongue margin. Consequently, Shenmen (H 7), the Yuan-source point of the Heart Meridian of Hand-Shaoyin, and Neiguan (P 6), the Luo-connecting point of the Pericardium Meridian of Hand-Jueyin, are the choice for the treatment. In consideration of the relation between blood stagnation and hepatic adjusting function, Taichong (Liv 3), the Yuan-source point of the Liver Meridian of Foot-Jueyin, was added in the third treatment for enhancing hepatic function in adjusting blood circulation.

Case 3: Breast tumour (multiple hyperplasia of mammary lobule)

Name, Cao x x; sex, female; age, 38; case No, 20-38953.

Complaints Since September 1982, she found tumours in her both breasts. She said the tumours were related to depression and anger. There was a tight sensation in her breasts and distending pain in the tumours, which was aggravated before menstruation. She improved with various Western medications. Treated with herbal medicine for one year, the symptoms decreased but the tumours did not diminish. The condition reoccurred in suspension of the herbal medicine. Intramuscular injection of testosterone proportionate could soften and slightly diminish the tumours. The patient had a history of hepatosplenomegaly, but with the normal hepatic functions. She had no history of malaria and schistosomiasis. The examination showed that there were teeth-marks in the tongue margin, thin and white tongue coating, string-taut and thready pulse and facial pigmentation. Hard, movable and tender nodes in different sizes (in grain or date size) could be palpated in both breasts. The syndrome was differentiated as liver qi stagnation and obstruction of qi and blood.

Prescription Main acupoints: Neiguan (P 6), Taichong (Liv 3), Xinshu (B 15), Geshu (B 17). Additional acupoints: Zusanli (S 36), Sanyinjiao (Sp 6), Xuehai (Sp 10), Yanglingquan (G 34), Ligou (Liv 5), Riyue (G 24), Qimen (Liv 14).

Treatment procedure The needles were punctured on acupoints bilaterally and retained for twenty minutes. After the needling technique, the Back-Shu points were followed by cupping therapy. Three treatments later, the tight sensation in the breasts decreased, but she still had pain in the left breast. After six treatments the distending pain was relieved. With forty treatments in five months, breast tumours, distending pain and facial pigmentation disappeared.

Explanation Starting with liver qi stagnation, the manifestations of obstruction of qi and blood developed afterwards. Therefore Neiguan (P 6) and Taichong (Liv 3) were used to regulate the Jueyin Meridians. Theoretically the heart dominates the blood and diaphragm and is described as the influential point of blood, so that Xinshu (B 15) and Geshu (B 17) were used to activate blood and to expel stagnation. Additional points activate blood and remove stagnation in the liver. The combination of both main and additional acupoints brought about the same effectiveness.

Case 4: Acute lumbar sprain

Name, Zhao x x; sex, male; age, 34; case No, 85-51.

Complaints He had lumbar sprain from improperly transporting a of heavy object. The patient had motor impairment and was unable to sit for a long time. Examination showed tenderness between the spinal processes of the fourth and fifth lumbar vertebrae, and obvious motor impairment in the lumbar region. The syndrome was differentiated as the obstruction of qi in the Du Meridian and injuries in the tendon and muscle. Therefore, the problem was advised to be treated for smoothing qi flow in the Du Meridian, and regulating collaterals and tendons.

Prescription Renzhong (Du 26).

Treatment procedure With the needle in place, lumbar pain decreased and movement improved. But there still was a little tight sensation in the left side of the lumbar region. Then the local puncture was done with an in-and-out technique, followed by cupping therapy. Three minutes later, lumbar symptoms disappeared and the patient could move freely.

EFFECT OF BACK-SHU POINT IN THE TREATMENT OF MENTAL DISORDERS

—Shao Jingming's Clinical Experience

Shao Jingming, a native of Xihua County, Henan Province, was born in February of 1911. He studied TCM from a famous veteran doctor Guo Yuhuang and started to practise medicine in 1932. In 1935, he attended the acupuncture correspondence course sponsored by acupuncturist Cheng Dan'an in Wuxi. From 1937 to 1951, he practised medicine by setting up a clinic called the Crane Longevity Hall. In August, 1954, he transferred to a municipal hospital where he served as doctor of internal medicine and acupuncturist. In 1968, he was a teacher in Henan College of Traditional Chinese Medicine. He took part in compiling the second and third edition of the textbook *Acupuncture and Moxibustion* for the national medical colleges. He has published twenty-nine principal theses and articles, including the *Clinical Observation and Experiment Research on Acupuncture Treatment of Asthma,* which won the third prize as the Excellent Thesis in 1982. Now, Shao is chief physician in Henan College of TCM, a board member of the China Acupuncture Association, and chairman of the Henan Acupuncture Society.

I. Academic Characteristics and Medical Specialities

1. Acupuncture with one hand and warm sensation under the needle

1) *Acupuncture with one hand*

a. Injecting: Hold the handle of a needle with the thumb and index finger of the right hand, quickly insert the needle to subcutaneous region. When a 3-inch filiform needle is used, hold the needle body wrapped with a sterilized dry cotton ball by the thumb and index finger of the right hand, leaving the needle tip 3 to 5 cm exposed, quickly insert it subcutaneously, and then further insert to the required depth by steps.

b. Rotational insertion with the finger pressure: Hold the needle handle with the thumb and index finger of the right hand, press the area of the point with the tip of the middle finger, rotate the needle with the thumb and quickly insert it subcutaneously.

2) *Warm sensation under the needle*

This is to use the required manipulation, based on the arrival of qi, in combination with tranquil qigong to send qi to the finger to quicken the warm sensation under the needle. According to clinical observation, the manifestations of such a warm sensation vary with the individual constitution. Some took place at the local area of the needling point; some travelled along the meridians; and some run over the whole body. Insert the needle to the required depth as the routine method and lift it to the subcutaneous region after the needling sensation is obtained, stay there for a while, and reinsert the needle to the original depth. After the needling sensation has arrived, tightly hold the needle with the thumb and index finger of the right hand in a fixed position with the thumb forward to expect the arrival of the warm sensation. At the same time, employ tranquil qigong to release qi to the needle body through the thumb and the index finger in order to promote the warm sensation. For instance, a female patient of fifty suffered from sciatica, accompanied with cold lower extremities which may be relieved by warmth. Dr. Shao was invited to give treatment because of her motor difficulty. Examination: Deep, slow and weak pulse, pinkish tongue proper with moist thin white coating, aversion to cold on the lower extremities. Diagnosis: Bi syndrome of cold type. Principle of treatment: Warm the meridians and dispel cold. Prescription: Huantiao (G 30), Weizhong (B 40), Yanglingquan (G 34), Zusanli (S 36). A warm sensation was induced on Huantiao (G 30) when the needle was inserted to a required depth with the appearance of the needling sensation. The patient felt a stream of warmth descending from the leg to the foot. After the needles were removed, the patient felt the pain greatly relieved and the cold sensation reduced. After being treated continuously for five days, the patient recovered.

2. Emphasizing differentiation according to the theory of zang-fu organs, and advocating the combination of the Front-Mu and Back-Shu points

1) *Selecting Feishu (B 13) as the principal point in the treatment of asthma* Dr. Shao began to treat asthma in the 1930s. Since then he has improved the methods of treatment and simplified the selection of the points. In recent years, it has been proved effective to apply Feishu (B 13), Dazhui (Du 14), and Fengmen (B 12) as the main points to treat asthma. From 1980 to 1982, 111 cases of asthma were treated, in which the seven pulmonary function determination index, such as vital capacity and the maximum respiratory capacity, are significantly different ($P<0.001$) before treatment. The total effective rate reached 98.2 percent. For instance, a girl aged thirteen had asthma for eight years, and asthma attacked with the change of the weather. In severe cases, asthma was associated with wheeze and purplish lips and the patient failed to lie down. Since she failed to respond to medication, she came for acupuncture treatment. Examination: Deep, thready and weak pulse, moist tongue proper with thin white coating, slight sallow complexion, cold hands and feet, and clear wheeze. Differentiation: Phlegm blocking the air passage due to deficiency of the spleen resulting from the retention of pathogenic cold and damp in the lung. Principle of treatment: Promote the dispersing function of the lung to resolve phlegm and relieve asthma. Prescription: Dazhui (Du 14), Feishu (B 13), and Fengmen (B 12). Perpendicular insertion 0.6 cun deep is needed on Feishu (B 13) and Fengmen (B 12) and 1 cun on Dazhui (Du 14). Retain the needles for fifteen minutes. After the needling sensation is obtained, even movement with lifting, thrusting and rotating is manipulated twice in between. Apply moxibustion for seven minutes after removing the needles. Treat once a day. Ten treatments constitute a course. After that asthma was relieved and normal respiration was restored. Treat once every other day after an interval for seven days. In winter of the same year, though very cold, in spite of stuffiness in the chest and unsmooth respiration because of a cold, the asthma didn't

attack. The next year, two courses of treatment were given with the same method, and in the third year, one more course was continued. Since then, she has never had asthma even though she sometimes had fever or aversion to cold during a cold. Now more than twenty years have passed and she still enjoys good health.

2) *The Back-Shu points in the treatment of difficulty in swallowing* Difficulty in swallowing, a disorder in the gastro-intestinal disgestive tract, mainly results from the depression of liver qi, stagnation of blood and retention of food. According to Dr. Shao's clinical experience, Geshu (B 17), Ganshu (B 18), Danshu (B 19), Pishu (B 20) and Weishu (B 21) are quite effective for such a condition. For instance, a female patient aged forty-nine had increasing difficulty in swallowing due to emotional depression and frustration with household affairs. For the last five years, she could only take liquid food. She was irritable, aggravated by emotional stimulation, accompanied with fullness in the chest and hyperchodrium, hiccup, which may be alleviated when in a good mood. She had been treated with various methods, but with no good results. A barium examination in a local hospital showed everything normal in exophagus and stomach. Examination: slight general edema, dark red tongue proper with thin white and moist coating, slow and string-taut pulse. Differentiation: Dysfunction of the stomach and stagnation of liver qi. Principle of treatment: Restore the harmony of spleen and stomach by removing stagnation of liver qi. Prescription: Geshu (B 17), Ganshu (B 18), Danshu (B 19), Pishu (B 20), and Weishu (B 21) in combination with Zusanli (S 36), Tanzhong (Ren 17), Zhongwan (Ren 12). Treat once daily with three to five points at a time and retain the needle for fifteen minutes. After the third treatment, edema disappeared, appetite improved and the patient even could swallow steamed bread. Another two treatments were given after an interval for three days. All the symptoms disappeared and appetite was restored to normal. A follow-up examination three months later found no relapse.

3) *Combination of the Front-Mu and Back-Shu points in the treatment of postoperative intestinal adhesion* Intestinal adhesion is mainly caused by abdominal incision for acute abdomen or trauma. The majority are postoperative cases. At an early stage after operation, the patient may feel tenderness around the incision but free from general symptoms, which is due to local blood stagnation, and easily treated with an appropriate diet. In case of improper treatment or failure of nourishment, the conditions may be aggravated later with appearance of abdominal pain, constipation, vomiting, difficulty in swallowing and even incomplete obstruction. According to Dr. Shao's experience, the principle of treatment should harmonize the stomach, moisten the intestines and regulate qi. For instance, a young male patient had an operation for the perforation of acute appendicitis. After that, the patient often felt dull stabbing pain on the lower abdomen. Because he did not pay any attention, later the pain became severe. Diagnosis by the local hospital: Intestinal adhesion. He was hospitalized twice and had intestinal adhesion decollement. The operation only relieved the abdominal pain, but the intestinal adhesion was not radically cured. In acute onset, abdominal pain, vomiting, and even vomiting with bloody water and syncope occurred. Several major hospitals diagnosed this case as three adhesions on colon ascendens accompanied with dudenal ulcer and considered that it was not suitable for the further operations. Then the patient came for acupuncture treatment. Examination: Weak constitution, deep, slow and weak pulse, abdominal

distending pain aggravated on pressure, constipation with bowel movement once every seven or eight days, and the feces the same as that of sheep. Pishu (B 20), Weishu (B 21), Dachangshu (B 25), Zhongwan (Ren 12), Tianshu (S 25), Zhangmen (Liv 13) were used in combination with Zusanli (S 36), Shangjuxu (S 37) and Neiguan (P 6) according to the pathological conditions. Treat once a day or every other day with five to seven points each. The patient was advised to take *wurenjupiwan* (Dried old orange peel) (Tangerine peel, peach kernel, hemp seed, bush-cherry seed, arborvitae seed, Chinese angelica root, white peony root, perilla fruit, self-made honeyed pill) two or three times a day with an average dosage of 6 g. After being treated for more than one month, the symptoms gradually improved. The observation for nearly ten years showed no recurrence and the effects remained stable.

4) *Selecting the Back-Shu points as the principal ones in the treatment of jaundice* Jaundice is mainly manifested by yellow discoloration of the sclera, skin and urine. Although it may be caused either by exogenous pathogenic factors or internal injury, the diseased organs are mostly the liver, gallbladder, spleen and stomach. Dr. Shao often applied reducing method for Yang jaundice, and acupuncture in combination with moxibustion for Yin jaundice. Prescription: Ganshu (B 18), Danshu (B 19), Pishu (B 20), Weishu (B 21). Secondary points: Zusanli (S 36) and Taichong (Liv 3). For instance, a middle school girl student aged sixteen suffered from jaundice for several months. She came for acupuncture treatment after failure to recover at her school clinic. Examination: Slow pulse, dark yellow skin and bulbar conjunctiva, accompanied with lassitude, poor appetite, abdominal distention, and loose stools. Diagnosis: Yin jaundice resulted from stagnant water passage due to hypoactivity of spleen yang. Principle of treatment: Strengthen the spleen and regulate the stomach function, reduce the liver and gallbladder, dispel cold and dampness by warmth. Prescription: Ganshu (B 18), Danshu (B 19), Pishu (B 20), Weishu (B 21) in combination with Zhongwan (Ren 12), Zhangmen (Liv 13), Zusanli (S 36) and Taichong (Liv 3). Apply acupuncture together with moxibustion once every other day. The jaundice disappeared after seven treatments.

3. Selecting Dazhui (Du 14) and Fengchi (G 20) as the main points for treating mental disorder

Dazhui (Du 14) is often used by the ancients in the treatment of febrile disease caused by exogenous pathogenic factors, convulsive diseases and malaria. From his clinical practice for several dozens of years, Dr. Shao found that Dazhui (Du 14) is effective for mental disorders because it is able to restore the balance of yin and yang, regulate qi and blood, invigorate yang qi and promote resuscitation and calm the mind.

1) *Dazhui (Du 14), Fengchi (G 20) in combination with Shenmen (H 7), Neiguan (P 6) for psychosis, hysteria and neurosis* Shenmen (H 7), the Shu-Stream and Yuan-source point of the Heart Meridian of Hand-Shaoyin has the function to subdue heat and calm the mind. Neiguan (P 6), the Luo-(Connecting) point of the Pericardium Meridian of Hand-Jueyin, connecting with Sanjiao Meridian of Hand-Shaoyang, also one of the eight Confluent Points, connecting Yinwei Meridian, is able to reduce

heart fire and promote the water passage of Sanjiao, regulate qi, relax chest, and sedate and tranquilize the mind. For instance, a woman from the countryside frustrated with household affairs suddenly acquired ravings and loud singing, violent behaviour such as hurting people no matter they were relatives or not. Strong stimulation was given on Dazhui (Du 14), (a 2.5-inch filiform needle is inserted 1 cun deep, then lift the needle subcutaneously after the arrival of qi. Press the needle handle downward in a 45° angle with the skin surface and puncture the needle upward obliquely 2 cun). As soon as the tip touches the marrow cavity, a general tremor associated with pallor occurred, then came lethargy. The medical examination showed no abnormality in her pulse, heart beat and respiration. Her relatives were asked to look after her. After sleeping for two hours, the patient noticeably improved. For the sake of consolidating the effect, routine acupuncture treatment was given once daily. Horizontally insert on Dazhui (Du 14) (first perpendicular insertion about 1.3 cun so as to obtain a needling sensation), Fengchi (G 20), Shenmen (H 7), and Neiguan (P 6). The patient recovered completely after five continuous treatments.

For another example, a male patient aged twenty-two came to the clinic on January 26, 1983 for the marked hypomnesia starting three months before. According to the patient's own account, he had dizziness, insomnia, excessive dreams, lassitude, palpitation and was easily frightened because of strain both in study and life at the beginning of that semester. Even though he was still able to keep on with his studies with some efforts. For the past three months the condition was aggravated so much that he could no longer concentrate during the class, and therefore, symptoms such as irritability, insomnia, marked hypomnesia resulted. The medication he took gave him no improvement. String-taut and thready pulse, pale tongue with thin white coating, lassitude, lustreless complexion, but with normal appetite. Diagnosis: Neurosis due to deficiency of blood in the heart and spleen. Prescription: Dazhui (Du 14), Fengchi (B 20), Shenmen (H 7), Neiguan (P 6) were needled for about five minutes, the patient had a fainting spell with symptoms of palpitation, nausea, sweating and pale complexion. The needles were withdrawn without delay and the patient was advised to rest in a prone position, and immediately the patient became normal. The next day, he said he had a sound sleep that night and was clear and calm in his mind. Five treatments were made and half a month later, the patient said he had restored the memory and resumed his classes.

2) *Dazhui (Du 14), Fengchi (G 20) in combination with Baihui (Du 20), Jinsuo (Du 8), Yaoqi (Extra) for epilepsy* Baihui (Du 20), a meeting point of all yang meridians, has the function of cultivating kidney yang, supplementing qi and dredging meridians, nourishing the head and tranquilizing the mind, and calming the liver to stop wind. Jinsuo (Du 8) is able to dredge the meridians, nourish the tendon, to check epilepsy and spasm. Yaoqi (Extra), a special point for epilepsy, is able, if used in combination with Dazhui (Du 14) and Fengchi (G 20), to reduce the attacks of epilepsy and to strengthen the late effect of a remission period. For instance, a woman aged sixty-one had epilepsy for over twenty years, and it was aggravated in the last two years, with two or three attacks daily, mostly occurring at night. During the attack the patient had convulsion of the extremities and coma. When she regained consciousness about one hour later, she had

mental confusion, sometimes accompanied with pale mucous sputum. No effects were obtained even though she had been treated by various methods. When she first came for acupuncture treatment, the patient could not tell the complaints. Examination: String-taut and retarded pulse, pale red tongue proper with thin white coating, dementia and thin body. Dazhui (Du 14), Fengchi (G 20), Baihui (Du 20), Jinsuo (Du 8) and Yaoqi (Extra) were needled continuously for three days, then the patient recovered and had an improved appetite. The condition remained stable after twenty treatments. The follow-up examination four months later found no relapse.

3) *Dazhui (Du 14) in combination with Huantiao (G 30) and Yanglingquan (G 34) for severe pain on the lumbar region and lower extremeties due to emotional factors* Huantiao (G 30), a meeting point of Foot Shaoyang and Taiyang Meridians, has the function of expelling wind and eliminating damp, dredging the meridians and strengthening the waist and lower extremities. Yanglinquan (G 34), a He-Sea point of Gallbladder Meridian and an influential point of the tendons, has the function of dispersing the depressed liver and gallbladder qi, relaxing muscles and tendons and activating the flow of qi, expelling the wind and alleviating the pain. The combination of these two points with Dazhui (Du 14) has a marked effect for severe back and leg pain due to emotional factors. For instance, a male patient aged twenty-four complained of pain on his left leg for twenty-two days. He could not stretch and flex the leg and felt a stabbing pain on exertion. He went to the local hospital for treatment, but failed to get any results. The patient was extremely nervous. He could not stretch the left leg and the pain was stationary on palpation. No pathological manifestations were found in the examination. Calm the patient's worries, and then puncture Dazhui (Du 14), Huantiao (G 30), and Yanglingquan (G 34), retaining the needles for twenty minutes, during which, manipulation was done three times. After the treatment, the patient could get up and walk by himself, and could stretch and flex his legs freely. Pain disappeared. Several days' observation found no relapse.

4) *Yamen (Du 15) and Dazhui (Du 14) in combination with Fengchi (G 20), Shenmen (H 7), Neiguan (P 6), Huantiao (G 30) and Yanglingquan (G 34) for hysterical paralysis* A female patient aged forty-two had paralysis on the lower extremities for seven years. At first, she had irritability, insomnia, melancholy and lacrimation. One year later, both legs became too weak to walk, and she was dizzy when looking up. For the last seven years, she had taken both herbal and Western medications but without any improvement. Examination: Facial complexion, urine and stools, tongue coating, and pulse were all normal. The free lifting and stretching of the legs proved free of organic disorder. Diagnosis: Hysterical paralysis. Acupuncture treatment was given with deep insertion on Yamen (Du 15) and Dazhui (Du 14) alternately in combination with Fengchi (G 20), Huantiao (G 30), Yanglinquan (G 34), Shenmen (H 7), Neiguan (P 6). After continuous treatment for five days, the patient could walk around the room with help. Dazhui (Du 14), Fengchi (G 20), Shenmen (H 7) and Neiguan (P 6) were punctured with even movement once every other day. After more than thirty treatments, all the symptoms disappeared, and the patient gradually recovered. More than ten years have passed and the follow-up visits showed no relapse.

II. Case Analysis

Case 1: Asthma

Name, Liu x x; sex, female; age, 11; date of the first visit, August, 1961.

Complaints Ever since she was one-year old, asthma attacked when catching cold, which became aggravated in winter. Repeated hospital treatment had not made any improvement. Attacks became frequent even in summer, accompanied with shortness of breath, girdling sound in the throat, difficulty in lying down, with purple lips and cold extremeties, deep thready and forceless pulse, pale red tongue proper with thin white and moist tongue coating, sallow complexion, and wheezing sound on the back and chest. Differentiation: Retention of phlegm in the respiratory tract due to dysfunction of the spleen in transportation and transformation caused by long-standing disorder of the lung in its dispersing ability resulting from an attack of wind. Principle of treatment: Alleviate asthma by promoting the dispersing function of the lung and resolving phlegm.

Prescription Feishu (B 13), Dazhui (Du 14), Fengmen (B 12).

Treatment procedure Retain the needles for fifteen minutes after the qi arrives and manipulate the needle two or three times. Apply moxibustion five to seven minutes after the needles are withdrawn. Asthma was immediately alleviated. Treat once every day. After ten treatments, asthma was brought under control. After a one-week interval, treat once every other day. Another ten treatments were given to strengthen the effect. The asthma did not attack in the winter, but instead a suffocating sensation in the chest and unsmooth breathing when she caught a cold appeared. Twenty treatments were given the next year, and ten treatments in the third year. She has remained healthy for more than twenty years.

Explanation This condition at its beginning stage is mostly the lung excess type. The long-standing illness may cause deficiency of lung, spleen, and kidney. The treatment during the attack is to dispel the exogenous pathogenic factors and soothe asthma. Feishu (B 13), Dazhui (Du 14) and Fengmen (B 12) are selected as principal points in combination with some supplementary points. Hegu (LI 4) is used to expel exogenous pathogenic factors in case common cold is associated; Guanyuan (Ren 4) and Taixi (K 3) are used to strengthen the kidney in receiving qi in case of deficiency asthma; Taiyuan (L 9) and Chize (L 5) are applied to regulate lung qi in case of cough; and Tiantu (Ren 22) and Tanzhong (Ren 17) are selected to reduce heat and resolve phlegm in case of excessive phlegm. Since asthma is not easy to completely cure, acupuncture in combination with moxibustion on Dazhui (Du 14) and Feishu (B 13) or cupping an area between these two points after acupuncture is quite effective. Avoid deep insertion on the Back-shu points. For adults, a one-inch filiform needle is inserted 0.5 to 0.8 cun deep, while for children, a 0.5-inch needle is inserted 0.2 to 0.3 cun deep without retaining the needle. The patient is required to avoid catching cold, and to do physical exercise, not to take cold and greasy food, and to give up smoking and drinking.

For the sake of strengthening the curative effect, ten to twenty treatments should be given the next summer or autumn no matter whether asthma attacks or not.

Case 2: Epigastric pain (gastroptosis)

Name, Zhang x x; sex, male; age, 40; date of the first visit, May 24, 1977.

Complaints The patient was hospitalized one day in September 1976, for the acute pain on the epigastric region and was diagnosed as having acute cholecystitis. After treatment the symptoms were improved. The patient had a medical examination for the discomfort on the upper part of the esophagus, but no exfoliated cells were found. An X-ray examination showed gastroptosis. After he was discharged from the hospital, paroxysmal epigastric pain attacked frequently. He lost his appetite gradually and his weight went down. On May 18, 1977, an X-ray revealed the lower part of the stomach was 11 cm below the intercristal connecting line. Examination: Pale red tongue proper with thin white and moist coating, deep, retarded and forceless pulse, thinner, scaphoid abdomen on supine posture, poor appetite, paroxysmal pain on the epigastric region. Differentiation: Qi deficiency in the middle jiao due to prolonged illness. Principle of treatment: Supplement qi and restore yang.

Prescription Zhongwan (Ren 12), Zusanli (S 36), Weishang (2 cun above Daheng (Sp 15)). Supplementary points: Pishu (B 20) and Weishu (B 21) for abdominal distension and stomachache. Treatment procedures: Treat once every day. Retain the needles for twenty minutes with manipulation for two or three times in between. The patient had a tense sensation of lifting and contraction when needling Weishang (Extra). After continuous treatments for five days, the pain was checked and appetite improved. Then, treat once every other day. By the beginning of July, two courses of treatment, about twenty times, were completed, and all the symptoms disappeared. An X-ray reexamination on July 11 showed that the stomach had returned to the normal position. For more than ten years no relapse was found.

Explanation Zhongwan (Ren 12) and Zusanli (S 36) are the toning points used to regulate stomach qi and ascend the clarity and descend the turbidity. Weishang, an extra point, is able to strengthen the spleen, supplement qi and check collapse. Needling depth and direction should be taken into account when puncturing this point. After inserting the needle subcutaneously, oblique insertion 3 to 4 cun in depth is applied with the needle tip directing the navel with even movement. Pishu (B 20) is the place where the spleen qi converges, and is able to strengthen the spleen function. Weishu (B 21) is the place where the stomach qi is infused, and is able to regulate the stomach qi and eliminate distension. All these points used at the same time are quite effective for gastroptosis and ulcer.

Case 3: Goiter (hyperthyroidism)

Name, Pang x x; sex, female; age, 22; date of the first visit, June 2, 1978.

Complaints One month ago the patient found swelling on both sides of the neck and palpitation. Examination on March 8, 1978: Obvious increasing of 131 I absorption test and the peak antedisplacement; 67.9 percent, for 2 hours, 69.0 percent for 4 hours and 64.8 percent for 24 hours. Scanning display of thyroid: Warm nodule on the right side of the thyroid, enlargement III (mixed type) and vascular murmur on the right side, heart rate 140 beats per minute, thythmia, trembling hand (+). Diagnosis: Hyperthyroidism. After taking tapazole for one week, palpitation was alleviated for a short time, but the swelling was growing bigger, with exophthalmus. Examination: String-taut rapid pulse, thin white tongue coating and tongue proper red on both sides, tumefaction of the neck with the right side more severe, exophthalmus, stuffy chest, palpitation, trembling fingers with both arms raising levelly, irritability, easily angered, and insomnia. Differentiation: Unsmooth flow of liver qi and spleen qi resulting in stagnation of qi and blood. Principle of treatment: Regulate qi circulation and remove stagnation.

Prescription Ashi point (0.5 cun above and below Renying (S 9) in combination with Hegu (LI 4), Neiguan (P 6) and Zusanli (S 36)).

Treatment procedure Treat once every day. Retain the needles for twenty to thirty minutes each time. After five continuous treatments, the patient felt relaxed on the neck and the palpitation was alleviated. Then treat once every other day and ten treatments constitute a course. Continue the treatment after five days interval. In the middle of August that year, three courses of treatment were completed and the size of the neck became normal and other accompanying symptoms disappeared. Isotope examination on October 24: 131I absorption test within normal range; 23.39 percent for 2 hours; 2.9 percent for 4 hours and 42.3 percent for 24 hours.

Now the hyperthyroidism was brought under control. No relapse was found after working for eight years.

Explanation Hyperthyroidism falls into aspect of goiter in TCM. The occurrence and development of the disease are mostly related to emotional factors. During the treatment, work should be done to free the patient from apprehension. Ashi points should be selected according to the size of the swelling with many needles at the local area, which functions to eliminate goiter. Hegu (LI 4) and Zusanli (S 36) may promote the free flow of qi along the Yangming Meridian, and remove stagnation of qi and blood. Neiguan (P 6), the Luo-connecting point of the Pericardium Meridian, is able to regulate sanjiao and heart qi and to relieve tachycardia. These four points used in combination have the function of eliminating swelling of the neck, regulating the heart rate and helping relieve the accompanying symptoms.

Case 4: Epilepsy

Name, Zhao x x; sex, female; age, 7.

Complaints The patient had epilepsy for three years, with frequent attacks for half a year, once in two or three days or several times a day. During the attack, there appeared convulsion in the extremeties, clenched jaws, strabismus of the eyes, general stiffness, and incontinence of urine. The attack lasts for three to five minutes. EEG examination: Epilepsy. Differentiation: Stirring up of deficiency-wind. Principle of treatment: Subdue wind and relieve spasm.

Prescription Dazhui (Du 14), Fengchi (G 20), Jinsuo (Du 8), Baihui (Du 20) and Yaoqi (Extra).

Treatment procedure Treat once a day. After three treatments, treat once every other day. Twenty treatments in all were given. No relapse was found for three years.

Explanation Epilepsy is mostly treated with acupuncture during remission period. In case of attack, puncture of Renzhong (Du 26), Baihui (Du 20), Hegu (LI 4), Neiguan (P 6) can alleviate the condition; however, these points are not significant for the treatment of epilepsy at remission period.

The points which are able to regulate the brain, calm the mind, pacify the liver to stop wind should be selected. In order to strengthen the late curative effects, Dazhui (Du 14), Fengchi (G 20), Baihui (Du 20), and Yaoqi (Extra) are clinically applied with satisfactory results.

Case 5: Metrorrhagia (uterine bleeding)

Name, Li x x; sex, female; age, 29; date of the first visit, March, 1981.

Complaints The patient started irregular menstruation after an induced abortion. She had continuous scanty dripping of blood from November 1980 at the menstrual onset until the next March, when she came for treatment. Examination: Slow and retarded pulse, thin white tongue coating, pale red tongue proper, pale complexion, emaciation and loss of appetite.

Differentiation Failure in controlling blood due to difficiency of spleen. Principle of treatment: Strengthen the spleen and kidney, check bleeding and regulate the menstrual cycle.

Prescription Yinbai (Sp 1), Guanyuan (Ren 4), Sanyinjiao (Sp 6), and Ciliao (B 32).

Treatment procedure The bleeding was checked after the first treatment, slight bleeding occurred again the next afternoon because of exertion. The treatment was given once every other day four times and there was no relapse.

Explanation Yinbai (Sp 1), a Jing-Well point of the Spleen Meridian of Foot-Taiyin, is quite effective for checking bleeding if used in combination with Guanyuan (Ren 4), and is able to strengthen the kidney qi. This point should be punctured 2 cun in depth so as to get the needling sensation radiating down to the perineum. Sanyinjiao (Sp 6), the meeting point of the Liver, Spleen and Kidney Meridians, has the function of strengthening the spleen, toning the kidney and nourishing the liver. This point should be punctured 1.5 cun in depth, and manipulated to keep the needling sensation radiating upward to the knees or downward to the heels. Ciliao (B 32) is an essential point for gynecological diseases. This point should be punctured about 2 cun in depth so as to lead the needling sensation forward to the anterior perineum. It is effective in the treatment of irregular menstruation or red-white leukorrhea. The four points used in combination can strengthen the spleen, tone the kidney and nourish the liver, control and check bleeding, they are therefore effective for uterine bleeding.

Case 6: Dysmenorrhea

Name, Wang x x; sex, female; age, 28.

Complaints The patient had dysmenorrhea with increasing severity. She had been married for eight years but was still unable to conceive. Each time at the onset of menstruation, she had severe pain in the lower abdomen, even associated with coma. When menstruation was over, the pain disappeared. String-taut rapid pulse, deep red tongue proper with scanty coating. Differentiation: Heat resulting from stagnation and depression of liver qi. Principle of treatment: Regulate menstruation by dispelling heat and regulating the flow of qi. Prescription: Three to five days before menstruation, select

Guanyuan (Ren 4), Zhongji (Ren 3), and Sanyinjiao (Sp 6) as the main points and add Ciliao (B 32) and Taichong (Liv 3) in case of pain.

Treatment procedure Treat once a day. Retain the needle for twenty to thirty minutes and manipulate two or three times in between. Continue the treatment in case of menstruation until disappearance of pain. The treatment was given continuously for three periods. After that, dysmenorrhea never reoccurred the patient got pregnant later.

Explanation For dysmenorrhea, Guanyuan (Ren 4), Zhongji (Ren 3) can regulate the Chong and Ren Meridians, and regulate the lower jiao, promote blood circulation and resolve blood stagnation. Sanyinjiao (Sp 6) is an essential point for genital and urinary disorders. Ciliao (B 32) and Taichong (Liv 3) are added in case of pain to promote the free flow of liver qi and regulate qi flowing, and more effective for regulating menstruation and checking pain. These five points used in combination produce satisfactory results not only for dysmenorrhea, but also for other gynecological diseases.

EFFECT OF MOXIBUSTION

—Luo Shirong's Clinical Experience

Luo Shirong, a native of Hefei, Anhui Province, was born in 1920. Starting from 1936, he learned acupuncture and moxibustion from his uncle, Dr. Luo Maoxun for five years. From 1943, he practised medicine in Hangzhou, and in 1958, he attended the United Clinic (the Present-day Hangzhou Special Hospital of Chinese Medicine, Acupuncture and Moxibustion). He has practised acupuncture and moxibustion for over forty years. He emphasizes the syndrome-differentiation and treatment of the Du Meridians. He published *Method of Spreading Moxibustion in Treating Bi-Syndrome of Cold-damp Type*. Now he is the honorary president of the Hangzhou Special Hospital of Chinese Medicine, Acupuncture and Moxibustion, the standing member of Zhejiang Association of Acupuncture and Moxibustion.

I. Academic Characteristics and Medical Specialities

1. Skilful in spreading moxibustion

"Spreading moxibustion," also called "long-snake moxibustion," is often used on the Du Meridian. It has the characteristics of being a larger moxibustion area, using bigger moxa cones, for more powerful fire and stronger warmth, and is more effective than normal moxibustion. It has the functions of warming up the toning yang of the Du Meridian, strengthening the Yuan (source) qi, regulating yin and yang and promoting the flow of qi and blood. This method is suitable for all the symptoms of the Du meridian and some chronic, deficient or cold conditions, for example, bi-painful syndromes (including rheumatoid arthritis, rheumatic arthritis, etc.), lumbago (including hyperplasia of lumbar, thoracic and cervical vertebrae; lumbar muscle strain, etc.), asthma (including chronic trachitis, bronchial asthma, pulmonary emphysema, etc.), deficient syndromes (including delayed hepatitis, hepatitis B, neurosis, etc.), chronic gastrointestinal conditions, etc.

1) *Time of spreading moxibustion* During the hot days of summer season.

2) *Acupoints* The acupoints of the Du meridian from Dazhui (Du 14) to Yaoshu (Du 2).

3) *Dressing* One to 1.8 g. of Banshe Powder (Banshe Powder is made of 50 percent Moschus, 20 percent Mylabris, 15 percent Flow Caryophylli and 15 percent Cortex Cinnamomi), 500 g. of mashed garlic, 200 g. of old moxa.

4) *Procedure* Ask the patient to lie down in a prone posture, give a routine sterilization on the spinal column, apply some garlic juice and then Banshe Powder on the midline of the spinal column, then apply mashed garlic from Dazhui (Du 14) to

Yaoshu (Du 2) of two inches in breadth and 0.5 inch in thickness. Afterwards, apply moxa on the mashed garlic as the shape of a snake, and then ignite the moxa on the upper end, lower end and middle point, and let it burn naturally. After burning out, another moxa cone should be reapplied (usually two to three moxa cones are applied). When moxibustion is finished, take away the smashed garlic slightly with a damp and warm towel. There will be blisters after moxibustion, so strict precautions should be taken against infection. On the third day, pierce the blisters to release fluid with a sterilized needle, dry the local area with absorbent cotton, apply gentian violet on the local area (once every other day), and then cover a layer of gauze and fix it with plaster until scar forms.

5) *Medical order* During one month after moxibustion, no raw, cold, pungent, greasy, sweet and strong-taste food, chicken, goose, fish are recommended, no cold shower (but warm shower can be applied) is advisable, the patient should avoid cold wind and sexual intercourse, but must rest for a month.

2. Skillful in using thunder-fire needle

Dr. Luo uses the thunder-fire needle to treat peripheral omarthritis, tennis-elbow, facial paralysis, hemiplegia due to apoplexy, pain in the joints of the limbs, etc. For instance, Dr. Luo has treated thirty-four cases of peripheral omarthritis, the effective rate reaching 92.3 percent.

1) *Method of making thunder-fire needle* The thunder-fire needle made by Dr. Luo is as hard as wood and durable in moxibustion. A waterpipe of 4 cm in diameter and 25 cm in length is sawn vertically into two pieces, and some vegetable oil is applied inside the two pieces of the waterpipe, and the herbal paste is put into the waterpipe. (The herbal paste is made of 150 g. of moxa, 3 g. of Flos Caryophylli, Cortex Cinnamomi, Gummi Olibanum, Myrrha, Rhizoma Currcumae Longae, Radix et Rhizoma Notopterygii, Radix Sileris, Radix Saussureae, Lignum Aquilariae, Squama Manitis respectively, which are ground into fine powder and added with 0.5 g. of Moschus and some paste after it is sieved.) The herbal paste should be stuffed in the waterpipe, and then the two pieces of waterpipe should be separated, a firecracker-shaped herbal stick appears finally. Afterwards, a layer of tissue paper is tightened over the herbal stick and then three to five layers of mulberry paper are added. It's ready for use after it is dry.

2) *Procedure* Ignite the thunder-fire needle with an alcohol burner, apply two to three layers of rough straw paper on the local region, and then press the acupoint rapidly and heavily with the ignited end of the thunder-fire needle for fifteen to thirty seconds. Every acupoint can be applied three times.

3. Emphasizing on suppurative moxibustion

The crux of suppurative moxibustion is to force to suppurate after moxibustion. Therefore, Dr. Luo pays great attention to the appearance of moxibustion blisters and emphasizes that during the application of medicinal extract after moxibustion, fish, fermented glutinous rice, and such rising foods should be taken for three to five days, so as to help bring about suppurating of blisters. If there is no suppuration, irritation food should be taken continuously and warm fomentation should be applied on the moxibustion blisters until suppuration occurs. This method is often used in some chronic gastrointestinal diseases, asthma, in prevention of apoplexy or for strengthening the constitution. For chronic gastrointestinal diseases, Dr. Luo often selects Zusanli (S 36), Zhongwan (Ren 12) and Mingmen (Du 4). For asthma, besides Fengmen (B 12) and Feishu (B 13), Dazhui (Du 14) and Shenzhu (Du 12) of the Du Meridian or Tanzhong (Ren 17) of the Ren Meridian should be added. For preventing apoplexy, besides Zusanli (S 36), Xuanzhong (G 39) and Yanglingquan (G 34) should be added. For strengthening the constitution, Zusanli (S 36) is a main acupoint, and Dazhui (Du 14) of the Du Meridian and Qihai (Ren 6) of the Ren Meridian should be used with great care. Dr. Luo thinks, suppurative moxibustion can be more effective than acupuncture if it is used appropriately. For instance, a male Patient Chen, fifty-six years old, had loose stool for a long time, two to three bowel movements a day, poor appetite, emaciation, white and greasy tongue coating. The patient had been treated in many hospitals, but with no results. Dr. Luo diagnosed it as yang deficiency of spleen and kidney, irregularity of transportation of transformation and accumulation of cold-damp inside the body. Moxibustion was thought to be the best therapy. Moxibustion was applied on Zusanli (S 36), Zhongwan (Ren 12) and Mingmen (Du 4) for three cones respectively. The patient was asked to put a medical extract on the moxibustion blisters (change every day), and to take fish for five days. After three months, appetite was better, bowel movement was normal, white and greasy tongue coating disappeared, and his weight increased three kilograms. After half a year, another treatment was given to consolidate the effect. For another instance, a patient, Shen, forty-three years old, had pain in the elbow and motor impairment of the arm for three months. Dr. Luo put an ignited thunder-fire needle on the most painful point on the patient's elbow five times. After two months, the patient recovered.

II. Case Analysis

Case 1: Bi-painful Syndrome (rheumatoid arthritis)

Name, Shen x x; sex, female; age, 28.

Complaints From 1978, soreness and pain appeared in the joints of the four limbs, and gradually the digital joints became enlarged. The clinical diagnosis was rheumatoid arthritis. After child birth in 1981, the condition became rapidly severe, and the patient had difficulty walking and moving. She had been treated with both traditional Chinese and Western medicine, but with no effect. On July 28, 1983, she came to our hospital to receive treatment. Symptoms were slightly yellow facial complexion, lassitude, poor appetite and tastelessness in the mouth, aversion to cold and preference of warmth, normal urination and bowel movement, small amount of menses, large amount of leukorrhea, enlargement on digital and ankle joints, no redness and swelling, but soreness and pain, and pain aggravated at night, warm preference in the painful area, more pain upon changes of weather, motor impairment in flexing and extending the limbs, pale tongue proper, thin, white and greasy tongue coating, deep, thready and string-taut pulse. Laboratory examinations: ESR (erythrocyte sedimentation rate) was 30 mm/hr; antistreptolysin "0" test showed normal; and rheumatoid factors were positive. The condition was diagnosed as rheumatoid arthritis in Western medicine, and as Bi-painful syndrome in traditional Chinese medicine. It was to be treated by warming up yang and strengthening the constitution, to warm the meridians and dispel cold, to promote qi circulation and activate blood.

Treatment procedure On August 9, 1983, two cones of spreading moxibustion were applied. On October 25, the movement of the four limbs were obviously improved, and soreness and pain disappeared. Examination on December 27 showed: ESR was 5 mm/hr.; antistreptolysin "0" test was normal; and rheumatoid factors were negative. A check-up on February 28, 1984 showed the patient could work and move normally. (During moxibustion treatment, no other medications were taken.)

Case 2: Asthma

Name, Zhou x x; sex, male; age, 16.

Complaints When he was five years old, he caught a cold and did not receive treatment. The cold developed into bronchial asthma gradually. In recent years there were frequent attacks, and only hormone, aminophylline and other medications can control the attack when the condition was serious. There was no results after various treatments. Symptoms: asthmatic sound; yellow facial complexion without lustre, symmetrical thoraces in bucket shape, pale tongue proper, white tongue coating, thready pulse with weak chi portion. X-ray examination: Lungs were clear, striae became wider and disordered, and bronchial shadow became wider. The condition was differentiated as exogeneous pathogenic factors which injured lung qi, which caused deficiency of spleen and kidney due to malnourishment. The unconsolidated wei (defensive) qi led to catching exogeneous pathogenic factors, so the patient was attacked with asthma frequently and his body resistance was injured. The condition was to be treated by warming yang and toning the middle jiao and benefit qi.

Treatment procedure On July 27, 1980, two cones of spreading moxibustion were given. The patient came to the hospital to tell the doctors on August 4, 1983, that there were no attacks of asthma during three years after a spreading moxibustion treatment.

Explanation Moxibustion is suitable to those conditions which cannot be treated by acupuncture. According to the principle of treating different diseases with the same method, those conditions can all be treated with moxibustion, so as to warm up yang and dispel cold, to promote qi circulation and activate blood, to strengthen the Yuan (source) qi and the constitution. "Spreading moxibustion," with the characteristics of a larger area, more powerful fire and stronger warmth, is suitable to some chronic conditions. The acupoints selected in spreading moxibustion are of the Du Meridian, which is "the sea of all the yang meridians," and regulates and controls the qi of all the yang meridians. Huatuojiaji points (Extra) bilateral to the spinal column, are related to the five zang and six fu organs, whose Back-shu points are also bilateral to the spinal column. Therefore, the spinal column and its nearby region can regulate the mechanical functions of the whole body. Garlic is selected to relieve poison and dispel cold, and Moschus is added as extra conductant ingredient to clear the meridians and strengthen the warmth of moxa, so as to guide the meridian qi to flow through the Du Meridian. The method can regulate the function of zang-fu organs and strengthen the body resistance.

Case 3: Wei-atrophy syndrome

Name, Wang x x; sex, female; age, 22.

Complaints After receiving dermoidectomy on the sacral region in a hospital on May 19, 1983, the patient had flaccid paralysis on both lower limbs, accompanied with fecal and urinary incontinence. There was no effect after being treated in many hospitals. On February 20, 1984, she came to our hospital to receive acupuncture treatment. Symptoms were pale facial complexion, pale lips, poor sleep, fecal and urinary incontinence, and an operation scar of 28 cm in length on the lumbosacral region. Examinations: Myodynamia of musculus psoas major was in degree IV; sensitivity existed in the medial aspect below the knees and medial aspect of the feet, and sensitivity disappeared in the lateral aspect below the knees and lateral aspect of the feet; myocynamia of both lower limbs was in degree 0, muscular tension decreased, muscles of the legs atrophied; movement of the area above the lumbar and both arms were normal; and red tongue proper with less fluid, thready and soft pulse. The course of the condition was longer, so qi and blood were deficient, and liver and kidney were also insufficient. An operation caused qi and blood stagnation in the local meridians, which caused weakness of the tendons and bones, flaccid paralysis in Western medicine. The condition was to be treated to benefit qi and blood, to tone the liver and kidney, to clear the meridians and to strengthen the tendons and bones. Choose the local acupoints first, and acupoints along the meridians secondly.

Prescription Huatuojiaji (Extra) from L3 to L5, Shenshu (B 23), Pangguangshu (B 28), Baohuang (B 53), Zhibian (B 54), Huantiao (G 30), Yanglingquan (G 34), Zusanli (S 36), Xuanzhong (G 39), Sanyinjiao (Sp 6), Jiexi (S 41), Yaoyangguan (Du 3).

Treatment procedure Even manipulation was applied on Huatuojiaji (Extra) from L3 to L5, and depth of needling was 1.2 to 1.5 cun, and the needling sensation should radiate to the sacrocossyx, Baohuang (B 53), Zhibian (B 54), Huantiao (G 30), Yanglingquan (G 34), Zusanli (S 36) and Xuanzhong (G 39) were punctured deeply, and the needling sensation should radiate downwards; the needling sensation of Zhibian (B 54) should reach the front and back private parts (i.e. the external genitalia, external urethral orifice and the anus); tonifying method was applied on Shenshu (B 23) and Sanyinjiao (Sp 6); and even manipulation was given on Pangguangshu (B 28) and Jiexi (S 41). Filiform needles were used to puncture the bilateral acupoints. Treatment was given once a day, and after 6-day treatments, the patient was asked to rest for a day. Needles were retained for fifty to sixty minutes when the needling sensation arrived. The patient was asked to do functional exercises for the diseased limbs and to take more nutrient food. After twenty treatments, the patient could walk with a stick in hand, and she could control her bowel movement, but sometimes she still had urinary incontinence. After forty-five treatments, she could control her urination, and myodynamia of both legs reached degree IV, she could walk for about thirty meters without a stick, and for over one kilometer with a stick in hand and she could take care of herself. (During acupuncture treatments, no other medications were taken).

Explanation According to the injured areas and loss of sensitivity, the problem was in the lumbosacral region where the Du Meridian, the Bladder Meridian of Foot-Taiyang and the Gallbladder Meridian of Foot-Shaoyang pass through. Therefore, we took the local acupoints first, and acupoints along the meridians secondly. Deep puncture on Huatuojiaji (Extra) from L3 to L5, Baohuang (B 53), Zhibian (B 54), Huantiao (G 30) and Yaoyangguan (Du 3) with needling sensation radiated downwards was to help promote local meridian qi and to regulate qi and blood. Puncture on Shenshu (B 23) and Sanyinjiao (Sp 6) was to tone the liver and kidney so as to benefit essence and blood. Puncture on Pangguangshu (B 28) to strengthen qi action. Zusanli (S 36) and Jiexi (S 41) support the source of nutrients for growth and development, to regulate and tone qi and blood. Puncture on Yanglingquan (G 34), the Influential Point of tendon and Xuanzhong (G 39), and the Influential Point of marrow to strengthen and benefit tendons and bones.

REGULATION OF THE SPLEEN, STOMACH AND QI

—Zheng Zhuoren's Clinical Experience

After several years' apprenticeship with Cheng Dan'an, an established traditional practitioner in the south of the lower reaches of the Yangtze River, Zheng Zhuoren (1904-1984), a native of Pujiang County, Zhejiang Province, learned his knowledge of traditional Chinese medicine from his teacher. He devoted his whole life to the study of traditional medical literature and acupuncture therapy, and was known as a specialist of traditional internal medicine with a profound knowledge of *Miraculous Pivot.* His works included *Miraculous Pivot in the Vernacular, Acupuncture Prose Interspersed with Verse,* etc. He was the deputy-director of the China Acupuncture Society, special research fellow of the China Academy of Traditional Chinese Medicine and senior consultant of the Hong Kong Acupuncture Association.

I. Academic Characteristics and Medical Specialities

1. Regulation of the spleen and stomach

Zheng greatly esteemed Li Gao or Li Dongyuan's (1180-1252) theory of the spleen and stomach, that "abundant original qi is a result of the absence of impairment of the spleen and stomach. When the stomach is weak, intemperance in drinking and eating naturally lead to injury of the spleen and stomach and less original qi, finally disease occurs." He held that the functions of the spleen and stomach were the basis of that of the meridians and lowered activity logically resulted in weak functioning of the meridians due to poor generation of qi, blood and the meridian qi, and finally diseases attack by taking advantage of their weakness. Based on the theory of "nourishment of the limbs guaranteed by the normal functioning of the spleen," he developed the views of "afflictions of limbs are caused by lowered meridian qi." In clinical treatment stress was laid on regulation of the spleen and stomach for psychomotor sufferings as well as for digestive disorders by needling Zusanli (S 36), Sanyinjiao (Sp 6) to strengthen the spleen —the basis of the acquired constitution, sometimes accompanied by such medicinal herbs as *Pericarpium Citri Reticulatae, Hemerocallis fulva, Folia Citri Reticulatae, Radix Codonopsis, Rhizoma Atractylodis Macrocephalae,* etc.

A female patient aged 68 was once consulted by him with complaints of painful shoulder joints and motion impairment for over two years. Acupuncture, Western drugs and medicinal herbs had been tried and no response was found. She was becoming emaciated, haggard with tight and thready pulse, pale tongue with thin, white coating, a manifestation of deficiency of qi and blood, failure of the meridians to be properly nourished and invasion of the meridians by exogenous pathogenic agents. Shoulder pain and motion impairment disappeared after twelve treatments. Needling was given to Zusanli (S 36), Yanglingquan (G 34) with the lift-thrust method, combined with moxibustion applied to Jiansanzhen (empirical point) and Quchi (LI 11).

2. Regulation of smooth flow of qi

"Abundant qi and normal flow of qi keep one healthy, whereas insufficient qi and perversive flow of qi bring about disease." Zheng's idea stressed the importance of smooth flow of qi to the zang-fu organs, limbs and even the body as a whole. In treatment he paid special attention to the normal flow of qi. In light of the travelling course of the meridian qi and the time passing through a certain point, he adopted the reinforcing and reducing methods by inserting the needle in the same direction as the meridians ran or in the opposite direction when two points of the same meridian were selected. He held that needling at Shanzhong (Ren 17) and Tiantu (Ren 22), Zhongwan (Ren 12) and Zusanli (S 36), Qihai (Ren 6), Guanyuan (Ren 4) and Sanyinjiao (Sp 6) regulated the upper, middle and lower energizers respectively. For particular cases, other points were added. For example, when disorders appeared in the Liver Meridian, Taichong (Liv 3), Zhangmen (Liv 13) were used; when disorders were in the Gallbladder Meridian, Qiuxu (G 40) and Jingmen (G 25) were used; when disorders appeared in the Heart Meridian, Neiguan (P 6) and Xinshu (B 15) were used; when disorders appeared in the Spleen Meridian, Yinbai (Sp 1) and Diji (Sp 8) were used; when disorders appeared in the Kidney Meridian, Shenshu (B 23) was used; when disorders appeared in the Lung Meridian, Lieque (L 7) was used; and when disorders appeared in the Stomach Meridian, Liangqiu (S 34) was used. Once a patient suffering from frequent vomiting for over one year came to be consulted. Physical examination showed stuffiness and fullness in the stomach, lassitude, pale tongue with white greasy coating, string-taut, tight and hesitant pulse. The patient said about ten days ago he had eaten too much popsicle. Zheng diagnosed it as obstruction of qi flow by accumulation of cold, failure of the middle energizer in descending qi and holding back of the spleen yang, resulting in dysfunction of the spleen in transporting and distributing nutrients and water. Treatment should aim at invigorating the vital function and dispersing the cold, regulating the flow of qi and bringing down the perverted flow of qi. Acupuncture was applied to Tanzhong (Ren 17), Neiguan (P 6) with needles obliquely inserted and the reducing method. Warm needling was applied to Zhongwan (Ren 12) and Zusanli (S 36). Vomiting stopped after one treatment and the patient became normal in three treatments.

3. Differentiation of excess and deficiency cases through the needling sensation

It is necessary to tell yin from yang. In treatment of a disease Zheng was good at detecting the condition of the genuine qi and differentiating excess or deficiency cases. He believed that it was most important to know the excess and deficiency conditions by needling sensations besides analysis of syndromes based on the eight principles, the state of the zang-fu organs, qi and blood. In his long clinical practice he concluded that "it is essential to obtain the desired needling reaction, differentiate the state of the needling sensation and its rate of coming." He pointed out that the needling sensation arrived quicker in patients with excess conditions, who had a far-spreading sore and distending feeling under the needles combined with tenseness around the needle. It was a case showing confrontation of the strong pathogenic factors and body resistance. But the needling sensation arrived slower in a patient with deficiency conditions, who had a short-spreading sore and numb feeling, accompanied by looseness around the inserted needle. In patients with great injury of the genuine qi the needle was very easily inserted without any resistance. In terms of the strength of the needling sensation in general, patients with excess conditions usually felt it from strong to weak, whereas patients with deficiency conditions felt it from weak to strong, which was considered the normal reaction. Except for the difference of the meridian qi—excess, deficiency, abundance and decline, Zheng thought patients with different extent of yin and yang would have different responses to acupuncture. Those with much yang were very sensitive; those with yin within yang were not so sensitive as the former; those with balanced yin and yang were neither sensitive nor slow, and response after acupuncture came at the right time in general; and in those with much yin and less yang, slow arrival of the needling reaction was seen, and response appeared only after withdrawal of the needle or after several treatments. In terms of the needling sensation, for patients with insufficient yang and abundant yin manipulation of "Tou Tian Liang" (an ancient reducing method) was employed to induce a cool sensation under the needle; but for the patient with insufficient yin and abundant yang the manipulation of "Shao Shan Huo" (an ancient reinforcing method) was used to bring about a hot sensation under the needle. Once a male patient with a mental disorder, aged fourteen, came for treatments. He was constantly restless for two months. In examination he was found to be red-cheeked and had a pale tongue with moist grey coating, thready, fainting pulse. Dazhui (Du 14) was needled, 1.2 cun in depth. Then the manipulation of "Tou Tian Liang" was applied. The patient said cold chilled him to the bone. After acupuncture treatment the patient was given the following herbs to be taken orally; *Radix Aconiti* 10 g (decocted first), *Cortex Cinnamon* 10 g, *Rhizoma Zingiberis* 10 g, *Rhizoma Arisaematis* 8 g, and *Radix Glycyrrhizae Praeparata* 10 g. After two decoctions were taken symptoms were relieved. After another three decoctions were given the patient recovered.

4. First-aid for carbon monoxide poisoning

Zheng held that carbon monoxide poisoning led to obstruction of the lung, impeding dispersal of the evil qi and entering of the pure qi. When the evil qi attacked the brain and screened yang outside coma and general red complexion appeared. The patient should be moved to fresh air and then Zanzhu (B 2), Renzhong (Du 26), Daling (P 7) were needled with the strong reinforcing method for five minutes. When the patient came to, he should be given some fresh radish juice. Since Zanzhu (B 2), a point of the Bladder Meridian of Foot-Taiyang, on which so many points effecting the zang-fu organs were distributed, selection of this point could promote smooth flow of qi and blood in the whole body and restore functional activities. Renzhong (Du 26), the Yuan-(source) point of the Pericardium Meridian worked to calm the mind and bring the patient back to consciousness from a coma. The fresh radish juice helped to dredge the Lung Meridian. Good results were achieved with the treatment.

5. The function of Zusanli (S 36), Shangjuxu (S 37), Xiajuxu (S 7) and their indications

Zusanli (S 36), Shangjuxu (S 37) and Xiajuxu (S 7) were points of the Stomach Meridian, with the function of regulating and strengthening qi, the function of the spleen and stomach and removing damp. Clinically they were used to treat disorders of the spleen and stomach. But Zusanli (S 36) was the He-(sea) point of the Stomach Meridian of Yangming, effecting on any disorders of the stomach and intestines. It was especially helpful to patients with weak spleen, stomach and lowered genuine qi. Shangjuxu (S 37) and Xiajuxu (S 39) were the lower He-(sea) points of the Large and Small Intestines Meridians respectively. "Lower He-(sea) points" meant the yang qi of the Large and Small Intestine Meridians went down together to the lower limbs and met the yang qi of the Stomach Meridian there. These two points both functioned to regulate qi flow, but the former was usually used to treat poor appetite and nausea due to accumulation of pathogenic damp, impeding the function of the spleen and stomach; the latter was often used to treat diarrhoea, vomiting, poor appetite, etc. due to failure of ascending of food energy and descending of the water.

II. Case Analysis

Case 1: Hemiplegia

Name, Liu x x; sex, female; age, 77; date of the first visit, February 22, 1984.

Complaints When she got up one day a month ago, she had a weak feeling of the left limbs with motion impairment and was diagnosed in a hospital as having cerebral thrombosis. After treatment, the symptoms were relieved. But ten days later she fell by accident and symptoms became worse. She was half-paralyzed, associated with a bitter taste in the mouth, disturbance of speech, pain in the back and legs.

Physical examination showed blood pressure: 150/90 mmHg, consciousness, sonorous voice, a 10 x 15 cm lump felt at the right groin, unmovable but painful on touch, string-taut, floating and deep pulse, red tongue with white, thin coating on the right side and no coating on the left.

Differentiation Invasion of meridians by pathogenic wind, impeded qi flow of the Liver and Gallbladder Meridians.

Method Regulating the flow of qi in the Liver and Gallbladder Meridians.

Prescription Juegu (G 39), Jingmen (G 25), Huantiao (G 30), Yanglingquan (G 34), Qiuxu (G 40) (all on the right side), Taichong (Liv 3).

Treatment procedure The reducing method, with retention of needles for twenty minutes was applied. On the second treatment pain was relieved, the lump at the right groin disappeared, the left arm was able to move a little since the patient had a formication. Treatment aimed at eliminating pathogenic wind and obstruction of the meridians, regulating qi and blood. Acupuncture and medicinal herbs were administered at the same time.

1. Fengchi (G 31), Jianyu (LI 15), Quchi (LI 11), Yangxi (LI 5), Huantiao (G 30), Yanglingquan (G 34), Jiexi (S 41), Jingmen (G 25), Zhangmen (Liv 13) on the left side were shallowly punctured. After the arrival of the needling reaction the needles were withdrawn immediately. Five cones of ignited moxa were applied to Quchi (LI 11) and Yanglingquan (G 34). Then the same points on the right side were deeply punctured with the reinforcing method and needle retention for twenty minutes.

2. Herbs prescribed: *Rhizoma seu Radix Notopteygii* 9 g, *Radix Ledebouriellae* 5 g, *Radix Angelicae Dahuricae* 5 g, *Lumbricus* 9 g, *Semen Coicis* 15 g, *Fructus Chaenomelis* 7 g, *Fructus Foeniculi* 6 g, *Rhizoma Cibotii* 15 g, *Radix Dipsaci* 15 g, *Radix Achyranthis Bidentatae* 9 g, *Ramulus Mori* 24 g, *Radix Polygoni Multiflori* 24 g (six doses).

On the third visit the patient felt that the lower back and leg pain were alleviated. The moyodynamia of the left limbs increased. The tongue was dull red with a thin, white coating. The pulse was thready and floating.

Then the same treatment was given and moxibustion was applied to Zusanli (S 36) and Sanyinjiao (Sp 6) besides Quchi (LI 11) and Yanglingquan (G 34).

In addition the following herbs were given too: *Radix Codonopsis Pilosulae* 15 g, *Poria* 10 g, *Rhizoma Atractylodis Macrocephalae* 18 g, *Radix Glycyrrhizae* 8 g, *Radix Ophiopogonis* 15 g, *Radix Angelicae Sinensis* 10 g, *Rhizoma Ligustici Chuanxiong* 5 g, *Radix Aconili Praeparata* 2 g, *Rhizoma Cibotii* 18 g, *Radix Dipsaci* 10 g, *Radix Polygoni Multiflori* 24 g, *Radix Achyranthis Bidentatae* 9 g, *Stigma Maydis* 24 g, *Lumbricus* 10 g (six doses).

On the fourth visit, symptoms were much relieved. The patient was able to walk a few steps with help. Disturbance of speech disappeared. After twenty-four treatments and thirty-six doses of herbs, the patient fully recovered.

Explanation In dealing with any disease it is essential to ascertain the causes or the affected organs and meridians and give treatment. In the above case hemiplegia and local pain presented owing to the meridian being attacked and obstruction of qi flow in the Liver and Gallbladder Meridians Zheng first managed to remove pains by selecting such points as Jingmen (G 25), and Huantiao (G 30). The former is the Mu-point of the Kidney Meridian. Because the liver and the gallbladder are interior-exterior related, and the liver and kidney have a common source, needling on Jingmen (G 25) regulates the qi and blood in the Liver and Gallbladder Meridians and may also invigorate the vital essence of the kidney. Puncturing Huantiao (G 30), Yanglingquan (G 34) helped bring about the effect. That is why local pain disappeared after acupuncture. The herbs administered functioned to eliminate the pathogenic wind and obstruction of the meridians. The reinforcing method was applied to the points on the affected side and the reducing method to the healthy side to regulate qi flow.

Case 2: Rubella

Name, Li x x; sex, female; age, 58; date of the first visit, November 28, 1983.

Complaints In the previous two months itching red patches appeared all over the body when she was caught in cold wind. Other symptoms included puffiness, scanty urine and constipation, poor appetite, floating and rapid pulse, red tongue with thin yellow coating.

Differentiation Pathogenic wind attacking the skin and growth of internal heat.

Method Removing pathogenic wind and heat.

Prescription Daling (P 7), Quchi (LI 11), Xuehai (Sp 10), Fengshi (G 31), Yangchi (SJ 4).

Treatment procedure Quchi (LI 11), Fengshi (G 31) and Xuehai (Sp 10) were punctured with strong stimulation and the needles were retained for twenty minutes. Then Daling (P 7), Yangchi (SJ 4) were needled, 0.5 cun in depth. The even movement was employed. Treatment was given once a day. After five treatments rubella and puffiness disappeared. Bowel movements and urination became normal. No relapse was found in the follow-up survey.

Explanation Quchi (LI 11) works to smooth a troubled lung and dispel external wind, and Yangchi (SJ 4), the Yuan-(source) point of the Triple Energizers Meridian can regulate qi flow in it; Fengshi (G 31) functioning to eliminate itching, together with Quchi (LI 11) and Xuehai (Sp 10) dispel wind and itching, remove excessive heat from the blood and rubella; and Daling (P 7) is often used to calm the mind and stop itching.

Case 3: Melancholia

Name, Zhao x x; sex, female; age, 24, date of the first visit, January 19, 1984.

Complaints Being usually depressed and reticent, she suddenly became insane half a month before, speaking incoherently and subject to changing moods. Sometimes she had a clear head but she complained of having a headache, an oppressed feeling in the chest, restlessness and fear. In physical examination she was found to have pallor, red cheeks, a sononous voice, deep and rapid pulse, pale and puffy tongue with white, moist coating.

Differentiation Preponderance of yin rendering yang impaired, derangement of qi and blood.

Method Warming up yang and regulating qi and blood.

Prescription Group 1: Shenshu (B 23), Danshu (B 19), Yaoyangguan (Du 3), Qianding (Du 21) with the shallow puncture and even movement; five cones of ignited moxa wool (the size of a grain of wheat) applied to Shenshu (B 23), Danshu (B 19) and Yaoyangguan (Du 3) respectively. Group 2: Zhaohai (K 6), Jianshi (P 5), Sanyinjiao (Sp 6), Neiguan (P 6), Quanliao (SI 18), with the strong stimulation of lifting and thrusting and retention of needles for twenty minutes.

Treatment procedure Treatment was given each day with the above two groups of points used alternately. After fifteen treatments symptoms were relieved and no relapse was seen in an examination half a year later.

Explanation Shenshu (B 23), Danshu (B 19) and Yaoyangquan (Du 3) function to invigorate the yang of the whole body, which helps dispel excessive yin; Zhaohai (K 6), Jianshi (P 5) and Sanyinjiao (Sp 6) were selected with the reducing method to remove excessive yin, regulate qi and blood and the meridians. In addition, Neiguan (P 6) and Zhaohai (K 6), the two of the Eight Confluent Points, served to eliminate depression and promote the smooth flow of qi. All in all, warming up yang, regulating qi and blood, dispelling pathogenic heat from the heart were taken into account simultaneously, then rapid results were obtained.

TREATMENT OF DIFFICULT DISEASES WITH "EIGHT METHODS"

—Zheng Kuishan's Clinical Experience

Zheng Kuishan, a native of Anguo County, Hebei Province, was born in December of 1918. He started to learn acupuncture from his father Zheng Yulin at the age of sixteen. In 1942, together with his father, he came to Beijing to practise medicine, and in 1947 he became a qualified doctor of traditional Chinese medicine. In 1951, together with Dr. Gao Fengtong, et al, he sponsored the acupuncture research course for the Beijing Association of Traditional Chinese Medicine and in July 1952, he established the Guanganmen United Clinic in Beijing. In March 1953, he assisted the Beijing Association of Traditional Chinese Medicine set up an acupuncture clinic and one year later he became an attending doctor of acupuncture in the North China Research Institute of Traditional Chinese Medicine. From 1955 to 1969, he worked as an attending doctor and the chief of the Third Research Office in the Institute of Acupuncture and Moxibustion of Academy of Traditional Chinese Medicine Affiliated to the Ministry of Public Health. In January of 1970, he was shifted to Gansu Province and has been working there up to now. He has published seven treatises and compiled two books, *Collection of Acupuncture and Moxibustion* and *Mid-night Ebb-Flow and Eight Methods of Magic Tortoise.* At present, he is the honorary dean and vice-chief-physician of Traditional Chinese Medicine in Gansu Province, a member of the council of the China Association of Acupuncture and Moxibustion, and the vice president of the Acupuncture Society of Gansu Province.

I. Academic Characteristics and Medical Specialities

In his fifty years of research, teaching, and clinical practice of acupuncture and moxibustion, Dr. Zheng has mastered the theories and traditional techniques of acupuncture. In addition, he has inquired into acupoint combinations and needling techniques under the guidance of the theories of traditional Chinese medicine, especially the theory of differentiation and the "eight methods," i.e. diaphoresis, emesis, purgation, mediation, warming, heat-reducing, reinforcement, and elimination. He prefers the double-hand manipulation and emphasizes the left hand. He considers the summary of the experience of treating refractory and complicated diseases important. Based on the traditional needling methods, he has simplified the manipulating techniques of "setting the mountain on fire" and "penetrating-heaven coolness." On the basis of the traditional theories of "mid-night and ebb-flow" and "eight methods of magic tortoise" and according to his understanding, he has revised the old chart of this method and has designed a new disc.

1. The application of the "Eight Methods"

1) *Diaphoresis* This is a method with a sweating technique in certain acupoints to open the pores so as to drive out the exogenous pathogenic factors, for example, the exterior syndrome due to the invasion of wind-cold is treated with techniques of "setting the mountain on fire" at Fengchi (G 20), Dazhui (Du 14), Hegu (LI 4) to make sweating, thus the pathogenic wind-cold is expelled and the syndrome relieved.

2) *Emesis* This is a method with an emetic technique to make the patient bring up certain pathogenic products to treat obstruction because of sputum in the throat. For example, to treat obstruction of excessive sputum in the throat appearing in apoplectiform stroke or infantile convulsion, the doctor should press hard on the bilateral Panglianquan (Extra), Tiantu (Ren 22) of the patient with the thumb and index finger of the left hand, and puncture the point swiftly just before the patient is ready to vomit, thus the reflex of the internal organs is induced and the sputum comes out.

3) *Purgation* This is the method to reduce the excessive heat, resolve the stagnation, eliminate the accumulation in the stomach and intestines and to relieve pain with the purgative technique at certain acupoints. For example, Zhongwan (Ren 12), Tianshu (S 25), Zusanli (S 36) are needled with the technique of "penetrating heaven coolness" for constipation due to accumulated heat in the stomach and intestines, therefore the heat is reduced and the bowels move.

4) *Mediation* This is the method with an even needling technique at some acupoints to regulate the excess or deficiency of the body, and to support the antipathogenic factors and to expel the evil pathogens. For instance, when the pathogenic factors reside at Shaoyang, Dazhui (Du 14), Yemen (SJ 2), Waiguan (SJ 5) can be selected and manipulated with the technique of hiding yin within yang to harmonize the Ying-Nutrient and the Wei-Defence for treating alternate chills and fever.

5) *Warming* This is the method to replenish yang qi and to eliminate the stubborn yin-cold at acupoints with a warming technique. For instance, for diarrhoea of the deficiency-type, Jianli (Ren 11), Qihai (Ren 6), Zusanli (S 36) are punctured with the warming reinforcing technique to produce the heat sensation to expel cold and arrest diarrhoea.

6) *Heat-reducing* This is the method using the cool-reducing technique at acupoints to reduce heat and to relieve dysphoria and promote the production of fluid in the body to quench thirst. For instance, in treating infantile convulsion, Renzhong (Du 26), Dazhui (Du 14) and Xingjian (Liv 2) are punctured with the water-entering-reducing technique to clear the heat for resuscitation and tranquility.

7) *Reinforcement* This is the method to tone the deficiency and debility of the body with the hot-reinforcing technique at acupoints. For example, when treating impotence resulting from deficiency of kidney yin, Shenshu (B 23), Guanyuanshu (B 26), Guanyuan (Ren 4) are manipulated with the hot-reinforcing technique to conduct the hot sensation down to the genitals to replenish the kidney essence and build up the primary source.

8) *Elimination* This is the method by applying acupoint and different needling techniques to resolve the lump and mass, to remove the stagnated qi and blood to promote

the circulation of blood, and to subdue swelling to alleviate pain. For example, to treat old intravitreous hematocele, Fengchi (G 20), Jiaosun (SJ 20) are punctured with the technique of "setting the mountain on fire" to promote the resolution and absorption of the blood stasis; and when treating thecal cyst, a three-edged needle is used to prick the cyst from the top and the colloid mucus can be squeezed out.

The above-mentioned are just a few examples which can be taken as reference for clinical treatment. Attention must be paid to the indications and contraindications of each of the methods.

2. Double-hand manipulation with emphasis on the left hand

1) *Feeling the point with the left hand assisted by the right hand* Either the thumb or the index finger of the left hand is used to feel the thickness of the muscles, and the width of the cleft or depression at the locus of the point to be punctured, in order to ensure the angle and the depth of insertion, and simultaneously to separate the tendons or vessels which may be the obstacles to the insertion. When feeling the points sheltered under the joints, bones or tendons, the right hand is used to hold the limb for rotation, swaying, flexion and extension, ascending and descending, thus the point can be exposed and the left hand fixes the point, while the right hand to insert the needle.

2) *Right hand inserting the needle while left hand waits for the arrival of qi* In order to obtain accurate and painless insertion and fast arrival of qi, the technique of "quick insertion with the aid of pressure of the finger of the assisting hand" is applied. The thumb or the index finger of the left hand presses hard the site to be punctured, while the right hand holds the needle and thrusts it swiftly 0.1 to 0.2 cun deep, and then the needle is slowly inserted further. The left hand stays on the point to feel the flow of qi beneath the needle and as soon as the qi arrives, the manipulation of certain needling techniques must be provided immediately. The moment must be grasped. To puncture Inner-Jingming (Extra), Doctor Zheng applies the method of "slow insertion by pressing the needle." The index and middle fingers or the thumb and index finger of the left hand are used to separate the upper and lower eyelids and the right hand presses the needle slowly 1 to 1.5 cun in the semilunar fold at the border of the lacrimal caruncle on the nasal side. No rotation, lifting and thrusting of the needle is manipulated.

3) *Closing the meridian with the left hand to direct the qi to the locus of the disease* After the needle is inserted by the right hand and once the left hand feels the flow of qi underneath the needle, the meridian is immediately closed by the left hand below the punctured point, and simultaneously the right hand thrusts the needle upward. By the cooperation of both hands, the needling sensation can be propagated up to the expected or the affected site. When the comfortable feeling is obtained with the manipulation of reinforcing or reducing technique, the "method of sustaining qi" should be employed, e.g. the needling sensation must be maintained so long as the treatment of the disease needs, this is one of the key points for acquiring satisfactory effects.

The above process of feeling the point, inserting the needle, waiting for the arrival of qi, conducting the qi to the locus of the disease and maintaining qi, cannot be performed with the right hand alone; otherwise, the points cannot be located accurately and the needling sensation cannot be easily controlled. Therefore, the double-hand cooperation with the stress on the left hand is essential in acupuncture treatment.

3. Simplifying the manipulating techniques

Dr. Zheng has put forward post-insertion techniques such as lifting-thrusting, twisting-rotating, closing, scraping, flying-pushing, plucking, flicking-trembling, swaying, massage along meridians, pad-moving, retaining, and pressing. During long practice, he has improved the techniques of "setting the mountain on fire" and "penetrating heaven coolness," simplified the old manipulation and invented manipulations of his own. The technique of "setting the mountain on fire" is manipulated by rotating-thrusting the needle, which is fixed by a pushing force for maintaining the arrival of qi, thus a tense heavy and hot sensation is produced underneath the needle, while the technique of "penetrating heaven coolness" is operated by rotating and lifting the needle, which is held by a pulling force for sustaining the qi, thus a light, slippery and cool sensation is obtained under the needle. Both the techniques can be manipulated for one minute and then the needle is withdrawn. The improved techniques have been verified not only clinically but also experimentally. Forty-one cases were punctured with the techniques of "setting mountain on fire" and "penetrating heaven coolness," after the manipulation of the former, the skin temperature was elevated from 1.4 to 1.9°C on average and the wave of the blood vessel capacity raised, while after the performance of the latter, the skin temperature dropped from 1.1 to 1.7°C on average and the wave of the blood vessel capacity lowered. The figures proved the significant difference between the two techniques ($P < 0.01$).

4. Revising the old chart and designing the new disc for clinical application

The recordings of "Ziwuliuzhu" (Midnight-noon Ebb-flow) and "Lingguibafa" (Eight Methods of Magic Tortoise) in acupuncture literature in the Yuan and Ming dynasties are mainly presented by literal recounting and calculating, so there is difficulty in studying and employing these methods. In addition, the calculation is complicated. This is the reason why these two methods of acupuncture were not popular a long time. In order to carry on this acupuncture therapy and to facilitate study, Dr. Zheng combined the experiences of ancient doctors with his own knowledge, and designed a pocket "disc of Midnight-noon Ebb-flow," and "Eight Methods of Intelligent Turtle for Clinical Application" by mixing "hour-prescription" method and "day-prescription" method of "Midnight-noon Ebb-flow" "Eight Methods of Intelligent Turtle" and 60-year "Huajiazi" in Gregorian calendar. This disc is characterized by portability and simplicity and it can be used to select points according to the hour-prescription method, the day-prescription method and "Eight Methods of Intelligent Turtle." Without calculation, the primary optimal point of any moment in any day and every day's "Huajiazi" in sixty years of the Gregorian calendar can be found. This disc has provided a simple but accurate tool for treatment, teaching and research work in acupuncture.

5. Treating refractory and complicated diseases with warming methods

When investigating the treatment for some refractory and complicated diseases, the warming methods are mostly used in clinic, while Fengchi (G 20) is the most used point. Warming methods include warming-reinforcing, warming-opening and warming-dispersing. For example, in treating retinal hemorrhage, Fengchi (G 20) is punctured with the technique of "setting mountain on fire" and the hot sensation is propagated to the eyeball to facilitate the resolution or absorption of the stasis of blood. In 1958, ninety-one cases of this disease were treated and the total effective rate was 90.2 percent. To treat optic atrophy, the technique of "setting mountain on fire" is manipulated at Fengchi (G 20) to clear the head and brighten the eyes, and to open the meridians for promoting the circulation of blood. In 1960, twenty-four cases of optic atrophy were treated with this technique and the total effective rate was 62.5 percent. To treat the exterior syndrome due to invasion of the exogenous pathogenic wind-cold, the technique of "setting mountain on fire" is used to induce perspiration for relieving the syndrome. In 1956, three patients suffering from tuberculosis of the spine and that of the sacro-iliac joint were treated with the technique of "setting mountain on fire" and the principle was stressed on reinforcing the kidney, toning the bones and strengthening the constitution. All three cases were cured.

The treatment of long-standing intractable diseases has achieved satisfactory results in the clinic through research and treatment. For instance, in treating poliomyelitis and its sequela, initially the hot reinforcing method was used, so the course of treatment was prolonged. In light of long clinical experience, except for the hot-reinforcing technique, heavy stimulation of the points should be applied, and the stimulating time should be prolonged to improve the nutritive status of peripheral nerves and blood vessels, thus the motoring functions of tissues and organs can be restored. Consequently, catgut embedding in acupoints and a ligation method are adopted. Among the 113 cases, the total effective rate was 99.1 percent. In addition, the full course of treatment with this method is shorter than that of acupuncture alone, therefore it is more convenient to patients from remote areas. It was also found that to treat patients with long-term muscular atrophy, the catgut-embedding and ligation method must be combined and then a satisfactory effect could be obtained.

The warming methods are also used in treating some common diseases in clinic. Early in the 1960 technique of "setting mountain on fire" was used to treat seventy-five cases of lumbago with satisfactory results. Warming methods are also used for Bi-syndrome and painful disorders. To treat flaccid limbs and muscular atrophy caused by malnutrition of muscles resulting from blockage of meridians, a warming-opening method is mainly used to warm and open meridians to facilitate the flow of qi and blood. When treating abdominal pain and diarrhoea due to cold and deficiency of the spleen and stomach and lumbar pain and impotence caused by kidney yang deficiency, the warming-reinforcing method is recommended to warm and tone the yang qi of the kidney. To treat the exterior syndrome due to the invasion of exogenous pathogenic factors the warming-dispersing method is used to expel pathogenic wind, cold and dampness so as to eliminate the exterior syndrome.

6. Treatment of infectious polyeneuritis

Infectious polyneuritis falls into the category of "Wei-syndrome" in traditional Chinese medicine. This disease is difficult to treat and is often fatal. The onset of this disease is manifested by paralysis of extremities, and its development results in respiratory paralysis which at length leads to death. This disease is differentiated as three syndromes.

1) *The syndrome of lung-heat consuming yin* "Lung-heat consuming yin interiorly will lead to Wei-Syndrome." This syndrome is represented by fever, dyspnea, profuse sputum which the patient fails to expectorate due to forcelessness, scanty and dark yellow urine, dry stool, yellow sticky tongue coating and thready rapid pulse. This is a critical syndrome which worsens quickly. Bed rest is needed and intensive care should be provided to save the patient. Dazhui (Du 14), Feishu (B 13), Lieque (L 7) and Shaoshang (L 11) can be pricked for bleeding to clear the heat, nourish yin and regain the normal flow of lung qi.

2) *The syndrome of damp-heat in the spleen and stomach* "Wei-syndrome must be related to the stomach trouble due to either damp-heat or damp phlegm." In this syndrome, there is paralysis of the limbs, fullness and stuffiness of the chest and epigastric region, slight swelling and numbness of lower extremities, dark yellow and dribbling urination, yellow sticky tongue coating and soft pulse. Quchi (LI 11), Shousanli (LI 10), Zusanli (S 36) and Sanyinjiao (Sp. 6) are punctured with the reducing technique or Liangqiu (S 34), Xuehai (Sp 10), Waiguan (SJ 5) and Hegu (LI 4) are manipulated with an even needling technique to eliminate the damp heat and to invigorate the spleen for strengthening its transportation and transformation.

3) *The syndrome of deficiency of both the liver and kidney* "When there is pseudo-heat in the liver, the bite may overflow, causing a bitter taste in the mouth; if the tendons fail to be nourished, Wei-syndrome of tendons results; when there is pseudo-heat in the kidney, the lumbar region and the spine cannot be straightened, bones wither and marrow diminishes, and the result is "Wei-syndrome of the bones." Lumbago, soreness and weakness of extremities, muscular atrophy, dizziness and vertigo, red tongue covered with scanty coating and thready rapid pulse are associated. Shenshu (B 23), Ququan (Liv 8) and Sanyinjiao (Sp 6) or Guanyuanshu (B 26), Xuehai (Sp 10), Liangqiu (S 34), Zusanli (S 36), Binao (LI 14), Shousanli (LI 10) and Ashi points can be recommended and needled with the hot-reinforcing method to replenish the kidney and liver, and to activate the flow of qi in the meridians and collaterals.

The above-mentioned three syndromes can be transformed into one another. The most critical or severe cases are initially manifested by the syndrome of lung-heat consuming yin and then transformed into the syndrome of damp-heat in the spleen and stomach or deficiency of both the liver and kidney after the disease is stabilized with treatment. On the contrary, those with slow onset are represented by the latter two syndromes; however, the improper treatment may worsen the diseases, so symptoms of lung heat syndrome may occur. Therefore, the treatment should be varied according to the change of disease.

The above mentioned treating methods were used in treating 24 patients, and the number of acupuncture treatments ranged from 2 to 50 sessions. A follow-up examination was done 3 months after the treatment had finished. The result revealed 9 cases cured, 6 markedly effectiveness, 9 improved, and 2 deaths.

7. Treatment of acupuncture for gastric and duodenal ulcer

In traditional Chinese medicine, this disease falls into the category of epigastric pain, stomach and chest pain, and heart pain. It is mainly caused by emotional disturbance, irregular food intake and stagnated qi and blood. The chief symptoms are dull, burning pain or megalgia in the upper abdomen, or abdominal distention, nausea and vomiting, belching and periodic acid regurgitation. Tenderness can be found by pressure at the epigastric region, Geshu (B 17), and Ganshu (B 18). The treatment is as follows:

1) *The syndrome of cold-deficiency in the spleen and stomach* This is represented by the symptoms such as dull pain of the epigastric region relieved by pressure and intake of food, indigestion, belching with foul gas, acid regurgitation, intolerance to cold and preference for warmth, lassitude, fatigue, pale tongue proper with thin white coating, and forceless pulse. Shangwan (Ren 13), Zhongwan (Ren 12), Liangmen (S 21), Tianshu (S 25), Zusanli (S 36), Sanyinjiao (Sp 6), and Shangqiu (Sp 5) are punctured with the hot-reinforcing method retaining the needles for ten to twenty minutes. This treatment aims at warming the Middle Jiao and alleviating pain, and benefiting the stomach and strengthening the spleen.

2) *The syndrome of stagnation of qi and blood* This syndrome is manifested by distention and fullness in the epigastric region, stomachache aggravated by pressure, bitter and acid regurgitation and vomiting, the pain excruciating after anger, hematemesis, dark stool, dark red tongue with a thick sticky coating, and string-taut pulse. Shangwan (Ren 13), Xianwan (Ren 10), Tianshu (S 25), Qihai (Ren 6), Zusanli (S 36), Neiting (S 44), Geshu (B 17), Ganshu (B 18) and Ashi points are manipulated with the even needling technique with retention of the needles from twenty to thirty minutes. The purpose of this treatment is to regulate the flow of qi, activate the circulation of blood, soothe the liver and relieve pain. Supplementary points: a. Neiguan (P 6) and Gongsun (Sp 4) are used in combination with the reducing method to control nausea and vomiting retaining the needles for twenty to thirty minutes. b. Needle-embedding is performed subcutaneously at Geshu (B 17) and Ganshu (B 18) for five to seven days in cases of belching, acid regurgitation, and recurrent stomachache to regulate the flow of qi and relieve the pain. c. Quchi (LI 11), Hegu (LI 4), Xuehai (Sp 10), Zusanli (S 36), and Sanyinjiao (Sp 6) are reduced with needles retained for twenty to thirty minutes in cases of hematemesis, tarrystool, and burning pain in the epigastric region so as to reduce the heat and stop bleeding. d. Stomachache associated with constipation is treated with reducing at Dachangshu (B 25), Tianshu (S 25), and Zhigou (SJ 6) and needles are retained for twenty to thirty minutes. So the intestines are moistened and stools moved. e. Pishu (B 20), Huiyang (B 35), Yaoshu (Du 2), and Qihai (Ren 6) are needled with reinforcing and moxibustion for ten to twenty minutes in the case of stomachache and diarrhoea to warm up the middle jiao and check diarrhoea.

Fifty patients were treated with the above-mentioned method. After 2 to 50 acupuncture treatments and a month's observation, 16 cases were cured, 17 were markedly effective, 16 improved and 1 failed. The total effective rate was 98 percent.

8. Treatment of scapulohumeral periarthritis by acupuncture and catgut embedding

This disease, known as frozon shoulder or shoulder wind in traditional Chinese medicine, is often caused by sprain, overstrain, or the invasion of pathogenic wind, cold and dampness. The main symptoms are pain of the shoulder and arm and functional impairment of the shoulder. Raising, abduction, adduction, moving-back and akimbo position of the arm are limited. The following treatments can be applied.

Since the disease is located at the shoulder, Jianyu (LI 15), Jianliao (SJ 14), Tianzong (SI 11) and Ashi points are selected as the primary points, and the catgut embedding method is employed. In case of the swinging of the shoulder and arm, tenderness in the depression at the acromion, and difficulty in backward movement of the arm, Jianfeng (Extra) and Chize (L 5) can be combined; in case of tenderness at the location of Jianyu (LI 15) with difficulty in raising the arm, Quchi (LI 11) and Jugu (LI 16) can be supplemented; in case of tenderness at the locus of Tianzong (SI 11) with impaired adduction, Jianzhen (SI 9) and Houxi (SI 3) are added; and in case of tenderness at the site of Jianliao (SJ 14) with the difficulty of abduction, the technique of "setting mountain on fire" is employed at Naoshu (SI 10) and Waiguan (SJ 5) and the needles retained for ten to twenty minutes to activate the blood circulation, remove the stagnation and benefit the joints.

After the needles are withdrawn, the penetrating method can be provided from Tiaokou (S 38) to Chengshan (B 57). The patient is required to do abduction, adduction, and raise the arm at the same time when the needle is manipulated so as to enlarge the motor range of the shoulder and to enhance the effect.

Catgut embedding can be done in 3 to 5 points for each treatment, one session for approximately 10 days. Five sessions constitute one course of treatment. If the disease is not cured, the embedding can be continued after ten days' interval. Five to eight days after each embedding, treatment can be performed with the above-mentioned points and techniques once or three times. A hundred and eleven patients were treated, among them, 29 cases were cured, 30 markedly improved, 50 improved, and 2 failed, making the total effective rate 98.2 percent.

9. Acupuncture treatment of thecal cyst

This disorder is categorized as injury of tendon in traditional Chinese medicine. It is a small localized lump which is hard and tough due to the expansion of the tendon sheath, mostly from trauma, contusion and sprain.

The chief symptoms: Lump located at the joint mainly on the dorsal aspect of the wrist, the anterior aspect of the ankle region, dorsum of the foot, and in the popliteal fossa, which looks like an apricot pit, different in size, hard and even, immovable with palpation (some are movable), absence of pain or mild soreness and pain, but the severe one can affect the daily life or work.

Treating method: The routine sterilization is made at the diseased area, and then a three-edged needle is inserted from the top of the cyst down to the middle and swiftly withdrawn. Mucus is squeezed out from the needled hole, and a sterilized cotton ball is placed on the hole fixed with adhesive plaster. Usually this problem can be cured with one treatment. If the mucus is not completely squeezed out, after four to eight days, encircling method with filiform needles can be offered, four needles are inserted transversely into the cyst each from one direction. The needles are retained for ten to twenty minutes. If the disease recurs, the same treatment can be repeated. Ninety patients were treated with this method 1 to 5 times, 2 to 3 times on average. The follow-up visit 3 months after the treatment showed that 78 cases were cured and 12 were markedly improved.

II. Case Analysis

Case 1: Windstroke (cerebrovascular accident complicated with pseudobulbar paralysis)

Name, Wang x x; sex, male; age, 54; date of the first visit, July, 2, 1979.

Complaints This patient started to suffer from hypertension in 1956, and in 1964 he got cerebrovascular spasm. Cerebral thrombosis occurred in 1972 and recurred in 1975 with complication of pseudobulbar paralysis. He was admitted to the hospital on April 9, 1979. During the treatment, salivation increased, speech was slurred, mouth opened, the tongue was inflexible and choking occurred when swallowing. He was irritable, cried and laughed insensibly, and he could not take care of his daily life since he was not able to complete any conscious action though his right extremities could move. Sticking out his tongue deviated to the right side, pharyngeal reflex could not be found, retinal hemarrhage alternated in the eyes. Because of the choking when eating or drinking, gastrogavage was used on June 5. Consultation concurred with the opinion that the worsening of the disease was the consequence of diffuse change of cerebrovascular lesion based on cerebral arteriosclerosis, causing the paralysis of 9, 10 and 12 cranial nerves, motoring aphasia, and pseudobulbar paralysis and no modern medicine was effective so far. Examination: Body temperature was 37.9°C, pulse 104 times per minute, respiration 24 times per minute, blood pressure 200/120 mmHg, consciousness was clear, voice slurred, bilateral pupils evenly big and round, light reflex sensation, frontal wrinkles symmetric, nasolabial groove on the right side shallow, stuck tongue in the middle; no abnormality in bilateral lungs, heart border expanded down to the left, heart rate 104 times per minute with arrythmia, systolic blowing murmur of II degree audile in the region of the heart apex, A2 › P2; spleen and liver nothing abnormal, the physiological reflex was normal, and the pathological reflex was not found; myodianamia of the extremities fair, radial arteriosclerosis positive, and retinal angiosclerosis in ocular fundus II to III degree. The patient had sluggish, sometimes crying sometimes laughing expression, the mouth partially opened, sticky saliva which could not be expectorated voluntarily. A tube was inserted in the nose for twenty-two days to feed him. The right wrist slightly dropped, muscles of the right arm slightly atrophic, and right limbs could extend and flex but could not do any other action. He could respond to questions only by saying "yin," and "yang." The tongue was stiff and short and not able to stick out. The tongue was red and covered with a yellow sticky coating and the pulse rolling and rapid. TCM differentiation regarded it as retention of dampness and phlegm which led to wind-stroke with aphasia and hemiplegia. Removing dampness and phlegm to open meridians and to resuscitate the patient was the principle of treatment. Prescription: According to "Ling Gui Ba Fa," it was *Bingzi hour-period Gengwu day*, Zhaohai (K 6) and Lieque (L 7) were punctured first retaining the needles, then Upper-Lianquan (Extra), Lianquan (Ren 23), Tiantu (Ren 22) were manipulated with an even needling technique without retention of needles, and Fengfu (Du 16), Fengchi (G 20), Tongtian (B 7), and Sanyinjiao (Sp 6) were reinforced and needles were retained for ten minutes.

Treatment procedure Before puncturing, the stomach tube was withdrawn and during needling, the patient was required to drink orange juice. He succeeded in drinking two spoons of juice, but failed to swallow a segment of orange because of choking. Then Yangxi (LI 5) on the right side was punctured and he could swallow two spoons of chicken soup with bakend wheat flour. Observation was continued on his swallowing and it was found that the patient had profuse and sticky saliva which he could neither spit nor swallow. The time was *Xinsi hour,* so left Lieque (L 7) and Yifeng (SJ 17) were punctured with the even needling technique, then saliva became thinner and swallowing was also getting better. He drank 500 ml of flour gruel. On July 3, the condition of the patient was slightly improved. He took 300 ml liquid diet, his pulse was 80 times per minute and body temperature was 37°C. The second treatment was performed at 10:20 a.m. Zhaohai (K 6), Lieque (L 7) (right alone), Baihui (Du 20), Tongtian (B 7), Fengchi (G 20), Upper-Lianquan (Extra), and Yangxi (LI 5) were punctured with the same technique as before and 1250 ml liquid diet was drunk in a whole day. The next day, swallowing became even better. At 7:10 a.m. the third treatment was undertaken with Linqi (G 41) and Waiguan (SJ 5) punctured first and Quchi (LI 11) (right side), Hegu (L 4), Huantiao, (G 30), Zusanli (S 36) and Xuanzhong (G 39) later to facilitate the flow in meridians and collaterals for remedying the hemiplegia. After the treatment the patient could eat semi-liquid and solid food. From July 5, on the primary points corresponding to an every hour period were selected with the same technique as before. Up to June 23, the patient could take a bowl of milk, two eggs, and two pieces of pastry for breakfast, two bowls of noodles mixed with fresh kidney beans and meat slice for lunch, and a bowl of rice gruel, a sugar cake and a cup of malted milk for supper. On the morning of June 25, the patient fell to the ground from a chair, so the tongue became shortened and the speech unclear. Jinjin (Extra) and Yuye (Extra) were punctured and the tongue could stick out and move all around after the needling. Up to July 28, the patient had twenty-five sessions of treatment, and he was able to hold the bowl for eating by himself, a quarter of a kilogram of food daily. Sometimes, he could also eat dumplings with meat filling, and he strolled outside by himself. The blood pressure was 140/100 mmHg. The tongue coating was thin and white and the pulse rolling. From that time, the treatment stopped and the patient was required to do exercise. On September 9, that year and October 20, 1980, he was followed up twice. He could take food normally, the motoring function of limbs on the right side was restored and he was able to speak three to four words. There was no recurrence of the illness.

Explanation Cerebrovascular accident complicated with pseudobulbar paralysis falls into the aspect of windstroke in traditional Chinese medicine. The symptoms of salivation, dysphagia, choking during drinking water, and nose feeding for twenty-two days are all critical, and the patient was debilitated. This is the syndrome of retained phlegm and dampness blocking the mind. Puncture at Zhaohai (K 6), Lieque (L 7), Yangxi (LI 5), with an even needling technique can eliminate dampness and phlegm, invigorate the flow of meridians and resurrect the patient, thus alleviating the disease.

Case 2: Windstroke (cerebral hemorrhage)

Name, Mo x x; sex, female; age, 61; date of the first visit; October 16, 1978.

Complaints She had a history of hypertension for more than two years. Eight days ago, she started to feel headache and dizziness. One day before, she had felt dizzy and had had syncope. Subsequently she lost her speech and motor function of the limbs on the left side and was lethargic all the time. The local clinic could help nothing, so she was shifted to our hospital. Examination: Somnolence, mental confusion, slurred speech, flushed face, the left pupil bigger than the right one, nasolibial groove on the left side shallower than that on the right side, and tongue deviated to the left; wheezing sound audible in the lungs, deep and rapid respiration, systolic blowing murmur of II degree audible in the region of heart apex, even heart rhythm, heart rate sixty times per minute, and accentuation of second aortic value sound; abdomen soft, liver and spleen impalpable, motoring function of right limbs possible, but inflexible, no motoring of the limbs on the left side, knee jerk reflex normal on the right, lowered on the left, but no pathological reflex found; body temperature 36.6°C, blood pressure 210/116 mmHg; blood routine examination: The total number of leukocyte 19600/mm , neutrality 91 percent lymph 9 percent cerebrospinal fluid sanguineous. The tongue coating was not visible, because the mouth could not be opened wide enough. The pulse was string-taut and forceful. Differentiation: Stirring-up of liver wind leading to reversed rising of qi and blood. The treating principle was to suppress the liver, reduce fire, eliminate wind and subdue yang.

Prescription According to the "Nazi" method, Taichong (Liv 3) was primarily selected in combination with Twelve Jing-Well points (bleeding) and bilateral Sanyinjiao (Sp 6) and Fenglong (S 40) at 2:00 p.m. October 16, 1978 (Yiwei hour-period, in Xinhai day).

Treatment procedure The reducing technique was used and needles retained for twenty minutes. The second treatment found the mind clear, but speech was slow and the voice weak, and an intake of a small amount of food, headache, involuntary movement of the left limbs, decreased grip strength of the left hand, blood pressure 190/70 mmHg, heart rate 64 times per minute, light red tongue with yellow sticky coating, and string-taut rapid pulse. At 4:00 p.m. of the 17th (Wushen hour-period in Renzi day), Jiexi (S 41) was prescribed as a primary point and Fengchi (G 20), Baihui (Du 20), Upper-Lianquan (Extra), Quchi (LI 11) (left), Hegu (LI 4) and Huantiao (G 30) were combined. Up to October 20, the fifth treatment, the headache was much relieved, speech became clear, eating was normal, pupils were equal, the tongue was still deviated to the left, the left nasolibial groove was shallower. She was able to raise the arm and leg of the left side but her grip strength of the left hand still weaker. Blood pressure was 150/60 mmHg, and tongue coating and pulse were the same as before. The corresponding primary point was selected first and Jianyu (LI 15) (left), Quchi (LI 11), Hegu (LI 4), Waiyuan (SJ 5), Huantiao (G 30), Fengchi (G 20), Yanglingquan (G 34), Zusanli (S 36), and Xuanzhong (G 39) were combined and manipulated with an even needling technique with needles retained for twenty minutes to facilitate the circulation of blood, suppress the wind, and invigorate the flow of meridians and collaterals. Until November 6, twelve treatments were given. The headache diminished, spirit was better, pupils were equal, the bilateral nasolibial grooves were free of difference, appetite increased, the grip strength of the left hand was enhanced, being able to grasp three fingers, the left hand could be lifted over the head. She was able to walk, but the left leg was not strong enough, not able to lift high. Blood pressure was 160/80 mmHg. The patient was eager to leave the hospital for home. Later, she went to the out-patient clinic for treatment. But the primary points corresponding to hour-periods were still selected and the combined points and needling technique were the same as before. After more than fifteen acupuncture treatments, the disease was basically stabilized, thus treatment stopped. On December 20, the follow-up visit showed that she recovered well, her left hand could be lifted above her head, her grip was fair, her gait was steady, and she was able to do some housework.

Explanation This disease is known as windstroke and hemiplegia. During the period of coma, oxygen inhalation should be supplemented. When it is becoming a bit milder, the hemiplegia should be treated timely. If the blood pressure is not very high and the patient is able to get up from the bed, appropriate exercise of the limbs should be added in order to heighten the effect. The above-mentioned method was used in treating twenty patients. Five cases were short-term cured, 10 markedly effective, 4 improved and 1 failed.

Case 3: Deafness

Name, Fu x x; sex, male; age, 58; date of the first visit, March 19, 1983.

Complaints In early January of 1983, the patient caught a cold, and in the middle of the month when he was attending a meeting in Xi'an, the cold was aggravated with symptoms of chills and aversion to cold because there was no indoor heating. He was injected with penicillin and streptomycin. In late January, he went back to Lanzhou and continued to have injection of penicillin and stroptomycin in combination with terramycin per os. On the morning of February 5, he attended a memorial meeting on Hualin Mountain. Due to the heavy heart and cold weather, he had cold sweating all over the body, subsequently, he was attacked by a general ache, and feeling hard to stand on his own. After coming back, severe nasal obstruction and dyspnea occurred and in the afternoon, his hearing decreased all of a sudden. On February 7, he went to see doctors in the department of internal medicine of a hospital, but the therapeutic effect was unsatisfactory. On the twelfth, he visited the ear, nose and throat department of an army hospital. The administration of terramycin, "Huanglianshangqingwan," (a Chinese medicine) nasal drip of ephedrin, and injection of Folium Isatidis injection caused him to have a dry mouth. On the seventeenth, he shifted to a civil hospital in Lanzhou where he was diagnosed as having nervous deafness and obstruction of eustachian tube. Injection of penicillin and fluid infusion were provided for ten days but little improvement was obtained. On March 11, incubation of the eustachian tube was undertaken in the right ear and the tube was opened; however, it was blocked again when the catheter was withdrawn. Moreover, the nose was bleeding, there was a loud sound in the ears which made no external sound audible, and the body temperature dropped down to 34.8 to 35.6°C. On the ninth, he moved to our hospital. Examination: The nasal mucosa was conjested and swollen, and the nasal tract was obstructed; bilateral otopiesis, both air and bone conduction decreased, hearing ability was lowered, severe deafness in both ears; increased lung markings; and nothing abnormal with the E.C.G, ultrasonic, X-ray of the nose, routine blood test, thrombcyte, biochemistry, bowel movement and urination, and liver function. The examination of traditional Chinese medicine found that the patient could not hear the voice of speech in front of his face, the nose was obstructed and there were harsh respiration with the mouth open, flushed face, pale tongue with white sticky coating and superficial forceful pulse beating seventy-four times per minute. In light of the differentiation, it was a syndrome of wind-cold disturbing the upper portion combined with retention of turbid dampness which blocks Shaoyang meridians and the sense organs, therefore the treatment aimed at dispersing wind and cold, eliminating dampness and regulating the flow of qi of the Gallbladder Meridian, and opening the affected organs to regain hearing.

Prescription According to the "Nazi" method, Hegu (LI 4), Fengchi (G 20) were selected as primary points with the technique of "setting mountain on fire" to conduct the hot sensation up to the forehead, thus sweating the whole body, and simultaneously Upper-Yingxiang (Extra) was pricked and Shangxing (Du 23) and Tinghui (G 2) were manipulated the even needling technique and needles were retained for thirty minutes.

Treatment procedure On the twenty-first, after the third treatment, when blowing his nose, the patient heard a sound in his ears and had a feeling like the ear drum was swollen, and immediately he could hear the talk in the room. On the twenty-third, the nose was opened and the hearing increased, so Upper-Yingxiang (Extra) and Shangxing (Du 23) were no longer used but Yifeng (SJ 17) was added, and the technique was the same as before. After thirty-one treatments, both the hearing and constitution recovered and the treatment ceased. On July 30, 1983 and January 20, 1984, he had a follow-up examination and everything was fine.

Case 4: Sudden loss of vision (retinal hemorrhage)

Name, Zhong x x; sex, male; age, 40; date of the first visit, November 18, 1953.

Complaints From 1944, the patient lost vision alternately in both eyes for nine years. The diagnosis was retinal hemorrhage. Various treatments were administered, but there was no remarkable improvement. He had blurred vision, emaciated and weak constitution, dizziness and shortness of breath, inability of walking, and cold sensation in the back and lumbar region. He had a history of rheumatic arthritis and gastric ulcer. There were also symptoms of arthralgia in the lower limbs, stomachache and gastric distress with food. Examination: thready and forceless pulse, beating sixty times per minute, blood pressure 100/60 mmHg, and emaciation. The blood test revealed erythrocyte 4,900,000, leukocyte 6,800, and thrombocyte 75,000. In fundus oculi, there was hyperplasia of connective tissues in the right eye and old hemorrhage in the left which had not been absorbed. The visual acuity was 0.8 of the right eye and 0.02 of the left. Differentiation: Yin deficiency in the liver and kidney. The principle of treatment: Regulate the liver and reinforce the kidney, and replenish the blood to brighten the eyes.

Prescription Dazhui (Du 14), Fengchi (G 20), Ganshu (B 18), and Shenshu (B 23) were recommended and the technique of "setting mountain on fire" was employed. Treatment procedure: After the eighteenth treatment, the patient felt eyes clearer and the cold feeling in the back, lumbar region and lower limbs diminished. Then Fengchi (G 20), Luxi (SJ 19) and Jiaosun (SJ 20) were punctured with the technique of "setting mountain on fire" and Zhongwan (Ren 12), Tianshu (S 25), Qihai (Ren 6) and Zusanli (S 36) were manipulated with even needling technique. In four months, fifty treatments were performed. The patient felt all the symptoms disappear, gastric ulcer and rheumatic arthritis cured, vision regained and health recovered. The examination of fundus oculi found the old hemorrhage absorbed and connective tissues reduced. The visual acuity was 1.0 of the right eye and 0.5 of the left one. There was 141,000 blood platelet. He gained 2.5 kilograms. Fengchi (G 20) and Jiaosun (SJ 20) were punctured continuously with the same technique and Inner-Jingming (Extra) was needled with the technique of "pressing the needle for slow insertion." Up to May 18, 1954, the patient had seventy treatments, his physical strength was restored and he put on five kilograms. In order to further observe the effect the patient was punctured once or twice a week as before. Twenty-eight more treatments were provided until November 1. The thrombocyte increased to 280,000. The visual acuity was still 1.0 of the right eye and 0.5 of the left eye. The patient resumed his work.

Explanation Generally Ganshu (B 18) and Shenshu (B 23) are selected and the technique of "setting mountain on fire" is employed in order to reinforce the liver and kidney and to replenish blood for brightening eyes. But when there is blood stasis in fundus oculi with severe blurring of vision, Fengchi (G 20) and Jiaosun (SJ 20) should be prescribed and hot sensation should be conducted inside eyes to facilitate the absorption of the stasis. Dazhui (Du 14), Geshu (B 17) and Ganshu (B 18) can be reinforced for thrombocytopenia since the constitution is strengthened and blood is nourished automatically. A hundred and eighteen cases with 188 affected eyes were treated and 50 eyes have been cured, 43 eyes markedly effective, 74 eyes improved, and 21 failed. The total effect rate was 88.83 percent. According to the result of treatment, the recurrence is high within less than twenty treatments. The majority of patients need the treatment more than 6 months, thus the therapeutic effect can be consolidated.

Case 5: Tuberculosis of sacro-iliac joint

Name, Guo x x; sex, female; age, 28; date of the first visit; November 4, 1953.

Complaints From November of 1950, the patient started to have painful swelling on the back and lumbar region and leg pain which was aggravated gradually. In 1951, she had an operation in a local hospital in Beijing for hysteromyomectomy and was hospitalized for twenty-eight days. On April 16, and May 5, 1952, she had abstraction of pus in the lumbar-sacral region in a hospital in Beijing. Her condition was getting worse, painful swelling on the lumbar-sacral region leading to the swelling on the back and the legs, pain of wrists, knees and joints of feet. Her spinal column was not able to curve laterally, and she could not sit, stand and turn her body over, lying motionless in bed for eighteen months. Menstrual period 3-5/24, and there was profuse leukarrhea. On May 19, 1951, the first X-ray film revealed osteoporsis is the lower part of bilateral sacro-iliac joints, arthrectasia, destruction of bone, which is worse on the right side, round and fairly dense shadow from the top of pelvic cavity down to the lower border of the fourth lumbar vertebra, looking like a tumour or dialated uterus, calcification shadow in the lower abdominal cavity and pelvic cavity. On April 10, 1952, the second film in A-P position revealed remarkable arthrectasia of the right sacro-iliac joint, notable destruction of the joint bone, a sharp border of the iliac bone, disappearance of the shadow in pelvic cavity, bilateral hip joint normal and destruction of bone not found in the fifth lumbar vertebra. Tuberculous focus in the right sacro-iliac joint was deteriorating more remarkably than before, and the left was looking abnormal. On May 23, 1953, the third and the fourth anterioposterior and lateral films revealed no destruction and hyperplasia of lumbar vertebrae, interspinal space not narrowing, the image of psoas muscle clear and no bulge visible, and the tuberculosis of the right sacro-iliac joint with no apparent change comparing that on April 10, 1952. Examination: The needle mark left by the abstraction of pus on the right sacro-iliac joint, bulge of soft tissues from the lumbosacral region up the back which was hard and tender on palpation, waist not able to bend, swelling on the lateral aspect of legs, the right one worse, excessive red-thread-like vessels, and appearance of stagnation of lymphocinesia. The patient could not sit and turn over her body, and her activities were limited. There were flushed face, thin and white tongue coating and thready pulse beating eighty-two times per minute. The diagnosis of Western medicine was tuberculosis of sacro-iliac joint, and TCM differentiation held that it was due to the deficiency of body resistance and the excess of pathogenic factors, decayed essence and blood, and flowing of turbid phlegm which accumulated in the lumbar and hip region. The treatment stressed trengthening the body resistance to expel the pathogenic factors, eliminating the phlegm and reducing the accumulation, and invigorating the flow of meridians to facilitate the circulation of blood.

Prescription Fengmen (B 12), Dazhui (Du 14), Pangguangshu (B 28) and Yaoyangguan (D 43) were punctured with even needling technique, and Shenshu (B 23) and Guanyuanshu (B 26) were manipulated with "fire-entering-reinforcing" technique. Needles were not retained.

Treatment procedure Treat twice a week. On February 4, 1954, the fifth and the sixth films in anterioposterior and lateral position revealed that after the two abstractions of pus the condition was the same as that in the film taken a year before, no pathological change occurred from the first to the fifth lumbar vertebrae. Up to March 14, 1954, the patient had thirty treatments, the pain and swelling were diminishing. She could get up and sit down. After two months (sixteen sessions), the swelling and pain on the back, the lumbar region and legs basically disappeared, and there was no obvious tenderness. But there was a fibrous hard nodule at the sacro-iliac joint (probably the scar resulted from the absorption of pus). At this time, the patient could get on and off the trolley bus with the assistance of a stick and could walk freely. In order to observe the change of disease, she continued to have reexamination and puncturing once for one or two weeks. Until March 20, 1955, the swelling and tenderness completely disappeared. The seventh film of A-P position for the right sacro-iliac joint showed that after two abstractions of pus from the tubercle, the joint cavity was broadened, the border of the joint cavity was sharp and well defined, and the left sacro-iliac joint was clear. On August 11, 1955, the reexamination found the condition was good. An X-ray film A-P position for the sacro-iliac joint showed bilateral tuberculous sacro-iliac arthritis which is spasticity-like is cured. The treatment stopped therefore. A follow-up examination was made one year after and no recurrence was found.

Explanation Tuberculosis of sacro-iliac joint falls into aspect of "bone and joint tuberculosis" in traditional Chinese medicine. Lying in bed for a long time made the patient weak and debilitated and the essence and blood became insufficient. Shenshu (B 23), and Guanyuanshu (B 26) with "fire-entering-reinforcing" technique can tonify the kidney to replenish essence and blood, thus body resistance is strengthened and the pathogenic factors are driven out, phlegm and stagnation resolved and the flow of qi and blood in meridians invigorated. The disease can be alleviated or even cured.

Case 6: Paralysis of ulnar nerve

Name, Shan x x; sex, male; age, 7; date of the first visit, July 21, 1964.

Complaints The boy suffered from toxic dysentery, associated with coma on May 18, 1964. He was hospitalized and treated with hibernation therapy, and fluid infusion continuously for three days. After the condition improved, it was found that there was motoring impairment, bradyesthesia and lowered skin temperature of the ring and little fingers of the right hand. He had physiotherapy for two months but with no marked effect. The examination found abducent flexion of the middle and ungual phalanges of the right hand, hypodynamic flexion, extension, adduction and abduction of the two fingers and forceless adduction and flexion of the right thumb not able to hold chopsticks. Thenar and hypothenar eminences were remarkably atrophic. Analgesia, apselaphesia, and thermoanesthesia were found on the ulnar side of the little and ring fingers. The skin temperature of the right little finger was 4.24°C lower than that of the left one and the right ring finger was 1°C lower than the left. The other three fingers were basically the same with those of the left hand. The tongue coating was thin and white and pulse thready. The diagnosis of modern medicine was paralysis of the ulnar nerve. Differentiation: High fever consumed qi and blood and injured the meridians and collaterals, resulting in deficiency of qi and blood and malnutrition of meridians, tendons and muscles. The treating principle was to regulate the flow of qi for facilitating the circulation of blood and to warm and open the meridians and collaterals.

Prescription Naohui (SJ 13), Xiaohai (SI 8), Quchi (LI 11), Waiguan (SJ 5), Wangu (SI 4), Houxi (SI 3), Zhongzhu (SJ 3), Shenmen (H 7), Yemen (SJ 2) and Hegu (LI 4) of the affected side were selected.

Treatment procedure All the points were punctured in the order from up to down

(Relaying the qi to open the meridians) with the hot-reinforcing method and the warm sensation propagating down to the fingers. The puncturing was given once every four days. After the treatment, the motor and sensory abilities were restored and the muscular atrophy improved. After six treatments, the amplitude of motor activity of the right ring and little fingers increased extension more obvious, and the extent of anesthesia lessened markedly. After one month of treatment, the extent of motor ability was further increased and the grip was notably improved and the boy could hold chopsticks to eat. The atrophy of thenar and hypothenar eminences also improved. The extent of analgesia was further reduced and the sense of touch was fully recovered. When the right little finger was needled or touched, a strong tingling sensation could be induced. After two months, the motor ability of the right hand was basically restored and it had no remarkable difference with the healthy side. The algesia also basically recovered, but was still duller than the normal places. From mid-October, the treatment was changed once a week to consolidate the effect. Until mid-November the treatment was stopped and everything restored to normal except slight hypoalgesia of the ungual portion of the right finger. Re-examination on January 29, 1965 found everything well.

Explanation Selection of Naohui (SJ 13), and Xiaohai (SI 8) with the hot-reinforcing technique and "relaying qi method" can conduct the warm or hot sensation down to the affected fingers, to warm and open the meridians and collaterals to improve or even restore the paralyzed and atrophic hand. The skin temperature recovered slowly, but not stably. At the beginning of the treatment, it was summer, and the temperature was fairly high, but the skin temperature of the right little finger was apparently lower than that of the healthy hand. Later on in the treatment, the weather was getting cold and the indoor temperature was 20°C. When the patient entered the room, the skin temperature was different on each side, but after rest for a period of time, the temperature was similar on both sides. This is evidence that acupuncture can also raise skin temperature.

HEAT-REINFORCING AND COLD-REDUCING AND THE EIGHT NEEDLING METHODS

—Dr. Zheng Yulin's Clinical Experience

Dr. Zheng Yulin (1896-1967) was from Beilou Village, Anguo County of Hebei Province. From his boyhood, he began to learn medicine and acupuncture from his uncle. As a disciple, he learned medicine from Dr. Cao Shunde and later from Dr. Huo Laoshun who was very good at acupuncture and qigong. In 1953, together with his eldest son, he opened an acupuncture clinic in Beijing. He was invited as an acupuncturist by the North China Research Institute in 1954. From October of that year until his death, he was the director of the third research division of the Acupuncture Institute, China Academy of the Traditional Chinese Medicine. Many famous doctors, such as Zheng Kuishan, Li Zhiming, Shang Guyu, Wang Deshen, Wu Xijing, Yang Renping, Wei Mingfeng, Jin Renqi, took him as their teacher. With their help, Dr. Zheng had more than ten papers published, such as *The Observation of the Therapeutic Effect on Treating the Retinal Vitreous Hemorrhage*, which was given an award in 1958 by the Ministry of Public Health and *The Summary of Therapeutic Effect on 102 Cases of Bi-Syndrome Treated by the Heat-Reinforcing and Cold-Reducing Method.*

I. Academic Characteristics and Medical Specialities

Dr. Zheng paid great attention to the manipulations of the heat-reinforcing and cold-reducing. On the basis of the ancients' experience, he put forward the "Eight Needling Methods." In needling, he emphasized the use of the left hand and advocated the coordination of both hands. He thought that the arrival of qi and qi reaching the diseased area were the key points to raise the therapeutic effect. He also advocated the combination of qigong and acupuncture and the selection of points according to the symptoms. He insisted that the principle of selecting the points should be smaller quantity, but better quality. The therapeutic effect on the treatment of windstroke, epigastric pain, asthma, uterine bleeding and infantile food retention was satisfactory. He developed special treatments of eye diseases.

1. Stressing the manipulations of heat-reinforcing and cold-reducing

According to the statement in *Plain Questions* that "needle withdrawal should be suspended in treating excess symptoms in order to bring about the conditions of deficiency, and the needle should be removed when the yin qi has arrived on a large scale; on the other hand, the needle should not be withdrawn until yang qi has arrived on a large scale and heat sensations are felt under the tip of the needle in order to bring about the conditions of excess," Dr. Zheng thought that the key point of acupuncture treatment was to find out whether the disease belonged to excess or to deficiency and then the reinforcing and reducing methods could be used respectively. In practice, he summarized a simplified method of heat-reinforcing and cold-reducing.

1) *Heat-reinforcing method* Press the point tightly with the left index finger and quickly insert the needle or twirl and rotate the needle into the point with the right hand from shallow to deep. Lift slowly and press heavily to promote the arrival of qi. Under the basis of the soreness and distention, insert the needle downward 0.1 to 0.2 cun, then twirl and rotate the needle with the thumb moving forward 3 to 5 times or 9 times, then there will be a heat-distention. If such a sensation fails to appear, use the same procedure once again two to three times. Most of the patients will feel the heat-distention. After the needle is withdrawn, knead and press the point. In the process of the needling, if the patient's sensation is dull, he can be ordered to inhale with his nose and to exhale with the mouth five to six times. Besides, the needle-scraping method can also be added, in which the needle handle is scraped downward with the thumb for one minute. Usually the heat sensation may be achieved. This method is applicable to deficiency and cold syndromes of zang-fu organs and meridians.

2) *Cold-reducing method* Press the point tightly with the left index finger and quickly insert or twirl and rotate the needle into the point with the right hand, first shallow, and then deep. Make the arrival of qi with heavy lifting and slow pressing. On the basis of a numbness and distension, lift the needle upwards 0.1 to 0.2 cun, and then twirl and rotate the needle with the thumb moving backward 2 to 3 times or 6 times, then there will appear a cold-numbness sensation. If such a sensation is not found, repeat the procedure two to three times. Most of the patients will have the cold numbness sensation. There is no need to knead and press the point after the needle is withdrawn. For the patient with a dull sensation, he should be ordered to inhale with the mouth and to exhale with the nose five to six times. Meanwhile, the needle-scraping method can also be added, that is, scrape the needle handle upward for one minute. This method is applicable to the excess and heat syndromes of the zang-fu organs and meridians.

2. The Application of the "Eight Needling Methods"

Of the reinforcing and reducing methods recorded in *Compendium of Acupuncture and Moxibustion,* many were named after the images of the animals, such as "the green dragon swaying the tail, the turtle exploring the cave, the white tiger shaking the head, fighting between the dragon and the tiger," and so on. Dr. Zheng had summarized eight needling methods of reinforcing and reducing, namely, two dragons playing with a pearl, the magpie climbing the plum trees, the old mule turning a mill, fishing with a gold hook, the white snake stretching out the forked tongue, the monster boa turning over the body, the golden rooster pecking at the rice and the mouse-paw needling.

1) *Two dragons playing with a pearl* When this manipulation is used, the needling sensation should be propagated along two routes, aiming at surrounding the eyeball. For example, when Taiyang (Extra 2) point is needled, press the point tightly with the left

index finger and insert or twirl the needle quickly into the point. After the needle reaches a certain depth and the qi arrives, lift and thrust or twirl and rotate the needle to make the needle tip direct to the upper eyelid and make the heat-distension or cold-distension transmit to the upper eyelid and further to the internal canthus. Then lift and thrust or twirl and rotate the needle to make the needle tip direct to the lower eyelid and make the heat distension or cold-distension transmit to the lower eyelid and further to the internal canthus, surrounding the eyeball. With this method Taiyang (Extra 2) can be needled to treat different kind of eye diseases. For the deficiency cases, the heat-reinforcing method is used, while for the excess cases, the cold-reducing method is applied.

2) *The magpie climbing the plum trees* The pushing manipulation is often used. For example, when Zanzhu (B 2) point is needled, press the point tightly with the right index finger and insert or twirl the needle into the point quickly. After the arrival of qi, hold the needle handle with the right thumb and push the needle body with the middle finger in order to keep the needle handle, needle body and needle tip sway up and down. For the reinforcing method, sway nine times and for the reducing, sway six times to make the heat distension or cold-distension travel continuously into the eyes. With this method, eye diseases can be treated by needling Zanzhu (B 2), Yuyao (Extra 5) and Sizhukong (SJ 23) points. Tinnitus and deafness are treated by needling Ermen (SJ 21), and toothache by needling Xiaguan (S 7). For the deficiency cases, heat-reinforcing method is used and for the excess cases the cold-reducing method is applied.

3) *The old mule turning the mill* When the needling is performed, the manipulation of "turning the millstone" is used. For example, when Touwei (S 8) is needled, press tightly the point with the left index finger, insert or twirl the needle into the point quickly. After qi arrives, lift the needle up to the subcutaneous region, turn the needle body like turning a millstone continuously for some time. For heat-reinforcing, turn the needle nine times at the small angle, while for cold-reducing, turn the needle six times at the large angle. With this method, Touwei (S 8) can be needled to treat headache, Qimen (Liv 14) is needled to treat the stagnation of the liver qi, Zhangmen (Liv 13) to treat masses in the abdomen. For the deficiency cases, the heat-reinforcing method is used and for the excess cases, the cold-reducing method is applied.

4) *Fishing with a gold hook* When the needling is performed, the manipulation of small-amplitude picking-up and shaking is used. For example, when Tanzhong (Ren 17) is needled after the arrival of qi, twirl and rotate the needle with the right thumb, index and middle fingers moving forward, then sticking the needle is achieved. This is very much like a swimming fish biting the bait. Hold the needle handle with the right hand and then pick up and shake the skin with the stuck needle slightly several times. For the reinforcing method, pick up the skin nine times and for the reducing method, pick up the skin six times. With this method, Yangbai (G 14), Jiache (S 6) and Taiyang (Extra 2) are needled to treat the deviation of the mouth and eyes; Tanzhong (Ren 17) and Zhongting (Ren 6) to treat the depression of liver and stagnation of the qi and obstruction of qi in the chest.

5) *The white snake stretching out the forked tongue* Two needles are inserted in line into the point, which is very much like the forked tongue of a snake. For example,

when Quchi (LI 11) is needled, press the point tightly with the left index finger and two needles held by the right hand are twirled into the point. After qi arrives, lifting and thrusting are performed. The two needles should be lifted or thrust at the same time. For the reinforcing, slow lifting and heavy thrusting should be done nine times, and the reducing, heavy lifting and slow thrusting six times. This method can be used to treat such diseases as hemiplegia, Bi-syndrome, and numbness of the four extremities. Jianyu (LI 15), Quchi (LI 11), Yanglingquan (G 34), Zusanli (S 36), Dazhui (Du 14), Pishu (B 20), Shenshu (B 23), Guanyuan (Ren 4) are needled. For the deficiency cases, the reinforcing method is used, while for the excess cases, the reducing method is applied.

6) *The monster boa turning over the body* In needling, the turning method is used. For example, when Ganshu (B 18) is needled, press the point tightly with the left index finger and quickly insert or twirl the needle into the point. After qi arrives, there appears numbness and distension. Turn the needle handle from below to above with the right thumb, middle and index fingers in order to rotate the needle body in a semi-circle, and turn the needle from left to right like a boa turning over its body. The cold-reducing method is used. Usually Ganshu (B 18) and Weishu (B 21) are needled to treat imbalance between the liver and the stomach.

7) *The golden rooster pecking at the rice* In needling, the method of small lifting and thrusting is performed. For example, when Quchi (LI 11) is needled, press the point tightly with the left index finger, insert or twirl the needle quickly into the point with the right hand. In order to promote rapid arrival of qi, the method of small lifting and thrusting is used to seek the needling sensation like a rooster pecking the rice. With this method, Quchi (LI 11), Hegu (LI 4), Zusanli (S 36), and Yanglingquan (G 34) can be needled to treat infantile paralysis, and Zhongwan (Ren 12), Guanyuan (Ren 4) and Qihai (Ren 6) are needled to treat incontinence of urine in children.

8) *The mouse-paw needling* After this method is used, there will be traces on the skin which are like the paw of a mouse. In needling, 3, 5, or 7 commonly used filiform needles which are either 1 or 1.5 cun long are used. The needles can be tied together or held by the right thumb, middle, and index fingers for pricking or for direct needling on the points or on the diseased area. After the needling, there will appear five or seven needling marks on the skin which are like the traces of a mouse's paw. This method is often used to treat children's diseases, such as retention of food, infantile dyspepsia and malnutrition. The points of Dazhui (Du 14), Ganshu (B 18), Pishu (B 20), Weishu (B 21), Zhongwan (Ren 12), Zusanli (S 36), Sanyinjiao (Sp 6) are often needled.

3. The combination of qigong and acupuncture

The key point of qigong is to regulate the heart and guard the mind so as to strengthen the real qi, while the key point of acupuncture is the concentration of mind. The operator should concentrate his mind on a definite part of the body and stimulate and arouse the body's antidisease function and regulate yin and yang with the Dantian qi. A qigong master can treat diseases by releasing the external qi to supplement the insufficient qi of the patient or to adjust the disturbed qi of the patient in order to balance the disturbed body and to treat the diseases. The effect of acupuncture on the Shu point is to adjust the balance of yin-yang of the zang-fu organs and meridians through the regulating function of the meridians (the meridian qi) so as to treat and prevent diseases. Many acupuncturists have experienced that the combined use of qigong and acupuncture can not only producc analgesia in inserting the needle and make it easier to observe the needling sensation, but also make it easier to obtain the needling sensation and make the qi easily reach the diseased area. The therapeutic effect is much better than that of pure needling. Dr. Zheng attached great importance to the combination of qigong and acupuncture. He insisted that practising qigong was one of the basic skills of an acupuncturist. He emphasized that an acupuncturist must practise the three passes, i.e. the shoulder, the elbow and the wrist, in order to ensure the passing of the qi. According to his experience of many years, he considered that the main point of the needling manipulation was the will-control. In clinical needling, he aroused the Dantian qi from his chest to the fingers through the shoulder, elbow and wrist and from the fingers to the body of the patient through the needle. This is the internal qi of the operator. By releasing the external qi, the dual purpose of qigong and acupuncture can be brought into play, which can mobilize the homeostasis of the patient's body. Therefore the therapeutic effect is often quick and satisfactory.

II. Case Analysis

Case 1: Optic atrophy

Name, Zhang x x; sex, male; age, 40; date of the first visit, March 16, 1958.

Complaints The patient began to have diminished vision ten years before. It was progressive and diagnosed later as optic neuritis and optic atrophy in a hospital. He was treated with both Chinese and Western medicines, but the effect was not satisfactory. Examination: Blurred vision, eyes easily tired, accompanied with headache, pain on the eyes, poor sleep, normal appetite, normal defecation and urination, clear mind, sallow complexion. Vision: right, 0.3, and left, 0.4, light yellow of the temporal side of both optic papillas in fundus examination, clear margin, normal physiological excavation and the blood vessels of the retina, central scotoma on visual field examination, white coating with greasy root of the tongue, retarded pulse and weak at "chi" region. Differentiation: Insufficient essence and blood in the liver and kidney leading to lack of nourishment of the eyes. The treatment is to nourish the liver and kidney and promote blood circulation to improve the eyesight.

Prescription Fengchi (G 20), Qubin (G 7), Tongziliao (G 1), Zanzhu (B 2), Ganshu (B 18) and Shenshu (B 23).

Treatment procedure The heat-reinforcing method was used. When Fengchi (G 20) was needled, the heat distension must be transmitted to the eye area. When Taiyang (Extra 2) was needled, the method of two dragons playing with a pearl was applied, to make the heat distension propagate along the upper and lower eyelids. After fourteen treatments, the eyesight was improved to 0.6 of the right and 0.5 of the left. Fifty-six treatments in all were given and the vision was restored to 0.9 of the right and 0.8 of the left. Both the fundus and visual field examinations showed no abnormal findings.

Explanation In traditional Chinese medicine, optic atrophy falls within the blurred vision which is caused mainly by both liver and kidney deficiency and insufficiency of qi and blood. Usually the therapeutic effect is not good with treatment using Western and Chinese medicine. However, after treating this disease with acupuncture, the effect is satisfactory. Fengchi (G 20), a point of the Gallbladder Meridian, is a crossing point of the Hand and Foot Shaoyang and Yangwei Meridians. As it is a very important point in treating eye diseases, it is selected as the main point. The method of heat-reinforcing was used to keep the heat distension transmitting to the eye region. Combined with other related points, satisfactory results are often achieved.

Case 2: Blindness

Name, Peng x x; sex, male; age, 27; date of the first visit, July 28, 1958.

Complaints The patient began to suffer from blurred vision four months before and the symptoms became worse gradually until his right eye became blind. He visited many hospitals, but the result was not good. He was diagnosed as having bleeding of the eyeground, retinal periphlebitis of the right eye. At the time when he visited the doctor, the symptoms were "blind right eye," distension, blurred vision of the left eye, deviation and deformity, normal sleep, appetite, bowel movement and urination. Examination: Listlessness, emaciation, right conjuctive congestion, right vitreous cloudiness and hemorrhage with large purple-brown floating substance, turbid fundus, the left vitreous slight cloudiness, blurred optic papilla in red, choroid atrophic arc on the lower margin. Vision: Right 0.01 and left 0.1, blood pressure 120/100 mmHg, thin white tongue coating, pale red tongue proper, deep and string-taut pulse. Differentiation: Yin deficiency of the liver and kidney, flaring-up of the deficiency fire leading to extravasation of the blood. The treatment should nourish the liver and kidney, cool the blood, promote the blood circulation and improve the vision.

Prescription Fengchi (G 20), Taiyang (Extra 2), Qubin (G 7), Zanzhu (B 2), Ganshu (B 18), Shenshu (B 23) and Neijingming (Extra).

Treatment procedure The heat-reinforcing method was used with retention of the needle for a few minutes. Treat once every other day. After the needling, the patient should have a heat sensation existing in the eyes for one or two hours. If it was too hot, Dazhui (Du 14) could be needled with the cold-reducing method. Ganshu (B 18) and Shenshu (B 23) were needled once a week with the heat-reinforcing method. After nine treatments, the vision was improved to 0.2 of the right and 1.2 of the left and the distension of the eyes disappeared. With the same prescription, the patient was treated 225 times. The interval between the courses was five to seven days. The vision further improved to 0.6 on the right and 1.5 on the left. Scars were found on the fundus and no bleeding was found for over one year.

Explanation For the vitreous opacity including the fundus hemorrhage in Western medicine, Fengchi (G 20), Taiyang (Extra 2), Zanzhu (B 2), Qubin (G 7) were needled with the heat reinforcing method according to the theory treating the acute symptoms first in an emergency case. The hot sensation was felt in the eyes for one or two hours to reduce the fire and stop the bleeding. However, if the hot sensation in the eyes was too strong, the cold-reducing method was used by needling Dazhui (Du 14) to lower the temperature, Ganshu (B 18) and Shenshu (B 23) were needled with the heat-reinforcing method in order to treat the root cause. Thus both the symptoms and the root cause were treated and the disease was cured.

Case 3: Epigastric pain (duodenal ulcer)

Name, Zuo x x; sex, female; age, 25; date of the first visit, September 8, 1955.

Complaints The patient began to have stomachache nine years before for an unknown reason. The disease was accompanied with nausea and acid regurgitation, which attacked repeatedly, especially in winter. She was treated by Western and Chinese medicine, but the result was poor. When she visited the doctor in this hospital, the symptoms were epigastric pain, which attacked two or three hours after a meal, severe pain, nausea and vomiting of acid water, pain worse on exertion or by irritability, accompanied by headache and vertigo, and brown stool. Examination: Sallow complexion, emaciation, body weight 45 kg liver and spleen, (-), obvious tenderness around Zhangmen (Liv 13) and Zhongwan (Ren 12) points. The feces examination: Green-brown stool, occult blood (++). She was diagnosed as having a duodenal bulbar ulcer by the barium X-ray. Differentiation: Depression of the liver and stagnation of qi and blood, insufficiency of the spleen and stomach qi. The treatment should soothe the liver and regulate the qi, remove the blood stasis and stop the pain, strengthen the spleen and replenish the qi.

Prescription Shangwan (Ren 13), Zhongwan (Ren 12), Zhangmen (Liv 13), Qihai (Ren 6), Neiguan (P 6), Zusanli (S 36), Gongsun (Sp 4), Neiting (S 44), Weishu (B 21), Pishu (B 20), Quchi (LI 11), Hegu (LI 4) and Xuehai (Sp 10).

Treatment procedure In each treatment, one or two points on the abdomen or on the upper or lower limbs were selected with the even reinforcing and even reducing method. The needling sensation was transmitted upward to the stomach region. Pishu (B 20) and Weishu (B 21) were needled with the heat-reinforcing method and the heat distension travelled to the stomach region. After three treatments, all the symptoms were basically attenuated, and after the sixth treatment, the epigastric pain diminished and the appetite improved greatly. After twenty-two treatments in two months, all the symptoms disappeared. Occult blood examination: (-). The total acidity and the free acidity were found normal by the gastric juice analysis. The barium meal films showed the bulbar ulcer had become less apparent and almost cured. It was reported several months later that the condition of the patient remained stable.

Explanation Epigastric pain is in most cases caused by the stagnation of liver qi, invasion of the stomach by deficiency cold and retention of the blood stasis. There are different kinds of methods of treatment. This case lasted for nine years and was treated many times by both the Western and Chinese medicine, but the conditions became aggravated. Dr. Zheng, according to the differentiation, thought that this disease was due to the stagnation of liver qi, retention of blood stasis and insufficiency of the spleen and stomach qi. This disease should be treated with the cold-reducing method. However, Dr. Zheng treated it with the even reinforcing and even reducing method for fear that the reducing method would injure the spleen qi because of the delicate constitution. At the same time the heat-reinforcing method was used.

Case 4: Uterine bleeding (functional uterine bleeding)

Name, Peng x x; sex, female; age, 30; date of the first visit, May 3, 1961.

Complaints The patient had been suffering from profuse and prolonged menstruation for eighteen years. She was diagnosed in hospital as having anovulatory menstruation, and was treated with Western and Chinese medicine, but with no effect. She had a menstruation every half a month and the amount was as much as urination. The colour of the blood was dark purple. There was abdominal distension, but without pain. Sometimes the menstruation could last for half a month. She also had palpitation, short breath, poor appetite, soreness and weakness of the leg and the lower back. She had not been pregnant since her marriage twelve years before. Her husband was healthy. Examination: Middle-leveled development and nutrition, sallow complexion, the white of the eye was green, pale lips, glossy tongue proper, peeling tongue coating, string-taut and thready pulse. The blood routine examination: Hematochrome, 6 to 8 g, RBC, $2800000/mm^3$. Differentiation: Deficiency of qi and blood, and failure of the spleen to control the blood. The treatment should strengthen the spleen, support the restraining, and regulate and reinforce the liver and kidney.

Prescription Pishu (B 20), Weishu (B 21), Ganshu (B 18) and Shenshu (B 23).

Treatment procedure The heat-reinforcing method was used every other day. After ten treatments, the mental condition became better, the appetite improved, the amount of menstruation was less than before, and the period lasted for ten days. Then the patient was treated with the same prescription, and warm-hot sensation was required after the needling. Twenty-five treatments in all were given and the amount of menstrual flow became normal and the period lasted only four days. The interval between the menstruations became thirty days. In order to consolidate the therapeutic effect, the patient was ordered to receive one treatment every week continously for the weeks. Clinically the patient was cured.

Explanation This disease is common in women. It is either due to deficiency of qi and blood and failure of the spleen to control the blood, or due to the insufficiency of the liver and kidney and retention of blood stasis. Usually, acupuncture treatment can obtain satisfactory therapeutic effect. For this case, the duration was long with deficiency of both qi and blood. According to the principle of treating the root cause in case of chronic case and the warm reinforcing may keep qi and blood return, Dr. Zheng selected Pishu (B 20), Ganshu (B 18), Weishu (B 21) and Shenshu (B 23) points with the heat-reinforcing method. The purpose was to invigorate qi and blood and to cure the disease.

Case 5: Asthma (Bronchial asthma)

Name, Fang x x; sex, male; age, 33; date of the first visit, October 23, 1958.

Complaints The patient had suffered from cough and asthma complicated with a wheezing sound in the throat and scanty white sputum since he was five years old. The attacks became more frequent in winter and were often induced by a cold. He had visited several hospitals and was diagnosed as having bronchial asthma. He had been treated with many kinds of drugs such as aminophylline, ephedrine, accessary adrenaline, and dexamethasone. After administration, the symptoms were controlled, and a few days were needed to relieve the symptoms. In recent days, the attacks became more frequent and the case became more severe, so he came to our hospital for treatment. The symptoms were asthma with wheezing sound in the throat, coughing with scanty white sputum, chest distress, dyspnea, and poor appetite. Examination: Clear mind, slightly red pharynx, scattered dry rales heard in the lungs, the heart, (-) glossy tongue without coating, string-taut and rapid pulse. The chest X-ray showed slightly thicker lung markings. Differentiation: Attack of the lung by wind-cold leading to failure of lung qi in dispersion. The treatment should strengthen the body resistance and the dispersing function of the lung, dispel the cold, resolve the phlegm and relieve asthma.

Prescription Dazhui (Du 14), Taodao (Du 13), Fengmen (B 12), Feishu (B 13), Pishu (B 20), Shenshu (B 23), Tiantu (Ren 22), and Tanzhong (Ren 17).

Treatment procedure When Dazhui (Du 14) and Taodao (Du 13) were needled, the even reinforcing and even reducing method was used. Fengmen (B 12), Feishu (B 13), Pishu (B 20) and Shenshu (B 23) were needled with the heat-reinforcing method. Three moxa-cones were applied with ginger at Tiantu (Ren 22), and five moxa-cones at Tanzhong (Ren 17). Immediately after the acupuncture and moxibustion, the patient felt better and the asthma was relieved. On his second visit, two more treatments were given and asthma was further alleviated and the patient could lie on his back. On the third visit, the patient told the doctor that his cough and asthma had become obviously lessened, only serious at night. The patient was still treated with the above-mentioned prescription. On his fourth visit, the moxibustion was removed, in addition to the above-mentioned points, Youmen (K 21) and Zhongwan (Ren 12) were added with the even reinforcing and even reducing method, and Qihai (Ren 6) was needled with the heat-reinforcing method. After the needling, his asthma became relieved gradually, the rales in the lungs disappeared, but there was still slight coughing at night. Then the treatment was given once every two or three days to consolidate the therapeutic effect. Altogether ten treatments were given and his asthma was completely cured clinically. The follow-up visit for two years showed that no big attacks were reported except for mild attacks once in a while when the weather changed greatly.

Explanation Asthma is a disease which is often caused by delicate constitution, attacked by the wind-cold and retention of phlegm-dampness. For a long time the disease will injure the kidney, then the disease will become difficult to cure. Dr. Zheng stressed that both the symptoms and the root cause should be treated at the same time, and strengthening the body resistance and eliminating the pathogenic factors should be taken into account. Fengmen (B 21) and Feishu (B 13) were needled with the heat-reinforcing method to strengthen the dispersing function of the lung, dispel the cold and relieve asthma; Zhongwan (Ren 12) and Fenglong (S 40) were needled to resolve sputum and stop coughing, both acupuncture and moxibustion applied at Tiantu (Ren 22) and Tanzhong (Ren 17) may resolve the sputum and stop the asthma. Needling Shenshu (B 23) and Qihai (Ren 6) with the heat-reinforcing method can nourish the kidney to treat the root cause. When all these points are used together, the functions of strengthening, dispersing and dispelling the cold, regulating the flow of qi and resolving the phlegm can be performed, so the asthma can be cured.

ACUPUNCTURE WITH MASSAGE TO INDUCE QI FLOW AND KILL PAIN

—Zhao Yuqing's Clinical Experience

Zhao Yuqing, a native of Daixian County of Shanxi Province, was born on March 11, 1918. Zhao Ji'an, her father, was a renowned traditional practitioner in Shanxi and she learnt traditional Chinese medicine from him. Afterwards Huang Zhuzai, an established traditional practitioner in Shanxi Province, was her teacher. Between the late 1930s and early 1940s she was appointed as an acupuncturist by the Central Institute of Traditional Chinese Medicine. In 1947 she was appointed professor of the North-China Institute of Traditional Chinese Medicine, teaching acupuncture and traditional medical history. She was admitted to the school of extensive studies of Chinese medicine, run by the Ministry of Public Health in 1950. In 1951 she began to work at the Institute of Traditional Chinese Medicine, Central Academy of Traditional Chinese Medicine, researching on acupuncture and medical history. Later she was transferred to work at the Beijing Xiyuan Hospital, China Academy of Traditional Chinese Medicine. Her works include *Essentials of Acupuncture* and *Essentials of Acupuncture and Ten Manipulations of Massage*. Now she is a member of the Acupuncture Commission, All-China Association for Traditional Chinese Medicine, member of Medical History Society, Chinese Medical Association, member of the Editorial Board of the *Journal of Traditional Chinese Medicine*.

I. Academic Characteristics and Medical Specialities

1. Laying Stress on Yin-Yang and Adjusting Moods

1) *Regulating yin-yang* It is stated in *Internal Classic* that "the chief function of acupuncture is to regulate yin and yang, ... bringing yang from yin or bringing yin from yang. In excess condition, get rid of the excessive part; in insufficient condition, replenish more to them." Based on this statement Zhao is good at harmonizing yin and yang, qi and blood to reach a state of equilibrium. A woman patient named Gai aged fifty was treated by Zhao. The patient had suddenly lost consciousness because of rage. Other symptoms included cold limbs, pallor, locked jaw, deep pulse, manifesting abundant yin and declining yang, imbalance of yin and yang due to stagnation of qi and blood. Both Neiguan (P 6) and Sanyinjiao (Sp 6) were punctured with the reducing method, and Renzhong (Du 26) and Baihui (Du 20) were needled with the reinforcing method. The patient came to after acupuncture therapy. In another example a woman named Han had been barren seven years after her marriage and suffered from painful menstruation. There was no response to any treatment. On the first visit she was found to have a bluish complexion, dark brown lips, a pale tongue with a white coating, and deep, retarded

pulse. Zhao believed that her sterility was due to stagnation of qi, cold accumulation in the uterus, impeding the smooth flow of qi and blood and causing disharmony of yin and yang, qi and blood. Hence, Zhongji (Ren 3), Guanyuan (Ren 4) and both Huangshu (K 16) were selected first with the reducing method to dispel the excessive cold. Then moxibustion was applied to the above points and Shenque (Ren 8), Qihai (Ren 6) to tonify pure yang. After three treatments the painful menstruation was gone. Later she had a baby boy and her menstruation became normal.

2) *Laying stress on moods* Zhao thinks that the body and mind are closely connected. An abnormal state of feeling leads to disease due to lowered body resistance. For this reason it is important to treat the disease and the mind at the same time. It is stated in *Plain Questions* that "no response to treatment in a seriously ill patient who had lost his qi and blood should be attributed to his failure of spirit and mind. Acupuncture therapy only stimulates the flow of qi and blood, so moods of the patient are very important in achieving the curative effect. Low spirited patients cannot be expected to be cured." In treatment Zhao pays special attention to the moods of a patient, and uses persuasive words to adjust the patient's moods. When the patient is free from bad moods, the smooth flow of qi and blood is obtained, then she massages along the meridians and does acupuncture. By using this approach she has cured many cases. For instance, in the early 1950s a Ms. Hu had hysteria because of bad relationship with her husband, who left home without saying goodbye. Zhao found the patient was in low spirits and anxious. Zhao started the treatment with comforting words to make the patient feel at ease. Then she managed to find her husband and asked him to attend to his wife. Afterwards, she first punctured Renzhong (Du 26) and both Waiguan (P 6) to calm the mind, then both Fengchi (G 20) to remove pathogenic heat from the Gallbladder Meridian. Juque (Ren 14) and Zusanli (S 36) were used to regulate the function of the spleen and stomach. The even movement was applied. Two treatments completely cured the case.

2. Carrying Forward the Inherited Good Acupuncture Techniques

1) *Inducing the meridian qi by massage and acupuncture* Zhao believes that acupuncture and massage have close ties. Acupuncture, moxibustion and massage can be used separately or in combination. Pressing the point before acupuncture can not only fix the place to be needled but also reduce pain on insertion of the needle. Rubbing maneuver may promote the flow of qi and relieve strong stimulation. After withdrawal of the needle, rubbing maneuver helps to close the point and invigorate the flow of qi and blood. For example, when you needle Zhongwan (Ren 12), you may feel tenseness around the needle after the arrival of qi, meanwhile the patient may have a strong unbearable needling sensation. At this moment, the operator should press the point with his left ring finger and hold the needle tightly with his left thumb, index and middle fingers, and then massage Jianli (Ren 11), Xiawan (Ren 10), Shuifen (Ren 9), Qihai (Ren 6), Guanyuan (Ren 4) and Zhongji (Ren 3) to promote qi flow and relieve the tense feeling around the needle. If Quchi (LI 11) is needled and there appears too strong reaction, massage is applied to Lieque (L 7), Hegu (LI 4), Erjian (LI 2) and Sanjian (LI 3) which helps promote qi flow and relieve pain. The same manipulation is applied to

Shangjuxu (S 37), Xiajuxu (S 39), Jiexi (S 41) and Xingjian (Liv 2) to alleviate the tense feeling around the needle when Zusanli (S 36) is punctured. Mild massage is used and the needle should not be touched.

Zhao attaches great importance to massage. Finger acupuncture is often used in patients who are afraid of acupuncture. She knows by experience that combined massage is more helpful. For example, once an old lady suffering from diarrhoea for about a year was given acupuncture to Zhongwan (Ren 12), Guanyuan (Ren 4) and Tianshu (S 25). At first no needling sensation was felt. By giving a massage the needling sensation quickly appeared. First the reducing method and then the reinforcing method were applied. Meanwhile finger acupuncture was given to Ganshu (B 18), Pishu (B 20) and Weishu (B 21). Afterwards moxibustion was used. After three treatments the woman was completely cured. Zhao successfully treated a baby with the same approach. The baby had had a cold, sore throat and vomiting. Zhao gave finger acupuncture to Zhongwan (Ren 12), Zusanli (S 36) and both Fengchi (G 20) and she used a three-edged needle to prick Shaoshang (L 11) until bleeding. Only one treatment cured the problem.

2) *Carrying forward her family's valuable acupuncture techniques* Zhao believes in the curative effect of acupuncture, but for some patients who are afraid of needling she thinks it's better to adopt the "painless puncture technique." The process is as follows:

a. Before the operation, she asks the patient to breathe evenly and then she rubs and taps the point to allow smooth flow of qi and blood.

b. On puncturing the filiform needle, Zhao strongly presses the point and slowly rotates the needle into the point. When a thicker or short needle is used, she presses the point heavily and quickly and rotates the needle in. On puncturing a small needle she uses the pricking technique to reduce pain.

c. After inserting the needle she applies the reducing or reinforcing method combined with massage. The reinforcing method is conducted in the following way. When the needle is lifted a little, she presses the handle tightly three times. When the needle is lifted to the superficial, she presses the handle three times to make qi go deep, or she shakes the needle tip to make qi reach the diseased part directly. On withdrawal of the needle, she asks the patient to breathe in and then straightly pulls the needle out straight. In using the reducing method, Zhao sometimes shakes the needle to widen the point or slowly lifts the needle and presses the handle. When the needling sensation appears she asks the patient to breathe out and pulls out the needle. A few seconds later she massages the point.

d. Zhao holds that when a strong needle sensation appears, acupuncture manipulations and massage should be conducted simultaneously. After the tense feeling around the needle is removed, the needle can gradually be pulled out. Massage is followed to make the flow of qi and blood smooth. After Fengchi (G 20) is needled and the problem of the temple or shoulder is not eliminated, massage may be given to Xuanli (G 6), Luxi (SJ 19) and Jianjing (G 21). After Sanyinjiao (Sp 6) is needled, massage may also be given to Xuehai (Sp 10), Yinlian (Liv 11), Zhongfeng (Liv 4), Zhaohai (K 6) and Dadu (Sp 2). Acupuncture of Neiguan (P 6) may be combined by massage of Laogong (P 8), Daling (P 7) and Quze (P 3). Acupuncture of Houxi (SI 3) may be combined by massage to Yanglao (SI 6), Xiaohai (SI 8), etc.

II. Case Analysis

Case 1: Windstroke (apoplexy)

Name, Ren x x; sex, male; age, 43; occupation, farmer; date of the first visit, April 10, 1960.

Complaints Two days before, the patient suddenly lost consciousness and when he came to, he had hemiplegia on the right side. A physical examination showed a yellow complexion, a pale red tongue with a thin white coating, string-taut pulse and blood pressure, 130/80 mmHg.

Differentiation Meridians attacked by pathogenic wind.

Method Dispelling pathogenic wind from the meridians.

Prescription Left Jianyu (LI 15), Jianliao (SJ 14), Quchi (LI 11), Hegu (LI 4), Huantiao (G 30), Fengchi (G 20), Yanglingquan (G 34), both Zusanli (S 36) and Juegu (G 39).

Treatment procedure The even movement and the reinforcing method were used successively. Fengchi (G 20) was for dispelling wind and Zusanli (S 36) for strengthening stomach qi. Juegu (G 39) was used to replenish essence. Acupuncture was applied to the left side since the diseased part was on the right. Treatment was given every two days, helped by taking herbal extracts. After four treatments the patient was cured.

Case 2: Arthritis with fixed pain and heaviness

Name, Yan x x; sex, female; age, 45; date of the first visit, October 12, 1959.

Complaints A month before she had a cold and fever. Since then she felt pain in the knee joints and a heavy sensation in the left knee. There was no satisfactory response to Western drugs. In the past few days the condition deteriorated. There was severe pain with motor impairment. It was diagnosed as rheumatic arthritis. Physical examination showed a swollen stiff right knee joint, pain on pressure, dry pale red lips, slightly red throat, deep and tight pulse, white greasy tongue coating. Erothrocyte Sedimentation Rate (ESR): 15 mm first hour, 33 mm second hour.

Differentiation Accumulation of wind and damp in the meridians.

Method Expelling wind and damp to regulate the meridians.

Prescription Both Dubi (S 35), Xiyangquan (G 33), Yanglingquan (G 34), Zusanli (S 36), Lianqiu (S 34), Chengshan (B 57), Weizhong (B 40), Weiyang (B 39), Heding (Extra 31), Hegu (LI 4), Xuehai (Sp 10), Ququan (L 8) and Tiantu (Ren 22).

Treatment procedure The above points were needled alternately every two days. The reducing method and even movement were applied successively. Nine treatments in total cured the case.

Case 3: Sequelae of cerebral concussion

Name, Lu x x; sex, male; age, 25; occupation, student; date of first visit, December 18, 1957.

Complaints In the summer of 1957 when he was doing a field study in an iron and steel works, he fell by accident and lost consciousness. When he came to after emergency treatment he could not recall what had happened. He suffered from amnesia and proxysmal dizziness. In September of the same year the condition became worse. Physical examination showed a 1.5 cm old wound on the right side of the head, red complexion, slow pulse, pale tongue without coating.

Differentiation Imbalance of yin and yang and breakdown of the normal physiological coordination between the heart and kidney.

Method Regulating qi and calming the mind, restoring the normal physiological coordination between the heart and kidney.

Prescription Both Fengchi (G 20), Tianzhu (B 10), Taiyang (Extra 2), Touwei (S 8), Baihui (Du 20), Tongtian (B 7), Shangxing (Du 23), Luxi (SJ 19), Qubing (G 7), Qucha (B 4), Fengfu (Du 16), Neiguan (P 6), Shenmen (H 7), Tanzhong (Ren 17) (pricking), Qiuxu (G 40), Xingjian (Liv 2), Shenshu (B 23) and Zhaohai (K 6).

Treatment procedure The above points were needled alternately every two days with the reducing method. Eight treatments in total cured the case.

Case 4: Amenia

Name, Wang x x; sex, female; date of the first visit, September 30, 1959.

Complaints Six months before she had amenia (pregnancy excluded) with symptoms of general cold sensation. Physical examination showed an uncomfortable feeling on pressure of the lower abdomen and around the umbilicus, retarded pulse, white thin tongue coating.

Differentiation Invasion of pathogenic cold leading to stagnation of qi and blood.

Method Removing blood stasis and pathogenic cold.

Prescription Huanshu (K 16), Guanyuan (Ren 4) and Sanyinjiao (Sp 6).

Treatment procedure Acupuncture was given with the reducing method and massage when the strong needling reaction appeared. After acupuncture, moxibustion was applied. Only three treatments cured the case.

Case 5: Hysteria

Name, Li x x; sex, female; Age, 18; occupation, student; date of the first visit, April 6, 1976.

Complaints Two weeks before she had been emotionally disturbed. Then there appeared dull-looking, weeping day and night, and fasting. A physical examination showed pallor, depression, weeping, fasting, deep pulse, and pale red tongue with thin white coating.

Differentiation Mind disturbed due to stagnation of qi.

Method Calming the mind and restoring the normal flow of qi.

Prescription Renzhong (Du 26), both Fengchi (G 20), Neiguan (P 6), Lieque (L 7), Zusanli (S 36) and Zhongfeng (Liv 4).

Treatment procedure Before acupuncture the operator tried to make the patient feel happy. Then the even movement was applied. After one treatment the condition greatly improved. All the symptoms were relieved except insomnia. On the third day acupuncture was given to Shenmen (H 7) and Fuxi (B 38) with the even movement. Retention of the needle at Shenmen (H 7) and Fuxi (B 38) for fifteen minutes and twenty minutes respectively. When the needles were twirled, the patient began to fall asleep. On withdrawal of the needles, the patient was already in a sound sleep. On the third visit, the patient was cured.

Case 6: Difficulty in swallowing (esophagospasm)

Name, Chao x x; sex, male; age, 30; date of the first visit, February 10, 1960.

Complaints The patient had had a feeling of a blocked esophagus for about a year. In the last few days the condition deteriorated with symptoms of sore throat, chest pain, insomnia. Doctors of Western medicine diagnosed it as esophagospasm. A physical examination showed bright complexion, red tongue without coating.

Differentiation Obstruction of qi flow and disharmony between the stomach and liver.

Method Calming the liver, normalizing the stomach and regulating qi.

Prescription Tiantu (Ren 22), Lianquan (Ren 23), Juque (Ren 14), Dazhui (Du 14), Dashu (B 11), Feishu (B 13), Ganshu (B 18), Jueyinshu (B 14), Geshu (B 17), Xinshu (B 15), Danshu (B 19), Weishu (B 21), Taichong (Liv 3), Zusanli (S 36) and Neiguan (P 6).

Treatment procedure Geshu (B 17) is the Confluent point of blood and Juque (Ren 14) is the Front-Mu point of the heart. Lianquan (Ren 23) and Tiantu (Ren 22) are located at the vicinity of the esophagus. Dazhui (Du 14) is the Confluent point of the three yang meridians of hand and foot and the Du Meridian. Points on the back may regulate the qi of the five zang organs. The above points were punctured alternately every other day with the reducing and even movement. After each treatment, massage and the plum blossom needling were applied along the line from Taodao (Du 13) to Xiyangguan (G 33). Moxibustion was given to Zusanli (S 36) by burning twenty-one cones of moxa wool. Nine treatments cured the case.

SELECTION OF POINTS BASED ON MINUTE DIFFERENTIATION OF SYNDROMES

—Zhao Erkang's Clinical Experience

Zhao Erkang, a native of Jiangyin County, Jiangsu Province, was born in July, 1913. In 1932, he began to learn acupuncture from Cheng Dan'an, an established acupuncture specialist. He worked as the acting head of the General Affairs and professor at the China Acupuncture Society, China Acupuncture School, Acupuncture Sanitorium run by Cheng Dan'an in 1935. In 1948 he established the All-China Acupuncture Society and opened an acupuncture clinic in Wuxi and started publication of *Contemporary Acupuncture* in 1952. Since 1959 he has successively served in the Acupuncture Institute, Medical Literature Research Section and the *Journal of Traditional Chinese Medicine.* He has published about a dozen works, including *Chinese Acupuncture*, *Acupuncture Therapy in Prose Poem,* etc. Now he is one of the senior editors of the *Journal of Traditional Chinese Medicine,* member of the Expert Consultative Committee of China Academy of Traditional Chinese Medicine.

I. Academic Characteristics and Medical Specialities

1. Selection of acupuncture approaches based on analysis of syndromes

For different syndromes Zhao adopts different acupuncture methods. He holds that for yang and exterior syndromes shallow needling without retention of needles or with little or without moxibustion is used; for yin or interior syndromes deep needling and retention of needles or more moxibustion are used; for deficiency and cold syndromes, acupuncture with the reinforcing method and more moxibustion are applied; and for excess and heat syndromes more acupuncture with the reducing method is applied. Without differentiation of syndromes acupuncture cannot obtain the desired effect.

2. Rules for the selection of points

Selection of points, Zhao believes, is in accordance with the meridians, the vicinity and locality. Points on the head, face and trunk usually function to treat local disorders or problems of the tissues and organs in the vicinity. Points on the four limbs are especially helpful in treatment of the general disorders besides the above-mentioned problems. It is demonstrated by clinical experience that selection of points in accordance with meridians is most helpful to general disorders. For instance, there occurred an epidemic of measles in Wuxi some years ago. Zhao treated the condition based on this approach and achieved great success. He usually selects three to five points in one treatment according to the condition of the disease.

3. Thorough training in basic skills

There are quite a number of acupuncture manipulations handed down by generations. Zhao thinks it necessary to have a thorough training in basic acupuncture skills first, then try to be good at a few special approaches. The following aspects should be noted for painless insertion of needles.

1) Patient persuasion should be done to those first consulting patients to free them from unnecessary worries and nervousness.

2) On treatment the patient should be in a comfortable posture and relax his muscles in the acupuncture area.

3) It is better to select points located at the thicker muscles and looser tissues.

4) On puncturing, the needle the operator wants to use should be inserted quickly and gently into the skin while pressing the point by other fingers.

5) When the needle goes through the skin and causes pain, the operator should move it a bit to avoid the tender spot.

6) If pain appears probably owing to the vessel or periosteum being pricked, the operator should lift the needle a little and insert it towards another direction.

7) On insertion of the needle, the operator should shift the patient's attention consciously by asking questions to avoid a painful feeling.

4. The needling sensation

Zhao believes that the key to having a desirable effect with acupuncture is the needling sensation besides correct differentiation of syndromes, selection of points and operations. The curative effect lies in the production of the needle sensation. For this reason he attaches great importance to the force of finger exertion. It is stated in the *Compendium of Acupuncture and Moxibustion* that in acupuncture, the appearance of the needling sensation is a priority. When he treats pain or spasms, Zhao usually gives strong stimulation to alleviate both symptoms. For elderly or weak patients, he often takes measures to promote the appearance of the needling sensation, sometimes by moxibustion.

For those who have a slow needling reaction Zhao uses the lift-thrust method or quick twirling, or he taps the needle handle to promote the appearance of the needling sensation. For some cases, manipulations are done in the period of needle retention to invigorate the needling sensation.

5. Prevention of possible accidents

It has been reported the accidents include bleeding of medulla, pneumothorax, heart rupture, spleen rupture, injury of the kidney and vessels, which are caused by too deep insertion of needles. Therefore, needles should not be punctured deep in the place where vital organs are located. Generally, according to the rules listed in the historic medical literature, depth of needle insertion should be taken into account or oblique puncture is used. For patients with severe asthma or asthma combined with pneumonectasis, it is better to avoid giving needling at the chest and back. In addition, for elderly and weak patients or patients who have overeaten or who are extremely hungry, acupuncture is not suggested. If necessary, the patient should lie down and receive shallow needling with gentle manipulation to avoid fainting. For pregnant women, it is strickly forbidden to puncture Hegu (LI 4), Sanyinjiao (Sp 6) and the points located at the lumbosacrum. For pregnancies less than five months, points on the lower abdomen should not be used and for pregnancies more than five months, points on the upper and lower abdomen should not be used to avoid miscarriage.

II. Case Analysis.

Case 1: Aphonia

Name, Wang x x; sex, male; age, 40.

Complaints The patient had taken too much pheniramine because of severe insomnia, then he could not utter a sound.

Prescription Yamen (Du 15) and Guanchong (SJ 1).

Treatment procedure At first no response was seen when Yamen (Du 15) was punctured. Then the left Guanchong (SJ 1) was needled and the patient surprisingly cried out: "I am all right."

Explanation The above two points are considered as the empirical points for aphonia.

Case 2: Carbuncle

Name, Xu x x; sex, female; age, 25.

Complaints At first she had a pain and swelling in the left lateral leg accompanied by aversion to cold and fever. Then it became worse, but no pus formed.

Prescription Ashi points.

Treatment procedure Moxibustion on garlic was applied to the affected area. On the following day the symptoms were considerably relieved. The same treatment was given and on the third day the swelling, pain and fever subsided.

Case 3: Chronic convulsions

Name, Yang x; sex, male; age, 4.

Complaints One night convulsion suddenly attacked with symptoms of pallor, closed eyes, cold limbs, absence of breath and pulse.

Differentiation Yang collapse.

Method Restoring yang from collapse.

Prescription Shenque (Ren 8).

Treatment procedure Salt was put in the umbilicus covered by a piece of ginger, to which moxibustion was applied to cause resuscitation. When about ten cones of moxa wool were burnt, the patient began to breathe, and after thirty cones of moxa wool were burnt the patient came to with warm limbs and normal breathing. Then moxibustion was applied to Zusanli (S 36) to strengthen the stomach and spleen qi.

Explanation It is held by Zhao that moxibustion is most helpful to collapse of yang when there is no complete loss of yang.

Case 4: Breast ulcer

Name, Wang x; sex, female; age, 29.

Complaints At first the patient had a movable mass as big as a plum stone in the right breast. Then it gradually became larger with dull pain. On operation pus was discharged. It seemed to heal afterwards, but some days later, an ulcer which produced thin pus was seen in the breast. The condition existed for four years and finally a fistula formed.

Prescription Ashi points.

Treatment procedure Moxibustion was applied to the ulcer covered by a mixture made of the powder of *Aconitum variagatum* and wine to invigorate yang. The treatment was given every other day. About thirty treatments in total cured the persisted case. A follow-up study for several years showed no relapse.

CONSISTENCY OF PATHOGENESIS, METHOD OF TREATMENT, PRESCRIPTION AND NEEDLING TECHNIQUES, AND CORRECT APPLICATION OF ACUPUNCTURE, MOXIBUSTION AND POINT INJECTION

—Jiang Shuming's Clinical Experience

Jiang Shuming was born in Tianjin in 1927. In 1940 when she was thirteen years old, she started her apprenticeship of acupuncture with Wang Jiaxiang, who was then working at the Dachengxiang Acupuncture Clinic. Three years later, she finished her apprenticeship and started working at the same clinic. In 1948, she studied in the Harbin Training Center of Traditional Chinese Medicine. In 1951, she received further training in the Harbin Traditional Chinese Medical School. The next year she was appointed director of the Dachengxiang Acupuncture Clinic. In 1956 she was transferred to the Harbin Hospital of Traditional Chinese Medicine. She treated liver diseases with point injection therapy and acupuncture in the early 1960s. She stressed the importance of gentle and swift insertion of the needle in combination with pressure of the skin with the fingers in order to reduce pain for the patient. She obtained marked therapeutic results.

Now she is an associate research fellow of the Heilongjiang Academy of Traditional Chinese Medicine, deputy director of Harbin Institute of Paralysis, member of the Standing Committee of Heilongjiang Acupuncture Association, deputy director of Harbin Acupuncture Association and a member of Council of Harbin Association of Traditional Chinese Medicine.

I. Academic Characteristics and Medical Specialities

Dr. Jiang attaches great importance to the application of acupuncture based upon differentiation of syndromes, lays stress on consistency of pathogenesis, method of treatment, prescription of points and needling techniques, and pays special attention to painless needling insertion with a gentle and swift technique.

1. Gentle and swift insertion of the needle in combination with finger pressure to reduce pain

1) *Insert the needle with both hands aided by the pressure of the fingers of the right hand* As the first step of inserting the needle, this method is similar to inserting the needle with the help of the puncturing and pressing hands. But there is a difference

between them, which lies in the fact that the middle, ring and small fingers of the right hand press the skin around the needle in this technique when the needle is inserted into the skin.

a. Hold the tip of the needle with the thumb and the index finger of the left hand to fix the needle body, and hold the handle of the needle with the thumb and the index finger of the right hand so as to insert the needle into the skin.

b. Press the skin around the needle with the middle, ring and small fingers of the right hand simultaneously when the needle is inserted. In this way, the pain scatters in various directions and is less severe or even disappears. This method is applicable for both short needles and long needles to be inserted at different angles.

2) *Gentle and swift insertion of the needle* This is the second step of inserting the needle. Gentle and swift insertion of the needle requires a deft and smooth manoeuvre of the thumb and the index finger of the right hand, which, additionally aided by the pressure on the skin with the other three fingers of the same hand, ensures rapid penetration of the skin by the tip of the needle without pain.

3) *Rotating the needle into the required depth and manipulating the needle to get qi* This is the third step of inserting the needle. After insertion into the skin, the needle is gently rotated back and forth with an amplitude of less than 90°. If the point is located accurately, qi generally arrives. In case qi fails to arrive, lift and thrust the needle three to five times with a moderate amplitude and frequency; then rotate the needle again. The operator can feel whether qi has arrived or not under the needle. As said in the book of *Ode to the Standard of Mystery*, "If a light, slippery and soft sensation is felt around the needle, qi hasn't arrived yet. A heavy, hesitant and tense feeling means the arrival of qi."

2. Two acupuncture points and three items for attention in the treatment of nocturnal enuresis

There are descriptions in medical classics of all ages concerning nocturnal enuresis. Its principal etiology and pathology are deficiency of the kidney qi, deficiency-cold of the lower jiao, or deficiency of qi in the spleen and lung. The method of treatment is to warm up the kidney, tonify qi and control urination. Based upon these descriptions, Dr. Jiang summarized the treatment as two acupuncture points and three items for attention. She has also paid much attention to the influence of the patient's psychological state on the disease.

Nocturnal enuresis is a pathological phenomenon of children over three years old. The patient may wet the bed once or twice a night. Some of the patients also have frequent urination at daytime, and bed wetting can not be avoided at night, even if the parents wake them up. When these children, especially girls, grow older, they feel ashamed to see the doctor.

1) *Two acupuncture points are Guanyuan (Ren 4) and Sanyinjiao (Sp 6)* The two points are needled with the reinforcing method. The needles are retained for fifteen minutes; meanwhile moxibustion with a moxa stick is applied to the two points.

Guanyuan (Ren 4) is the meeting point of the three yin meridians of foot and the Ren Meridian, and Sanyinjiao (Sp 6) is the meeting point of the Liver, Spleen and

Kidney Meridians. Needling and moxibustion at the two points are able to warm up the liver, spleen and kidney, to tonify qi and control urine.

2) *Three items for attention*

a. The patient should drink fluid and eat fruits as little as possible at dinner time.

b. The patient shoul keep in mind that he or she should wake up and go to the toilet at night.

c. The parents should wake up the patient before bed-wetting occurs.

These above three items should be carried out for more than one month. Generally, with three acupuncture treatments recovery can be expected. The curative rate is 100 percent.

3. Stress on warming method with moxibustion

When Dr. Jiang was young, the patients she treated were mostly suffering from long-standing diseases with the symptoms of cold, deficiency and weakness. The warming method was applied in the treatment. Since then, she has been inclined to apply moxibustion to such syndromes as deficiency of yang of the spleen and kidney, long-standing retention of wind-cold, deficiency of qi and blood, cold and deficiency of the epigastium and abdomen. Over the past forty years, she has applied and studied moxibustion carefully and obtained satisfactory therapeutic results in the treatment of various diseases.

1) *Uterine bleeding* Uterine bleeding may result from heat in the blood, stagnation of blood, deficiency of the spleen, or deficiency of the kidney. There is one thing in common: All of them subsequently cause weakness of the Chong and Ren Meridians, thus impairing their function in controlling blood. As acupuncture is less effective in the treatment of uterine bleeding due to heat in the blood or blood stagnation, herbs of clearing heat, cooling blood, removing blood stasis and checking bleeding should be used in combination with acupuncture in order to improve the therapeutic effects. If uterine bleeding is due to deficiency of yang of the spleen and kidney, the method of choice is acupuncture and moxibustion, especially moxibustion.

Pishu (B 20) and Shenshu (B 23) are needled first with the reinforcing method by rotating the needle. The needles are retained for fifteen minutes. Meanwhile, moxibustion using the moxa stick is applied to the points. After the withdrawal of the needles from these points, do Qihai (Ren 6), Guanyuan (Ren 4) and Sanyinjiao (Sp 6) in the same way.

Pishu (B 20) is the Back-Shu Point of the spleen; needling this point with the reinforcing method tonifies the spleen qi and controls blood. Shenshu (B 23) is the Back-Shu Point of the kidney; the application of the reinforcing method tonifies the kidney qi. Qihai (Ren 6) is from the Ren Meridian, functioning to tonify qi of the middle jiao and regulate the Chong and Ren Meridians. Guanyuan (Ren 4) is the meeting point of the three yin meridians of the foot and the Ren Meridian, functioning to regulate the three yin meridians of the foot and strengthen the Chong and Ren Meridians. Sanyinjiao (Sp 6) is the meeting point of the three yin meridians of foot, functioning to regulate and tonify these meridians. Acupuncture and moxibustion are used in combination to warm up the yang of the spleen and kidney, tonify qi and and control blood.

Dr. Jiang has treated 250 cases of uterine bleeding with a success rate of more than 90 percent.

2) *Windstroke* The sequelae of windstroke such as hemiplegia and aphasia due to rigid tongue should be treated with acupuncture and moxibustion as early as possible. Flaccidity or contracture of the muscles and tendons in a prolonged case is due to obstruction of qi and blood in the meridians, which deprives them of nourishment. The warming method should be applied in order to clear the meridians. In the treatment of weak limbs and trunk due to long-term deprivation of nourishment, the warming method is even more important. The local points of the diseased limbs and trunk are combined with Ganshu (B 18) and Shenshu (B 23). The needles should be retained, and moxibustion should be combined to tonify the liver and kidney, to remove the obstruction from meridians to promote ample qi and blood and restore the functions of the limbs and trunk.

4. Fluid injection at the acupuncture points in the treatment of chronic diseases

1) *Chronic hepatitis* Chronic hepatitis is due to either stagnation of qi and blood or deficiency of the antipathogenic factors complicated with retention of the pathogenic factors. When combined with acupuncture and moxibustion, fluid injection at the acupuncture points relieves enlargement of the liver and spleen, restoring the liver's function and improving symptoms and signs. Three hundred and eight cases of chronic hepatitis were treated with the total effective rate reaching 96 percent.

a. Fluid injection at the acupuncture points. One ml of Vitamin B_{12} (0.015 mg) is injected into Ganshu (B 18) on one side one day and another side the next day. Put the syringe needle into the point; rotate the syringe gently to cause soreness, numbness and distention; then inject the fluid into the point slowly. Twenty treatments constitute one course. The patient rests for one or two weeks before the second course of the treatment begins.

b. Acupuncture and moxibustion. Pishu (B 20), Hunmen (B 47), Zhongwan (Ren 12), Zhangmen (Liv 13) and Yanglingquan (G 34) are used as the main points.

Add Zusanli (S 36) in cases of epigastric distention and poor appetite; Geshu (B 17) and Shenshu (B 23) in cases of pain at the lumboback region; Daheng (Sp 15) in cases of abdominal distention and constipation; Tianshu (S 25) and Gongsun (Sp 4) in cases of diarrhoea and loose stools; Qihai (Ren 6) in cases of shortness of breath and lassitude; Fengchi (G 20) and Touwei (S 8) in cases of dizziness and tinnitus; and Neiguan (P 6) and Shenmen (H 7) in cases of insomnia and palpitations.

If chronic hepatitis is due to stagnation of qi and blood, reducing needling technique is applied, and moxibustion is not advisable. If it is due to deficiency of the antipathogenic factors complicated with retention of the pathogenic factors, reinforcing needling technique is used with the needles retained for fifteen to twenty minutes, during which moxibustion with the moxa stick is applied.

c. In the therapeutic results of 308 cases, the longest duration of treatment was 13 courses, the shortest 1 course, 3 courses was the average. One hundred and twenty-three cases, or 40 percent, were cured; 78 cases, or 25.3 percent, improved; 96 cases, or 31 percent, were relieved; 9 cases, or 2.9 percent, failed; and 2 cases, or 0.64 percent, deteriorated. The total effective rate was 96 percent (the effective standard was formulated in a national conference of hepatitis).

2) *Pain in the shoulder, arm, hip and thigh (radiculitis)* Injection of Vitamin B_1 and B_{12} into local and adjacent points of the diseased area is a method of choice if radiculitis fails to respond to other methods of treatment. Half to one ml is injected to each point either once a day or once every other day.

For the pain in the shoulder, Jianliao (SJ 14), Jianzhen (SI 9) and Jianyu (LI 15) are selected.

For the pain in the arm, Binao (LI 14), Quchi (LI 11) and Shousanli (LI 10) are used.

For the pain in the hip, Zhibian (B 54) and Huantiao (G 30) are applied.

For the pain in the thigh, Yinmen (B 37) and Fengshi (G 31) are chosen.

3) *Sequelae of infantile paralysis* Sequelae of infantile paralysis may manifest as muscular atrophy and unsteady walking. Injection of Vitamin B_1 and B_{12} and galanthamine into acupuncture points on the diseased limb helps restore its function. The points are selected according to symptoms and signs. Half to one ml is injected to each point once a day or every other day. The patient should receive treatment continuously for a period of time before treatment takes effect.

5. Combination of main points and secondary points

1) *Combination of Feishu (B 13) and Zhongfu (L 1) in the treatment of cough and asthma* Feishu (B 13), the Back-Shu Point of the Bladder Meridian of Foot-Taiyang, regulates the lung qi, tonifies deficiency, clears heat of the deficiency type and relieves cough. Zhongfu (L 1), the Front-Mu Point of the Lung Meridian of Hand-Taiyin, regulates the lung qi, clears heat from the lung, checks cough and soothes asthma. The combination of the two points is effective for cough and asthma.

If cough is due to invasion by wind-cold, Feishu (B 13) and Zhongfu (L 1) are combined with Lieque (L 7) to promote the lung's function in dispersing and relieving exterior syndromes. If cough is due to retention of fire and heat in the lung, they are combined with Yuji (L 10) with the reducing needling technique to clear heat from the lung. If asthmatic breathing is due to dysfunction of the lung qi in dispersing and descending, they are combined with Dingchuan (Extra 17). If cough and asthma are due to deficiency of the kidney which leads to dysfunction of the kidney in receiving qi, they are combined with Qihai (Ren 6) and Shenshu (B 23). Qihai (Ren 6) tonifies the qi of the middle jiao and Shenshu (B 23) tonifies the kidney qi. When the lung and kidney are well nourished, the ascending and descending function of qi will be normal.

In January, 1986, a man named Wang came to Dr. Jiang's clinic with a thirty-eight year history of asthma since his childhood. He had asthma attacks every winter, for which he had to be hospitalized. The patient had asthmatic breathing with raised shoulders, shortness of breath and wheezing.

Feishu (B 13) and Dingchuan (Extra 17) were needled first. The needling sensation at

Dingchuan (Extra) was caused to spread to the shoulder or back region. Cupping was also applied there after the withdrawal of the needles. Then Zhongfu (L 1) was pricked with a three-edged needle, cupping was applied there immediately to cause slight bleeding. The patient felt more relaxed in breathing at once. But he still had stuffiness in the chest. So Neiguan (P 6) was then needled. Treated once a day, ten treatments were given in all. After that he was almost free of symptoms and able to work for the whole winter.

2) *Combination of Chize (L 5) and Zhaohai (K 6) to clear the lung and ease the throat* As the He-Sea Point, water point and sun point of the Lung Meridian, Chize (L 5) is indicated in fullness of the chest, asthmatic breathing, cough and sore throat due to heat, and functioned to regulate qi of the lung, nourish yin of the lung, clear heat from the lung and soothe cough and asthmatic breathing. Zhaohai (K 6), a Confluent Point, is indicated in dryness of the throat, insomnia and frequent urination, nourishing both yin and yang of the kidney and regulating the lower jiao. The combination of the two points moistens the lung, nourishes the kidney and eases the throat.

The lung is a delicate organ, and likes moisture but dislikes dryness. If dryness of the lung results from consumption of body fluid by deficiency fire due to deficiency of the lung yin, Chize (L 5) is selected. If it results from flaring up of deficiency fire due to deficiency of the kidney, Zhaohai (K 6) is used.

A man named Sun, aged sixty, complained of dryness and a hot sensation in the throat, both of which were more pronounced at night, and had been going on for several years. The diagnosis was chronic pharyngitis.

The patient had dryness of the tongue, inflamed throat, and a rapid pulse of the deficiency type, which were differentiated as dryness of the lung due to yin deficiency.

Chize (L 5) was reduced with lifting and thrusting maneuver to relieve dryness of the lung. Zhaohai (K 6) was reinforced with rotation movement to nourish the kidney yin. The ear apexes on both sides were pricked to cause bleeding to clear heat from the lung. After being treated for several days, the symptoms improved markedly.

3) *Combination of Lieque (L 7) and Fengchi (G 20) to eliminate wind and relieve pain* Lieque (L 7), the Luo-(Connecting) Point of the Lung Meridian, connecting with the Large Intestine Meridian, and also a Confluent Point, functions to clear meridians and eliminate pathogenic wind. Fengchi (G 20) is the meeting point of the Gallbladder Meridian and Yangwei Meridian. It is also one of the important points for eliminating wind. Its other functions include: relieve exterior syndromes, clear heat, clear fire of the liver and gallbladder, and brighten the eyes. The two points are combined to treat headache due to invasion of the pathogenic wind-cold.

One early summer evening in 1986, a man named Chen, aged fifty, came to Jiang for the pain on the left side of the head and neck. The patient held the painful area with his hand, eyebrows knitted and teeth clenched. A family member said the patient was normally healthy except for headaches. One week before, another strong attack of pain suddenly occurred on the left side of the head and neck, intermittent at first and continuous over the past two days. He couldn't fall asleep at night because of the pain, although he took pain killers. For fear that he might not fall asleep again, he came to see the doctor for help.

Fengchi (G 20) was punctured with the reducing method by rotating the needle and

Lieque (L 7) was penetrated towards Pianli (LI 6). As soon as the needling sensation arrived, the pain was much relieved. The needles were retained for thirty minutes and manipulated twice during this period. The pain disappeared when the needles were removed.

4) *Combination of Neiguan (P 6) and Shenting (Du 24) to soothe the heart and calm the mind* Neiguan (P 6), the Luo-(Connecting) Point of the Pericardium Meridian, one of the Eight Confluent Points and the representative point of the Yinwei Meridian, functions to promote mental resuscitation, tonify the qi of the heart, ease the chest and diaphragm and relieve fever. Shenting (Du 24) is indicated in mental disorders such as palpitations, insomnia, mania and depression. The two points are combined to tonify the heart and calm the mind.

In winter of 1985, an old couple came to her clinic. The wife said that a few months before her husband had got frightened, which resulted in palpitations, mental restlessness and fear as if he were going to be arrested by the police. He hated to be seen by other people, including doctors. Therefore treatment of the disease was delayed. Recently the symptoms became worse, and he could not fall asleep at night, so he was persuaded by his wife to consult the doctor.

He had a red tongue with little coating and a thready, rapid pulse. Since the disease was due to fright, the method of treatment was to suppress fright and calm the mind.

Shenting (Du 24) was needled towards Shangxing (Du 23); and Neiguan (P 6) towards Waiguan (SJ 5) by reinforcing method with rotation technique. Considering his age, the mental restlessness and insomnia must be related to deficiency of the kidney yin. So Sanyinjiao (Sp 6) was needled with the reinforcing method. The symptoms improved greatly after the first treatment, and disappeared after three treatments in succession.

5) *Combination of Tianshu (S 25) and Shangjuxu (S 37) to consolidate the intestines and check diarrhoea* Tianshu (S 25), the Front-Mu Point of the large intestine, is located lateral to the umbilicus and functions to promote smooth circulation of qi of the intestines, check diarrhoea, warm intestines, regulate the lower jiao, assist digestion and relieve distention and fullness. It is indicated in abdominal pain around the umbilicus, abdominal distention, borborygmus, diarrhoea and constipation. Shangjuxu (S 37) is a point where the qi of the Stomach Meridian starts, and the Lower He-Sea Point of the Large Intestine Meridian. It is indicated in diarrhoea, borborygmus and abdominal pain. The two points are combined to consolidate the intestines and check diarrhoea.

A patient aged fifty had chronic diarrhoea for several years. The diagnosis of the Western medicine was chronic enteritis. The clinical manifestations included two or three bowel movements with loose stools a day, lassitude, abdominal discomfort which was alleviated by warmth, cold limbs and aversion to cold. Bowel movements increased after eating oily food. As the disease didn't respond to medication, he wanted to try acupuncture.

Differentiation: Cold and deficiency of the intestines due to prolonged diarrhoea.

Treatment was to warm and tonify the intestines and check diarrhoea.

Tianshu (S 25) and Shangjuxu (S 37) were needled with the reinforcing method. The needles were retained for twenty minutes, during which moxibustion with the moxa stick was applied. Soon after the treatment, the patient felt warmer and more comfortable in the abdomen. Convinced by the result of the first treatment and encouraged by the doctor, the patient came for treatment every day. After one week of treatment, the frequency of bowel movements was reduced and other symptoms were alleviated greatly. The treatment continued for three weeks, after which all the symptoms and signs disappeared.

6) *Combination of Guanyuan (Ren 4) and Jiaoxin (K 8) to warm the uterus and assist pregnancy* Guanyuan (Ren 4) is the meeting point of the three yin meridians of foot and the Ren Meridian, and the Front-Mu Point of the small intestine. It is indicated in infertility due to menstrual diseases, postpartum dizziness due to excessive loss of blood, lingering lochia, impotence, nocturnal emission, retention of urine, nocturnal enuresis, weakness of the body due to overstrain and flaccid syndrome of windstroke. Its action is to regulate and invigorate the Chong and Ren Meridians, regulate qi and blood, warm the kidney, and restore yang from collapse.

Jiaoxin (K 8), the Xi-(Cleft) Point of the Yinwei Meridian, is indicated in irregular menstruation, uterine bleeding and leukorrhea. Jiaoxin (K 8) means monthly onset of menstruation, and functions to regulate the Chong and Ren Meridians, invigorate the spleen and kidney, activate blood circulation, regulate menstruation and clear the lower jiao. The two points are combined to regulate menstruation and assist pregnancy.

A few months before, a woman named Su, aged thirty-two, came to the clinic, complaining of infertility for six years after marriage. Her menstrual cycles used to be delayed, and at present each cycle consisted of several months. She was menstruating at that time. The flow was scanty and pale in colour. She was also having a dull pain and a cold feeling in the lower abdomen, which was alleviated by warmth. The other symptoms included cold limbs, sallow complexion, emaciation, and a deep and tense pulse.

Differentiation: Cold and deficiency of the uterus.

The principle of treatment was to warm and tonify the uterus.

Guanyuan (Ren 4) and Jiaoxin (K 8) were reinforced with rotation needling technique. The needles were retained for twenty minutes, during which moxibustion with the moxa stick was applied to the points. Moxibustion relieved the pain immediately. The following day, the patient told the doctor that the menstrual flow had increased. She continued the treatment until the end of the menstrual period. She was advised to resume treatment before the next menstrual period.

The next menstrual period arrived on time with an increased amount of flow. The colour was also redder; the cold sensation in the abdomen was much reduced. The same treatment was given and continued for three months.

A few days before, she came to the clinic again. She looked plump, healthy and happy. It was fifty days since the last menstrual period finished. She was choosy for food and felt reluctant to move. The pulse was slow and rolling. All these signs showed that she was pregnant.

7) *Combination of Jiaosun (SJ 20) and Sidu (SJ 9) in the treatment of dizziness and vertigo* Jiaosun (SJ 20) and Sidu (SJ 9) are combined to treat dizziness and vertigo by regulating the qi of the Sanjiao Meridian.

There are different divisions of sanjiao in medical classics. In terms of location, the area above the diaphragm is upper jiao, the area between the diaphragm and umbilicus is middle jiao and the area below the umbilicus is lower jiao. In terms of zang-fu organs, the upper jiao includes the heart and lung; the middle jiao includes the spleen and stomach; and the lower jiao includes the liver and kidney. *The Thirty-Second Problem of Classic on Medical Problems* says: "Sanjiao is the pathway of water and food, the starting and terminating point of qi." So sanjiao includes the meridian qi and blood vessels of the whole body.

Dizziness and vertigo may result from many factors such as liver yang rising, retention of phlegm-damp in the middle jiao, deficiency of the kidney essence and deficiency of qi and blood. In short, retardation of the qi circulation in the meridians due to pathological changes of any zang-fu organs may cause the disease. Since the combination of Jiaosun (SJ 20) and Sidu (SJ 9) circulates the qi of the Sanjiao Meridian, it is effective for dizziness and vertigo.

A man named Wei, aged 30, had dizziness and vertigo for two years. During each attack of the disease, he developed nausea, poor sleep with dreams and dizziness. The disease had not responded to any previous treatment.

Jiaosun (SJ 20) was needled horizontally, and Sidu (SJ 9) needled with the even method. The needles were retained for thirty minutes and manipulated once every three to five minutes during retention. The patient felt better soon after the treatment.

The treatment was given once daily. After one week, dizziness and vertigo disappeared. The patient has been free from attacks since then.

8) *Combination of Ermen (SJ 21) and Waiguan (SJ 5) in the treatment of deafness*

Ermen (SJ 21) is located in the depression anterior to the supratragic notch, and is indicated in deafness and tinnitus. Its action is to ease the ear and assist hearing.

Waiguan (SJ 5) is indicated in deafness, tinnitus, febrile diseases due to invasion of external pathogens, headache, lymphatic tuberculosis of the neck, hypochondrial pain and hemiplegia, and functions to clear meridians, eliminate wind, relieve exterior syndromes, clear heat from the upper jiao, resolve masses, promote the liver's function in maintaining free flow of qi, and harmonize qi and blood. It is also one of the Eight Confluent Points, communicating with the Yangwei Meridian, and its own meridian runs from the dorsal aspect of the hand to the ear.

The two points are combined to treat deafness and tinnitus effectively.

Deafness may result from the upward disturbance of wind and fire of the liver and gallbladder due to anger, fear and fright, or from failure of essential qi to reach the ear due to deficiency of the kidney qi. Acupuncture is effective if treatment is based upon the causative factors. But deafness complicated with mutism resulting from a congenital factor, a severe disease or drug poisoning are intractable. Deafness should be treated first for deaf-mutism. Ermen (SJ 21) and Waiguan (SJ 5) are selected, with Ermen (SJ 21) penetrated downward towards Tinggong (SI 19) and Tinghui (G 2) with the even method. The needle is retained for twenty to thirty minutes and manipulated for a few times during retention. Treat once a day. When hearing improves, treat once every other day.

In winter, 1976, a deaf-mute boy was treated with the above method for a whole season. His hearing greatly improved. He went to school the following year, and could hear the teacher from the front seat.

9) *Combination of Geshu (B 17) and Zhongwan (Ren 12) in the treatment of hiccup*
Geshu (B 17) is the Influential Point dominating blood, and is indicated in hiccup, regurgitation, poor appetite, cough, dyspnea, spitting blood, spontaneous sweating, night sweating and blood extravasation. Its action is to ease diaphragm, harmonize the stomach qi, regulate the nutrient blood and tonify deficiency.

Zhongwan (Ren 12), the Influential Point dominating the fu organs and the Front-Mu Point of the stomach, is indicated in epigastric pain, abdominal distention, acid regurgitation, vomiting, diarrhoea and weakness of the spleen and stomach. Its action is to circulate qi of the fu organs, and conduct the clear upward and the turbid downward.

The combination of the two points is effective for easing the diaphragm and conducting rebellious qi downward.

Six years before, Dr. Jiang came across a female patient of nearly forty, who complained of hiccup for several months. The herbal treatment she had received did not work.

The frequent hiccup was accompanied with distention and fullness of the chest and diaphragm, poor appetite, a pale tongue and a string-taut pulse.

The case history showed that the disease was due to mental depression which led to stagnation of the liver qi. The invasion of the stomach by the liver qi did not allow the stomach qi to descend. The ascending of the stomach qi gave rise to hiccup.

Geshu (B 17) was punctured perpendicularly with reducing technique by rotating the needle, which was retained for ten minutes and manipulated for several times during retention. Cupping was applied after the withdrawal of the needle for easing the diaphragm. Then Zhongwan (Ren 12) was needled with the even method for circulating stomach qi, pacifying the stomach and conducting the rebellious qi downward. After that, Yanglingquan (G 34) was needled with the reducing method. The needling sensation spread to the foot for suppressing the rebellious qi of the liver and gallbladder.

After several treatments, the hiccup disappeared.

10) *Combination of Zhongji (Ren 3) and Diji (Sp 8) in the treatment of dysmenorrhea*
Zhongji (Ren 3), the Front-Mu Point of the Bladder Meridian, is located in the lower abdomen and is indicated in dysmenorrhea, irregular menstruation, retention of lochia, nocturnal emission and impotence. Its action is to regulate the Chong and Ren Meridians, clear meridians, activate blood circulation, remove blood stasis, relieve pain, consolidate the reproductive gate and regulate the lower jiao.

Diji (Sp 8), the Xi-(Cleft) Point of the Spleen Meridian, is effective for relieving pain.

The two points are combined to activate blood circulation, regulate menstruation, clear meridians and relieve pain.

Dysmenorrhea is mainly due to retardation of qi circulation, which blocks the blood in the uterus.

A female patient once got angry during menstruation, resulting in distending pain in the lower abdomen which was aggravated on pressure, scanty dark-red menstrual flow mixed with clots, and distended pain in the chest and hypochondrium. From then on, pain was present during each period, getting worse little by little. She also developed pain in the lower back region. The tongue was dark-purplish with purple spots; the pulse appeared deep and string-taut.

Zhongji (Ren 3) and Diji (Sp 8) were reduced with rotation needling technique. When the needles were retained in place, moxibustion was applied. Both needling and moxibustion aimed at clearing meridians, circulating qi, activating blood circulation, removing blood stasis and relieving pain. As lower back pain was present, Shenshu (B 23) was also needled with the even movement, and moxibustion was also applied.

The same treatment was continued for three months until dysmenorrhea disappeared.

II. Case Analysis

Case 1: Uterine bleeding

Name, Wang x x; age, 18; occupation, student; date of the first visit, March, 1980.

Complaints In November last year, she noted profuse dark menstrual flow mixed with clots. Then the flow turned pale, dilute and odourless. But the amount of flow remained profuse. Meanwhile, she suffered emaciation, lassitude, shortness of breath, dizziness, blurring of vision, lower back pain, cold limbs, stuffiness in the chest, poor appetite and loose stools. Abdominal pain was not present.

The disease was diagnosed as functional uterine bleeding in Western medicine, and did not respond to Western and Chinese medication. She gave up her studies because of the illness.

Her face was pale and puffy; the tongue was pale and moist and covered with a white coating. Her voice was low, without foul breath. The pulse was thready and weak.

Differentiation Deficiency of the spleen impaired its function of controlling blood; the resultant sinking of the clear yang and weakness of the Chong and Ren Meridians gave rise to excessive loss of blood. Deficiency of the kidney yang caused deficiency of the spleen yang; the resultant deficiency of the qi of the middle jiao failed in controlling blood.

The method of treatment was to invigorate the spleen qi, warm the kidney and check bleeding.

Prescription Pishu (B 20), Shenshu (B 23), Qihai (Ren 6), Guanyuan (Ren 4), Sanyinjiao (Sp 6).

All the points were reinforced with rotation technique. The needles were retained for fifteen minutes, during which moxibustion with the moxa stick was applied.

Bleeding reduced after the second treatment. The same treatment was continued five times until bleeding stopped and all the symptoms improved except lower back pain, for which Shenshu (B 23) and Zhishi (B 52) were then reinforced with rotation needling technique. The needles were retained for fifteen minutes, during which moxibustion was applied. Another three treatments later, the lower back pain also disappeared.

Explanation As the disease is due to deficiency of yang of the spleen and kidney, Pishu (B 20) and Shenshu (B 23) are used as the main points for tonifying the spleen and kidney. Qihai (Ren 6) invigorates the qi of the middle jiao. Guanyuan (Ren 4) strengthens the Chong and Ren Meridians. Sanyinjiao (Sp 6) nourishes the liver, spleen and kidney. Moxibustion warms up the yang of the spleen and kidney and consolidates the Chong and Ren Meridians. All these are aimed at checking bleeding.

Case 2: Hoarse voice

Name, Tan x x; sex, female; age, 21; occupation, worker; date of the first visit, September 21, 1980.

Complaints The patient suddenly noticed she had a hoarse voice after quarrelling one year before. The disease was alleviated with medication, but was never cured. The hoarse voice became worse fifteen days before due to anger. She also had stuffiness in the chest and distention in the hypochondrium. She was admitted to the hospital with the diagnosis of acute laryngitis. The examination showed slight congestion of the membrane and anterior and posterior walls of the pharynx, edema and incomplete occlusion of the anterior juncture of the vocal cord, and slight edema of the laryngeal membrane. She received antibiotics and hormone intravenously and orally for two weeks, but the symptoms did not improve. So an acupuncture doctor was asked for help.

The patient had mental depression, red cheeks, a red and dry tongue and a string-taut, rapid pulse, in addition to a hoarse voice.

Differentiation Sudden hoarseness of voice was due to anger, which injured the liver and gave rise to liver qi stagnation. It then turned into fire over a period of time and produced hyperactivity of the liver fire above and deficiency of the kidney water below. The accumulated heat ascended and disturbed the throat.

The method of treatment was to promote the liver's function, suppress the fire, nourish the kidney and ease the thorat.

Prescription Ganshu (B 18), Hegu (LI 4) and Taichong (Liv 3) were reduced with rotation needling technique; Zhaohai (K 6) was reinforced with rotation needling technique; Yuji (L 10), Shaoshang (L 11) and the ear apexes were pricked to cause bleeding.

The patient was able to make vocal sounds after the first treatment. The voice became normal after the third treatment.

Explanation Ganshu (B 18) promotes the liver's function and suppresses the liver fire; Zhaohai (K 6) nourishes water for controlling fire; Taichong (Liv 3) and Hegu (LI 4), the "Four Gates," circulate qi; bleeding Yuji (L 10) and Shaoshang (L 11) clear lung fire and heat of the upper jiao; bleeding the ear apexes on both sides eases the throat.

Case 3: Plum stone qi

Name, Cao x x; sex, female; age, 32; occupation, accountant; date of the first visit, June 29, 1986.

Complaints The patient complained of the sensation of a foreign body in the throat two months before after a quarrel with her husband. The sensation could not be relieved by spitting or swallowing. She also developed a stifling sensation in the chest. The chest X-ray was normal. Her tongue was white and sticky, and the pulse was string-taut and rolling.

The disease was differentiated as liver qi stagnation, leading to the disorder of the chest and diaphragm.

The method of treatment was to promote the liver's function in maintaining the free flow of qi and relieve depression.

Prescription Ganshu (B 18), Neiguan (P 6), Tiantu (Ren 22), Zhongwan (Ren 12), Qianjin (Extra) (in the depression lateral to Xiawan (Ren 10) when breathing in), Yanglingquan (G 34).

Ganshu (B 18) was reduced with rotation needling technique. The needle was retained for twenty minutes, and cupping was applied after the withdrawal of the needle. Even method was applied to Neiguan (P 6), Tiantu (Ren 22) and Zhongwan (Ren 12). Qianjin (Extra) and Yanglingquan (G 34) were needled with the reducing method, and the needles were retained for twenty minutes.

Explanation Ganshu (B 18) is used as the main point for promoting the free flow of qi of the Liver Meridian; Neiguan (P 6) relieves the stagnant qi in the chest and diaphragm; Tiantu (Ren 22) conducts the rebellious qi downward and eases the throat; Zhongwan (Ren 12) regulates the qi of the middle jiao and conducts the clear upward and the turbid downward; Qianjin (Extra) is an important point of regulating qi and treating qi disorders; and Yanglingquan (G 34) promotes the liver's function and conducts the rebellious qi downward.

The symptoms improved after the first treatment and disappeared after the third treatment.

Case 4: Contusion of the right ankle joint

Name, Zhang x x; sex, female; age, 27; occupation, worker; date of the first visit, January 10, 1980.

Complaints Six years before, she had a contusion on her right ankle joint, and the pain resulting from the contusion lasted for a period of time. When the pain was relieved, she was symptom free except on rainy and cold days. Over the past year, she had noted spasm of the toes on the right side, which caused contracture and pain of the right lower extremity, and spasm of m.gastrocnemius. The symptoms had been getting worse, especially in winter. She often walked with a limp, or even couldn't move if the symptoms were bad. Neither Western nor Chinese medication from different doctors could help her.

The examination showed that the right foot was deformed like a claw, and that the lower leg on the right side was 1.5 cm thinner than on the left side.

The disease was due to contusion, which resulted in retardation of qi and blood circulation, thus depriving the meridians and tendons of nourishment.

The method of treatment was to clear the meridians and activate the blood circulation.

Prescription Three sets of points are prescribed.

1) Heyang (B 55), Zhubin (K 9), Xuanzhong (G 39), Taichong (Liv 3);
2) Yanglingquan (G 34), Feiyang (B 58), Kunlun (B 60), Fuliu (K 7);
3) Chengshan (B 57), Fuyang (B 59), Zhongdu (Liv 6), Xingjian (Liv 2).

All the points were selected on the right side.

The three sets of points took turns with one of them needled every day. All the points were needled with even method. The needles were retained for twenty minutes, during which moxibustion was applied. The spasm of the toes could be relieved slightly during the treatment, but came back soon after the withdrawal of the needles. So fluid injection at these points was decided. Five hundred micrograms of Vitamin B_{12} was diluted into 3 ml with distilled water. To each point 0.5-1.0 ml was injected a day. The three sets also took turns with one of them injected daily. The symptoms and signs started improving a few days later. The patient was able to extend the toes, and spasm, contracture and pain of the lower leg disappeared after twenty days of treatment. The same treatment continued another ten times in order to consolidate the therapeutic results. After that, the patient could go to work. A follow-up visit one year later showed full recovery.

Explanation The points from the Bladder Meridian and the Kidney Meridian are used as the main points, because these two meridians pass through the diseased area. The selection of the points from the Liver Meridian and Gallbladder Meridian is due to the fact that the liver dominates the tendons, and Yanglingquan (G 34) is the Influential Point dominating tendons.

Case 5: Paralysis of the lower limbs

Name, Wang x x; sex, male; age, 22; occupation, worker; date of the first visit, December, 1980.

Complaints Four months before, the patient suddenly developed abdominal pain when he was in the factory. The pain was soon followed by paralytic weakness of the lower limbs. He was immediately sent to the hospital. The pain was diagnosed as bleeding of the spinal cord. After four months of hospitalization, he still could not stand erect with frequent spasms of the lower limbs. Incontinence of urine and difficulty in bowel movements were still present. He was then referred to the acupuncture department.

He had a sallow complexion, painful expression, paralyzed lower limbs with frequent spasms, a clear but low voice, and a deep and slow pulse. He still had a catheter.

The disease was differentiated as blockage of the meridians, which deprived the tendons of nourishment.

The method of treatment was to clear the meridians, activate the blood circulation and relax the tendons.

Prescription Injection of Vitamin B_1 (100 mg) and B_{12} (500 ug) into the acupuncture points of Shenshu (B 23), Qihaishu (B 24), Dachangshu (B 25), Huantiao (G 30), Zhibian (B 54), Yinmen (B 37), Heyang (B 55), Chengshan (B 57), Feiyang (B 58), Xiyangguan (G 33), Yanglingquan (G 34), Zusanli (S 36), Yinlingquan (Sp 9), Xuanzhong (G 39), and Sanyinjiao (Sp 6).

Two or three points were selected each time with 0.5-1.0 ml of fluid injected to each point. Twenty treatments comprised a course. There was one week's interval between two courses of treatment.

After one week's treatment, the spasms started improving; the patient could stand erect against the railing and his incontinence disappeared. After two courses, the patient could walk with crutches. He was hospitalized for three months, but continued the treatment after discharge from the hospital. After six months, he could ride a bicycle. After one year, he recovered fully. He got married in 1985.

TREATMENT OF DISEASES WITH THE FIVE ANCIENT ACUPUNCTURE TECHNIQUES

—Jiang Yijun's Clinical Experience

Jiang Yijun, a native of Xinghua County, Jiangsu Province, was born in 1922. He started learning traditional Chinese medicine from Jiang Ziwei, his uncle, in 1938. His medical career began in 1943 in his hometown. In 1952 he organized a united clinic with his colleagues and started studying Western medicine in 1954. In 1956 he went to work in the Jiangsu School of Traditional Chinese Medicine and in 1957 he served as a clinical teacher of acupuncture in the Affiliated Hospital of Beijing College of Traditional Chinese Medicine. He is good at selection of the special points and the Eight Confluent Points. His chief works include *Concise Acupuncture*, *Acupuncture*, *Essentials of Chinese Acupuncture*, *Meridians and Collaterals*, *Clinical Application of the Five Ancient Acupuncture Techniques* and *Clinical Application of the Eight Confluent Points*. Now he is an associate professor at the Affiliated Hospital of Beijing College of Traditional Chinese Medicine.

I. Academic Characteristics and Medical Specialities

1. Clinical application of the Eight Confluent Points

The Eight Confluent Points of the eight extraordinary meridians and the twelve regular meridians are located at the hands and feet. In ancient times acupuncturists used them according to the change of day, hour, heavenly stems and earthly branches, but Jiang selects them based on syndromes without considering these changes.

1) *Gongsun (Sp 4) and Neiguan (P 6)* They are used in combination to treat heart pain, stomachache, dysentery and other digestive disorders. For instance, Mr. Xu about 30 years old had frequently suffered from nervous vomiting. When it attacked he was not able to eat anything and became emaciated. Finally he was cured by acupuncture applied to Gongsun (Sp 4) and Neiguan (P 6). Another patient named Yang suddenly had severe abdominal distension one day due to overeating. These two points were used and alleviated the condition. Fifteen minutes later the abdominal distension completely disappeared. Neiguan (P 6) was punctured 1 cun in depth, or punctured deep at first and then lifted a bit and the needle was retained for some time. Gongsun (Sp 4) was punctured 1 cun in depth. Care must be taken not to harm the meridian.

2) *Houxi (SI 3) and Shenmai (B 62)* These points are selected in combination to treat hemiplegia, motion impairment of limbs and mental disorders. In treating schizophrenia Jiang often uses these two points. Houxi (SI 3) is usually penetrated towards Laogong (P 8). Shenmai (B 62) is needled about 1 cun in depth. For those who are afraid

of acupuncture, slow deep puncture is applied with retention of the needle and less manipulations. For severe conditions Shenmen (H 7) is selected too and penetrated towards Daling (P 7). An elderly patient who had schizophrenia for three years was treated by selection of these two points and gradually cured.

3) *Zulinqi (G 41) and Waiguan (SJ 5)* They are often used to treat ringing of the ears, deafness, eye troubles, puffy legs, migraine, hypertension, etc. They are perpendicularly punctured together with Fengchi (G 20) and Sizhukong (SJ 23). Horizontal puncture with continuous mild rotating is applied to cases of stiff neck and apoplexy. For cases of eye trouble, the needle must be inserted towards the direction of the other eyeball, 1 to 1.5 cun in depth with the needling reaction transmitted to the head. Sometimes Taichong (Liv 3) is the secondary point, used to invigorate qi and blood flow and check hyperactivity. Deep puncture is not allowed for Zulinqi (G 41) and it is usually punctured 0.5 to 0.6 cun in depth, the most shallow puncture point among the Eight Confluent Points. Ms Zeng, 32, had had migraine for years. It attacked before menstruation as a rule. She had thin tongue coating and string-taut pulse. Thirty treatments with the two points cured the case.

4) *Lieque (L 7) and Zhaohai (K 6)* These points are used to treat speech troubles, laryngitis, climacteric syndromes and globus hystericus. Lieque (L 7) is closely related to the Du Meridian and Chong Meridian and used to treat reproductive disorders in men and women. An elderly patient with Parkison's disease, mental disorders and speech troubles was treated with success by Lieque (L 7) and Zhaohai (K 6), accompanied by Lianquan (Ren 23) and Fengfu (Du 16).

Puncture techniques are as follows Perpendicular puncture is applied to Neiguan (P 6), Waiguan (SJ 5) and Zhaohai (K 6), 1.2 cun in depth. Lieque (L 7) is punctured 0.8 cun in depth.

Manipulations are usually done alternately from left to right, up to below or vice versa. For weak patients slight lift-thrust is conducted, but for cases of excess syndromes 360° rotation is used with more lift manipulation.

2. Five ancient techniques for varied cases

1) *Extreme shallow puncture* The needle is inserted very superficially, 0.05 cun in depth so that the muscles are not injured, good for lung disorders, patients of qi deficiency and those who are afraid of acupuncture. For instance, 42-year-old Ms Ma came for a consultation on October 14, 1980. She complained that she fell off a bicycle on June 12, 1980. She had lost consciousness for half an hour. She was diagnosed as having a minor cerebral concussion. Since then she became emaciated with symptoms of lassitude, nausea, poor memory and appetite, slow reaction, dizziness, insomnia, thin white coating, thready, deep and string-taut pulse. Her blood pressure was 112/80 mm Hg. This was a syndrome of qi and yin deficiency. Extreme shallow puncture was given to Sishenchong (Extra 6), Touwei (S 8), Sanyinjiao (Sp 6), Taixi (K 3) because she was weak and emaciated. Ten treatments alleviated dizziness and nausea. Then Touwei (S 8) was replaced by Anmian (Extra 9), Sizhukong (SJ 23) and Daling (P 7). Thirty treatments cured the case except for occasional dizziness on exertion.

2) *Leopard-spot puncture* Small blood vessels around the affected area are pierced to bleed so as to evacuate the sludged blood or local numbness and carbuncles. Infection must be prevented on treatment. For example, 62-year-old Mr. Liu came for a consultation on July 25, 1984. He complained that he had had a numb sensation in the left thigh and hypertension for five months. Two years ago he had minor hemiplegia. After treatment his condition improved, yet he had weakness in the arms. His blood pressure was 160/100 mmHg and he had a string-taut, slippery and rapid pulse, white, smooth and greasy tongue coating. It was a case of disturbance of the nutrient and defensive systems and invasion of the meridians by pathogenic wind. At first Huantiao (G 30), Fengchi (G 20), Yanglingquan (G 34), Weizhong (B 40), Kunlun (B 60) and Taichong (Liv 3) were selected in combination, with the plum-blossom needling applied to the lateral left thigh with a little success. Then the leopard-spot puncture was given to the numb area until it bled to remove obstruction of qi and blood stasis. Three treatments alleviated the condition and another ten treatments cured the case.

3) *Hegu puncture* This puncture is to directly puncture the muscles of the affected area, obliquely right and left for treating painful muscles, rheumatic muscles, muscular spasm and stiffness. For example, 52-year-old Ms Jiao came for a consultation on October 23, 1980. The patient complained that she had headache, hypertension (230/130 mmHg) and apoplexy. Physical examination showed right hemiplegia, speech trouble, blood pressure of 180/120 mmHg, dark red tongue with greasy coating. It was a case due to hyperactivity of liver yang and obstruction of the meridians. Quchi (LI 11), Zusanli (S 36), Lianquan (Ren 23) and Tongli (H 5) were used. Hegu puncture was applied to Lianquan (Ren 23). After one treatment the tongue could be moved out a little. Treatment was given every other day. About twenty treatments in two months alleviated the condition.

4) *Joint puncture* It is to directly puncture the muscles around the joints of the limbs without bleeding. The indications are disorders of tendons and tendon sheaths, and problems around the joints. For example, 59-year-old Mr. Quan came to be consulted on August 12, 1980. He complained that he had a pain in the metatarsophalangeal joints for three years. In 1979 there were many attacks. Dark grey skin colour and tenderness were seen in the first metatarsophalangeal joint. He could not walk properly because of the pain. Other symptoms included neck and lower back pain, hyperplasia of the lumbar vertebrae and wandering pain in the costal region. Physical examination showed liver (-), less urine discharge, dark red tongue, deep and irregular pulse. This was a case due to obstruction of qi and blood stasis. Joint puncture and Shu-point puncture were applied to Taichong (Liv 3), Taixi (K 3), Gongsun (Sp 4), Dadu (Sp 2) and Sanyinjiao (Sp 6) with the local plum-blossom needling. Three treatments were given each week. Two weeks later the skin colour of the first metatarsophalangeal joint turned to normal and tenderness was relieved.

5) *Shu-point puncture* This technique thrusts the needle deeply to the bone to treat osteal pain, spur chondritis, etc. due to kidney problems. For example, 53-year-old Ms Zhang came to be examined on October 9, 1980. The patient complained that he had had lower back pain for five years. There was no response to Western drugs,

herbs and physical therapy, and he was found to have a deformity of the spinal column and hyperplasia of the vertebra. Other symptoms included thin, white tongue coating, string-taut pulse, loose stools, poor appetite. It was a case of affliction of pathogenic cold in the bones. The Shu-point puncture and joint puncture were applied to the paravertebral points (from the 1st lumbar vertebra to the 5th lumbar vertebra) and Shenshu (B 23), Dachangshu (B 25). Six treatments alleviated the lower back pain. Fifteen treatments completely relieved the pain. Four months later the patient visited again, complaining that she had minor pain in the lower back, left foot and right palm. Five of the same treatment removed the lower back pain and other symptoms.

The nine acupuncture techniques and the twelve acupuncture techniques recorded in the *Miraculous Pivot* were also employed by Jiang. For instance, 41-year-old Mr. Liu came for examination on October 13, 1980. He complained that he had had a pain in the left tarsus for two days due to being caught in the rain. He also had a history of left traumatic knee arthritis for about ten years. Other symptoms included thin, greasy, yellowish tongue coating, slippery and rapid pulse. Laboratory tests showed a white blood cell count $16200/mm^3$; neutrophils, 70 percent; lymphocytes, 26 percent; and major monocytes, 4 percent. This was a case due to accumulation of heat in the meridians resulted from damp. The Shu-point puncture was applied to Zusanli (S 36), Yanglingquan (G 34), Sanyinjiao (Sp 6), Kunlun (B 60), Taixi (K 3), Gongsun (Sp 4), Jinggu (B 64) and Bafeng (Extra 36) with deep insertion and slow withdrawing. On the second day after the acupuncture, the pain was alleviated. White blood cell count showed $11100/mm^3$; neutrophils, 72 percent; and lymphocytes, 28 percent. After two treatments the patient could walk properly without any pain. White blood cell count showed $8200/mm^3$; neutrophils, 64 percent; lymphocytes, 32 percent; and oxyphil cells, 4 percent. Three treatments cured the case. Here is another example. Mr. Mi, 74, came for treatment on October 3, 1980. He said that he had trigeminal neuralgia for some years. There was no severe attack after the acupuncture therapy. Now he was suffering from a gingival abscess. A physical examination showed swollen gums, yellow tongue coating, and a rapid, string-taut pulse. It was a case due to accumulation of heat in the Stomach Meridian. A three-edged needle was used to prick the abscess and discharge the pus. The Shu-point puncture was applied to Hegu (LI 4), Quchi (LI 11) and Neiting (S 44). The needles were withdrawn slowly and the points were not pressed after acupuncture. Borneol powder was for external application. On the second day the swelling and pain were relieved. After the third visit the case was cured.

3. Differentiation of syndromes based on three pathogenic factors

1) *Exogenous affection of pathogenic wind and cold* Dazhui (Du 14) and Hegu (LI 4) are punctured, 1 cun in depth with the reducing method to bring about perspiration. After appearance of qi by the lift-thrust method, the needle is rotated to cause sweating. In case of absence of perspiration, the manipulation is done again or the needle is retained for some minutes. Dazhui (Du 14) is selected to invigorate the yang of the whole body and Hegu (LI 4), the Yuan-(source) point of the Yangming

Meridian, is for perspiration. (Hot boiled water is given to weak patients tending to have fainting spells during acupuncture to induce perspiration). If it is due to wind and heat with less perspiration, Quchi (LI 11) is added. For example, 62-year-old Ms Liu came for treatment on October 26, 1984. She had had a cold for two days with the symptoms of nasal obstruction, itchy throat, cough with thin, white phlegm, aversion to cold, fever, absence of perspiration, congestive throat, swollen tonsils (I°-II°), dark red tongue with thin, white coating, string-taut and tight pulse. This was a case due to exogenous invasion of pathogenic wind and cold. Dazhui (Du 14) and Hegu (LI 4) were selected with the reducing method and Zusanli (S 36) was used with the reinforcing method. The patient had perspiration all over the body and other symptoms were relieved after acupuncture therapy.

2) *Endogenous cause of diseases* This refers to excessive emotional changes harming the internal organs, of which the liver is often the most injured in anger. For a prolonged case acupuncture is given to Taixi (K 3), the Yuan-(source) point, with the even movement method for one or two minutes. For excess condition Dadun (Liv 1), the Jing-(well) point, or Xingjian (Ren 2), the Ying-(spring) point, is used with the rotation and the lift-thrust methods. Taixi (K 3) and Sanyinjiao (Sp 6) are added with the reinforcing method for the deficiency condition. Furthermore, points on the related meridians such as Daling (P 7) and Baihui (Du 20) are often selected. For instance, 36-year-old Ms Gao came for treatment on September 13, 1984. She complained that she had been very angry one day, and on the following day she had a tic on the right side of her face. The condition was relieved a little after a dozen of acupuncture treatments. But it became worse because of anger. Menstruation was delayed for ten days, with a discharge of a large amount and dark red clots. Physical examination showed thicker skin of the right side of the face, pale red tongue with thin white coating, deep and string-taut pulse. This was a case due to stagnation of liver qi. Daling (P 7), Dadun (Liv 1), Hegu (LI 4), Taichong (Liv 3), Chengjiang (Ren 24) and Fengchi (G 20) were selected to regulate qi flow in the Liver Meridian. Treatment was given once a day and the needle was retained for thirty minutes. The tic ceased with the acupuncture treatment. Two treatments cured the case. Then Daling (P 7), Taichong (Liv 3), Chengjiang (Ren 24) and Baihui (Du 20) were punctured to strengthen the effect.

3) *Strains* This is a condition due to neither endogenous factors nor exogenous affection of pathogenic factors. Local points or points on the opposite side are selected when a disease occurs at one side. Sometimes the patient is instructed to move his body during treatment, known as "puncture on body movement." If the strain covers a larger part of the body, distant points along the meridians are usually selected. Yanglinquan (G 34) is most helpful in treatment of strains. The point should be punctured 1 cun in depth with the reducing method. Zhigou (SJ 6) is also used to relieve pain because the Sanjiao Meridian controls qi. When this meridian is injured, pain occurs. For example, 63-year-old Ms Gao came for treatment on November 21, 1984. She complained of a pain in the right costal region for three days. The condition became worse on breathing and coughing. A physical examination showed mild tenderness, red tongue with dry yellow coating and a string-taut pulse. This was a case due

to impeded flow of qi and blood caused by the strained muscles. Zhigou (SJ 6), Yanglingquan (G 34) and Neiguan (P 6) were selected with needle retention for thirty minutes. The first treatment relieved the pain. Four treatments cured the case.

4. Combining acupuncture with herbs

Here is an example of how to cure a case of meningitis by Jiang. A 5-year-old boy with meningitis came to be consulted in 1964. Symptoms were high fever (41°C), severe headache, vomiting, restlessness, occasional convulsion, opisthotonos, abdominal pain, red cheeks and tongue, and rapid pulse. Fengchi (G 20) and Fengfu (Du 16) were punctured first, then Hegu (LI 4) and Zusanli (S 36) were needled with the reducing method without needle retention. Headache immediately disappeared. Afterwards, the patient was advised to take the following decoction known as Prescription of Powder of *Lonicera* and *Forsythia (Flos Lonicerae, Fructus Forsythiae, Fructus Arctii, Herba Menthae, Herba Schizonepetae, Semen Sojae Praeparatum, Radix Plalycodi, Radix Glycyrrhizae, Herba Lophoretic and Rhizoma Phragmitis),* to which *Radix Puerariae* and *Radix Isatidis* were added. The dosage of *Flos Lonicera Radix Puerariae* was doubled. Two doses cured the case. For this case acupuncture must be given first to check the severe condition, then herbs administered to strengthen the effect.

5. Lower He-(sea) points to be used to treat intestinal infarction

Each of the twelve regular meridians has a He-(sea) point, which is used for treating diseases of the six fu organs. Shangjuxu (S 37), Xiajuxu (S 39) and Zusanli (S 36) are often used by Jiang to treat muscular atrophy of the legs, myasthenia and abdominal problems. For instance, an 8-year-old child had intestinal infarction one day in 1963. It was suggested he should be operated on, but this was refused by his parents. Jiang treated him with acupuncture applied to both Zusanli (S 36), Shangjuxu (S 37) and Xiajuxu (S 39) with needle retention for one hour. When Zusanli (S 36) was needled, pain immediately reduced and vomiting ceased. On the second morning the patient could eat his breakfast. Another two treatments cured the case. To use several points lined one after another on a meridian is one of the ways to continuously strengthen the needling reaction and alleviate abdominal pain. Generally, local points are selected for chronic conditions and distal points for acute cases.

6. Cross selection of points

It refers to puncturing the left to treat the right or vice versa, or puncturing the left or right upper limb and the right or left lower limb. For instance, a patient who had thigh-bone and neck fracture was given 50 mg of dolantin. An hour later the pain was still there. Then Taichong (Liv 3) of the diseased side and Hegu (LI 4) of the healthy side were punctured. Strong stimulation of needling was given. A few minutes later the pain was relieved. After an interval the manipulations were conducted again and the pain finally ceased. The needle was retained for an hour and the patient slept well that night without feeling any pain.

7. Puncturing Yinbai (Sp 1) to stop hemorrhage

On the Eve of the Spring Festival of 1963 Jiang was invited to see a patient suffering from functional uterine bleeding. Yinbai (Sp 1) was selected for moxibustion. But he couldn't find moxa wool cones so he had to give acupuncture to both Yinbai (Sp 1) and finally the bleeding stopped. Then the patient was administered *Rehmannia Decoction with Artemisia* and the case was cured.

II. Case Analysis

Case 1: Hiccup (hiatal hernia)

Name, Wang x x; sex, male; age, 71; date of the first visit, September 5, 1980.

Complaints The patient had had hiccup and stomach distension for seven months. Barium meal examination showed a hiatal hernia. When he came for treatment his symptoms were distending pain in the stomach, worse after meals, hiccup, loose stools, occasional incontinence of urine, white and greasy coating on the tongue, string-taut pulse.

Differentiation Deficiency of spleen qi, failure of the stomach to send the food contents downwards.

Method Regulating the function of the spleen and stomach to make qi flow smoothly.

Prescription Neiguan (P 6) and Gongsun (Sp 4).

Treatment procedure Gongsun (Sp 4) and Neiguan (P 6) were selected as the chief points, and the secondary points used were Tanzhong (Ren 17), Zhongwan (Ren 12), Qihai (Ren 6), Tianshu (S 25), Zusanli (S 36) and Taichong (Liv 3). Treatment was given two or three times a week. Four months later the case was cured.

Explanation Although hiccup may be divided into cold, heat, deficiency and excess types, perverted flow of qi is the common cause. Gongsun (Sp 4) is used to bring down the perverted flow of qi and relieve pain because the Spleen Meridian connects with the stomach. Neiguan (P 6) is selected to regulate qi of the whole body since it is a point where the Yangwei Meridian runs through and the branch of the Pericardium Meridian connects with the Sanjiao Meridian. Tanzhong (Ren 17), Zhongwan (Ren 12) and Qihai (Ren 6) can regulate the pectoral qi, stomach qi and genuine qi of the elixir field. Tianshu (S 25), the Front (Mu) point of the Large Intestine Meridian, is used to promote transmission. Zusanli (S 36) is punctured to regulate qi in the fu organs and invigorate qi flow in the whole body. Taichong (Liv 13) is needled to alleviate pain and ease the liver.

Case 2: Depression (Schizophrenia)

Name, Liu x x; sex, female; age, 19; date of the first visit, September 1980.

Complaints She was very angry one day. Afterwards she did not like to speak or go to sleep at night for four months. Her condition was better after she was administered perphenazine, artane and other sedatives. Symptoms included dizziness, dull-looking impression, slow mind, absence of emotion, poor appetite, nightmares, weak, painful legs, white and greasy tongue coating, slow and forceless pulse.

Differentiation Mental disturbance due to stagnation of liver qi and obstruction by phlegm.

Method Invigorating yin and calming the mind.

Prescription Hegu (LI 4), Taichong (Liv 3), Houxi (SI 3), Shenmai (B 62), Shenmen (H 7), Kunlun (B 60) and Baihui (Du 20).

Treatment procedure At first there was no response to acupuncture therapy. Since this was a case due to disorders of Yangqiao Meridian, Houxi (SI 3) and Shenmai (B 62), two of the Eight Confluent points, were selected as the chief points, together with Taichong (Liv 3), Shenmen (H 7) and Sanyinjiao (Sp 6). The dosage of Western drugs was suggested to be reduced. After two treatments her puffy legs were cured and she began to cheer up. Forty treatments made her sleep well at night and her mood returned to normal. In the later stage of treatment she did not take any drugs for four months, then acupuncture ceased.

Explanation It is stated in the classic medical literature that "mania is due to yang excess, and general mental disorder is due to yin excess." Therefore the latter is caused by problems in the Liver, Gallbladder and Stomach Meridians. Houxi (SI 3) and Shenmai (B 62), two Confluent points, were used to restore normal sleep. Taichong (Liv 3), Shenmen (H 7) and Sanyinjiao (Sp 6) were needled to invigorate yin and calm the mind. Sedatives were suggested to be gradually reduced and finally ceased to prevent relapse and too much suppression of the nerves.

Case 3: Headache

Name, Sun x x; sex, male; age, 17; date of the first visit, August 7, 1980.

Complaints The patient had had frontal and temporal headache for over two months. On attack his complexion was red associated with nausea and vomiting. He was allergic to Western drugs and there was no response to about twenty decoctions of herbs. The condition became worse in the afternoon. Symptoms included poor appetite, yellow urine, red tongue border with white coating, string-taut, slippery and rapid pulse. His blood pressure was 108/60 mm Hg.

Differentiation Headache due to problems in the Shaoyang Meridians.

Method Removing problems from the Shaoyang Meridians.

Prescription Zulingqi (G 41), Waiguan (SJ 5), Hegu (LI 4), Taichong (Liv 3), Fengchi (G 20) and Taiyang (Extra 2).

Treatment procedure The first treatment eased the headache immediately. On the second visit he still had the headache. Acupuncture was given to Zulingqi (G 41) and Waiguan (SJ 5) with the cross manipulations with success. Another ten treatments cured the case. A follow-up study two years later showed there was no relapse.

Explanation Types of headache are usually divided according to the affected meridians. The present case was due to abundant heat in the Yangming Meridian, which was partly removed by acupuncture. Then Zulinqi (G 41) and Waiguan (SJ 5), the Confluent Points of Yangwei and Dai Meridians, were used to eliminate excessive heat in the Shaoyang Meridian. Meanwhile, they regulate the qi of the whole body and alleviate pain.

Case 4: Cerebral psychosis

Name, Li x x; sex, female; age, 56; date of the first visit, January 3, 1980.

Complaints The patient had had dull expression for a year which became worse. She was diagnosed as having cerebral psychosis. When she came for treatment, her intelligence was poor. She had a thin tongue coating and slippery pulse.

Differentiation Obstruction of meridians by phlegm, leading to mental disorder.

Method Removing phlegm and calming the mind.

Prescription Shenmen (H 7), Houxi (SJ 3), Zhaohai (K 6) and Lieque (L 7).

Treatment procedure After seven weeks' treatment she was willing to have stronger acupuncture stimulation. She began to know where to go and took medicine in time. She could answer questions normally and did cooking for the family. Three months later when she came to visit again, she was in good mental condition.

Explanation Lieque (L 7) and Zhaohai (K 6) function to dispel phlegm and invigorate the kidney function. Houxi (SI 3) and Shenmen (H 7) were added to calm the mind. Besides, phlegm-removing bolus was taken to strengthen the effect.

SKILLFUL NEEDLING TECHNIQUE AND EFFECTIVE METHODS FOR SAVING THE DYING AND CURING THE SICK

—Shi Jimin's Clinical Experience

Shi Jimin (1888-1973), also named Xiaoxian, was born in Liyang County, Jiangsu Province. He learned medicine handed down from the older generation, and took Dr. Zhang Zhongjing as his model, and followed over ten teachers. He started to practise medicine in 1937 in Shanghai and went to Chongqing in 1947. He took the combination of acupuncture and herbal medicine. Among his twelve books are *On Febrile Disease*, *Acupuncture Clinical Case Examples*, *Treatments for the Dying* and *Essentials of Auscultation and Olfaction*.

I. Academic Characteristics and Medical Specialities

1. Experience in differentiation and treatment of critical diseases

He accumulated much experience in the treatment of critical diseases. For example, when there appears pallor with cyanosis of lips, corediastasis, incontinence of urine and stool, fading pulse, running nose and flaccid hands, the patient is incurable. If the patient has pale complexion, but without incontinence of urine and stool, lips contracted, but the tongue free of stiffness and rolling, the cold four extremities over the elbow and knee joints but not icy cold, staring eyes but free of astigmatism, the eyes closed but with froth in the mouth and strong snoring, hidden or fading pulse but Fuyang pulse (the pulse of arteria dorsalis pedis) and heart beating available, he is curable. Emergency management should be given by prying open the mouth and touching the tongue with a finger. If it is slippery with much fluid, it reflects the direct attack by pathogenic cold. When profuse sweating and cold limbs appear, it reflects the pathogenic cold in the interior blocking the qi circulation and collapse of yang. In this case, strong moxibustion is advisable to Baihui (Du 20) superiorly to strengthen the yang qi of the Du Meridian, and to Yongquan (K 1) inferiorly to strengthen the primary qi of the Shaoyin Meridian so as to collect the floating yang. At the same time, moxibustion at Shenque (Ren 8) and Guanyuan (Ren 4) is applied to eliminate the pathogenic cold in the abdomen by invigorating yang. The dying could also be saved by applying direct moxibustion with three slender medicinal paper rolls to Renzhong (Du 26). In addition, decoctions for cold extremities and for restoring yang from collapse are applied to dispel pathogenic cold and support yang. If there is salivation with stagnation of phlegm in the throat, which reflects the pathogenic cold affecting the throat, moxibustion at Tiantu (Ren 22) and

Tanzhong (Ren 17) is applied and decoction for cold extremities with ginger juice and Fructus Euodiae, or decoction of Fructus Amomi and Fhizoma Pinelliae, decoction of Fructus Euodiae, are taken. All these are the effective methods to rescue the deficiency and cold.

Dr. Shi was also experienced in dealing with heat syndromes. For the syndrome which is difficult in differentiation of cold or heat. If the tongue is not moist, but thorny, it is certainly a heat syndrome. In the treatment of heat syndrome, Dr. Shi emphasizes pricking the twelve Jing-Well points, Weizhong (B 40) and Baihui (Du 20) (three points around Baihui) to cause bleeding, and puncturing Renzhong (Du 26) shallowly and Chengjiang (Ren 24) deeply. This management is known as yin-yang needling method. In case of syncope with sudden fall, loss of consciousness, pallor and normal lips, it is considered to be caused by temporary obstruction due to stagnation of liver qi which is mingled with sudden invasion of exogenous pathogenic factors, or obstruction of clear passage by phlegm leading to imbalance of yin and yang. Treatment should be given to regulate yin and yang, restore their functions to free the qi activity. It is not advisable to purge crudely. Needle Daling (P 7) and Jianshi (P 5) to promote the circulation of qi of the pericardium, and needle Xingjian (Liv 2) to harmonize the liver qi, and needle Zusanli (S 36) to pacify the stomach qi.

2. Light and skillful technique by needling both Front-Mu and Back-Shu points, and by applying the reinforcing and reducing method without needle retention

Dr. Shi was good at applying the skillful and light technique with short needles to few points, and reinforcing or reducing method without retaining the needle. He often inserted two needles with both hands at the same time, one Back-Shu point and one Front-Mu point or one point from the upper body and one from the lower part. He considered that the qi of the zang organs accumulates in the Front-Mu points and is transmitted into the Back-Shu points. The simultaneous needling of Back-Shu and Front-Mu points may dispel pathogenic factors from yin via yang for excess syndromes, and help promote the distribution of qi and blood for deficiency syndromes. Simultaneous selection of the points from the upper and lower boby may help to connect the circulation of qi in the meridians mostly for excess syndromes. There was a patient who had suffered from a postauricular tumour for half a month. Many doctors believed that the tumour could be eliminated, but should take a long period. Dr. Shi said, "Immediate effect can be expected and the patient can be cured in a few days." He punctured Waiguan (SJ 5) and Yifeng (SJ 17). When the needling sensation arrived, he reduced Waiguan (SJ 5) first and then reinforced Yifeng (SJ 17). The tumour was much reduced after fifteen minutes and disappeared the next day. There was another patient suffering from cough for months, which was diagnosed as exhaustion of lung qi. Dr. Shi needled Back-Shu and Front-Mu points by reinforcing Feishu (B 13) and reducing Zhongfu (L 1). The cough stopped when the needles were removed. There was a female patient suffering from lower abdominal pain (diagnosed in Western medicine as adnexitis), leading to inguinal tuberculosis (enlargement of limph node) and she had difficulty walking. Dr. Shi punctured Ququan (Liv 8) with the needles retained for thirty minutes.

The mass dispersed and she walked normally after the treatment.

3. Acupuncture fainting saved by moxibustion and moxibustion fainting treated by acupuncture

It is a therapeutic method created by Dr. Shi to cure fainting caused either by acupuncture or by moxibustion. He considered that acupuncture fainting was caused by much reducing of yang qi, while moxibustion fainting was caused by upward movement of yang qi. He said: "My colleagues often have fainting cases. Although most of them were cured by needling, there did exist some cases who were not cured. It is perfect to apply moxibustion for acupuncture fainting and needling for moxibustion fainting. I have travelled many places to practise medicine and teach students. The same management was adopted whenever I had such a case and an accident has never occurred. Points are selected from three parts of the body: the upper, the middle and the lower. Select the points in the lower body for the fainting caused by the upper points needled, the points in the upper body for the fainting caused by the lower points needled, and the points in the both upper and lower body for the fainting caused by the middle points needled. For example, select the points on the lower extremities for the fainting caused by the points needled on the head and upper extremities, select the points on the upper extremities for the fainting caused by the points needled on the lower extremities, and select the points on the upper and lower extremities for the fainting caused by the points needled on the trunk. Points can never be selected from the same area as the points needled that have caused fainting. The following are the effective points: Head, Baihui (Du 20); upper extremities, Neiguan (P 6), Jianshi (P 5); lower extremities, Zusanli (S 36), Yongquan (K 1); and loss of consciousness, Renzhong (Du 26). In mild cases, moxibustion is applied with a medicinal fuse, and in severe cases, heavy indirect moxibustion with several layers of paper is adopted. The same principle is taken when needling is used for fainting caused by moxibustion with mild stimulation." In 1969, a case of fainting caused by needling was managed by puncturing Renzhong (Du 26) and Baihui (Du 20), but no response. Dr. Shi used an ignited cigarette end to give the patient indirect moxibustion with paper, and the patient regained consciousness at the end of treatment. Another example. In 1956, a female patient from a coal mine had a reaction to an injection of penicillin, and acremaline and coramine injection did not help her, Dr. Shi applied moxibustion to Baihui (Du 20), Renzhong (Du 26) and Hegu (LI 4) and the patient was cured.

II. Case Analysis

Case 1: Food fainting

Name, Ran x x; sex, male; age, 48; date of the first visit, August 6, 1962.

Complaints The patient was tired and wanted to get some medicine from the dispensary, but he suddenly fell on the ground with such symptoms as pallor, clenching of teeth, foul breath, cold limbs, string-taut and rapid pulse, and thick and sticky tongue coating.

Differentiation Food fainting due to stagnation in the middle jiao, leading to dysfunction of the qi activity in ascending and descending and dysfunction of yin and yang, giving rise to cold limbs, food retention turning into phlegm which clouds the mind and hence loss of consciousness. Treatment was given to resuscitate, resolve phlegm, pacify the stomach and regulate the liver.

Prescription Neiguan (P 6), Zusanli (S 36), Fenglong (S 40) and Xingjian (Liv 2).

Treatment procedure Puncture Neiguan (P 6) with even method and Zusanli (S 36), Fenglong (S 40) and Xingjian (Liv 2) with reducing method. The patient regained consciousness after the treatment.

Case 2: Heat fainting

Name, Yang x x; age, 45; date of the first visit, March 10, 1962.

Complaints The patient suddenly lost consciousness at midnight with such symptoms as lacrimation, bleeding in the mouth, cold limbs, slight sweating and flapping of the ala nasi, dry stool, hidden pulse and full Fuyang pulse. The tongue was dry with thin coating. Although the patient had hidden pulse on the hand, the Fuyang pulse was full, the tongue was dry, as well as the stool, and bleeding in the mouth presented, it was therefore a heat syndrome, in which the extreme heat looked like yin, the fire-heat in the liver and stomach misted the pericardium, indicating a heat syncope. Treatment was given to restrict yang, restore yin and activate the heart qi.

Prescription Zhongchong (P 9), Neiguan (P 6), Xuehai (Sp 10), Zusanli (S 36) and Xingjian (Liv 2).

Treatment procedure Prick Zhongchong (P 9) to cause bleeding, puncture Neiguan (P 6) with even method, and Zusanli (S 36), Xingjian (Liv 2), Xuehai (Sp 10) with reducing method. The patient regained consciousness three minutes after the treatment.

REINFORCING AND REDUCING WITH MOXIBUSTION AND SIMPLE SELECTION OF ACUPOINTS

—Zhong Yueqi's Clinical Experience

Zhong Yueqi (1900-1981) was a native of Anqiu County, Shandong Province. He graduated from Wuxi Chinese Acupuncture School run by the famous acupuncturist Cheng Dan'an in 1937. From 1946 to 1956, he practised medicine in Qingdao. In 1956, he attended Shandong Research Class on Traditional Chinese Medicine. In 1957, he was appointed as a teacher working in the Acupuncture Teaching and Research Section in Shandong School for Advanced Studies of Traditional Chinese Medicine. In 1960, he was transferred to Shandong College of Traditional Chinese Medicine and worked in the Acupuncture Teaching and Research Section. He spent all his life teaching, in clinical practice and researching ancient classics of acupuncture. He helped compile the books *Explanation on Plain Questions of Internal Classics with Modern Chinese*, *Check and Translation of Systematic Classic of Acupuncture*, *Explanation on Miraculous Pivot*, *Simple Acupuncture*, *Charts of Acupuncture Meridians and Points*, etc. He also published some academic articles such as Discussion on Selection of Acupuncture Points and Divergence in Proportional Measurement.

I. Academic Characteristics and Medical Specialities

1. Precise selection of points and proper depth of needling

Dr. Zhong selected points precisely. He followed the principle given in the book *Ode to the Standard of Mystery*: One good point from one meridian is better than five points from three meridians. He selected points precisely and summed up a lot of simple and accurate methods for locating points in his clinical practice. For example, when locating Xiabai (L 4) in male, ink the two nipples and then ask the patient to attach the two arms on the chest. The dyed points on the arms by the nipples are the required points. When locating Yangxi (LI 5), ask the patient to place the hand on the lateral side, extend the thumb and index fingers, stick up the thumb forcefully and there will appear a depression posterior to the divergent bone where the required point is located. When locating Pianli (LI 6), ask the patient to place the arm on the ulnar side with the elbow joint flexed, draw a line connecting Yangxi (LI 5) and Quchi (LI 11); the point is located in the depression 3 cun superior to Yangxi (LI 5) and a little lateral to the line. When locating Wenliu (LI 7), flex the arm and make a tight fist, which will give rise to a muscular prominence and the point is located at the lower end of the prominence. When selecting Daying (S 5), ask the patient to close the mouth and blow air in the cheek until it bulges. There will appear a groove at the border of the palatine bone where an artery can be felt on pressure, thus the point is found. When locating Liangqiu (S 34), ask the patient to sit with both legs flexed, and the point is 2 cun superior to the middle of the knee and 1 cun lateral to it. When locating Zusanli (S 36), ask the patient to sit with the legs flexed and place his hand on the knee with the index finger touching the tibia below the knee. Where the tip of the middle finger reaches is the point which is 3 cun below Xiyan (Extra) and between the two tendons lateral to the tibia. Gongsun (Sp 4) is located at the junction of the first metatarsal bone and first cuneform bone. When locating this point, push downward with the finger from the highest portion of the dorsum of the foot and there is a depression on the medial side of the bone, in which the point is located. When locating Fuhai (Sp 16), let the patient sit or lie on the back with the arm spread, it is the crossing point directly below the nipple which levels with Jianli (Ren 11). When selecting Shaofu (H 8), ask the patient to flex the fingers towards the palm. Where the tip of the small finger reaches is the point, which is between the first and second metacarpal bones and levels with Laogong (P 8). Tinggong (SI 19) is in the depression anterior to the ear tragus. When heavily pressing the point, there may be ringing in the ear. When locating Chengshan (B 57), ask the patient to stand with the two arms raising upward towards a wall and the heel apart from the floor, there will appear a depression below the muscle gastrocnemius where the point is located; or ask the patient to take a prone position with the lower limbs extended and the sole facing upward, there will be a depression where the point is located. When locating Tianjing (SJ 10), ask the patient to flex the elbow and the point is in the depression 1 cun above the tip of the elbow (olecranon). When locating Xiaoluo (SJ 12), ask the patient to take a front-sitting position, it is directly below the lateral end of the shoulder and 4.5 cun superior to the tip of the elbow; or ask the patient to make a loose fist and stretch the arm with the palm side facing downward, then make the fist tight and twist the forearm counterclockwise and there will appear a muscular prominence, the lower border of which is where the point is located. When locating Jiaosun (SJ 20), fold the ear forward and the ear apex will point to the therapeutic point; or press where the ear apex reaches and ask the patient open and close the mouth. The point is located at the place where one can feel the movement of the mouth. When locating Tongziliao (G 1), ask the patient to close the eye and the point is at the end of outer canthus. Jianjing (G 21) is located in the depression posterior to the acromion. When pressing the shoulder with three fingers (index, middle and ring fingers), the point is located in the depression felt by the middle finger. When locating Tiantu (Ren 22), let the patient lie down, the point is located in the depression 0.5 cun superior to the upper semilunar border of sternum. When locating Mingmen (Du 4), the doctor may press the umbilicus with the both hands, then move the fingers laterally to the spine where the point is located. Yaoyan (Extra) is located in the depression on either side of the lumbus when the lumbar muscle is relaxed. The above mentioned methods are simple, accurate and easy to practise, and are the experiences obtained from his long-standing clinical practice.

2. Application of moxibustion for reinforcing and reducing

Based on differentiation of syndromes, Dr. Zhong thinks that moxibustion often works when acupuncture does not and the therapeutic effect is often better than that of acupuncture. Moxibustion can be applied to reinforce qi and blood when they are deficient, lift the qi of the meridian when it sinks, remove obstructions from meridians when they are blocked, and lift the qi in the middle jiao when it sinks.

1) *Prevention of windstroke* If a patient had numbness of the fingers, dizziness and vertigo, temporal stiffness of the tongue and dysphasia before an attack of apoplexy, we can use moxibustion with moxa cones to Baihui (Du 20), Fengchi (G 20), Jianjing (G 21), Quchi (LI 11), Fengshi (G 31), Zusanli (S 36) and Xuanzhong (G 39) for prevention.

2) *Treatment of cough* Moxibustion with moxa cones on Taodao (Du 13) can be used for coughs in either deficiency or excess. For a fresh case, three to seven cones should be given and for a chronic case, treat once a day. The therapeutic effect can be expected in a few days.

3) *Treatment of nausea and vomiting* Moxibustion at Tanzhong (Ren 17), Qihai (Ren 6), Neiguan (P 6), Weishu (B 21) and Sanyinjiao (Sp 6) with five to seven cones each should be applied. Secondary points: Tianding (LI 17), Zhongkui (Extra), Danshu (B 19) and Hegu (LI 4).

4) *Treatment of headache* In case of deficiency of qi, apply moxibustion at Baihui (Du 20), Dazhui (Du 14), Zhongwan (Ren 12), Qihai (Ren 6) and Zusanli (S 36) with moxa sticks. In case of deficiency of blood, use moxibustion at Touwei (S 8), Taiyang (Extra), Quchi (LI 11), Hegu (LI 4) and Ganshu (B 18). Secondary points: Fengchi (G 20), Geshu (B 17), Pishu (B 20), Shenmen (H 7) and Zusanli (S 36). Apply moxibustion at each point for three to five minutes.

5) *Treatment of dizziness and vertigo* In the case of deficient blood, indirect moxibustion with ginger is applied to Baihui (Du 20), Shangxing (Du 23), Shenzhu (Du 12), Zhiyang (Du 9), Ganshu (B 18) and Pishu (B 20). Each point is treated with one date-pit-sized moxa cone per day and good result can be expected in one month.

6) *Treatment of abdominal pain around the umbilicus* In case of abdominal pain around the umbilicus caused by deficiency and cold, moxibustion is given to Shenque (Ren 8) and Qihai (Ren 6) for about one hour until the pain is arrested.

7) *Treatment of lumbar muscle strain* Apply direct moxibustion to Shenshu (B 23), Yaoyangguan (Du 3), Mingmen (Du 4), Zusanli (S 36) with five to seven cones each. Frequent treatments may reduce attacks.

8) *Treatment of diarrhoea due to deficiency and cold* Apply moxibustion to Tianshu (S 25), Qihai (Ren 6), Zhongwan (Ren 12) and Zusanli (S 36) with moxa sticks. Each point should be treated for five minutes.

9) *Treatment of toothache* The lower toothache often has a tenderness on Pianli (LI 6) and the upper toothache on Jiexi (S 41). Indirect moxibustion with ginger may be applied to the tenderness with ten to twenty cones each time.

10) *Treatment of uterine bleeding* Shimen (Ren 5) is selected for moxibustion with seven cones, Guanyuan (Ren 4) with seven cones, Yinbai (Sp 1) with five cones, and Sanyinjiao (Sp 6) with five cones. Secondary points: Pishu (B 20), Shenshu (B 23), Qihai

(Ren 6), Dadun (Liv 1). Five to seven cones should be used for each point.

11) *Treatment of throat disorders* During attacks, apply moxibustion at Dazhui (Du 14) with three to seven grain-size moxa cones. Moxa sticks can also be used to Zhaohai (K 6) bilaterally for four to five minutes on each side. Good results may be expected after three treatments (once a day).

12) *Treatment of morbid leukorrhea*

a. Select Sanjiaoshu (B 22), Shenshu (B 23), Zhongliao (B 33), Qihai (Ren 6), Zhongji (Ren 3), Xuehai (Sp 10) and Sanyinjiao (Sp 6) for moxibustion with seven grain-size moxa cones each. Moxa sticks are also applicable.

b. Select Daimai (G 26), Guanyuan (Ren 4), Yaoyangguan (Du 3) and Sanyinjiao (Sp 6) for moxibustion with moxa stick for five minutes each time. Treat once a day.

13) Treatment of chronic infantile convulsion Apply moxa sticks to Dazhui (Du 14), Pishu (B 20), Weishu (B 21), Guanyuan (Ren 4), Qihai (Ren 6) and Zusanli (S 36). Each point should be treated for five minutes.

14) *Treatment of morbid night crying*

a. Prepare one bundle of green garlic and two bundles of moxa leaves into small pieces, mix up and put them into two small white cloth bags to be steamed. When the two bags are hot, squeeze out the excessive fluid. Put one of them on the umbilicus when it is not burning to the skin. Replace with another one when it is getting cold. The two bags are used alternately.

b. Moxibustion is given to Ganshu (B 18), Mingmen (Du 4) with three half-grain-size moxa cones each.

15) *Treatment of common cold* Feishu (B 13) and Xinshu (B 15) are selected for moxibustion with three cones each. Prevention: Apply indirect moxibustion with ginger to Shenzhu (Du 12), Ganshu (B 18), Pishu (B 20), Shenshu (B 23), Zhongwan (Ren 12), Qihai (Ren 6) and Tianshu (S 25) with three cones each, and Zusanli (S 36) with moxa sticks for fifteen minutes every morning on either side alternately.

16) *Treatment of malaria*

a. Dazhui (Du 14) is selected for direct moxibustion, indirect moxibustion with ginger, or moxibustion with moxa sticks with good therapeutic results;

b. Crush pepper into powder and spread it on a piece of plaster. Puncture Dazhui (Du 14) retaining the needle and stick the plaster on the point when the needle is removed. This could be done two hours before an attack.

17) *Treatment of deep-rooted boil*

a. Deep-rooted boil at the angle of the mouth. Moxibustion is applied at the top of the boil with five small cones, then at Shousanli (LI 10) with twenty cones. Treatment must be given for three days and generally three treatments may cure a case.

b. Deep-rooted boil at the frontal eminence. Method for locating point: Take a piece of string which is as long as the circumference of the abdomen around the umbilicus, attach the midpoint of the string on the lower border of the laryngeal prominence, drop and spread the two ends of the string along both sides of the nape of the neck and back; the place where the two ends meet on the midline of the back is the point for moxibustion. Treat once a day with five cones each time.

c. Red thready deep-rooted boil. Ignite a piece of lampwick (rush) soaked with plant oil and give a flash burning to the distal end of the red thread, and it can be found that the red thread is shortened slowly. Repeated practice may make the red thread shortened and localized at the root of the boil. Finally do it once again at the original distal end of the red thread.

d. In case of deep-rooted boil located on the hand, foot or face, early moxibustion is advisable. Apply moxibustion at the point 4 cun above the palm and between the two tendons (1 cun above Jianshi (P 5)) with fourteen cones on the left side in male and right side in female; or apply moxibustion at the point 2.5 cun above and 0.3 cun medial to Lingdao (H 4) with fifty cones and repeat the treatment for two to three days; or at Yanglao (SI 6), Shousanli (LI 10) and Hegu (LI 4) with thirty to a hundred cones.

18) *Scorpion bite of the wrist* Take a piece of thread as long as the girth of the wrist, place it straight with one end attached to the tip of the middle finger and the other end the midpalm, measure the width of the mouth of the patient. Locate the point one width of the mouth above the other end on the palm. Apply moxibustion at this point with seven cones and good therapeutic result can be expected.

Dr. Zhong's clinical practice proved the above mentioned methods highly effective.

3. Principal and secondary points to be selected and the order of therapeutic methods to be used

Dr. Zhong followed the principle given in the book *Internal Classic* in his practice. He considered that points should be selected less and better. For this, a doctor should first have a keen understanding of the action and indication of each point, and then he can get twice the result with half the effort. For example, when treating hemiplegia caused by windstroke, Quchi (LI 11) is the principal point for the upper limbs and Yanglingquan (G 34) the principal one for the lower limbs. Jianyu (LI 15), Waiguan (SJ 5) and Hegu (LI 4) are selected in combination for the upper limbs and Huantiao (B 30), Xuanzhong (B 39) in combination for the lower limbs. When treating insomnia, Shenmen (H 7), Neiguan (P 6) and Zusanli (S 36) are taken as the principal points and Ganshu (B 18) (for moxibustion), Xingjian (Liv 2) and Sanyinjiao (Sp 6) (for acupuncture with retaining of the needles) are selected in combination. When treating facial paralysis, Jiache (S 6), Dicang (S 4), Hegu (LI 4), Taichong (Liv 3) and Sizhukong (SJ 23) are taken as the main points and Renzhong (Du 26), Yangbai (G 14), Quanliao (SI 18) are selected in combination. When treating tense syndrome of windstroke, it is advisable to select the twelve Jing-well points as the principal ones for bleeding and select Renzhong (Du 26) and Jiache (S 6) in combination. In case of windstroke of the flaccid type, it is advisable to apply big-cone moxibustion to Qihai (Ren 6) and Guanyuan (Ren 4). When treating vertigo of the deficiency type, moxibustion is used mainly to Baihui (Du 20), Shenting (Du 24), Taiyang (Extra) and Zusanli (S 36), and to Ganshu (B 18), Shenshu (B 23), Guanyuan (Ren 4) and Qihai (Ren 6) in combination. When treating vertigo caused by phlegm-fire, mainly puncture Fengchi (G 20), Hegu (LI 4), Fenglong (S 40), Shangxing (Du 23), prick Taiyang (Extra) to cause bleeding, and select Xingjian (Liv 2), Xiaxi (G 43) and Daling (P 7) in combination. For abdominal pain, puncture Zhongwan (Ren 12), Zusanli (S 36), Gongsun (Sp 4), and select Liangmen (S 21) in combination (moxibustion should be applied for cold syndrome and needling for heat syndrome). For sciatica, mainly penetrate Tiaokou (S 38) towards Chengshan (B 57), retain the needle for ten minutes, then remove the needle and puncture Huantiao (B 30), Yanglingquan (B 34) and Xuanzhong (G 39).

Dr. Zhong paid much attention to the order of the points to be selected during treatment, since he considered it to be closely related to the therapeutic effect. For example, when treating tense syndrome of windstroke, the twelve Jing-well points should be needled first and points Renzhong (Du 26) and Jianche (S 6) second. When treating sciatica, puncture Tiaokou (S 38) towards Chengshan (B 57) on the diseased side first with ten minutes retaining of the needle, and then needle Huantiao (G 30), Yanglingquan (G 34) and Xuanzhong (G 39). For facial paralysis, puncture the points on the healthy side first, then three to five points are used for moxibustion on the affected side such as Jiache (S 6), Dicang (S 4), Yangbai (G 14), Sizhukong (SJ 23) and Renzhong (Du 26), and finally select one or two points on the hand and foot. When dealing with the points on the face, if moxibustion follows acupuncture, better results will be obtained. When treating deep-rooted boil, first prick Lingtai (Du 10) to cause bleeding, then select other points according to the area affected. For example, select Hegu (LI 4) for the deep-rooted boil on the face and Weizhong (B 40) for that on the back. With this method, good therapeutic results will be obtained for every treatment.

II. Case Analysis

Case 1: Aura of apoplexy

Name, Gao x x; age, 49.

Complaints She suffered from sudden attack of twisting of mouth, vertigo and distending pain in the head. The blood pressure was 185/110 mmHg. Diagnosis made by the Acupuncture Department in the hospital was aura of apoplexy. After twelve acupuncture treatments, the blood pressure was lowered to 158/90 mmHg. Later, treatment was given once every three to five days. Recently she had a quarrel with a family member, which gave rise to the right hemiplegia, aphasia, twisting of mouth, dizziness and headache, and she came to the clinic. Examination: She remained mentally clear, her speech was difficult, the mouth was twisted to the left side, the tongue coating was sticky and pulse string-taut and rolling. Blood pressure: 230/125 mmHg. The movement of the right limbs was limited. Diagnosis: Stirring-up of liver wind in the interior. Principle of treatment: Soothe the liver, dispel wind and remove obstruction of the meridians.

Prescription Jiache (S 6), Dicang (S 4), Jianyu (LI 15), Quchi (LI 11), Hegu (LI 4), Tongli (H 5), Zusanli (S 36) and Yanglingquan (G 34). In addition, twelve Jing-well points to be pricked for bleeding.

Treatment procedure After one treatment with reducing method, the deviation of the philtrum was alleviated and the pulse was still string-taut and rolling. Blood pressure: 200/110 mmHg. Treatment was continued with the above points ten times and the blood pressure was lowered to 140/85 mmHg, deviation of mouth disappeared, speech was clear and the right leg was fine. However, the movement of the right arm was still poor. Then the points Waiguan (SJ 5), Shousanli (LI 10) were added and she was cured after twenty-one more treatments.

Explanation This is a case of hyperactivity of liver yang due to deficiency of kidney yin in which the liver yang stirred up the endogenous wind because of anger. Complicated with phlegm-fire, the blood followed the perversion of qi, affecting the meridians, giving rise to facial paralysis, hemiplegia and aphasia. Therefore Jiache (S 6) and Dicang (S 4) were selected to regulate the qi of the meridians on the face to cure facial paralysis. Jianyu (LI 15), Quchi (LI 11) and Hegu (LI 4) were needled to activate the qi and blood of the Yangming Meridian. The twelve Jing-well points were pricked to cause bleeding to regulate the yin and yang in general. Tongli (H 5) is the point from the diverging meridian of Hand-Shaoying which may activate the circulation of collaterals on the tongue to cure aphasia. Zusanli (S 36) and Yanglingquan (G 34) can not only regulate the qi and blood to soothe the perversion of qi of the liver and gallbladder, but also activate qi and blood circulation of the lower limbs. The above-mentioned points selected together may soothe the liver, dispel wind and remove obstructions from the meridians.

Case 2: Enuresis

Name, Wang x x; sex, female; age, 7.

Complaints The girl suffered from whooping cough complicated with pneumonia when she was five. She was cured after hospitalization, but had suffered from enuresis once or twice each night since then. It was worse and occurred even during the day when affected by a cold and cough. Examination: The tongue was pale with thin and white coating, the pulse was deficient and thready, and the facial complexion pale. Diagnosis: Deficiency of lung and kidney qi. Principle of treatment: Tonify the lung and warm the kidney.

Prescription Select Pangguangshu (B 28), Shenshu (B 23), Guanyuan (Ren 4) and Sanyinjiao (Sp 6) for both needling and moxibustion, and Fengmen (B 12) and Feishu (B 13) for moxibustion only.

Treatment procedure Cough was alleviated and frequency of enuresis reduced after three treatments. Same points except Feishu (B 13) and Fengmen (B 12) were selected for eight treatments and the patient was cured.

Explanation It is a case of deficiency of lung qi leading to weakness of water passage. Therefore, Pangguangshu (B 28) and Shenshu (B 23) were selected to strengthen the kidney qi so as to invigorate the function of the bladder. Guanyuan (Ren 4) is located in the lower jiao where the bladder is, and it is the Front-Mu point of the small intestine and the crossing point of the three yin meridians and Chong and Ren Meridians as well. It can warm and tonify the primary qi in the lower jiao to strengthen the controlling function of the bladder. Sanyinjiao (Sp 6) is the crossing point of the three yin meridians of foot. It has the function to strengthen the spleen, warm the kidney and nourish the liver. Moxibustion applied to Fengmen (B 12) and Feishu (B 13) can tonify the qi of the lung and strengthen the function of the water passage.

Case 3: Heat Bi syndrome

Name, Wu x x; sex, male; age, 28.

Complaints At the initial stage, the patient had fever, aversion to wind, sweating, spinal pain and redness and swelling in the joints of the shoulder, elbow, wrist, knee and ankle. The pain became worse after exertion. Diagnosis made by a hospital was rheumatic arthritis. Western medicine was given for the treatment without a marked therapeutic effect. Finally he came for the acupuncture treatment.

Examination Red tongue with slightly yellow and sticky coating, spiritlessness, tychypnea, groaning, feeble speech, redness and swelling of the elbow and knee joints, rapid and superficial rapid and soft pulse.

Diagnosis Obstruction of the meridians caused by wind-damp turning into heat.

Principle of treatment Clear heat, resolve damp, remove obstruction from the meridians and arrest pain.

Prescription Dazhui (Du 14), Fengmen (B 12), Quchi (LI 11), Neiguan (P 6), Shenmen (H 7), Sanyinjiao (Sp 6), Yanglingquan (G 34) and Kunlun (B 60).

Treatment procedure After the first treatment with reducing method, the fever was lowered and joint pain alleviated, but the patient still had sweating, palpitation and shortness of breath. Treatment was given again with the above points, Yinxi (H 6) and Daling (P 7), the fever then subsided and the redness and swelling were alleviated. The patient was cured after eight treatments.

Explanation This is a case of Heat Bi syndrome caused by long-time accumulation of wind and damp which have turned into heat. Therefore, select Dazhui (Du 14), Fengmen (B 12), and Quchi (LI 11) to dispel wind and clear heat, Neiguan (P 6) and Shenmen (H 7) to activate the heart qi and nourish the heart and mind, Sanyinjiao (Sp 6) to strengthen the spleen and resolve damp, Yanglingquan (G 34) and Kunlun (B 60) to relax tendons and activate the circulation of the collaterals so as to arrest pain. All the above points selected together have the function to clear heat, dispel wind, resolve damp, remove obstructions from the meridians, nourish the heart, calm the mind and arrest pain.

STRESS ON DIFFERENTIATION OF QI, TONING THE SPLEEN AND PURGING THE LIVER OF PATHOGENIC FIRE

—He Huiwu's Clinical Experience

He Huiwu (1900-1979) was a native of Weixian County, Shandong Province. He began studying the medical classics in childhood and obtained his medical training in the apprenticeship system. He started his medical career in his native town when he was 18 years old. In 1927 he went to Japan and learned acupuncture techniques from two established Japanese acupuncturists. From 1932 to 1936 he studied at an acupuncture college in Japan. When he returned to China he settled down in Beijing. In 1939 and 1950 he passed twice the examination for a licence to practise Western medicine. He had not only knew ancient Chinese, but also had a good command of English and Japanese, a solid grounding with which to inherit and develop acupuncture therapy. Since 1964 he served as the Deputy Director of the Acupuncture Department, Beijing Hospital of Traditional Chinese Medicine. His works included *New Understanding of Acupuncture*, *Two Newly Found Meridians*, *Note on Acupuncture*, *Explanation of How to Treat Ten Kinds of Diseases* and *My Understanding of Meridians.*

I. Academic Characteristics and Medical Specialities

1. Regulating qi as the source of force and the fundamental aspect in treating diseases

In differentiating syndromes Dr. He emphasized qi, pointing out qi is not only the source of force of life, but also the material basis of nutrition, because qi is derived from the vital essence of the parents and food nutrients. No one can survive without qi, which nourishes the zang-fu organs and at the same time is generated by them. Heart qi controls the mind; lung qi cleanses the inspired air and keeps it flowing downward; liver qi helps the normal flow of qi and blood; spleen qi works for digestion and transportation; kidney qi controls and promotes inspiration; stomach qi serves to receive food and water; qi of the small intestine controls transportation and transformation; qi of the large intestine functions to pass the content on; qi of the bladder helps to restore urine; qi of the sanjiao functions to regulate water metabolism, production and transformation of food essence, etc. In terms of pathological changes, external affection often brings about disorders of qi, e.g. an attack of the lung by exogenous pathogenic factors leads to stagnated lung qi; disturbance of the stomach and spleen qi results from invasion of the stomach and intestines by pathogenic cold; and pathogenic heat invading the pericardium leads to disturbance of the heart qi. Perverted flow of the liver qi is present in anger, smooth flow of the liver qi is seen in happiness, grief causes qi loss, mental anxiety brings about depression of the spleen qi, and fear causes the kidney qi to sink. On the other hand, disorders of qi naturally reveal problems of the zang-fu organs. Disturbance of the heart qi (excess condition) results in mania, and insufficient heart qi (deficiency syndrome) leads to palpitation. Impediment of the lung qi (excess condition) brings about cough and asthma, and insufficient lung qi (deficiency condition) leads to shortness of breath. Stagnated spleen qi (excess condition) causes puffy limbs; failure of normal transportation of the spleen (deficiency condition) causes diarrhoea; perverted flow of the stomach qi (excess condition) leads to belching and nausea; insufficient stomach qi (deficiency condition) results in poor appetite; stagnated liver qi (excess condition) leads to fullness feeling in the chest and costal regions; and insufficient liver qi (deficiency condition) causes fear. Excessive heat in the kidney (excess condition) brings about scanty dark yellow urine and urethral pain. Instability of the kidney qi (deficiency condition) causes spermatorrhoea and premature ejaculation. Blood impaired by stagnated qi leads to hemoptysis and dysmenorrhea. All these cases are embraced in two types—excess or deficiency.

2. The spleen to be treated in deficiency cases, the liver in excess cases

1) *The spleen is to be treated in deficiency cases* Dr. He followed the theory developed by Li Dongyuan or Li Gao (1180-1252) that fullness of the primary qi results from normal qi of the spleen and stomach, which nourishes the former. When the stomach qi is weak and food is taken as usual, the qi of the spleen and stomach must be injured, which affects the primary qi, then disease occurs. The theory considers stomach qi as the fundamental aspect. He strongly believed the following explanation recorded in the *Miraculous Pivot*: Motion impairment of limbs and problems of the zang-fu organs are caused by insufficient spleen qi. Problems of the spleen and liver are often combined with such symptoms as abdominal distension, poor appetite, borborygmi, diarrhoea, white greasy tongue coating, string-taut and slow pulse, manifesting deficiency in the spleen and stagnated qi in the liver. Problems of the spleen and heart are usually associated with symptoms of yellow complexion, shortness of breath, amnesia, less intake of food, lassitude, disturbed sleep, pale tongue coating, thready pulse, showing deficiency in the heart and spleen. Problems of the spleen and lung often cause lassitude, poor appetite, loose stools, cough with profuse phlegm, white, thin and greasy tongue coating, soft, weak pulse, manifesting deficiency in the spleen and lung. Problems of the spleen and kidney are often connected with lassitude, aversion to cold, abdominal distension, poor appetite, loose stools with indigested food, pale tongue, deep and slow pulse, showing deficiency in the spleen and stomach. The excess condition of the spleen together with other zang organs is rarely seen clinically. For this reason, he often selected Zhongwan (Ren 12), Weishu (B 21), Zhangmen (Liv 13) combined with Pishu (B 20), and Zusanli (S 36) as the primary group of points with modifications in treatment of different kinds of diseases. For example, Quchi (LI 11), Xuehai (Sp 10) and Xingjian (Liv 2) were added to invigorate the spleen, soothe the liver and regulate qi. Shenmen (H 7), Neiguan (P 6), Sanyinjiao (Sp 6) were added to calm the mind by treating the spleen and heart. Mingmen (Du 4), Dachangshu (B 25) and Guanyuan (Ren 4) were added to strengthen

the spleen and kidney and invigorate yang. Gaohuang (B 43), Feishu (B 13) and Zhongfu (L 1) were added to treat the spleen and lung and remove asthma. Dabao (Sp 21), Gongsun (Sp 4) and Neiting (S 44) were added to regulate the function of the spleen and stomach. Dachangshu (B 25), Zhigou (SJ 6) and Xingjian (Liv 2) were added to promote urination. Tianshu (S 25), Qihai (Ren 6) and Dachangshu (B 25) were added to invigorate yang. Xuehai (Sp 10), Fuliu (K 7) and Yinlingquan (Sp 9) were added to treat the spleen and bring down fire to nourish yin. All the above methods brought successful results.

In treatment of bi syndromes or rheumatic or rheumatoid arthritis, Dr. He did not use the reinforcing or reducing method alone; he used the even movement based on the case and its features. He said, "Wind moved quickly, and the meridian qi was stirred up on invasion of wind. It easily wandered everywhere and caused unfixed pain, which was known as arthritis with migratory pain." In this case, the most important thing was to stabilize the qi flow. The even movement was necessary with light stimulation. The needle was slowly rotated in 180° for thirty seconds and not retained. Severely painful arthritis was another example. Pain was at the fixed spots and aggravated by cold. This was caused by an accumulation of cold, which prevented smooth qi flow. In this case, the quick even movement was applied to break the obstruction in the meridians. The needle was quickly inserted, lifted and rotated in 240° to 360° for one minute and retained for ten to fifteen minutes. Soreness and numbness felt at the main point must transmit along the meridian. Arthritis due to dampness was marked by a heavy sensation in the joints and fixed or localized pain. In this case the moderate even movement was applied to regulate qi. Needle rotation within 180° to 240° was advised. The needling reaction was decided by the patient's condition and tolerance. For bi syndromes Dr. He usually selected Fengchi (B 20), Zhongwan (Ren 12), Weishu (B 21) and Zusanli (S 36) as the main points. For arthritis with migratory pain Waiguan (SJ 5), Xuehai (Sp 10) were added. For arthritis with severe pain, Dazhui (Du 14) and Mingmen (Du 4) were added. For arthritis due to damp, Fuliu (K 7) and Sanyangluo (SJ 8) were added. For problems in the upper limbs, Jianyu (LI 15), Quchi (LI 11) and Hegu (LI 4) were added. For problems in the lower limbs, Huantiao (B 30) , Quchi (LI 11), Yanglingquan (Sp 9) and Juegu (B 39) were added.

2) *The liver is to be treated in excess condition* Dr. He believed that disorders of qi was related to the emotions. The condition of the liver qi was an important factor effecting on the pathogenesis of qi disorders. For instance, stagnancy of liver qi causes a full sensation and pain in the costal region, anorexia, abdominal pain, belching and a bitter taste in the mouth—manifestations of disharmony of the liver and stomach, dysfunction of the liver and spleen. Stagnated liver qi may cause fire, which attacks the lung; the descending function of the lung is impaired and the lung yin is injured. Then the symptoms are a bitter taste in the mouth, dry throat, cough without expectoration of phlegm or bloody coughing, a full sensation in the chest, costal distension, etc. Since the liver and lung are of the same source, there may appear other symptoms such as dizziness, dry eye, weak legs, red cheeks, sore throat—manifestations of deficiency in the kidney. When the liver fire attacks the heart, one may see irritability and restlessness, mania, loss of consciousness, delirium, dream-disturbed sleep, bitter taste in the mouth, fullness

feeling in the costal region—manifestations of exuberance of fire in the liver and heart. All in all, stagnated liver qi tends to cause fire. That is why growth of fire due to abnormal activity of the seven emotional factors may find a root cause in the liver. He held that tympanites was caused by the impaired liver due to stagnation of qi. Abdominal distension and less food intake due to deficiency in the spleen and its poor transportation were only the secondary symptoms, whereas a spasm of dull pain below the heart, irritability and restlessness due to stagnated liver qi were the main symptoms. He believed it was proper to treat the liver first by eliminating the stagnated qi, strengthening the spleen yang and regulating the stomach and spleen. In treatment he selected Qimen (Liv 14), Taichong (Liv 3) with the reducing method to remove stagnancy of qi; Zhigou (SJ 6) and Yanglingquan (B 34) were needled with the reducing method to regulate qi and break obstruction; Zhangmen (Liv 13) and Taibai (Sp 3) were punctured with the reinforcing method to invigorate the yang of the stomach and spleen; and Zusanli (S 36) was punctured with the even movement to regulate the stomach and spleen qi. Before the attack of wind-stroke the patient often has dizziness, distending pain and heaviness in the head, numb limbs, weak legs, incoherent speech, string-taut pulse, slightly red tongue with thick coating, a manifestation of hyperactivity of yang and deficiency of yin. The location of the disease is in the kidney but it seems in the liver. It is said in *Miraculous Pivot*, "In cases of exuberance of yang due to deficiency of yin, it is advised to invigorate yin and then remove excessive yang." Following the principle in emergency cases, treat the acute symptoms first. Dr. He thought deficiency of yin was the root cause while exuberance of yang was the manifestation. He made efforts to eliminate the hyperactivity of yang first, and then to invigorate the kidney yin by selecting Baihui (Du 20), Taiyang (Extra 2), Xingjian (Liv 2) with the reducing method. Half ml bloodletting was also applied to the former two points. The twelve Jing-(well) points were punctured with bloodletting for severe cases suffering from loss of consciousness. Then Yongquan (K 1) and Fuliu (K 7) were needled with the reducing method. Finally Quchi (LI 11) and Huantiao (B 30) were selected with the even movement to regulate qi.

3. Seven operating techniques and five reinforcing and reducing approaches

Dr. He laid special stress on manipulations, which were considered as the key link in regulation of qi. Precise puncture of needles, depth of insertion are quite important in acupuncture therapy. He used a tube, 6 cm in length as the holder in which a needle was fixed and punctured.

1) *Seven operating techniques* Operating techniques include the puncturing method, direction, angle, depth, frequency and force. It is not only a kind of approach to insert the needle, but also an approach to find, induce and promote the flow of qi in the meridians, which is the basis of the reinforcement and reduction. The detailed information of the seven operating techniques is as follows:

a. Method to regulate qi: Yang Jizhou (1522-1620) and Zhang Jiebin (about 1563-1640), two ancient practitioners, stressed that the patient should make a cough when the needle was punctured. He thought that a cough might induce the flow of qi in the abdomen by relaxing the muscles and tendons, and invigorate the qi circulation. He transformed the ancient approach into the method to regulate qi. After insertion of the needle just into the skin, he asked the patient to breathe naturally while he twirled the needle evenly five to six times within a range of 240°. Then he inserted the needle into the muscle. In this way he made qi and blood spread, relaxed the muscle and reduced the painful feeling when the needle was going through the skin.

b. Sparrow-pecking technique: It is done by lifting and thrusting the needle with quick frequency, the same amplitude and force after the needle reached a desired depth. It works to promote the flow of qi in the meridians, and the transmission of the needle sensation. But for some points it is improper to lift or thrust the needle. Then the needle is kept unmoved, but the needle handle is pecked at by the thumb and index finger to promote the qi flow. The needling sensation is not as strong as the former.

c. Method of twirling: The needle should be twirled repeatedly with the even force and appropriate angle. It can make the qi arrive quickly and the needling sensation transmit steadily to the diseased part. In operation, sometimes the needle is twirled evenly with the same angle and force. Sometimes the needle is twirled counterclockwise with stronger force and a bigger angle, while it is clockwise twirled with weaker force and smaller angle or vice versa. The above approach is often used in reinforcement.

d. Lifting and thrusting technique: The force, speed and depth of lifting and thrusting should be even. It is different from the sparrow-pecking technique because the needle is inserted deep with slow frequency and strong force in rotation. In operation more varied manipulations are employed, e.g. thrusting the needle with stronger force and lifting it slowly when the even movement is applied; or lifting the needle quickly and strongly and thrusting it slowly with stronger force when the even movement is applied. Any kind of lifting and thrusting techniques may bring stronger needling sensation suitable for slow reaction patients.

e. Round twirling technique: It means to twirl the needle clockwise or counterclockwise with only moderate force and speed to strengthen and prolong the transmission of the needling sensation. The rotating angle is within 360°. Usually two to three rotations are enough.

f. Needle-vibrating technique: It is conducted by vibrating the needle handle slightly in moderate frequency and with even force by the thumb and index finger when it is quickly inserted to the desired depth. It has a function of eliminating heat, often used together with the reducing method to treat excessive heat in the yang meridians.

g. Needle-snapping technique: It is done for reinforcement by snapping the needle handle slightly once everyone or two seconds to invigorate the flow of the meridian qi, usually employed to treat problems in the eye, ear, face or mouth.

2) *Five reinforcing and reducing approaches* They include reinforcement, reduction, needling along or against the direction of the meridians and the even movement. Reinforcement and reduction refer to different stimulations, to which varied reactions of the body are found. Qi regulation is achieved and then disease is cured.

a. Reinforcing method: Three steps of insertion of the needle are conducted. First the needle is inserted through the surface of the skin, sparrow-pecking technique or the lifting and thrusting manipulation is applied to promote the flow of qi in the meridians. Afterward the needle is rotated to cause the needling sensation, which transmits along the meridians. At this moment the needle is inserted deeper and the same manipulation is repeated. When stimulation appears the needle is inserted to the deepest place. After the arrival of the needling reaction, the needle is rotated clockwise two or three times to strengthen the stimulation. When the patient is breathing in, the needle is quickly pulled out and the point is pressed with one of the fingers to prevent qi from releasing.

b. Reducing method: First the needle is inserted to the desired depth and twirled to induce the flow of qi in the meridians. Then the lifting and thrusting techniques are used when the operator first feels tenseness and then looseness around the needle. The needle should be gradually lifted to the deeper part and the same manipulation is conducted. The third step is to lift the needle to the superficial part and the same manipulation is repeated. At this moment the needle-vibrating technique is used and the needle is pulled out gradually. The point is not pressed to allow pathogenic factors going out.

3) *Needle-puncturing along the direction of the meridians* It refers to a needle quickly inserted to the desired depth along the travelling course of the meridian. Vibrating and lift-thrust techniques are used in combination for two to three times. When the operator feels tenseness around the needle and the patient feels the needle sensation transmitting to the terminals of the meridian, the needle is gradually pulled out. The point is not pressed to allow pathogenic factors going out. This is included in the reducing method, but is usually applied in the limbs instead of in the abdomen and back.

4) *Needle-puncturing against the direction of the meridian* It is conducted by a needle inserted just through the skin against the travelling course of the meridian. Then the needle is thrust a little deeper and the lift-thrust technique is applied for half to one minute. When the operator feels tenseness around the needle and the patient has numb and sore reactions, the needle is thrust deeper. The same manipulation is repeated until presence of the needle sensation. Then the needle is thrust to the deepest place and the same manipulation is done for 1 to 1.5 minutes. When the patient feels the needle sensation transmitting to the terminal of the meridian, the needle is quickly withdrawn. The point should be pressed to prevent qi from release. This is included in the reinforcing method, but is usually used in the limbs and in cases of both deficiency and exccess instead of in the abdomen and back.

5) *Even movement* This is performed by inserting the needle to the desired depth. The sparrow-pecking and lift-thrust techniques are employed to promote the flow of the meridian qi. The needle is again rotated until arrival of the needle sensation. At this moment the needle may be gently withdrawn. It is a kind of moderate reinforcement and reduction to invigorate the meridian function.

II. Case Analysis

Case 1: Gastroptosis

Name, Wang x x; sex, male; age, 49; occupation, worker; date of the first visit, November 11, 1964.

Complaints He had had stomach problems for years with a distended bearing-down sensation in the gastric region. In the past two years the condition became worse. In October, 1964, he was diagnosed as having gastroptosis accompanied by gastric ulcer after barium meal examination. No positive response was seen on medication. When he came for treatment, he complained that he had a distended feeling in the stomach and abdomen after meals with occasional gastric pain. He had aversion to cold. Other symptoms included poor appetite, lassitude, dizziness, slightly dry stools, emaciation, enlarged lower abdomen, yellow complexion, pale red tongue with thick white coating, string-taut and slippery pulse.

Differentiation · Yang deficiency and lowered functioning in the spleen and stomach and failure of transportation.

Method Strengthen the function of the spleen and stomach.

Prescription Shangwan (Ren 13), Zhongwan (Ren 12), Xiawan (Ren 10), Burong (S 19), Chengman (S 20), Weishu (B 21), Zusanli (S 36) and Qihai (Ren 6) (moxibustion applied).

Treatment procedure After ten treatments the distended feeling in the abdomen and the pain were markedly alleviated. He could eat more. After sixteen treatments the major complaints were gone. Absence of gastroptosis was shown by the barium meal examination on December 9, 1964. Six months later another barium meal examination showed no abnormality.

Acupuncture technique Shangwan (Ren 13), Xiawan (Ren 12), Zhongwan (Ren 10), Burong (S 19), Chengman (S 20), Liangman (S 21): After the needles were inserted just through the skin, he rotated them gently with a small amplitude to relax the muscle. Then the needles were punctured 0.5 cun in depth and the sparrow-pecking technique was applied to promote the flow of the meridian qi. Afterwards the needle was rotated clockwise with stronger force and a wider amplitude, and counterclockwise with less force and a smaller amplitude to wait for the arrival of qi. When the operator felt tension around the needle and the patient had sore and numb feelings, which spread to the upper and lower abdomen, the needle was thrust 0.8 cun in depth (don't insert deeper in patients with an enlarged spleen). The same acupuncture technique was applied. When the patient had a strong needling sensation, the needle was inserted 1.2 cun in depth and the same manipulation was repeated. Now the patient felt a sore and contracting sensation of the stomach and peristalsis sped up. The needle was then twirled clockwise two or three times with a range of 180° to 240° to strengthen the needling sensation. When there was tension around it, the needle was twirled a little and withdrawn in moderate speed.

Zusanli (S 36) and Sanyinjiao (Sp 6): The needles were inserted with the tip slightly upward. For Zusanli (S 36) the depth was 1 cun, while for Sanyinjiao (Sp 6), the depth was 0.5 cun. The sparrow-pecking technique was used to wait for the arrival of qi. The needles were slowly and gently rotated to make the needle sensation spread upward (better to the abdomen) along the running course of the meridians. The needles were rotated clockwise two to three times with a range of 240° to 360° to strengthen the needling sensation. Afterwards the needles were quickly withdrawn.

Weishu (B 21): It was perpendicularly punctured to a depth of 0.5 cun and the sparrow-pecking technique was applied to wait for the arrival of qi. The same rotating manipulations were done until the patient had a local soreness, which spread downward along the running course of the meridian. The needle was lifted to the subcutaneous part that was obliquely punctured, 0.5 cun in depth (reaching the part between Weishu (B 21) and Sanjiaoshu (B 22).) Then the needle was perpendicularly punctured, 0.8 cun in depth and the same manipulations were repeated. When the patient felt the gastric peristalsis speed up, the needle was rotated a little and withdrawn in moderate speed.

Explanation He believed that gastroptosis was caused by looseness of the ligaments due to lowered functioning of the spleen and stomach. Two hundred and sixty-seven cases of gastroptosis shown by the barium meal examination were treated by strengthening the function of the spleen and stomach. Out of the cases 141 were male and 126 were female, aged from sixteen to seventy years old, among which, the majority were from twenty-one to fifty years old, amounting to 231 cases. The success rate was 95.8 percent, of which seventy-seven cases were markedly effective, thirty-eight cases were improved and eleven cases failed.

Case 2: Gastric torsion

Name, Mu x x; age, 34; sex, male; occupation, worker; date of the first visit, September 17, 1972.

Complaints On September 9, he had a big lunch and went to do physical labour immediately afterwards. At about 2 p.m. he had sudden gastric pain, aggravated a few minutes later. He was sent to a hospital for emergency treatment and was thought to suffer from a gastric spasm. In the following eight days he had prolonged gastric pain, a full sensation in the chest, abdominal distension, irritability, shortness of breath and disturbed sleep. Other symptoms were yellow complexion, lassitude, a hard painful eminence at the right side of the abdomen, a red tongue with yellow greasy and thick coating, poor appetite, string-taut and rapid pulse. The barium meal examination showed gastric torsion.

Differentiation Stagnation of qi in the stomach and obstruction of stomach yang due to improper diet injuring the stomach.

Method Break the stagnation of qi to regulate the function of the stomach and spleen, and invigorate stomach yang.

Prescription Shangwan (Ren 13), Xiawan (Ren 10), Zhongwan (Ren 12) (the even movement being applied), Jiuwei (Ren 5), Tanzhong (Ren 17) (the reducing method being applied), Burong (S 19), Chengman (S 20), Liangmen (S 21), Taiyi (S 23), Tianshu (S 25), Wailing (S 26) (in each treatment points on both sides are selected with the reducing method applied to those on the left and the reinforcing method to those on the right in turn), Weishu (B 21) (moxibustion being applied).

Treatment procedure One treatment alleviated gastric pain and abdominal distension. The patient was able to take food and there was no pain after two treatments. Symptoms completely disappeared after seven treatments. The barium meal examination showed a normal stomach.

Explanation Although it is a rarely seen problem of the digestive system, about a hundred cases were treated by Dr. He. It is thought that the cause of the problem is not complicated only due to eating too much at one meal, but also doing physical labour immediately afterward. It is important to eliminate the stagnated qi in the stomach meridian, for which reason Zhongwan (Ren 12), the Mu-point of the Stomach Meridian, Weishu (B 21), and Tanzhong (Ren 17), the Confluent point, were selected to regulate the stomach qi. In comparison with other gastric disorders, more forceful manipulations were applied.

Case 3: Prolapse of the uterus

Name, Chen x x; sex, female; age, 48; occupation, office worker; date of the first visit, December 17, 1963.

Complaints She had not had a good rest after childbirth in August, 1949. In the winter of that year she began to feel soreness and pain in the lower back, legs, shoulders, elbows and knee-joints, and a bearing-down sensation appeared in the lower abdomen. There was no response to herbal medicine. In 1958 she was diagnosed as having a prolapse of the uterus. On the first visit she had symptoms of lassitude, dizziness, palpitation, weakness in the lower back and legs, a bearing-down sensation in the lower abdomen, prolapse of the uterus, pale complexion, pale tongue with thin coating, and thready and weak pulse.

Differentiation Qi injured after childbirth, sinking of qi of the spleen.

Method Tone qi and blood to invigorate the qi of the spleen.

Prescription Qihai (Ren 6), Zhongji (Ren 3), Zigong (Extra 16) (penetrating towards Henggu (K 11)), Daimai (B 26), Zhiyin (B 67), Mingmen (Du 4) (the reinforcing method being applied).

Treatment procedure After one treatment the bearing-down sensation was markedly alleviated. There was no uncomfortable feeling when she walked slowly. After three treatments, dizziness, palpitation, soreness and pain of the lower back were relieved. No uncomfortable feeling was found when going up or down stairs. After nine treatments the uterus returned to the normal position.

Explanation Dr. He thought prolapse of the uterus was only the sign, but the real cause of the illness was deficiency of qi. For this reason he toned qi and blood, invigorated yang to support qi. Qihai (Ren 6), the Confluent point of qi and blood where essence is stored, was punctured with the reinforcing method to invigorate the function of the five zang organs, strengthen the spleen qi to warm up the kidney qi and invigorate kidney yang. Other points were used as the secondary ones to bring about good results.

Case 4: Continuous dripping of urine

Name, Guo x x; sex, male; age, 14; occupation, student; date of the first visit, November 19, 1977.

Complaints The patient's lower back had been injured five years before. Half a year later he was injured in the head in a car accident and was diagnosed as having a mild cerebral concussion. Four years ago he began to suffer from continuous dripping of urine. There was no response to any treatment. On the first consultation he still had continuous dripping of urine with urethral pain. Other symptoms were distended and painful lower abdomen, painful lower back, dizziness and lassitude, yellow complexion, pale tongue, string-taut and thready pulse, foul urine, a hard lump of 30 cm x 10 cm by 0.7 cm to 1.2 cm was found on the right side of the lower abdomen. A cystography showed the bladder was four fifths displaced. X-ray diagnosis of the lumbar vertebra suggested overgrowth of right processus transversus of the fifth lumbar vertebra and pyelograph gave signs of hydrops.

Differentiation Qi deficiency of the stomach and spleen, damp and heat in the kidney causing failure of water metabolism, obstruction of the water passage by blood stasis.

Method Strengthen qi to remove damp and stasis.

Prescription 1) Qihai (Ren 6), Guanyuan (Ren 4) (the reinforcing method being applied), Shuidao (S 28) (the reducing method being applied), Qugu (Ren 2) (the even movement being applied), Sanyinjiao (Sp 6), Shenshu (B 23), Pangguangshu (B 28) and Yanglingquan (B 34) (the reinforcing method being applied). 2) Qugu (Ren 2), Henggu (K 11), Sanyinjiao (Sp 6), Shenshu (B 23), Ashi, 4.5 cm away from Zhongji (Ren 3), and Huantiao (G 30), the reinforcing method being applied. 3) Guanyuan (Ren 4) penetrating towards Qugu (Ren 2), Sanyinjiao (Sp 6) (the reinforcing method being applied), Shuidao (S 28) and Guilai (S 29) (the reinforcing method being applied to those on the left and the reducing method being applied to those on the right), Shenshu (B 23) and Pangguangshu (B 28) (the reinforcing method being applied to those on the left and the reducing method being applied to those on the right).

Treatment procedure After points of Group 1 were done fifteen times the continuous dripping of urine was alleviated, but the urine passed was turbid and smelled foul. The first group of points was replaced by the second group. After six treatments the interval of urination became longer and the patient was able to control a little water in the bladder and the urine was less turbid. Then the first and second groups were used in turn. Another twenty treatments were given, the abdominal eminence disappeared and the patient was able to control water in the bladder during the day, but the urethral pain remained. Then points of Group 3 were used to help the bladder turn to the normal position. After twelve treatments no bed-wetting was seen at night. At this moment the three groups were alternately used every other day. After thirty treatments he recovered. A cystorgraphy showed the normal position of the bladder. Treatments amounted to eighty-eight in total.

Explanation Dr. He believed that disorders of water metabolism was the chief cause of the problem due to qi deficiency in the spleen. Hence Qihai (Ren 6) was selected as the main point associated with Guanyuan (Ren 4), Shenshu (B 23) and Sanyinjiao (Sp 6). He used both the reinforcing and reducing methods with the stress on the former and finally good results were obtained.

THREE METHODS TO REMOVE STAGNATION OF QI—CHIEF CAUSE OF A DISEASE

—He Puren's Clinical Experience

He Puren, a native of Laishui County, Hebei Province, was born in 1926. At the age of fourteen he began to learn acupuncture from Niu Zehua, a famous acupuncture specialist. Eight years later he practised acupuncture by himself. In 1956 he went to work in the Beijing Hospital of Traditional Chinese Medicine and in 1976 he joined the medical group to work in the Upper Volta. He was awarded a knight medal for his devoted service to the local people by the President of that country. His works include *Acupuncture Techniques*, *Pain Treated by Acupuncture*, *A Study of Points*, etc. Now he is one of the members of the standing committee of the Beijing Society of Traditional Chinese Medicine, Director of the Acupuncture Commission and Vice-Chairman of the China Acupuncture Society.

I. Academic Characteristics and Medical Specialities

1. Stagnation of qi—the main cause of a disease

Dr. He believes that stagnation of qi is the pathogenesis in traditional Chinese medicine. In light of the pathological changes due to stagnation of qi, he has designed three approaches to deal with various symptoms with success. Although the pathological factors, which include overactivity of the seven emotional factors, untimely working of the six natural factors, improper diet and trauma, injuries, etc. are varied, stagnation of qi is universal in leading to disorders. For instance, exterior stagnation of qi brings about aversion to cold and fever while interior stagnation of qi results in pains. Stagnated qi in the upper jiao leads to stomachache and pain of the costal regions; and stagnated qi in the lower jiao may cause lumbosacral pain. Stagnation of qi in the liver may induce costal pain, jaundice, eye troubles, spasm, dizziness, etc. Stagnation of qi in the heart is manifested by worry, insomnia, itching and pain. Stagnation of qi in the lung leads to cough with expectoration of phlegm. Stagnated qi in the spleen brings about poor appetite, diarrhoea, abdominal pain, a distended feeling in the abdomen, edema, etc. When there is stagnation of qi in the kidney, there may be lumbago, blurring of eyes, difficulty hearing, and ringing of the ears. From all these examples, we can see that nearly all of the diseases are caused by stagnation of qi. Removal of stagnation of qi can cure any kind of disease.

In fact, the acupuncture technique is the approach to regulate the flow of qi and blood and eliminate stagnation. The three approaches developed by Dr. He, in a word, are methods to invigorate the body resistance and expel pathogenic factors.

2. Moderate stimulation

It refers to gentle, painless and moderate stimulation in acupuncture therapy to promote the smooth flow of qi and blood and adjust the function of the internal organs. In operation Dr. He has summarized three important aspects.

1) *Quick insertion of the needle* It is quite important to puncture the needle through the skin without pain. In addition to the skillful technique of the operator it is necessary to shift the patient's attention if he is too nervous. The operator may ask the patient to make a cough and in the instant thrust the needle into the skin.

2) *Appearance of the needling reaction* In general, when the needle reaches a certain depth, the patient may feel soreness, numbness or distension around the needle, while the operator at the same time may feel tenseness around the needle. This is fine as the result is good. Sometimes the patient does not have a marked needling reaction, but the effect is still good. Dr. He thinks that effectiveness means the appearance of a needling reaction.

3) *Intensity of stimulation* Dr. He believes that the intensity of stimulation is decided by the reaction of the patient, which may be divided into three degrees—mild, strong and moderate.

a. Mild stimulation means the patient has a comfortable feeling after the insertion of the needle.

b. Strong stimulation means the stimulation is too strong and beyond the tolerance of the patient.

c. Moderate stimulation: It is between the degrees of mild and strong. There is a strong needling reaction the patient can tolerate. Besides, stimulation is closely related to the number of points selected, size of needles, depth of insertion, manipulations and time of needle retention. Patients with hypertension often show excess in the upper and deficiency in the lower; it is better to select more points and give moderate stimulation. But for points of the Liver Meridian, mild stimulation is more helpful because strong stimulation tends to stir up wind and cause deterioration of hypertension. He thinks only moderate stimulation can relieve hypertension. However, for some disorders, it is better to employ strong stimulation, e.g. inflammation, spasm and acute pains. For paralysis, numbness, tuberculosis, pneumocardiac disease, indigestion, bed-wetting and any disorders due to insufficient primary qi, mild stimulation is more helpful. Stimulation intensity of acupuncture not only depends on conditions but also on age, profession, sex, physical condition, climate, season, habit, locality of points, etc. Generally speaking, those who are engaged in industrial and agricultural production often have tight muscles, strong constitution and abundant qi and blood. Disorders they have are usually of excess type. Practice shows that strong stimulation is good for them. But for mental workers it is better to give mild stimulation because they are not as strong as physical workers. Moderate stimulations are applied to trade workers and semiphysical workers.

3. Warming approach

It refers to the fire needling or moxibustion applied to a point or an area to expel cold and invigorate the flow of qi and blood.

Fire needle therapy is a heated red hot needle inserted into the point or the diseased part immediately and withdrawn at once (in an instant of half a second). After withdrawal of the needle the point is covered by a swab. Shallow needling is usually applied to a new disorder, and deep needling is often used in prolonged cases. For instance, for scrofula or lumps, the needle must be punctured into the center of the lesion and shallow needling is not helpful. Furthermore, depth is relied on the locality of points and the size of the body. Generally, points on the head, chest, the back of the hand and foot need to be punctured shallowly, but points on the thick muscles should be punctured deeply. The second puncture should not be done at the very place of the first puncture, to which a very small space is left.

Pricking puncture and retention of needles: Sometimes Dr. He retains the needle for five to thirty minutes for prolonged cases, or conducts manipulations in the period of needle retention. The needle burnt hot red must be quickly inserted into and withdrawn from the point to avoid giving pain to the patient.

Indications:

1) *Pain* Pain may be due to a number of causes—cold or heat pathogenic factors, but cold is a possibility more than heat. It is held by traditional Chinese medicine that obstruction of meridians brings about pain because of impeded flow of qi and blood. For example, 64-year-old Ms, He had a right shoulder pain for six days, afterwards the condition deteriorated and she couldn't move the right arm properly. Other symptoms were yellow complexion, white coating, string-taut and slow pulse. This was a case due to the failure of defensive qi, leading to cold and damp accumulation in the meridians and stagnation of qi and blood. He applied fire needling to five tender spots. On the second day when the patient came, she told Dr. He that she was markedly improved except for the motion impairment of the right arm. The pulse became less tense and slow; it means pathogenic cold had not been completely eliminated. He gave ten punctures around the affected shoulder with the fire needle. Five days later most of the symptoms were alleviated and she began to do household chores. But the pulse was still slow and string-taut. He again punctured locally with the fire needle. Finally the patient recovered.

2) *Numbness* Many causes may bring about numbness, which is found in various conditions, e.g. patients of qi deficiency are apt to have general numbness. One-side numbness is an omen of apoplexy; deficiency in the liver and spleen causes hand and foot numbness; primary qi impaired by heat induces numbness, frequently seen in summer; and injury of vessels or meridians causes local numbness. No matter how complicated the case is, it is chiefly due to obstruction of the meridians, leading to failure of the qi to command blood and nourish muscles. For this reason, the fire needling is used to invigorate yang and remove obstruction. When the smooth flow of qi and blood is restored, numbness is relieved naturally. For instance, 43-year-old Mr. Liu felt numbness in the left leg for half a month. Other symptoms included yellow complexion, white tongue coating and string-taut, slippery pulse. The condition was caused by an abnormal flow of qi and blood. Dr. He cured the case in three treatments with the prompt prick technique.

3) *Lump* It is usually caused by stagnation of qi and blood stasis. Fire needling

therapy may eliminate the problem. For instance, 38-year-old Ms. Tang had had a miscarriage eight years before and she had not been pregnant since. She was first diagnosed as having an ovary follicle by a gynecologist of a hospital, and an operation was suggested. But she refused. Then she went to a hospital for obstetrics and gynecology and was diagnosed as multiple pseudymyxoma on the left side and secondary sterility. An operation was again suggested, but she refused again and came to an acupuncturist. Physical examination showed two hard, unmovable lumps of 16 x 16 cm and 14 x 14 cm in the left lower abdomen. It was a condition due to stagnation of qi and stasis of blood, resulting in lumps in the uterus. The fire needling was applied to the lumps with the needle puncturing the center of them. Treatment was given every three days. After three treatments the lumps became smaller and thirteen treatments completely cured the case. Gynecological examination showed the lumps had disappeared.

4) *Scrofula* It is often caused by deficiency and cold in the spleen and stomach and accumulation of body fluid. The fire needling therapy may invigorate yang and eliminate stagnation. Mr. Zhang, 31, had had a hard lump on the left side of the neck for over a year. At first it was as big as a soybean. Gradually it grew to the size of a walnut, about 4 cm x 5 cm, and there were several small hard lumps around it. He was diagnosed as having tuberculosis of cervical lymph nodes in a hospital. Since he was allergic to streptomycin, he was treated by other antituberculotics without marked success. He had yellow complexion, emaciation, pale tongue with white coating, thready pulse, manifestations of stagnated qi and blood in the meridians due to stagnancy of qi in the liver. Three fire needles were applied to the center of the lump vertically. A two-month treatment cured the case.

4. Bloodletting

This is an important approach in acupuncture therapy, which is done with a three-edged needle or the like to prick the superficial vessels until bleeding. The amount of blood let is depended on the pathological condition.

1) *Apparatus* Three-edged needle, plum-blossom needle or filiform needle.

2) *Method*

a. Slow puncture: It is used in venous bloodletting, e.g. applied to Quze (P 3), Weizhong (B 40) and Taiyang (Extra 2). First tie tightly the upper part near the point with a piece of adhesive plaster, and then prick the protrusive vein on the point, 0.05 to 0.1 cun in depth. Dark blood flows out, and when the colour turns red, loose the adhesive plaster and press the point with a swab.

b. Quick puncture: On operation pinch the point to be pricked and thrust a three-edged needle or a filiform needle, 0.05 to 0.1 cun in depth. Squeeze the point to let blood out quickly. For instance, it is applied to Shaoshang (L 11) for sore throat, to Shixuan (Extra 30) for sunstroke, to the twelve Jing-(well) points for apoplexy.

c. Prick: It is usually applied to the points on the chest, abdomen, head, face and thin muscles clinically for treatment of sycosis and stye, etc. On operation pinch the red-spotted muscle and prick it with a three-edged needle.

d. Puncture in circle: It is usually applied to carbuncle, rheumatoid arthritis and to pestilence by giving a few or dozens of prick to the affected area with a three-edged needle. Then squeeze the pricked area or apply cupping to it to discharge the toxic blood and relieve swelling and pain.

e. Dense puncture: It is often applied to dermotosis such as persisted tinea with a plum-blossom needle to tap the affected area until slight bleeding.

3) *Contraindications of bloodletting* Bloodletting is especially effective to excess and heat syndromes, but special precautions must be taken.

a. Contraindications of patients: It is not permitted to use bloodletting for patients of deficient yin and blood, edema, faint pulse, and far too weaker patients (coma patients excluded), obstetric and traumatic patients, patients susceptible to hemorrhage; or on patients who have overeaten, who are hungry, thirsty, drunk or in a rage. For these patients one has to wait for some time to allow them to calm down their qi and blood and then use bloodletting. Otherwise it would do more harm than good.

b. Contraindications of points: About twenty points are not permitted for bloodletting listed in the classic medical literature. They are Naohu (Du 17), Shenting (Du 24), Yuzhen (B 9), Luoque (B 8), Chengling (G 18), Luoxi (SJ 19), Shendao (Du 11), Lingtai (Du 10), Shuifen (Ren 9), Shenque (Ren 8), Huiying (Ren 1), Henggu (K 11), Tanzhong (Ren 17), Qichong (S 30), Qimen (L 14), Chengjin (B 56), Wuli (LI 13), Sanyanluo (SJ 8), Qingling (H 2), etc. Besides, the following points should not be punctured deeply. They are Yunmen (L 2), Jiuwei (Ren 15), Kezhuren, Jianjing (G 21), Xuehai (Sp 10), Hegu (LI 4), Sanyinjiao (Sp 6), Shimen (Ren 5). Points in the lumbosacrum of pregnant women should not be punctured to prevent accidents. Other points located at the chest, abdomen and crown should not be punctured deep or allowed to apply acupuncture.

II. Case Analysis

Case 1: High fever

Name, Luan x x; sex, female; age, 8.

Complaints She had had a body temperature of 39°C for five days with symptoms of headache, stiff neck, and poor appetite. She was suspected to have meningitis by a children's hospital and lumbar puncture was suggested, but her parents refused. When she was transferred to our hospital she still had a high fever of 39.6°C. Other symptoms were lassitude, severe frontal headache, irascibility, bitter taste in the mouth, yellow urine, thin yellow tongue coating, floating and rapid pulse.

Differentiation Affection of both the exterior and interior by pathogenic wind and heat.

Method Eliminate wind and heat from the exterior and interior.

Prescription Shixuan (Extra 30) and Zanzhu (B 2) were punctured until bleeding appeared. Dazhui (Du 14) was pricked to bleed and cupping was applied to it.

Treatment procedure On the second day the temperature lowered to 38°C and other symptoms were relieved. The same treatment was given and afterwards she was completely cured.

Case 2: Lumbago

Name, Li x x; sex, female; age, 32.

Complaints For a number of days she had had lumbago. But on the day before consultation the condition suddenly became worse. She could not move her waist. No trauma and deformity were seen on physical examination. She had thin white tongue coating and deep tight pulse.

Differentiation Obstruction of the meridians by pathogenic wind and cold and malnourishment of the kidney by blood.

Method Eliminate wind and cold from the meridians.

Prescription Weizhong (B 4) and Renzhong (Du 26) were punctured to bleed.

Treatment procedure After one treatment the patient could move her waist and walk with a stick. Five treatments completely cured the case. Shenshu (B 23) was used in the last two treatments.

Case 3: Suppurative infection in the nape

Name, He x x; sex, male; age, 30.

Complaints He had had suppurative infection in the nape for about two years. There was no response to any treatment. Physical examination showed diffused suppurative infection covered with pus and blood scar, yellow complexion, slippery pulse, white tongue coating.

Differentiation Heat in the blood system and affection of pathogenic wind.

Method Subside wind and remove toxity.

Prescription Slow puncture was applied to Weizhong (B 40) to bleed and the red spots on the back were pricked until bleeding.

Treatment procedure Four treatments nearly cured the case. A follow-up survey showed no relapse.

Case 4: Migraine

Name, Zong x x; sex, male; age, 41.

Complaints The patient had had hypertension for years. Two years ago he often had intolerable migraines. In the previous week migraine on the left side occurred. Physical examination showed obesity, dark complexion, dry stools, yellow urine, red tongue with thin white coating, deep and string-taut pulse.

Differentiation Insufficient kidney yin, hyperactivity of fire in the liver and gallbladder and invasion of external pathogenic wind.

Method Dispel fire and wind.

Prescription Slow puncture was applied to Taiyang (Extra 2) to bleed.

Treatment procedure Three treatments cured the case and a follow-up study showed no relapse.

Case 5: Numbness of the fingers

Name, Xu x x; sex, male; age, 30.

Complaints He had had numbness of the left thumb and index finger. Recently numbness recurred because he had been caught in wind in sleep. He usually disliked cold and preferred heat. The tongue coating was thin white, and the pulse was thready and slow.

Differentiation Deficiency of yang and invasion of the meridians by pathogenic wind.

Method Invigorate yang and dispel wind from the meridians.

Prescription Shaoshang (L 11), Shangyang (L 1), Quchi (LI 11), Hegu (LI 4).

Treatment procedure Shaoshang (L 11) and Shangyang (L 1) were quickly punctured to bleed, and Quchi (LI 11) and Hegu (LI 4) were needled. Marked effect was seen in the first treatment and the second treatment cured the case.

Case 6: Dizziness (hypertension)

Name, Yin x x; sex, male; age, 62.

Complaints After a banquet he had felt lassitude and dizziness. On the second day he came to be consulted. The condition became worse with cold sweats, vomiting, restlessness and cold limbs. Physical examination showed central yellow and greasy tongue coating, string-taut, slippery pulse. Blood pressure was 190/110 mmHg.

Differentiation Deficiency of yin in the lower and yang hyperactivity in the upper.

Method Remove heat and invigorate qi to calm the mind.

Prescription Renzhong (Du 26), Quze (P 3), Weizhong (B 40), Sishencong (Extra 6), twelve Jing-(well) points, Zusanli (S 36).

Treatment procedure First Renzhong (Du 26) was quickly punctured to bleed. Then Quze (P 3) and Weizhong (B 40) were slowly punctured to bleed. The third step was to puncture quickly the twelve Jing-(well) points until bleeding. Then Neiguan (P 6) and Zusanli (S 36) were punctured with filiform needles. After acupuncture, blood pressure decreased to 170/70 mmHg, the symptoms were relieved and the dizziness disappeared.

SKILLFUL USE OF ACUPOINTS IN DU MERIDIAN AND CONFLUENT POINTS OF EIGHT EXTRA MERIDIANS, PIONEERING IN "NEEDLE-SUBSTITUTE HERBAL PLASTER" AND "MOXIBUSTION WITH HERBAL PAD"

—Qin Liangfu's Clinical Experience

Qin Liangfu, a native of Shanghai, was born in December, 1924. He studied medicine from his father Qin Zhicheng since his childhood. In 1946, he got the certificate of the first national examination for higher TCM doctors and the license of TCM doctor. He has assisted in the research of the Infectious Route of Meridians and the Observation on Physiology and Biochemistry Under Acupuncture Anesthesia. At present, he is the director of TCM department in Renji Hospital affiliated with the Shanghai Second Medical University, a councillor of China Acupuncture Association and a committee member of the Shanghai Acupuncture Association.

I. Academic Characteristics and Medical Specialities

1. Selecting acupoints of the Du Meridian to treat problems of the limbs

There are a lot of clinical manifestations of problems of the four limbs, such as soreness and pain, numbness, redness and swelling on the joints of the four limbs, muscular atrophy of the four limbs, spasm of the four limbs, even paralysis of the four limbs, which are usually caused by rheumatic arthritis, retromorphosis of cervical and lumbar vertebrae, sequelae of apoplexy, sequelae of cerebral injury, syringomyelia, progressive muscular atrophy, etc. In traditional Chinese medicine the problems of the four limbs are considered as meridian problems. In the treatment, the method of selecting local acupoints is often used, which, however, is not so effective in some conditions.

In traditional Chinese medicine, the Du Meridian, one of the Eight Extraordinary Meridians, is the gathering site of all the yang meridians of the human body, so it is called "the sea of the yang meridians." In modern medicine the peripheral nervous system is the peripheroneural part from brain and spinal marrow. When certain pathogen causes disorders of the peripheral nerves, symptoms such as abnormal sensation, motor disturbance or muscular atrophy will appear. According to the above theory, Dr. Qin changed the simple method of selecting local acupoints and put forward the viewpoint of selecting acupoints from the Du Meridian to treat the problems of the four limbs, which is more effective as proven by clinical practice.

The principle of selecting acupoints from the Du Meridian is to select Dazhui (Du 14) as a main acupoint for the problems of the upper limbs and to select Mingmen (Du 4) as a main acupoint for the problems of the lower limbs. Dazhui (Du 14), the gathering site of the three Hand-Yang Meridians, three Foot-Yang Meridians and Du Meridian, is to treat all kinds of deficient and strain problems, so it is also called the point of hundreds of strains. Mingmen (Du 4) is an important point for tonifying the Yuan (source) qi and kidney, and strengthening the lumbar and spiral column. When the essence and qi of the kidney are sufficient, the lower limbs will be strong and forceful. For example, a patient Li, male, had paralysis of the right lower limb for half a year due to a traffic accident. Diagnosis in the department of neurology was paralysis of nervus peroneus communis and neruogenic injury. In acupuncture treatment, the main acupoints are Mingmen (Du 4) penetrating towards Yaoyangguan (Du 3), Shenshu (B 23) towards Dachangshu (B 25), and the supplementary acupoints are Huantiao (G 30), Fengshi (G 31), Futu (S 32), Yanglingquan (G 34), and Taichong (Liv 3), etc. The method of Hegu Puncture was applied with electro-stimulation and cupping therapy. After twenty treatments, the myodynamia of the right lower limb increased from degree IV to V, and sensitivity turned to normal.

2. The indications of the Confluent Points of the Eight Extraordinary Meridians

The Confluent Points of the Eight Extraordinary Meridians are eight acupoints of the twelve regular meridians, which are related closely to the Eight Extraordinary Meridians. Dr. Qin often combines two acupoints as a group: Gongsun (Sp 4) and Neiguan (P 6) are for problems of heart, chest and upper abdomen; Houxi (SI 3) and Shenmai (B 62) for problems of inner canthus, neck, ears, shoulder and upper limbs; Waiguan (SJ 5) and Zulinqi (G 41) for problems of outer canthus, posterior region of ears, cheeks, neck and shoulder; and Lieque (L 7) and Zhaohai (K 6) for problems of throat, chest and diaphragm.

Selecting the Confluent Points of the Eight Extraordinary Meridians is one of the commonly used methods in clinic. Dr. Qin has found that the Confluent Points of the Eight Extraordinary Meridians have a large scope of treament. For instance, in addition to the problems of heart, chest and upper abdomen, Gongsun (Sp 4) and Neiguan (P 6) can also treat problems of the lower abdomen, such as chronic diarrhoea and irregular menstruation. Because Gongsun (Sp 4), the Luo-connecting point of the Spleen Meridian of Foot-Taiyin, which meets the Ren Meridian in the lower abdomen, has the functions of regulating spleen and stomach, benefiting qi and producing blood; Neiguan (P 6), the Luo-connecting point of the Pericardium Meridian of Hand-Jueyin, which has an exterior-interior relationship with the Sanjiao Meridians of Hand-Shaoyang and meets the Liver Meridian of Foot-Jueyin, has the functions of helping qi action of sanjiao, removing stagnancy of liver qi and regulating menstruation; the combination of Gongsun (Sp 4) and Neiguan (P 6) can strengthen spleen in transportation and transformation, and regulate menstruation and blood. For instance, a woman who had postpartum deficiency of qi and blood, had a small amount of menses in pale colour and a dull pain in the lower abdomen. Acupuncture had been applied on Guanyuan (Ren 4) and

Sanyinjiao (Sp 6) for her, but no effects occurred. Therefore warm needling treatment was given on Gongsun (Sp 4) and Neiguan (P 6) three to four times one week before menstruation came. After three-period treatments, the condition became normal. For another instance, a patient with diarrhoea for several years had two to four bowel movements a day, accompanied with distension in the lower abdomen. The distension did not decrease after bowel movements. Needling on Zusanli (S 36) and Tianshu (S 25) did not bring about any effect. Therefore Gongsun (Sp 4) and Neiguan (P 6) were added in this case. After five treatments, bowel movement became normal and there was no more abdominal distension.

Besides the problems of chest, diaphragm and throat, Zhaohai (K 6) and Lieque (L 7) can treat profuse leukorrhea in women. Lieque (L 7) connects the Ren Meridian, which is "the sea of all the yin meridians," and mainly treats the internal qi stagnation in males and leukorrhea in females. Zhaohai (K 6), connecting with the Chong Meridian which distributes at the lower abdomen, and the emerging site of the Yinqiao Meridian, can treat kidney qi deficiency and consolidate the Yuan (source) qi. These two acupoints arranged in a pair can tonify kidney and consolidate the body constitution, so they can treat leukorrhea due to deficiency and cold. For instance, a lady about thirty years old had large amount of leukorrhea-like urine, a white colour as clear water, odourless, pruritus vulvae. She had been treated with some medication but with no effect. Therefore warm needling technique was applied on Zhaohai (K 6) and Lieque (L 7), moxibustion with ginger on Guanyuan (Ren 4). After six treatments, the leukorrhea turned thicker, the volume decreased, and pruritus vulvae also improved. After the second course of treatments, the volume of leukorrhea decreased obviously and there was no pruritus vulvae.

3. Moxibustion with herbal pad for stagnant pain due to deficiency and cold

There are a lot of heat sources in moxibustion. In ancient times, there were fire-chopstick moxibustion, tobacco moxibustion, sulphur moxibustion, Moschus moxibustion, Lignum Aquilariae moxibustion, charcoal moxibustion, and moxa-stick moxibustion, etc. Now in the clinic, moxa-stick moxibustion, moxa-cone moxibustion, moxibustion with ginger, moxibustion with herbal cake and warm-needling moxibustion are often used. Dr. Qin assimilates the strong points of Taiyin Needle, Thunder-fire Needle and of external application with herbal extract, and creates moxibustion with herbal pad on the basis of moxibustion with herbal cake and moxibustion with ginger. Moxibustion with herbal pad has a large scope of indications. Besides Xu (deficient) syndromes, cold syndromes and painful syndromes due to stagnant blood, moxibustion with herbal pad is also used in those who are not suitable to acupuncture, such as the aged, the weak and babies, or in those regions not suitable to acupuncture, such as finger, toes, small joints, lateral epicondule of humerus, external and internal malleolus, ribs, and spinous processes, or in those regions where acupuncture may cause severe pain, such as the palm, sole, and heel. Moxibustion with herbal pad is so easy to operate that the patients can do it at home themselves.

Principle of the functions: Dr. Qin thinks that the warmth of both moxa stick and herbal pad, penetrating to the muscles and bones, makes blood flow freely in the meridians, so as to warm up the meridians and dispel the cold, to ventilate the meridians and remove stagnancy, to open the aperture and relieve pain.

1) *Tools* A moxa stick, and a Chinese herbal pad.

2) *Procedure* Mix 300 ml of herbal decoction, which is cooked with 15 g of ginger and some other herbs with heat nature and functions of activating blood and opening aperture, with wheat flour into a paste. Apply the paste on five to six layers of cotton cloth, which are put together as a pad. Dry the pad under the sunlight and cut it into small pieces about 10 cm square. During the treatment, the herbal pad is put on certain acupoint or diseased areas by the left hand, and then the ignited moxa stick is applied on the pad by the right hand. After about five minutes, when the area applied with moxibustion has a burning sensation, take away the moxa stick, lift the pad a little and put it on the original area again, and then give another moxibustion as mentioned above. Moxibustion should be applied five times on each point.

3) *Precautions* a. The method cannot be used for patients with hypertension, on the upper part of the body and the head; b. The method cannot be used on the eye region and the pudendal region; and c. The method cannot be used on pregnant women.

Dr. Qin has treated a patient in Morocco who had pain in the costal region for three months after an injury, which was aggravated by coughing. The pain was not relieved after taking pain-killers. Acupuncture was given three times, but pain in the costal region was still not relieved. Therefore, moxibustion with the herbal pad was applied once every day. After five treatments, the pain was relieved a lot, and no more pain occurred after eight treatments.

Dr. Qin has observed 393 cases of thirteen diseases treated by moxibustion with herbal pad. The average success rate was 83.1 percent.

4. "Needle-substitute herbal plaster" used for special patients

For babies, the weak and those who will faint when acupuncture is applied, Dr. Qin gives them the Qin's needle-substitute herbal plaster, which can stimulate acupoints and ventilate meridians so as to regulate qi and blood, yin and yang of the body.

1) *Tools* Medical plaster, Semen Sinapis Albae, Cortex Cinnamomi, Borneolum and other hot and spicy herbs with the function of opening aperture.

2) *Procedure* Cut the plaster into small pieces about 3 cm square. Smash the herbs and mix them well with vaseline, and make into small pills about 1.5 cm in diameter. The pill is put in the center of a piece of plaster which is applied on certain acupoints for six to eight hours. If an itching sensation occurs in the skin of a local region, the time of the treatment is cut short.

3) *Indications* The method of needle-substitute herbal plaster can be applied on the old, the weak, babies and those who are afraid of needling or those who will faint when acupuncture is given. The method is effective for vascular headache, chronic colitis, bronchial asthma, impotence, and enuresis. For instance, a patient Wu, male, 35 years old, had chronic diarrhoea for nearly ten years. No effects occurred after he was treated with both traditional Chinese medicine and Western medicine. Therefore the needle-

substitute herbal plaster was used. After the first course of treatments the symptoms improved and bowel movements decreased to once a day. After one more course of treatments, the patient was cured.

II. Case Analysis

Case 1: Hemiplegia

Name, Jiang x x; sex, female; age, 44.

Complaints She had a history of hypertension. Then paralysis and weakness of the legs appeared. She could not walk, accompanied with dizziness, and even vomiting. Examination by the department of neurology, an EEG and ECG showed normal. So she was treated as intracranial hypotension with infusion, but the condition did not improve. After that, acupuncture and moxibustion were applied. The pulse was deep, thready, rolling and string-taut; tongue coating was thin and slightly yellow; blood pressure was 110/70 mmHg. The condition was differentiated as flaring-up of liver fire due to kidney yin deficiency which resulted in the Wei-atrophy syndrome of excess in the upper body and deficiency in the lower body, which was treated by tonifying the liver and benefiting the kidney yin, and by regulating qi and blood of the Taiyang Meridians and the Du Meridian.

Prescription Renzhong (Du 26), Taichong (Liv 3), Hegu (LI 4), Mingmen (Du 4), Yaoyangguan (Du 3), Shenshu (B 23), Dachangshu (B 25), Feiyang (B 58), Zusanli (S 36), Taixi (K 3).

Treatment procedure Reducing method was applied on Taichong (Liv 3), warming needle technique on Shenshu (B 23), even manipulation on the other acupoints, and cupping method on the Du Meridian for five minutes afterwards. After five treatments, the symptoms were relieved, and the patient could walk. She was cured and went to work after eight treatments.

Case 2: Glossocoma

Name, Li x x; sex, male; age, 40.

Complaints In recent three months, he could not stretch his tongue out of the mouth, accompanied with distension of the head, dry mouth, and string-taut and rapid pulse. The condition was differentiated as kidney water deficiency which caused flaming-up of liver fire, which was treated by nourishing the kidney water to suppress the liver fire.

Prescription Lianquan (Ren 23), Jinjing, Yuye (Extra 9), Fengfu (Du 16), Fuliu (K 7), Xingjian (Liv 2).

Treatment procedure Penetrating method was used on Lianquan (Ren 23). The patient recovered after three treatments.

Explanation Glossocoma is not a common disease in clinic. According to the theory of meridians and collaterals, the Kidney Meridian of Foot-Shaoyin goes to the root of tongue, and its small collaterals are scattered on the back of the tongue; and the Liver

Meridian of Foot-Jueyin goes upwards to the throat. Because of the kidney water deficiency which results in flaming-up of liver fire, the symptoms as distension of the head, dry mouth, motor impairment of tongue occur. Needling on Lianquan (Ren 23), Jinjing, Yuye (Extra 10) and Fengfu (Du 16) is able to open the aperture, so as to arouse the meridian qi in tongue region, especially for stiff tongue and aphasia. Fuliu (K 7) and Xingjian (Liv 2) are selected to nourish the kidney water and reduce the liver fire.

ANALYSIS OF THE DISEASED AREA WITH THE COMBINED APPROACHES OF WESTERN AND TRADITIONAL CHINESE MEDICINE, DEPTH ON PUNCTURING THE POINTS OF THE DU MERIDIAN AND THE SHU-POINTS

—Yuan Shuo's Clinical Experience

Yuan Shuo, a native of Shenyang, was born in October 1934. At the age of nineteen he was admitted to the Department of Medicine, Beijing Medical College. In 1958 after graduation he began to work as a pediatrist in the Third Affiliated Hospital of Beijing Medical College. Meanwhile, he started learning Chinese medicine from Jiao Yongqun. His diagnosis is usually made by a Western approach with differentiation of syndromes guided by traditional Chinese medicine, and selection of points according to the meridians. Since May 1969 he has done acupuncture therapy. His works include *A Dictionary of Chinese Medicine and Herbs* (acupuncture section), *Selected Proved Recipes for the Common Cold and Bronchitis.* In the past twenty-eight years he had served as a teacher at the Beijing Medical University (the former Beijing Medical College). Now he is an associate professor in medicine.

I. Academic Characteristics and Medical Specialities

1. Analysis of the diseased area and meridian for nervous disorders

It is important to know the diseased area, whether in the brain, spinal cord or in the peripheral nerves, for a nervous disorder.

1) *Pathological changes in the brain, points on the Du Meridian being selected* When pathological changes occur in the brain, such as mental disorders, windstroke (cerebral thrombosis, cerebral hemorrhage), etc., points on the Du Meridian are selected because this meridian ascends posteriorly along the interior of the spinal column to Fengfu (Du 16) at the nape, where it enters the brain. For this reason the Du Meridian is closely related to the brain and the spinal cord. When it is diseased, puncture of the points on this meridian may replenish the spinal cord, benefit the brains, calm the mind and stop convulsions. Since it controls the yang meridians and limb motion is motivated by yang qi, in case yang qi fails to reach the limbs, a cold feeling in the four limbs will occur. Blocked flow of qi and blood causes weak limbs or motion impairment because of failure to nourish them. Puncturing points on the Du Meridian can invigorate yang qi, promote qi flow in the meridians, so as to cure weak limbs or motion impairment. In operation, shallow puncture with multiple needles is necessary, to a depth of about 1 cun.

Since the shallow puncture brings about mild stimulation, more points are selected at a time. The group of points commonly used are Sishencong (Extra 6), Baihui (Du 20), Fengfu (Du 16), Yamen (Du 15) and Dazhui (Du 14). They function to invigorate yang qi, resuscitate, benefit the brain, calm the mind and relieve convulsion. Penetrating puncture is applied to Sishencong (Extra 6) towards Baihui (Du 20). Horizontal puncture is applied to Baihui (Du 20) and perpendicular puncture is given to Fengfu (Du 16), Yamen (Du 15) and Dazhui (Du 14). After appearance of qi, manipulations are done for one or two minutes, and then retain the needle for twenty minutes. In the duration of needle retention do the manipulations once or twice.

If the needle is inserted through the ligament, the needle reaction must be strong. Only one point is enough to be used, either Yamen (Du 15) or Dazhui (Du 14). This method is often used to treat such cases as encephalopathy, epilepsy, sequelae of encephalitis, and intractable hysterical paralysis, etc., which have no response to general acupuncture techniques. However, it is dangerous to use this method. When an electric shock-like feeling appears, the needle must be withdrawn immediately. Needle retention and the lift-thrust manipulations are forbidden. The following are some examples of this method. In October 1969, a 12-year-old girl named Liu came to be consulted because she often had dull-looking eyes for about a year. One year before she had had a virus cold with high fever (39°-40°C) for four days. The case was cured by herbs. Since then dull-looking eyes appeared two or three times a week, lasting one or two minutes for each time. She said what she saw was enlarged. Meanwhile she had incontinence of her urine. After the attack, she felt all right. An EEG was normal at the Capital Hospital. Physical examination showed her mind was clear, pale red tongue with thin white coating, string-taut pulse, normal motion of limbs and normal reflexes. She was diagnosed as having temporal lobe epilepsy. The brain is responsible for the mental activities so Fengfu (Du 16), Dazhui (Du 14), Yamen (Du 15), Baihui (Du 20) and Sishencong (Extra 6), were selected. Twenty treatments cured the case completely. A follow-up study sixteen months later showed no relapse. Here is another example. In the winter of 1972 a 32-year-old woman peasant named Tian quarrelled with her neighbour. The neighbour kicked her on the buttock and she fell to the ground and found her legs paralysed. She was carried to the treatment. No fracture of lumbar vetebra or pelvis was seen on an X-ray. She was diagnosed as hysterical paralysis due to stagnation of liver qi and disturbance of tendons. At first strong electro-acupuncture was given to Yanglingquan (G 34) and Huantiao (G 30) for twenty minutes, but failed. Then Yamen (Du 15) was tried with deep insertion. When an electric shock-like sensation spread to the legs, she felt she was able to move them, and she walked home after the acupuncture treatment.

2) *Pathological changes in the spinal cord (myelitis, hemiplegia due to trauma), points on the Du Meridian and Jiaji points being simultaneously selected* It means that when the pathological changes occur in the spinal cord, the points on the Du Meridian at the diseased area and the corresponding Jiaji points are punctured strongly to lead the meridian qi running from the diseased part downward and to make the qi in the Du Meridian travel smoothly. Here is an example. Three days before, a 26-year-old male had had a low fever. Then lumbago appeared. At first he had a heavy feeling in the legs. On the following day the two legs were paralysed associated with incontinence of urine and

feces. His mind was clear, but he lost sensation below the second lumbar vertebra. Physical and laboratory tests showed: myodynamia (I), monocyte $48/mm^3$, protein 49 mg percent, weak reflex. He was diagnosed as acute myelitis. The following two groups of points were selected. Group 1: Jiaji points located at the place, one vertebra above and below the level of the diseased part and Huantiao (G 30), Yanglingquan (G 34) and Xuanzhong (G 39). Group 2: Jiaji points located at the place two vertebrae above and below the level of the diseased part, and Zhibian (B 54), Weizhong (B 40) and Kunlun (B 60). Electro-acupuncture was applied to the two groups alternately every other day for twenty minutes. After fifteen treatments he had markedly improved and the myodynamia increased. After thirty-five treatments the patient could walk slowly for a distance of ten meters. Then he was discharged from the hospital.

3) *Pathological changes in the pheripheral nerves, points along the meridians being selected* Points selected along the meridians refer to two approaches: One is to select the points near the diseased nerve, e.g. Yifeng (SJ 17), which is posterior to the ear lobe in the depression between the mandible and mastoid process, is selected for facial peripheral paralysis; the other is to select the points along the meridians, e.g. Hegu (LI 4) on the healthy side is used for left facial peripheral paralysis because the Large Intestine Meridian of Hand-Yangming runs through the cheek and enters the gums of the lower teeth, curves around the upper lip and the two branches cross at the philtrum and stop at Yingxiang (LI 20). An example of treatment is as follows: In November 1985, there was a 23-year-old woman whose right eye and the right corner of her mouth were twisted to the left side. She felt a slight pain in the posterior of the right ear, and the right eye could not be closed. She had excessive flow of saliva, pale red tongue with thin white coating, floating and tight pulse. This was a case due to invasion of the meridians by pathogenic wind and cold. Fengchi (G 20), Yifeng (SJ 17), Jiache (S 6) towards Dicang (S 4), Yangbai (G 14), Sibai (S 2) and left Hegu (LI 4) were used. Treatment was given every other day and ten treatments constituted a course. After appearance of qi, the reducing method was applied and the needle was retained for thirty minutes, during which manipulation was done two or three times. Fifteen treatments in total cured the case.

2. Pathological changes in the zang-fu organs, the Back-Shu points being selected

When there are disorders in the zang-fu organs, it is important to know what organ and meridian are affected. Afterwards, based on their relationship, the points are selected. The Back-Shu points are located on the Bladder Meridian at both sides of the spinal column, 1.5 cun lateral to the central line of the back, which is the place where the qi of the zang-fu organs is transmitted.

1) *Feishu (B 13)* Accompanied by Taiyuan (L 9), Zusanli (S 36) and Qihai (Ren 6), puncture with the reinforcing method for treating asthma due to insufficient lung qi. When it is used together with Dazhui (Du 14), Waiguan (SJ 5), Fengchi (B 20), Hegu (LI 4), Chize (L 5) and Lieque (L 7) (by needle retention or moxibustion), cough due to affection of wind and cold or wind and heat (by quick puncture) may be cured. Feishu (B 13) selected with Zusanli (S 36), Fenglong (S 40) and Lieque (L 7) may cure block

of the lung by phlegm and heat, or with Sanyinjiao (Sp 6), Taixi (K 3), Zhaohai (K 6) and Tiantu (Ren 22) may cure cough due to deficiency of yin and heat in the lung. Here is an example of the treatment. A 43-year-old female had a cough for five days. Two days before the consultation she had a low fever (37.5°-37.6°C). Physical examination showed a bubble in the lung, red tongue with thin yellow coating, slight rapid pulse, yellow urine and dry stools. X-ray examination showed more striation on the lung. It was a syndrome of cough due to wind and heat. Feishu (B 13), Fengchi (G 20), Hegu (LI 4), Lieque (L 7) and Tiantu (Ren 22) were selected with the reducing method. Treatment was given every other day. Five treatments in total cured the case. No more abnormal condition was seen in an X-ray examination.

2) *Xinshu (B 15)* When it is used with Shenmen (H 7), (Tongli (H 5)), Neiguan (P 6) and Sanyinjiao (Sp 6), insomnia and other deficiency syndromes due to insufficient blood and malnourishment of the heart may be cured. When it is used with Neiguan (P 6), (Ximen (P 4)), Tanzhong (Ren 17), Juque (Ren 14), coronary heart disease may be cured. Zusanli (S 36) is added in case of qi deficiency, and Geshu (B 17) added to promote smooth blood flow in case of stagnation of qi and blood. For example, in April 1979, a 64-year-old professor Zhao came for treatment. He complained that one day when he was going upstairs he suddenly felt stuffiness in the chest, associated with two attacks of stabbing pain, lasting one or two minutes. He was diagnosed as having coronary heart disease due to insufficient heart qi and a block of the Heart Meridian. Neiguan (P 6) was punctured first with the reducing method for twenty minutes, and then Tanzhong (Ren 17) was quickly needled with the reducing method. Afterwards, the needle tip was directed up and down, right and left for one or two minutes. Zusanli (S 36) was needled with the even movement and the needle was retained for twenty minutes, during which manipulation was done once or twice. After five treatments symptoms were relieved and twenty minutes later all the symptoms disappeared. Xinshu (B 15) and Geshu (B 17) were perpendicularly punctured, 1 cun in depth with manipulations for one or two minutes. The needle was retained for twenty minutes. Then the ECG turned to normal.

3) *Ganshu (B 18)* It is used with Yanglingquan (G 34), Zhigou (SJ 6), Tanzhong (Ren 17) to treat costal pain occurring in liver trouble or neurosis. When it is selected with Sanyinjiao (Sp 6), Yinlingquan (Sp 9) and Taixi (K 3), numbness of the limbs, dryness of the eyes due to insufficiency of liver yin can be cured. When it is used with Yanglingquan (G 34), Taichong (Liv 3), Xingjian (Liv 2) and Quchi (LI 11) by the reducing method, hypertension due to hyperactivity of liver yang may be cured. It is used with Zusanli (S 36), Yanglingquan (G 34) and Neiguan (P 6) to treat disharmony of the liver and stomach. For instance, Mr. Guo came for treatment in winter, 1974. He complained that his left breast had enlarged in the past twenty days with tenderness. In the previous six months he sometimes had stuffy chest. Physical examination showed a 2 x 3 cm movable lump at the upper part of the breast. He was diagnosed as having male mastoplasia by an X-ray examination, due to stagnation of qi. He was first given acupuncture to Ganshu (B 18) perpendicularly, 1 cun in depth. After appearance of qi, manipulations were done for one or two minutes and the needle was withdrawn. Then two groups of points were alternately selected. They were Yanglingquan (G 34), Fenglong (S 40), Yingchuan (S 16) and Zusanli (S 36), Tanzhong (Ren 17) and Rugeng (S 18).

Treatment was given every other day. Twenty-eight treatments cured the case.

4) *Pishu (B 20)* It is used with Zusanli (S 36), Sanyinjiao (Sp 6), Qihai (Ren 6) by the reinforcing method to treat general debility due to insufficient qi. It is used with Weishang (Extra 14), Zhongwan (Ren 12) and Zusanli (S 36) to treat gastroptosis. In October 1978 a 43-year-old woman patient came for treatment. She complained that in the previous two years she had had a distended feeling in the stomach, worse after meals and a bearing-down sensation. She was diagnosed as having gastroptosis by barium meal examination. A physical examination showed puffy tongue with thin white coating and tooth-prints on the border of the tongue. Electro-acupuncture was applied to Weishang (Extra 14) with a four cun needle. The needle was penetrated towards Tianshu (S 25) with manipulations for twenty minutes. Then Zhongwan (Ren 12) and Zusanli (S 36) were applied with the reinforcing method and retention of the needle for twenty minutes. With acupuncture the patient had a contracting sensation in the stomach. The bearing-down sensation disappeared after seven treatments. On the fourteenth treatment she did not feel uneasy in the stomach after meals. Barium meal examination showed the stomach had returned to the normal position. Then another seven treatments of warm acupuncture were given to Pishu (B 20) and Weishu (B 21) to strengthen the effect.

5) *Shenshu (B 23)* It is used with Qihai (Ren 6), Zusanli (S 36) and Guanyuan (Ren 4) to treat incontinence of urine due to insufficient qi. When it is punctured with Mingmen (Du 4), Zhishi (B 52) and moxibustion is applied to Guanyuan (Ren 4), pain and cold feeling in the lower back due to insufficient kidney yang, female sterility due to cold in the uterus and impotence can be treated. When it is used with Sanyinjiao (Sp 6), Taixi (K 3) and Zhaohai (K 6) or Jiaoxin (K 8), ringing in the ears due to deficiency in the kidney and male sterility due to less sperm can be treated. For instance, 30-year-old Mr. Liu came for treatment. He complained that after three months of his marriage he was impotent. Symptoms included lassitude, weak lower back and legs, yellow complexion, puffy tongue with thin white coating, deep and thready pulse. This was a case of impotence due to insufficient kidney yang. Two groups of points were used alternately with the reinforcing method. They were a. Shenshu (B 23), Mingmen (Du 4), and Zhishi (B 52) and b. Guanyuan (Ren 4), Qihai (Ren 6), and Sanyinjiao (Sp 6). Treatment was given every day. Twenty treatments in total cured the case. Then further treatment was given to strengthen the effect. Eight months later he told the doctor that his wife was pregnant.

3. Deep needling of Yamen (Du 15)

Yamen (Du 15) is located at the midpoint of the nape, 0.5 cun below Fengfu (Du 16) in the depression 0.5 cun within the hairline. This is a point where the Du Meridian and Yangwei Meridian meet. The indications of the point are epilepsy, mental disorders, stiffness of tongue and post-apoplexy aphasia, stiff neck, back headache. In the past fifteen years Yuan has studied the method and depth of acupuncture for intractable epilepsy, sequelae of encephalitis, mental disorders and hysterical paralysis.

1) *Deep puncture* Ask the patient to sit straight and lower his neck as far as he can to allow the nape to be straight and widen the space between the cervical vertebrae. A

3-cun-long needle is inserted into the center of the upper border of the second cervical vertebra in the direction of the mouth. When it reaches the ligamentum supraspinale and ligamenta interspinalia there is a tight feeling around the needle, and when it reaches the yellow ligament there is a flexible feeling around the needle. At this moment the needle is thrust 1.5-5 mm in depth. When a loose feeling around the needle and an electric shock-like sensation appears it should be withdrawn at once.

2) *Depth of puncture* Acupuncturists through the ages had varied opinions about the depth of puncture for Yamen (Du 15). It is stated in *A Classic of Acupuncture and Moxibustion* that the depth is 0.4 cun, but the *Compendium of Acupuncture and Moxibustion* says the depth is 0.3 cun. The *New Acupuncture and Moxibustion* points out the depth is 0.3-0.4 cun at most. There are some reasons for the above arguments in terms of anatomy. Because Yamen (Du 15) is located above the spinal cord and close to medullary bulb, a too deep puncture may damage the spinal cord or medullary bulb, causing bleeding or death. But since the shallow puncture does not produce desirable effects for intractable diseases, some acupuncturists say the point can be punctured 1-2 cun or even 2-3 cun in depth according to their own clinical experiences. Yuan believes deeper puncture of Yamen (Du 15) is better than shallow puncture in treatment of hysterical aphasia, paralysis, and attack of hysteria. He says puncture of 2-3 cun in depth does not bring any harmful effect. It is demonstrated by his experience that deeper puncture of Yamen (Du 15) produces better effects in treatment of epilepsy, hysterical paralysis, sequelae of encephalitis. But he also points out care must be taken to avoid accidents because of its special anatomical position. Only by complete understanding of the acupuncture technique, depth of puncture, indications and strict sterilization, can good effects be produced without any accidents. (The beginner must be cautious to do acupuncture in this point because accidents tend to happen—editor).

3) *Shallow and deep puncture of Yamen (Du 15)* Up to now there is no marked standard to differentiate the depth of puncture. Generally speaking, 0.5 cun in depth is shallow and 2-3 cun in depth is a deep puncture. Yuan holds that the dividing line lies in the yellow ligament. If the needle does not go through the yellow ligament yet at a depth of two cun and there is a local needling reaction, it is known as the shallow puncture. On the contrary, if the depth is not beyond 2 cun but it has already got through the yellow ligament and there is an electric shock-like sensation, it is known as the deep puncture. The reason is as follows:

a. When the needle tip does not touch the yellow ligament, no matter how deep it is inserted there always occurs a local needling reaction, which is different in nature from the reaction produced when the needle tip has got through the yellow ligament. Varied needling sensations bring different therapeutic effects.

b. Shallow puncture is safe because the needle tip will not go into the canalis vertebralis and damage the spinal cord and medullary bulb. Care must be taken to do deep puncture because it is dangerous.

4) *Indications for deep puncture of Yamen (Du 15)* Because it is dangerous to do deep puncture of the point, one must know clearly about its indications. Deep puncture is only to be used when shallow puncture or other approaches are not effective. Yuan holds that the indications are as follows:

a. Frequent attack of epilepsy;
b. Hallucinatory paranoid form of schizophrenia;
c. Sequelae of encephalitis;
d. Hysterical paralysis; and
e. Aphasia.
5) *Contraindications for puncture of Yamen (Du 15)*
a. Coagulation disorders due to various reasons;
b. Deformity of the cervical vertebra, causing difficulty to locate the point;
c. Patients of restlessness; and
d. Patients who have inflammation on or around the point.

II. Case Analysis.

Case 1: Diarrhoea

Name, Zeng x x; sex, male; age, 20 months; date of the first visit, June 16, 1959.

Complaints A month before the baby had had a low fever (37.2°-37.5°C) for two days together with diarrhoea, ten to twenty times a day and was hospitalized. Pathogenic colibacillus was found in the laboratory test. After given infusion neomycin and pepsin for 4 days the body temperature became normal, diarrhoea decreased to six to eight times a day associated with nausea and poor appetite. Twenty days later the baby showed lassitude, crying in low voice, pallor, cold limbs, moderate prolapse of rectum, puffy pale tongue with thin white coating, deep and thready pulse.

Differentiation Diarrhoea due to insufficient yang of the spleen and kidney.

Method Strengthen yang of the spleen and kidney.

Prescription Group 1: Pishu (B 20) and Shenshu (B 23).

Group 2: Tianshu (S 25) and Zusanli (S 36).

Treatment procedure Moxibustion was applied to the two groups of points alternately for three minutes, twice a day. After five treatments diarrhoea was markedly reduced to three to four times a day. Other symptoms were alleviated too. On the ninth day bowel movements became normal, yet with loose stools. Moxibustion was given once every day. Twenty-four treatments given in fifteen days cured the case.

Explanation At first the case was manifested by major loss of body fluid due to abundant heat that injures yin. After infusion, yin was balanced but yang deficiency was seen. Then moxibustion was applied to Pishu (B 20) and Shenshu (B 23) to invigorate yang. Meanwhile, moxibustion is also given to Zusanli (S 36) and Tianshu (S 25) to regulate the function of the intestines and stop diarrhoea.

Case 2: Epilepsy

Name, Tian x x; sex, female; age, 12; date of the first visit, January 10, 1969.

Complaints Six months before she often had had dull-looking eyes with no sense of what happened to her, ten to twenty times a day. The attack lasted for thirty seconds. There was no convulsion and incontinence of urine and feces. After the attack nothing was wrong with her. On October 17, 1968 she was diagnosed as having a minor attack of epilepsy based on an EEG. Then she was given antiepileptics and the attacks were reduced to seven or eight times a day. But three months later the attacks increased to ten times a day. When she came for treatment she was clear-minded. She had pale red tongue with thin white coating and slippery pulse.

Differentiation Upward attack of liver wind.

Method Calm the mind to remove epilepsy.

Prescription Yamen (Du 15), Neiguan (P 6) and Anmian (Extra 9).

Treatment procedure Deep needling was applied to Yamen (Du 15). After insertion of the needle there was an electric shock-like sensation radiating to the head and limbs. The needle was withdrawn without delay. After appearance of the needling reaction, the reducing method was given to Neiguan (P 6) and Anmian (Extra 9) for one minute and the needle was retained for twenty minutes. After six treatments, two or three attacks were seen a day, each lasting for a few seconds. Thirty treatments cured the case. But ten months later she again had epilepsy followed by a fever (41°C) due to upper respiratory tract infection. Another twenty acupuncture treatments finally cured the case again. A follow-up survey of twenty-six months showed no relapse.

Explanation Epilepsy was called "children's serious disease" by the ancient Chinese. It often has a long disease course and is not easy to be cured. Now it is held that the pathological changes occur in the brain, that is why points of the Du Meridian is selected since this meridian runs to the brain. Yamen (Du 15), Neiguan (P 6) and Anmian (Extra 9) were needled to calm the mind and stop convulsions. Thirty-two cases were treated by our department with the above method from 1968 to 1972, the total effective rate was 87.5 percent, 53 percent of which vastly improved.

Case 3: Mammary hyperplasia

Name, Shi x x; sex, female; age, 51; date of the first visit, November 6, 1969.

Complaints A lump in the left breast had been removed four years before and the pathological test showed lobular hyperplasia. Since then she often bound her breast with a piece of thick cloth, which led to breathing difficulty. Two months ago there suddenly appeared a paroxysmal distending pain in the right breast, lasting a few seconds each time. In the past twenty days it deteriorated. The pain spread to the right armpit. On examination a lump as big as a peanut was found in the upper part of the right breast and an operation was suggested. She refused and asked to be treated by acupuncture. Physical examination showed a tenderness at the right Ganshu (B 18), dark red tongue with swollen sublingual veins and thin white coating and string-taut pulse.

Differentiation Stagnation of qi and blood stasis.

Method Relieve stagnancy of liver qi and blood stasis.

Prescription Group 1: Tanzhong (Ren 17), Geshu (B 17), and Rugen (S 18).

Group 2: Yanglingquan (G 34), Xuehai (Sp 10) and Yingchuang (S 16).

Treatment procedure The two groups of points were used with the reducing method alternately every other day. After appearance of qi the lift-thrust and rotation were done for one or two minutes. Horizontal puncture was applied to Yingchuang (S 16) and Rugen (S 18). The needles were retained for twenty minutes.

Explanation It is stated in the *Orthodox Manual of Surgery* that "mammary hyperplasia is caused by grief or worry, leading to injury of the liver and spleen, and lumps formed in the meridians." Yuan believes it is often caused by stagnation of qi, phlegm and blood stasis. For this case it was due to stagnation of liver qi and failure of smooth flow of blood. That is why Tanzhong (Ren 17), Yanglingquan (G 34) were needled to regulate qi flow in the liver. Rugen (S 18) can regulate qi, blood and remove obstruction. The case was cured when smooth flow of qi and blood was achieved.

Case 4: Asthma

Name, Wang x x; sex, female; age, 47; date of the first visit, November 10, 1981.

Complaints In the previous nine years asthma often attacked on weather changes, common cold or inhalation of odours. Two weeks ago she had an attack of asthma due to upper respiratory tract infection and it became worse day by day. Symptoms included moderate cough with expectoration of runny yellow phlegm. Physical examination showed a clear mind, respiratory rate: 32/m., wheezing sound, red tongue with yellow coating and slippery rapid pulse. There was a tenderness at Feishu (B 13).

Differentiation The lung obstructed by heat and phlegm.

Method Remove heat and phlegm.

Prescription Feishu (B 13), Dingchuan (Extra 17) or Tanzhong (Ren 17), Chize (L 5), Fenglong (S 40).

Treatment procedure Acupuncture was given to Feishu (B 13) and Dingchuan (Extra 17) with the reducing method. The needles were quickly punctured and rotated for one or two minutes. When the patient felt better the needles were retained for twenty minutes, during which manipulations were done one or two times. Then Chize (L 5) and Fenglong (S 40) were needled. After appearance of qi the needles were retained for twenty minutes. Ten treatments relieved the condition and twenty treatments cured the case. The function of the lung was examined before and after acupuncture. See the following table:

Functional Changes of the Lung Before and After Acupuncture

Item	Before	Immediately after	After ten treatments	After twenty treatments
FEV 1.0	1.40 L	1.72 L	2.60 L	2.68 L
FEV 1.0%	6.604%	78.18%	82.28%	80.24%
FEV 1.0/VCPR	49.8%	61.2%	92.5%	95.4%

Explanation This case was due to obstruction of the lung by heat and phlegm. Therefore, Feishu (B 13), Dingchuan (Extra 17), Tanzhong (Ren 17) and Chize (L 5) were selected to remove obstruction of heat and phlegm. Fenglong (S 40) is on the Stomach Meridian, a branch of which runs to the spleen. Needling Fenglong (S 40) may invigorate the spleen and eliminate damp and phlegm because growth of phlegm is due to deficiency in the spleen. Since asthma is a prolonged condition, it is necessary to give further treatment in the easing period. Moxibustion was applied to Pishu (B 20) and Shenshu (B 23) for two months to strengthen the body resistance. A follow-up study for one year showed no relapse.

Case 5: Hiccup

Name, Wang x x; sex, female; age, 30; date of the first visit, July 9, 1986.

Complaints She had grieved deeply for the loss of her son five years before. Afterwards she had a stuffy chest, distended abdomen and hiccup. After sixty-seven doses of herbal decoctions, the symptoms were relieved. But for about a year she was quite depressed because of a miscarriage and the condition became worse. Hiccup occurred from morning till night. She could not get out of bed due to lassitude, accompanied by costal pain and poor appetite. She was diagnosed as chronic gastritis by gastroscopy. No response was seen to Western drugs. The symptoms were relieved six months later after herbal treatment. She was found to have dry stools, yellow urine, red tongue with thin yellow coating and string-taut pulse.

Differentiation Invasion of the stomach by liver fire and dysfunction of the stomach in sending down food content.

Method Soothe the liver and remove fire, regulate the vital function of the stomach and bring down the food content.

Prescription Group 1: Ganshu (B 18), Weishu (B 21) and Taichong (Liv 3).

Group 2: Tanzhong (Ren 17), Yanglingquan (G 34), Neiguan (P 6) and Zhigou (SJ 6).

Treatment procedure The two groups of points were selected alternately with the reducing method once a day. Manipulations were done for two minutes and the needles were retained for twenty minutes. Ganshu (B 18) and Weishu (B 21) were obliquely punctured, 1.5 cun in depth. Tanzhong (Ren 17) was horizontally needled.

Explanation Hiccup may be of excess and deficiency types. Hiccup due to stomach cold and fire is considered to be the excess syndrome. The former is usually caused by intake of too much cold food, leading to stomach inhibited yang and disturbance in upward and downward functional activities. But the present case was due to invasion of the stomach by liver fire and dysfunction of the stomach in sending down food content. Ganshu (B 18), Yanglingquan (G 34) and Taichong (Liv 3) were used to eliminate fire. Tanzhong (Ren 17), Weishu (B 21) and Neiguan (P 6) (penetrating towards Zhigou (SJ 6)) to regulate qi flow and the function of the stomach. Four treatments relieved the condition markedly. The attack was reduced to three to four times a day. Acupuncture was also given to Zusanli (S 36) with the even movement. Ten treatments cured the case.

CLINICAL APPLICATION OF THE THEORY OF SPLEEN AND STOMACH IN ACUPUNCTURE TREATMENT

—Yuan Jiuling's Clinical Experience

Yuan Jiuling, a native of Qingpu County, Shanghai, was born in a well-known family which practised traditional Chinese medicine. He loved Chinese medicine since childhood and at the age of twenty he started learning acupuncture from his mother. In 1956 he was admitted to the advanced acupuncture class for teachers of the Jiangsu School of Traditional Chinese Medicine (the predecessor of the Nanjing College of Traditional Chinese Medicine). Afterwards he worked as a teacher and acupuncturist at the school. He joined the group to compile textbooks of acupuncture and has been invited to present lectures and give treatment in Poland, Thailand, the Philippines and Japan. He was invited to attend the Seventh World Acupuncture Conference held in Sri Lanka in 1981, on which he made a presentation about the Midnight Noon Ebb and Flow. Now he is an associate professor and the deputy-director of the Teaching Section in the Beijing International Acupuncture Training Center.

I. Academic Characteristics and Medical Specialities

1. Regulating the function of spleen and stomach

In the treatment of wind-stroke, insomnia, dizziness, facial paralysis, tic of the facial muscles, Yuan often deals first with the spleen and stomach, the source of qi and blood, because abundant qi and blood guarantee good health. Points that regulate the spleen and stomach are Zusanli (S 36), Zhongwan (Ren 12), Pishu (B 20), Weishu (B 21), Yinlingquan (Sp 9), Neiguan (P 6), Gongsun (Sp 4), etc. A patient over sixty years old suddenly felt dizzy one morning. He was found half paralyzed on the right side, with left-wryed tongue, incoherent speech, string-taut pulse, pale red tongue with thin white coating. Zusanli (S 36) and Neiguan (P 6) of both sides were selected. On the second day he could speak clearly. A week later the paralysis of the right side was gone. The case was due to hyperactivity of liver yang, which turned into wind, causing dizziness, incoherent speech and hemiplegia when the pathogenic wind invaded the meridians. It would be thought that soothing the liver and removing wind was the routine way to treat this condition, but Yuan thought the spleen was the material basis of the acquired constitution. Only when the spleen and stomach function well could yin and yang be balanced. For this reason he selected Zusanli (S 36) and Neiguan (P 9), and the desired results were obtained.

For severe or critical cases Yuan is also experienced in application of moxibustion to regulate the function of spleen and stomach. He cured a case of paralysis due to hypokaliamie. The story is as follows: A patient had suffered from paralysis of the legs for four days. Other symptoms included cool lower limbs, poor appetite, loose stools, palpitation, insomnia, pale tongue, thready and weak pulse, which was diagnosed as paralysis due to hypokaliamie by medical doctors. Potassium venous transfusion for forty-eight hours did not bring any improvement. In the consultation, Yuan thought it was caused by deficiency in the spleen and stomach and suggested to treat the Stomach Meridian. Pus-forming moxibustion was applied to Zusanli (S 36) on both sides. After the first cone of moxa wool was burnt, the part receiving moxibustion turned pale; after the second cone of moxa wool was burnt, the part receiving moxibustion turned brown. Small blisters appeared in the vicinity. Seven cones of moxa wool in total were used in fifty minutes. On the morning of the following day the patient jumped out of bed and walked normally. There was no relapse afterwards. Later on it was known that people in that district had had vegetable oil containing cotton acid, which affected the absorption and use of potassium by the body.

2. Treatment given at the right time

For paroxysmal diseases Yuan first finds the rule of the attack, then treats it before the attack. For instance, an epileptic woman patient usually had an attack just before menstruation in the past ten years. When the period was coming she felt quite nervous, and had no desire to eat. During menstruation she had severe distending pain in the lower abdomen, sometimes even causing loss of consciousness. Other symptoms and signs were purple menstruation flow with blood clots, string-taut pulse and violet tongue. Yuan gave treatment seven days before the periods. Points selected were Taichong (Liv 3), Xuehai (Sp 10), Guanyuan (Ren 4) and Qihai (Ren 6) to regulate the liver qi and the Du and Ren Meridians. After a course of treatment on the evening of the sixth day the menstrual flow came with slight abdominal pain. When the blood clots were discharged, abdominal pain was relieved, and it was surprising that no relapse of epilepsy was found. Treatment ceased on the following day. Then repeated treatment was given successively for five months. Dysmenorrhea and epilepsy were removed. The successful treatment of this case proves the importance of treatment given at the right time based on precise differentiation of syndromes.

3. Different acupuncture techniques applied to the same kind of disease

Clinically, the same kind of disease may be treated with different acupuncture techniques and approaches because treatment should be based on case types—excess or deficiency, physical conditions and age. For example, Yuan cured two cases of herpes zoster with quite different approaches. The first patient had had left costal pain for five days and nights. In the space of the fourth rib the skin was red with transparent herpes, extending over an area of 8 x 2 cm. Besides, he had red tongue and string-taut pulse. In treatment, one needle was punctured in the centre of the affected area with four needles superficially punctured around it. The reducing method was applied. Three treatments relieved the pain and after six treatments the herpes were gone. The second patient had had herpes zosters for two months. External application of drugs cured some, but there was stubbing pain on the right costal region and no response to any treatment. Symptoms seen were lassitude, emaciated constitution, pale tongue and weak pulse. Needling was applied to Zusanli (S 36), Qihai (Ren 6) and Yanglingquan (B 34) with the reinforcing method. Small needles were embedded underneath the affected area. Pain and herpes completely disappeared after twelve treatments.

The above two cases had the same problem. The first case was an excess condition due to accumulation of pathogenic damp and heat in the skin, so stress was laid on clearing pathogenic heat and damp, and removing obstruction of the local vessels. For this purpose quintuple puncture was used. The second case was an excess condition associated with deficiency due to lowered vital function. So Zusanli (S 36) and Qihai (Ren 6) were selected to strengthen the vital function. The subcutaneous embedded needles were used to regulate the meridian locally.

4. Treating the left side of the body for disorders on the right, and vice versa

In dealing with hemiplegia, facial paralysis, tic of the facial muscles, shoulder and leg pain, he often treats the left side of the body for disorders on the right and vice versa. The approach is especially conducted for patients who have got treatment on the affected part without improvement. Puncturing the healthy side may regulate yin and yang. For example, a patient of facial paralysis had been given electro-acupuncture therapy for eight months. Afterwards he improved somewhat, but there was tic of the facial muscles, worse in the lower jaw. Points on the right side were continuously punctured and no positive response was seen. Yuan believes the meridians on the left and right are connected, and when points on one side were selected without success, points on the other side should be tried. He selected Quanliao (SI 18), Sibai (S 2), Dicang (S 4), Jiache (S 6) and Chengjiang (Ren 24) on the left side as the main points, and Hegu (LI 4), Taichong (Liv 3) on both sides as the secondary points. After five treatments tic of the facial muscles was markedly relieved and in twenty treatments tic and facial paralysis were removed.

5. Importance of shallow and deep needling

Yuan holds that shallow needling is helpful to patients of insomnia as well as to weak patients, the elderly and children. No matter what physical condition and types of the disorder are, Yuan uses shallow needling. For instance, a patient had suffered from insomnia caused by overexcitement due to playing cards until midnight. In the following three weeks he had relied on sedatives to fall asleep. On the consultation, symptoms seen were dizziness, poor appetite, pale tongue with thin white coating, slightly rapid and string-taut pulse. Yuan gave shallow puncture to Wangu (SI 4), Neiguan (P 6), Shenmen (H 7) and Sanyinjiao (Sp 6), 1 cun in depth, with moderate stimulation. Needles were retained for twenty minutes. At the night that day, although the patient took a half dosage of the sedatives he usually had taken, he slept quite well. After five treatments he slept soundly without sedatives. Then treatment ceased.

The deep needling technique is mostly applied to the excess condition, strong and fat patients. Alongside the deep needling technique, Yuan retains the needle for some time to cure some difficult cases. For example, one day a patient came with a burning sensation on the right cheek, associated with foul breath, dry throat, irritability, brown urine, constipation, red tongue with yellow, greasy coating, string-taut and rapid pulse —and manifestations of excessive heat. He had been diagnosed as having trigeminal neuralgia, and there was no response to about a month's treatment. Using 2-cun needles Yuan punctured the right Xiaguan (S 7), and Quanliao (SI 18) with the lift-thrust and rotating, reducing methods to dispel pathogenic damp and heat. After manipulations he fixed the needles at the points for six hours to promote qi flow in the meridians. Meanwhile he punctured Neiting (S 44) and Xingjian (L 2) on both sides. Pain was relieved after one treatment and seven treatments completely killed the pain.

II. Case Analysis

Case 1: Abdominal distention (acute ascris intestinal obstruction)

Name, Wang x x; sex, female; age, 7.

Complaints For seven days the patient had been in a coma, high fever and convulsion, accompanied by clenched jaw, stiff limbs, shortness of breath and rapid pulse. After hospitalization she was diagnosed as having encephalitis B. She was given hibernation therapy because of high fever. But one hour later a swollen abdomen was found. It was thought that she had acute enteroparalysis and measures were taken to reduce the pressure in the stomach and abdomen. No improvement was seen, then acupuncture was resorted to.

Differentiation Obstruction of the abdomen due to the unsmooth flow of qi.

Method Regulating the qi in the fu organs.

Prescription Tianshu (S 25), Qihai (Ren 6) and Zusanli (S 36).

Treatment procedure Using 1.5 cun needles Yuan gave a deeper puncture. When there was tenseness around the needle, he applied the reducing method. Manipulations first were given to the left Tianshu (S 25), then to the right Tianshu (S 25) and Qihai (Ren 6) for three minutes each. In an interval of five minutes, manipulations were repeated. In thirty minutes borborygmi appeared. At this moment the frequency of twirling was speeded up. Fifteen minutes later a large amount of black stools was discharged and abdominal eminence quickly became smaller. On the following day fever subsided and the patient came to. With treatment given by both traditional and Western medicine the child was finally cured and discharged without any sequela.

Case 2: Male sterility

Name, Li x x; sex, male; age, 34.

Complaints Li had been married for seven years without being able to have children. In examination, the amount of seminal fluid was 3 ml and the survival of spermatozoa was 10 percent. The survived spermatozoa could not move straight. Symptoms were pallor, lassitude, cold sensation of the limbs, weak lower back and legs, pale tongue with tooth print on its border, thready pulse.

Differentiation Insufficient kidney yang, decline of Mingmen fire.

Method Warming the kidney and invigorating yang.

Prescription Group 1: Mingmen (Du 4), Shenshu (B 23), Zhishi (B 52) and Taixi (K 3). Group 2: Guanyuan (Ren 4), Qihai (Ren 6), Zusanli (S 36) and Sanyinjiao (Sp 6).

Treatment procedure Treatment was given every day and the two groups of points were punctured alternately and superficially with the reinforcing method. During the process the patient was advised to stop sexual activity to preserve the kidney qi. After a two-month treatment sperm examination showed increased sperm count, the surviving rate and activity improved, but still below the normal level. Another two-month treatment was given. On the third examination it was found that the sperm count was 23.60 million, the surviving rate of sperm was 60 percent and the shape of half of the spermatozoa was normal. At this time treatment ceased and the patient was instructed to have moxibustion on Guanyuan (Ren 4) and Qihai (Ren 6) for twenty minutes every day by himself. Six months later his wife was pregnant and they had a girl.

Explanation This problem was caused by innate insufficiency and indulgence of sexual activities. Moxibustion was applied to Mingmen (Du 4) and acupuncture to Shenshu (B 23), Zhishi (B 52) and Taixi (K 3) to warm kidney yang. Moxibustion applied to Guanyuan (Ren 4), where sperm is stored and menstruation originates, may help to invigorate the original qi. Needling at Qihai (Ren 6), Zusanli (S 36) and Sanyinjiao (Sp 6) strengthens the spleen and stomach qi, the source of growth of qi and blood. Because it was a prolonged case, shallow puncture was used with the reinforcing method.

Case 3: Asthma

Name, Qian x x; sex, Female; age, 27.

Complaints At the age of seven the patient had asthma induced by measles and pneumonia. When the weather changed the asthma attacked. In the last four days asthma occurred frequently because of the common cold. She was found to have shortness of breath, asthma with expectoration of thin white phlegm, a pale red tongue with thin white coating, floating and tense pulse.

Differentiation Invasion of pathogenic wind and cold.

Method Ventilating and smoothing the lung and solving phlegm, stopping cough and asthma.

Prescription Tiantu (Ren 22), Dingchuan (Extra 17), Feishu (B 13), Kongzui (L 6), Fenglong (S 40), Fengmen (B 16), Geshu (B 17).

Treatment procedure Perpendicular puncture with short needles was given to Tiantu (Ren 22). After the arrival of qi, the needle was twirled and spasm of trachea was quickly relieved. Then Dingchuan (Extra 17), Feishu (B 13) and Kongzui (L 6) were punctured with 1 cun needles. After the arrival of qi, the reducing method was used. Treatment was given every day with retention of needles for thirty minutes. Cupping was applied to Geshu (B 17). Ten days later asthma and other symptoms were alleviated. At this time Dazhui (Du 14), Taiyuan (L 9), Feishu (B 13) and Zusanli (S 36) were needled to strengthen lung qi. Besides, moxibustion was applied to Fengmen (B 12) and Geshu (B 17) too. Treatment was given every other day successively for four months. Afterwards, when weather changed greatly no relapse of asthma was seen.

Explanation Tiantu (Ren 22) and Dingchuan (Extra 17) are important points to cure asthma. Feishu (B 13), Kongzui (L 6) and Fenglong (S 40) function to ventilate the lung and eliminate phlegm. Moxibustion was applied to Fengmen (B 12) and Geshu (B 17) as an experienced approach to dispel pathogenic wind from the lung.

STUDY AND APPLICATION OF THE LIGHTNING POINT

—Xu Bin's Clinical Experience

Xu Bin, a native of Suizhong County, Liaoning Province, was born in 1928. At the age of fourteen he began to learn traditional Chinese medicine and he has been practising acupuncture for over forty years. He joined four medical teams to work in Albania, North Yemen and Kuwait and received about 100,000 patients. He has written over twenty papers on acupuncture. Now he is a member of the Liaoning Society for Traditional Chinese Medicine, Vice-Chairman of the Jinzhou Society for Traditional Chinese Medicine, President of the Suizhong County Hospital of Traditional Chinese Medicine and associate chief doctor.

I. Academic Characteristics and Medical Specialities

1. The upper lightning point

This point was discovered by Dr. Xu. Marked effects have been achieved with this point and the needling sensation transmits as fast as lightning, hence the name.

1) *Location* Three cun away from the median of the larynx nodule (Futu (LI 18)), one cun obliquely and laterally downward, i.e. the posterior margin of the sternocleidomastoideus, corresponding to the meeting place of the vertical line from the lobulus auriculae and sternocleidomastoideus. The point is used in sitting position.

2) *Puncture techniques* Shallow puncture of a 1.5 cun needle No. 32 is conducted to a depth of 0.5 cun. Then manipulation of sparrow-pecking is applied with the needle point towards the diseased part. Transmission of the needling sensation to the finger tips suggests success. Retention of the needle is unnecessary.

3) *Precautions*

a. Patients should be reassured to free them from nervousness and fear of the strong needling sensation.

b. Local (the diseased part) swelling tends to occur. It is not used in patients of bone fracture and muscle injury.

c. It is not advisable to be used for pregnant women and patients with rheumatic heart disease.

d. The needling sensation which causes breathing difficulties would remain in the chest and back of some patients after acupuncture. Needling is repeated at the same point and when the new needling sensation reaches the place where the first needling sensation rests, the needle is pulled out at once and the first needling sensation would disappear immediately.

e. Avoid heavy physical labour, exercises and catching cold of the hand and foot.

4) *Clinical application* Two hundred and sixty-four cases of shoulder, chest and back pain, and strained arms were treated by using this point from 1967, when the point was discovered, to 1981. A hundred and thirty-three cases were cured, 122 cases were markedly effective and nine cases were effective. For example, 56-year-old Mr. Wang had suffered from right arm pain and motor impairment for over two years and there was no response to any treatment. Two treatments cured his condition.

2. The lower lightning point

It is also discovered by Xu and named on the above reason. The only difference is the location of this point at the lower limbs.

1) *Location* Six cun away from the 21st spinal vertebra (or 4 cun away from the 4th sacral vertebra), or 3 cun laterally away from Zhibian (B 54), forming a triangle with Zhibian (B 54) and Huantiao (B 30).

2) *Body posture in using the point* The patient is asked to stand and arch his back. The feet are separated with a distance of 30 cm. The patient's hands must rest on something hard. Ask him to relax his muscles and insert the needle in. Sometimes prone posture is used.

3) *Puncture techniques* Slightly inward and obliquely deep puncture to a depth of three or four cun is done with a four to six cun needle. The lift-thrust method is given to cause a strong needling reaction. It is effective when the needling sensation transmits to the heel and toes. Retention of a needle is unnecessary.

4) *Precautions*

a. First reassure the patients about the strong needling sensation.

b. Local (diseased part) swelling tends to occur. It is not used in patients with bone fracture and muscle injury.

c. It is not advisable to be use for pregnant women and patients with severe heart disease.

5) *Clinical application*

a. Five hundred and eighteen cases of lower back strain were treated by using this point from 1967, when it was discovered, to 1981. Most of the cases were cured by two or three treatments. It is also effective for paralysis, numbness of the lower limbs, rheumatism and sciatica.

b. It is an extraordinary point, located on the travelling course of the foot three yin and yang meridians. Clinical observations show Xinhuantiao, Huantiao (B 30), Zhibian (B 54) cannot replace the lower lightning point. For instance, 30-year-old Mr. Weng once fell and hurt his lower back severely on a big stone. He was hospitalized for four days and there was no response to any treatment. On September 14, 1971 he was sent to the county hospital by carriers. An X-ray showed no abnormality and he was diagnosed as having a strained lower back. One treatment by using this point cured the case. A follow-up survey ten years later showed no relapse.

II. Case Analysis

Case 1: Windstroke (Cerebral thrombosis)

Name, Men x x; sex, male; age, 49; officer.

Complaints One day when he was making a speech he suddenly had slurred speech, deviated mouth and eyes, numbness of the left limbs and loss of consciousness. Hospital examination showed: Blood pressure, 140/100 mmHg, mild slurred speech, wry tongue, salivation, 10 cm raise of the left arm, hemiplegia of the left leg, hyperactive deep reflex and dull shallow reflex of the left limbs.

Differentiation It is a case of windstroke or cerebral thrombosis due to long deficiency of the pectoral qi, disturbance of qi flow and malnutrition of the limbs.

Method Promote qi flow in the meridians and eliminate wind.

Prescription The upper and lower lightning points, Quchi (LI 11), Hegu (LI 4) (penetrating towards Houxi (SI 3)), Yanglingquan (G 34), Yinlingquan (Sp 9), Zusanli (S 36), Sanyinjiao (Sp 6) and Jiexi (St 41).

Treatment procedure Deep perpendicular or oblique puncture was applied with the lift-thrust and sparrow-pecking techniques. Strong manipulations were given to the upper and lower lightning points to transmit the needling sensation to the toes and finger tips. Generally the needle was retained fifteen to twenty-five minutes. Treatment was given once a day, ten treatments made a course. After the first course with an interval of three days the second course followed. After the first course of treatment the patient was able to raise his hand over his head and walk normally. The second course of treatment removed all the symptoms and restored the function of the left limbs. A follow-up survey showed that he was entirely recovered.

Explanation The upper and lower lightning points were selected to treat hemiplegia with strong stimulation and reducing method to get rid of the pathogenic factors in the three yin and yang meridians. Physical build varies and for weak, hypertensive or nervous patients moderate stimulation is suggested.

Case 2: Wei syndrome (Sequelae of polio)

Name, Ali (of North Yemen); sex, male; age, 5.

Complaints The patient was not able to walk after a high fever. He had mild atrophy of the buttock and right leg with a cold sensation, curved knee joint, pes pronatus, and muscular flaccidity.

Differentiation Injury of body fluid by pathogenic heat, yin deficiency and internal heat resulted in malnutrition of the tendons and muscles.

Prescription The upper and lower lightning points, Quchi (LI 11), Waiguan (SJ 5), Hegu (LI 4), Biguan (S 31), Zusanli (S 36), Yanglingquan (G 34), Yinlingquan (Sp 9), Yinmen (B 37), Qimen (Liv 14), Jiexi (S 41), Sanyinjiao (Sp 6), Jianliao (SJ 14), Luodi, Taixi (K 3), Kunlun (B 60), Heyang (B 55) and Dazhui (Du 14).

Treatment procedure The reinforcing, reducing and even movement methods were used without or with needle retention for twenty minutes. Sometimes electro acupuncture was employed. Treatment was given once a day. Ten treatments constituted a course.

After eight courses of treatment the case was cured.

Explanation Fifty cases of the sequelae of polio were treated by Xu. Five to eighty treatments were given. The total effective rate was 94 percent, failure was three cases. For cases of flaccid upper limbs, the upper lightning point, Jianliao (SJ 14), Quchi (LI 11), Hegu (LI 4) and Waiguan (SJ 5) were used. For flaccid lower limbs, Zusanli (S 36), Yanglingquan (G 34), Yinlingquan (Sp 9), Heyang (B 55), Sanyinjiao (Sp 6), Xuanzhong (G 39), Yinmen (B 37), Qimen (Liv 14), Biguan (S 31), Kunlun (B 60) and Taixi (K 3) were selected. Five to six points were punctured in each treatment and electro-acupuncture was more effective.

Case 3: Bi syndrome

Name, Zhang x x; sex, female; age, 65.

Complaints The patient had had a common cold a month before. Afterwards she felt soreness of the knee joints, lower back pain and difficulty in walking.

Differentiation Obstruction of the meridians by wind and cold.

Method Dispel wind and cold to invigorate smooth flow of qi and blood.

Prescription The lower lightning point, Yanglingquan (G 34), Yinlingquan (Sp 9), Yinmen (B 37) and Shenshu (B 23).

Treatment procedure The even movement method was applied. Then electricity was connected. When the pain was relieved, electricity ceased. Treatment was given once a day. Seven treatments cured the case.

Explanation A hundred cases of Bi syndromes were treated by Xu. The effective rate was 91 percent, among which thirty-five cases were cured, twenty-five cases were markedly effective, thirty-one cases were effective and nine cases failed.

Case 4: Bi syndrome (sciatica)

Name, Houssain (of North Yemen); sex, male; age, 66.

Complaints The patient had suffered from sciatica and was treated by several local hospitals without success. Physical examination showed intolerable pain in the left lateral buttock and leg.

Differentiation Accumulation of wind, cold and damp in the Foot-Shaoyang and Foot-Taiyang Meridians, obstruction of meridian qi.

Method Restore smooth flow of qi to kill pain.

Prescription The lower lightning point, Wangu (G 12), Yanglingquan (G 34), Kunlun (B 60).

Treatment procedure Deep (perpendicular or oblique) puncture was done with the reducing method and needle retention for twenty to thirty minutes. One treatment alleviated the pain. Ten treatments cured the case.

Explanation Forty-eight cases of sciatica were treated by Xu. The total effective rate was 92 percent, among which eighteen cases were cured, twelve cases were markedly effective, fourteen cases were effective and four cases failed.

QUICK NEEDLING TECHNIQUE AND NEW WAYS FOR SELECTING ACUPOINTS

—Xu Benren's Clinical Experience

Xu Benren, a native of Changtu County, Liaoning Province, was born in 1928. He graduated from the Harbin Medical University in 1950 and served as a doctor of Western school of medicine. From 1958 to 1961 he studied Chinese medicine at the Hubei College of Traditional Chinese Medicine. Then in 1962 he began to work as a doctor of traditional Chinese medicine in the Shenyang Air Force Hospital. He shows great interest in acupuncture and a book entitled *Quick Needling Technique* was written by him. Another book *Clinical Acupuncture* was written by him together with Ge Shuhan. He has written more than thirty papers, among which the *Observation of 225 Cases of Primary Trigeminal Neuralgia by Acupuncture* won the first prize of Air-Force Scientific Achievements in 1982. He has developed an apparatus known as the Portable Electric Fire Needle in 1983. Now he is a member of council of the China Acupuncture Association, Director of the Army Acupuncture Therapeutic Group, Member of the Air-Force Health Committee, Director of the Acupuncture Department at the Shenyang Air Force Hospital.

I. Academic Characteristics and Medical Specialities

1. Quick needling technique

The quick needling technique is invented by Xu, inspired by the statement recorded in the *Complete Works of Acupuncture* by Xu Feng in the Ming Dynasty. The main aspects are as follows:

1) *Less points selected* In treatment of disease he often first finds out the chief cause and chooses one or two points to cure it.

a. Hemiplegia: He believes that a good acupuncture effect is decided by getting the desired needling sensation. He usually selects Futu (LI 18) and Huantiao (B 30) and makes the needling sensation quickly radiate to the hand and foot. Hemiplegia is often caused by cerebral thrombosis and obstruction of the meridians. Futu (LI 18) is on the Large Intestine Meridian of Hand-Yangming, which is full of qi and blood. Huantiao (B 30) is a confluent point of the Gallbladder Meridian of Foot-Shaoyang and Bladder Meridian of Foot-Taiyang. These two points function to regulate the flow of qi and blood in the meridians. In terms of anatomy, puncturing Futu (LI 18), in fact, means puncturing the nerves of the plexus brachialis, inducing excitement of the nerves of the upper extremities. Puncturing Huantiao (B 30) means puncturing ischium nerves, inducing excitement of the nerves of the lower extremities. Hence the function of the upper and lower extremities can be restored. He has treated 104 cases of cerebral thrombosis with an effective rate of 91.3 percent.

b. Hysterical aphasia: It is caused by an abnormal flow of qi due to overactivity of the seven emotions. Xu treats this condition only with one point—Futu (LI 18), making the needling sensation radiate to the hand. It is very effective and some patients regain the ability to speak quickly. Futu (LI 18) can regulate qi and blood, and remove troubles in the throat.

c. Epilepsy: Xu only uses one point—Dazhui (Du 14) to treat it. Dazhui (Du 14) is on the Du Meridian, which runs to the brain and back, meeting the Liver Meridian of Foot-Jueying at the crown. This meridian is considered as the meeting place of the yang meridians, that is why when Dazhui (Du 14) is needled, yang qi of the whole body is regulated. He thinks that a good result is obtained only when a shock-like needling sensation radiates to the limbs. If a patient feels local soreness and numbness, it is not the desired effect. He has treated ninety-five cases of epilepsy with an effective rate of 72.6 percent.

2) *Quick insertion of needles* On operation he insists on using the finger force to puncture a needle through the skin quickly, then goes further deeper to reduce the pain.

3) *Deep insertion and joint puncture of needles* Some of the points should be punctured deeper than usual, e.g. Sibai (S 2), Xiaguan (S 7), and Quchi (LI 11) are expected to puncture deeper to induce prolonged stimulation. He also makes stress on joint puncture of needles to improve effects and reduce the sufferings when many needles are used. For instance, Quchi (LI 11) is penetrated towards three points—Chize (L 5), Quze (P 3) and Shaohai (H 3); Ermen is penetrated towards two points—Tinggong (SI 19) and Tinghui (B 2); or left Fengchi (B 20) penetrated towards the right Fengchi (B 20), Neiguan (P 6) penetrated towards Waiguan (SJ 5), Hegu (LI 4) penetrated towards Houxi (SI 3).

4) *Strong stimulation and absence of retaining needles* When the patient feels marked soreness and numbness or an electric shock-like sensation, the needle is immediately pulled out. The effects are greatly enhanced by inserting the needles deeper (unsafe parts excluded) with strong stimulation.

Of course, it is necessary to make a special analysis for concrete conditions. For weak patients, moderate stimulations are given. Retention of needles is suggested when pain remains on withdrawal of the needle for pain cases.

2. Selection of points by combining the theory of meridians with local anatomy

Dr. Xu combines the theory of meridians with local anatomy when he treats intractable diseases.

1) *Primary trigeminal neuralgia* It is not satisfactory to use acupuncture, block therapy and surgical operation. Thinking of the theory of meridians and the distribution of nerves in the affected area, Dr. Xu finds out puncturing Xiaguan (S 7) may directly stimulate the branch of trigeminal nerves with quick arrival of qi and a strong needling sensation. According to this principle, he selected Yuyao (Extra 3), Sibai (S 2), Chengjiang (Ren 24) as well as Xiaguan (S 7) to treat trigeminal neuralgia. For example,

when the first branch is affected, puncture Yuyao (Extra 3) in an angle of 30° downward and inwardly. When an electric shock-like sensation radiates to the forehead, do the lift-thrust method twenty to fifty times. When the second branch is affected, obliquely puncture Sibai (S 2) in an angle of 45° upward and backward. When an electric shock-like sensation radiates to the upper lip, lift and thrust the needle twenty to fifty times. When the third branch is affected, puncture Xiaguan (S 7) upward towards the back. When an electric shock-like sensation radiates to the lower jaw or the root of the tongue, lift and thrust the needle twenty to fifty times. If it is not satisfactory, puncture another point —Chengjiang (Ren 24) in an angle of 30° forward down. When an electric shock-like sensation radiates to the lower lip, lift and thrust the needle twenty to fifty times. For example, a patient named Zhang had a tearing pain at the upper part of the right orbit, which attacked fifty to sixty times a day in 1974. All year round he had aversion to wind, and even snow falling on the affected area caused severe pain. He was diagnosed as having primary trigeminal neuralgia in fourteen hospitals. Treatments over eight years were not satisfactory and in 1982 he came for acupuncture. Two treatments with the above approaches killed the pain and after a course of treatment (in 10 days) he was cured. A follow-up survey of four years did not show any relapse. In 1983 in a follow-up survey of a thousand cases the curative rate was 49.6 percent and the marked effective rate was 99.1 percent.

2) *Intractable belching* This is a condition of phrenospasm due to stimulation of nervus phrenicus, which is unable to be cured by simple treatments such as holding one's breath, swallowing food or quick drinking and common acupuncture technique. In combination with the theory of the traditional Chinese and Western medicine, anatomy and points, acupuncture is directly applied to inhibit the nervus phrenicus and to stop abnormal belching. Prescription: Futu (LI 18), horizontally puncture towards the cervical vertebra, 0.5 to 0.8 cun in depth with a one-cun needle. When the needling sensation radiates to the fingers, lift and thrust the needle a few times and withdraw it. Nervus phrenicus is located at the deep part of the posterior margin of the sternocleidomastoideus and lateral upper musculus scalenus anterior, formed by three to five cervical nervus ramus anterior. Since the four to five cervical nervus ramus anterior pass Futu (LI 18), selection of this point directly inhibits excitement of nervus phrenicus and stop spasms.

3) *Chronic prostatitis* This condition is usually treated with antibiotics. But action of antibiotics cannot affect prostatitis. Besides, the vicinity of the lesion becomes sclerotic, which prevents the drug action from dissemination in the lesion. Dr. Xu selects Huiyang (B 35) in combination with Shenshu (B 23) to treat this problem. Huiyang (B 35) is punctured perpendicularly with a two-cun needle, and when the needling sensation reaches the perineum, the needle is pulled out after lifting and thrusting three to five times. A two-cun needle is inserted at Shenshu (B 23) obliquely towards the spine. When there is a local needling sensation, a lift-thrust is done three to five times, then the needle is withdrawn. Huiyang (B 35) and Shenshu (B 23) are located on the Bladder Meridian of Foot-Taiyang. Needling them may regulate qi flow in the meridians and strengthen kidney qi. In terms of anatomy, puncturing Huiyang (B 35) means stimulation of the pelvic plexus of prostate or its prostatic nervus plexus. The pelvic plexus is made of vegetative nerves formed by parasympathetic fibers and sympathetic fibers. When the

pelvic plexus is stimulated, the regulating function of nerves is improved, which invigorates the local circulation of blood and absorption of inflammation. Sixty-five cases of prostatitis have been treated by this approach and the curative rate is 80 percent.

3. Treatment of skin disease by improving the Portable Electro-Fire Needle

In 1985 Dr. Xu improved the apparatus Portable Electro-Fire Needle to replace the fire needle heated by a primitive alcohol burner. It is simple to use, small, easy to carry and effective, especially good in treatment of dermatosis. For instance, a patient named Cui had grown a black eminence at the right lateral eyebrow ten years before. At first it was as big as a grain of millet, but later on it enlarged to the size of a soybean. Meanwhile two small eminences appeared in the vicinity. They were diagnosed as pigmented nevi, which failed to respond to any external application of drug or cold therapy. Then the fire needling was applied to the base of the pigmented nevi. Two months later the follow-up survey showed they disappeared. Six hundred and twenty-seven cases of common wart, flat wart and pigmented nevus have been treated by the electro-fire needling, the curative rate was 100 percent. It has also been used to treat corn with success.

4. Skillful application of tectonic method to treat inflammation of costal cartilage

Swollen and painful costal cartilage is often caused by qi stagnation and blood stasis due to malposition of the joints of costal cartilage and rib by violence or strains. Dr. Xu usually adopts tectonic method to cure this condition. In treatment the patient is asked to sit on a chair with the back to the operator and two hands crossed on the head. The operator stands behind the patient with his arms under the armpits of the patient. The patient is instructed to breathe deeply and hold his breath. At this moment the operator raises the patient's arms backward and upward with the shoulder joints forming an angle of 150° to 160°. First the operator separates the joints and then reduces them to allow smooth flow of qi and blood. For example, a patient named He had had a stroke on the left side of the chest in 1973. Since then he had taken many analgesics. In 1980 he was diagnosed as having inflammation of the costal cartilage. On physical examination there was an eminence as big as a yoke at the fourth and fifth costal cartilages with local tenderness (++). The white blood cell count was normal. After being treated by the above mentioned method, pain disappeared immediately. Two years later the follow-up study showed no relapse. He has treated seventy-one cases of costal cartilage, the curative rate is 49.3 percent, and the marked effective rate was 88.7 percent.

II. Case Analysis

Case 1: Vomiting (cardiospasm)

Name, Zhang x x; sex, male; age, 52; occupation, office worker; date of the first visit, August 10, 1973.

Complaints In 1972 he found a block sensation at the lower part of the esophagus and vomiting occurred after meals. There was a paroxysmal pain in the upper abdomen and he was diagnosed as having cardiospasm. In the same year after he received cardiodiosis the symptoms were mostly removed. He had a relapse in May 1973. A barium meal examination showed a 1 cm stenosis at the lower esophagus and he was diagnosed as having cardiospasm.

Differentiation Perverted attack of stomach qi.

Method Bring down the perverted flow of the stomach qi and stop vomiting.

Prescription Futu (LI 18) and Neiguan (P 6)

Treatment procedure Three courses of treatments were given in total (ten treatments constituted a course). After that the patient could take meals normally.

Explanation A relapse after the treatment was cured by acupuncture on Futu (LI 18). When an electric shock-like sensation radiated to fingers, the lift-thrust technique was done for a while and the needle was withdrawn. The point on one side was chosen. The secondary point Neiguan (P 6) was used to remove the pervertedly flowing qi.

Case 2: Bluish blindness (optic atrophy)

Name, Cui x x; sex, female; age, 30; occupation, worker; date of the first visit, April 27, 1970.

Complaints She had blurring of vision after a high fever in February, 1972. The diagnosis was the first stage of opticatrophy. She took a large amount of Vitamin and intramuscular injection of ATP without success. Eye examination showed pale optic papilla of the temporal side, paler than that of the nasal side, and the vessels were smaller.

Differentiation Insufficient kidney yin and failure of the eyes to be nourished.

Method Nourish kidney yin to restore the eye function.

Prescription Main points: Both Qiuhou (Extra 4) and Yiming (Extra 12). Secondary points: Sanyinjiao (Sp 6).

Treatment procedure After five courses of treatment her eyesight was restored to 1.0. A follow-up study eight years later showed her eyesight was 1.2.

Explanation When Qiuhou (Extra 4) was punctured, the needling sensation must reach the eyeballs. At this moment the needle was pulled out. Sanyinjiao (Sp 6) was for invigorating the liver and kidney yin and regulating qi flow in the meridians.

Case 3: Dry eczema (neurodermatitis)

Name, Wang x x; sex, female; age, 38; occupation, teacher; date of the first visit, November 25, 1966.

Complaints In 1964 she had dermatitis on the left and back side of the nape. It was so itchy that she could not sleep well. Later on dermatitis occurred in the right elbow and the back of the left knee. It was diagnosed as neurodermatitis. There was no response to any oral or externally applied drugs, to radiation therapy for a few months. The patient came to be consulted because the white blood cell count decreased. Physical examination showed there were several patches of dermatitis in the left nape (5 x 8 cm), left lateral knee (5 x 5 cm).

Differentiation Invasion of the meridians by pathogenic wind, imbalance of blood and qi.

Method Dispel pathogenic wind, regulate qi and blood.

Prescription Quchi (LI 11), Zusanli (S 36); plum blossom needle therapy applied to the affected area.

Treatment procedure After six courses of treatment the dermatitis was gone. In 1986, eighteen years later, a follow-up survey showed no relapse at all.

Explanation The affected area was tapped with the plum blossom needle until slight bleeding to strengthen the spleen and eliminate damp, nourish blood and dispel wind. Both Quchi (LI 11) and Zusanli (S 36) were used with the reducing method to regulate qi and blood.

Case 4: Flaccid paralysis of limbs (syringomyolia)

Name, Lu x x; sex, male; age, 20; occupation, soldier; date of the first visit, October 14, 1972.

Complaints In 1970 he found a frequent numb feeling of the right hand, then he felt weakness of the right arm. A month later the right hand was burned by boiling water, but he did not feel pain. Physical examination showed hypalgesia in one or two right cervical vertebrae, analgesia on the right 3rd cervical vertebra and the seventh thoraxic vertebra and muscles near the thumb were atrophic.

Differentiation Qi deficiency and blood stasis, malnutrition of tendons and vessels.

Method Invigorate qi and promote blood flow to restore the function of tendons.

Prescription Dazhui (Du 14), right Quchi (LI 11).

Treatment procedure After seven courses of treatment, analgesia disappeared except slight hypalgesia in the back. No deterioration of muscular atrophy was seen.

Explanation Dazhui (Du 14) is the Confluent point of the three yang meridians of hand and foot, which serves to regulate qi in the yang meridians and qi in the body. The needle was pulled out at once when the needling sensation reached the limb concerned without any lift-thrust manipulation. Quchi (LI 11) is a point on the Large Intestine Meridian of Hand-Yangming in which abundant qi and blood flow. This point was used to strengthen the function of tendons.

Case 5: Headache (pain of the nervus occipitalis major)

Name, Xu x x; sex, female; Age, 26; occupation, worker; date of the first visit, April 24, 1975.

Complaints In the past week she had a paroxysmal pain in the area of the occipitalis major. Every several minutes there was an attack and it became worse in the afternoon. No response was seen when four tablets of analgesic were taken at a time. She was diagnosed as having pain in the nervus occipitalis major.

Differentiation Stagnation of qi and blood.

Method Remove stagnation of qi and blood and 'pain.

Prescription Left Fengchi (G 20).

Treatment procedure After four treatments pain completely disappeared.

Explanation Fengchi (G 20) is a point on the Gallbladder Meridian of Foot-

Shaoyang, located at both sides of the head. Strong stimulation was given to cause the needling sensation radiating to the crown and remove the pain.

INSERTING NEEDLES IN SEQUENCE, WITHDRAWING NEEDLES IN PARTICULAR CONDITIONS

—Gao Yuchun's Clinical Experience

Gao Yuchun, a native of Beijing, was born into a well-known family for traditional Chinese medicine in 1930. From 1946 she began to learn traditional medicine and acupuncture from her father. In 1953 she passed the examination and became an acupuncturist. From 1958 to 1960 she was sent to do advanced study of traditional medical education at the Beijing College of Traditional Chinese Medicine. In 1969 she began to work at the Hebei College of Traditional Chinese Medicine. Her chief works include *Teaching Materials for Midnight-Noon Ebb-Flow in Clinical Application, Questions and Answers of Traditional Chinese Medicine,* (Second Volume, part of acupuncture) and about a dozen papers. Now as an associate professor she is the chief of the Department of Acupuncture and Moxibustion, of the Hebei College of Traditional Chinese Medicine, as well as the director of the Acupuncture Department of the Affiliated Hospital, a member of the Board of the China Association of Acupuncture and Vice-Chairman of the Hebei Acupuncture Society.

I. Academic Characteristics and Medical Specialities

1. Left hand manipulation in acupuncture treatment

Generally speaking, in acupuncture the left hand is known as the pressing hand while the right hand is called the needling hand. In operation the two hands should be coordinated, i.e. on puncturing, the left hand presses the meridian concerned along its running course and the point to allow the needle to be quickly inserted. The right hand helps to puncture at the right place by avoiding a sudden movement on the part of the body. In addition, pressure exerted by the left hand may induce temporary numbness of the muscles and relieve the pain being felt at the moment of the thrust of the needle. When a long needle is used, the left hand may help to keep the needle straight in the thrust. Dr. Gao insists different left hand manipulations be employed on varied conditions, e.g. on puncturing Jingming (B 1), a point at the eye region, one of the left finger tips is pressing the inner canthus and the needle is straightly inserted in front of the fingernail to prevent the eye from injury. This manipulation is also used when acupuncture is applied to Renying (S 9), Taiyuan (L 9) and Jiexi (S 41). When long needles are used to puncture Huantiao (G 30), or Chengfu (B 36), the left hand manipulation helps to keep the needle from bending.

2. The reinforcing and reducing methods

1) *Reinforcing method* Dr. Gao believes that better effects can be achieved by twirling and rotating the needle associated with lift-thrust manipulations. She says, after the arrival of the needling reaction, twirl the needle to the extreme and thrust it 0.05-0.1 cun in depth and retain the needle for a while. Before withdrawal of the needle another reinforcing technique should be conducted.

2) *Reducing method* In acupuncture therapy the reducing method is more often used than the reinforcing method as a whole. But in extreme excess cases the force of the routine reducing method is often not enough. Dr. Gao thinks for better effects different reducing methods should be used for varied conditions, e.g. in cases of stagnation of qi and blood stasis with symptoms of distending and painful breast, distending feeling in the chest and hypochondriac region, the needle is inserted into Tanzhong (Ren 17) against the running course of the Ren Meridian, which runs from below to above, to get good result. If there is a sharp pain or a manifestation of attack by strong pathogenic factors the reducing method is applied in coordination with the breathing of the patient. Breathing infers the ascending and descending of qi, in which exhalation means qi ascending, whereas inhalation refers to qi descending. When the manipulations used by the operator are coordinated with the respiration of the patient, the desired result is achieved. In operation after the arrival of the needling reaction, the patient begins to breath deeply, in exhalation the needle is withdrawn a little and rotated clockwise, in inhalation the needle is inserted deeper and rotated counterclockwise. The operation is done five to seven times, followed by retention of needles for ten to fifteen minutes. Afterwards the same operation is conducted three to five times. If the patient cannot do deep breathing, no curative effect is seen.

3. Puncturing the main points first, secondary points second

In acupuncture therapy the prescription should follow the treating principle, the main points should be needled first, the secondary points second. For instance, for dizziness due to exuberance of yang of the liver, the purpose of treatment is to soothe the liver and remove excessive heat by bringing downward the perverted flow of qi. Taichong (Liv 3) is the main point for quenching the liver fire; the secondary points are Baihui (Du 20) and Fengchi (G 20) for subduing hyperactivity of the liver and the endogenous wind and Waiguan (SJ 5) for eliminating heat from the upper jiao. Then puncture Baihui (Du 20) first and other points from above to below in order to bring down the pathogenic factors, finally retain the needles for some time. Another example is stomachache due to improper diet and stagnant indigested food in the stomach. Treatment should be aimed at clearing stagnation of food and relieving pain by restoring the stomach function. Zusanli (S 36) is needled first with the reducing method to invigorate digestion and kill pain. The secondary points include Zhongwan (Ren 12), the Front-(Mu) point of the Stomach Meridian and Tianshu (S 25), the Front-(Mu) point of the Large Intestine Meridian to regulate the function of the stomach and intestines. Then puncture again Zhongwan (Ren 12), Tianshu (S 25) and Zusanli (S 36) successively to drive pathogenic factors downward. Since points automatically open at right times, first puncture the point which opens at the time, and then puncture the diseased and secondary points. For example, in treatment of epilepsy due to exuberance of yang of the liver, it is essential to soothe the liver, regulate the function of the gallbladder and calm the mind. In this case, puncture Zulingqi (G 41)—the main point first, then Waiguan (SJ 5)—the secondary point, Fengchi (G 20)—the diseased point and the meeting point of the Gallbladder and Yangwei Meridians to ease the mind and regulate the function of the gallbladder; Tanzhong (Ren 17), the Front-(Mu) point of the Pericardium Meridians or the Converging point to calm the mind. The reducing method is applied; after that, puncture the same point from above to below in order and retain the needles. This is the technique frequently used by Dr. Gao.

4. The sequence to withdraw needles

It is held by Dr. Gao that different methods to withdraw needles correspond to varied conditions to improve effects and reduce side-effects. Gao believes that improper withdrawal of needles may cause sticking of the needle and pain, or affect the curative effect. The commonly used methods to withdraw a needle by Dr. Gao are as follows:

1) *The common method* It is used in stable cases with no marked evidence of excess or deficiency conditions. The sequence of withdrawal of the needles is from above to below or from the side of the body close to the acupuncturist to the other side when the patient is in decubitus.

2) *How to withdraw the needles in cases of deficiency* When a weak patient complains of lassitude, weak or numb legs and loose muscles after withdrawal of the needle, the point is first pressed by a swab and then kneaded for a while. If the patient has a slow reaction, manipulations are conducted and the needle is quickly pulled out to increase stimulation. The sequence of withdrawal of the needles is the same as above.

3) *How to withdraw the needles in cases of excess* Patients resorting to acupuncture therapy mostly have an excess condition, e.g. severe headache, leg pain, toothache, sore throat or abdominal pain, etc. After the application of the reducing method, twirl the needle handle slightly to make sure that no needle sticking is found before withdrawal of the needle. It is no good to rotate the needl strongly to avoid the appearance of the needling sensation. If it does appear, retain the needle for some time before it is pulled out. After withdrawal of the needle never press or knead the point. In this way the pathogenic factors may completely be brought out, or squeeze the point until slight bleeding to obtain better results.

4) *Withdrawal of the needles from below to above in sequence* For prolapse of organs or tissues, such as gastroptosis, prolapse of the uterus or rectum and hypotension, the sequence of withdrawal of the needles should be from below to above to lead the meridian qi upward. For instance, for prolapse of the rectum, Changqiang (Du 1) and Baihui (Du 20) are needled successively. Before the needles are pulled out, twirl and rotate them again to induce the needling sensation, then withdraw them from Changqiang (Du 1), then Baihui (Du 20). The same is done in moxibustion.

5) *Withdrawal of the needles from above to below* It is used to bring pathogenic

factors downward. Cough, hypochondriac pain, dizziness and hypertension are disorders due to perverted flow of the lung or liver qi. Therefore, on withdrawing of the needles it should be borne in mind that it should be done from above to below. For example, for hypertension with symptoms of headache, dizziness due to exuberance of yang of the liver, puncture Xuehai (Sp 10) first, then Zusanli (S 36) and Xingjian (Liv 2) with the reducing method. After retention of the needle for some minutes withdraw the needle from Xuehai (Sp 10), Zusanli (S 36) and Xingjian (L 2) one after another. If needles are withdrawn from below to above, the desired effects cannot be achieved.

6) *Special methods to withdraw the needles* After manipulations, a needle must be withdrawn immediately. But sometimes a stuck needle may present owing to nervous tension of the patient or improper operation of the acupuncturist. It can be removed by shallow puncture of one or two points in the vicinity. Retain the needles for a while and the stuck needle can be easily withdrawn. If a strong needling sensation is felt at this moment, the needle should be pulled out two thirds. Only after disappearance of soreness can the needle be pulled out without leaving any uneasy feeling.

5. Selection of points at the time when they open or based on differentiation of syndromes

Midnight-Noon Ebb-Flow—an ancient acupuncture theory of selecting points and the Eight Magic Turtle Techniques—one of the ancient theories to select points originated from the *Internal Classics,* are related to the day and hour in terms of Heavenly Stems and Earthly Branches to select appropriate points. Midnight-noon Ebb-flow includes the *Jia* method, the *Zi* method and the *Yangzi* method, and the Eight Magic Turtle Techniques. By point opening, Gao holds it is the place to which abundant qi and blood flow at a certain time in a day. Several points open at the same time. In accordance with the theory of Midnight-noon Ebb-flow, several points open in every two-hour period, but point selection is still important. The point selected should work for the corresponding cases to get twice the result with half the efforts. For instance, a female patient, age twenty, came to visit at 11:15, August 20, 1986. She complained in the previous three days of a distending and painful feeling in the stomach. She had normal appetite, bowel movements and urination, but overtaking of food would cause stomach distension, bitter taste in the mouth and foul breath. Physical examination showed thready string-taut pulse, pale red tongue with thin white coating. It was analyzed as deficiency in the stomach and hyperactivity of the liver. In terms of time the attack occurred at 11 p.m. in summer or 9 p.m. to 11 p.m., which was the time when the abundant qi and blood flowed along the Sanjiao Meridian. Since the stomach disorder appeared successively at the time in three days, it was diagnosed as the obstruction of the Sanjiao Meridian. According to the Jia method and Zi method, on that day from 9 p.m.-11 p.m. Yinlingquan (Sp 9), Zhongchong (P 9) and Tianjing (SJ 10) opened. In accordance with the Yangzi method and the Eight Magic Turtle Techniques, Yinbai (Sp 1), Zhaohai (K 6) and Lieque (L 7) opened. So in this case Yinlingquan (Sp 9) or Tianjing (SJ 10) could be selected.

II. Case Analysis

Case 1: Infantile malnutrition

Name, Lu x x; sex, female; age, 4 months; date of the first visit, June 20, 1954.

Complaints After she was born, the baby could not be fed well because of inadequate lactation of her mother. Fifty-six days later she was sent to a nursery. On the first visit she was thin and weak, and did not know how to smile. Physical examination showed lassitude, pale complexion, scaly dry skin, thin yellow hair, hard potbelly and thin limbs, pale tongue, frequent discharge of loose stools, unclear finger print. She was diagnosed as having infantile malnutrition.

Prescription Sifeng (Extra 29) (peck needling is applied until discharge of some light yellow mucus); Zhongwan (Ren 12), Guanyuan (Ren 4), Zusanli (S 36), Sanyinjiao (Sp 6) (for moxibustion).

Treatment procedure On the second visit of the next day less bowel movements were found. The same treatment was given. On the third visit abdominal distension was relieved. Slight moxibustion was applied to Zhongwan (Ren 12), Guanyuan (Ren 4), Zusanli (S 36) and Sanyinjiao (Sp 6). On the fourth visit, the baby was in good spirits and bowel movements were two to three times a day. Slight moxibustion was again applied to the same points. Four treatments were given in total. Several months later she had a normal development with a red complexion. Appetite and bowel movements both became normal.

Case 2: Difficult labour

Name, Li x x; sex, female; age, 24; occupation, peasant; date of the first visit, summer, 1971.

Complaints She was a peasant woman in good health. A local midwife was called in when the signs of delivery appeared. Since it was a bigger fetus she exerted too much strength at first and on the second day when the orifice of the uterus widely opened she was completely tired, with weak uterine contractions. After oxytocin was administered uterine contraction stopped. Then she was transferred to one of the big provincial hospitals. Many oxytocic approaches were tried with failure. The heart beat of the fetus ceased. It was to be taken out surgically.

Differentiation Great loss of qi and blood.

Prescription Hegu (LI 4), Sanyinjiao (Sp 6) and oxytocic points.

Treatment procedure Before the operation, acupuncture was tried to speed up the delivery. First, both Hegu (LI 4) was punctured with the reinforcing method since the pulse and qi were weak. Then both Sanyinjiao (Sp 6) was selected with the reducing method. Afterwards the two oxytocic points (three cun away from Guanyuan (Ren 4)) were used, 0.5 cun in depth with the reinforcing method. Uterine contraction reappeared and increased. About one minute later the dead fetus was delivered. Not too much blood was lost and the mother was all right.

Case 3: Herpes zoster

Name, Zhao x x; sex, male; age, 24; date of the first visit, June, 1974.

Complaints Three days before patches of blisters had appeared in the left hypochondriac region and waist. The blisters quickly spread to the right side and the whole waist with a sharp burning pain. Symptoms were poor appetite, disturbed sleep, dry stools, yellow urine, string-taut, rapid and forceful pulse, red tongue with yellow coating.

Differentiation Accumulation of pathogenic heat in the Sanjiao and strong pathogenic factors in the liver and gallbladder.

Method Clear pathogenic factors from the liver and gallbladder and the Sanjiao.

Prescription Zhigou (SJ 6), Zhangmen (Liv 13), Yanglingquan (G 34).

Treatment procedure Perpendicular puncturing was applied to Zhigou (SJ 6), 0.6 to 0.8 cun in depth with the reducing method in coordination with respiration to eliminate the pathogenic heat from the Sanjiao. After manipulations the needle was retained for fifteen minutes. Then another manipulation was conducted and the needle was retained for an hour. Zhangmen (Liv 13), the secondary point, was needled perpendicularly, 0.5 to 0.7 cun in depth with the reducing method. Retention of the needle was the same as above. Yanglingquan (G 34) was punctured with the reducing method in coordination with respiration, the needle was retained for an hour to eliminate pathogenic factors from the liver and gallbladder. On withdrawal of the needles pain was greatly relieved. On the second visit the following day, after acupuncture the patient did not feel any sharp pain. He had a sound sleep that night and good appetite. There was no presence of new herpes and the old ones became dry and shrivelled. The pulse was still string-taut and rapid, the tongue was red with thin yellow coating. The same treatments were given with success.

Case 4: Chronic pharyngitis

Name, Liu x x; sex, male; age, 50; occupation, engineer; date of the first visit, July 10, 1982.

Complaints The patient had worked hard and seldom drunk water. When he was anxious he had a pain appearing in the throat, as if something had stuck in it, but there was no difficulty in swallowing. Esophagograms showed no abnormality. At 5 o'clock every afternoon in the previous year he had felt increased pain in the throat. Other symptoms were dislike of drinking water, depression, disturbed sleep, poor appetite, string-taut thready and rapid pulse, red throat, pale puffy tongue with scanty coating.

Differentiation Deficiency of yin of the lung and kidney, stagnated liver qi and insufficient kidney yin.

Method Strengthen the function of the lung and kidney and select the opening points in treatment.

Prescription Lieque (L 7), Zhaohai (K 6), Zhongwan (Ren 12), Zusanli (S 36) and Sanyinjiao (Sp 6).

Treatment procedure Treatment was given at 8:30 a.m. when Lieque (L 7) opened. It was needled to a depth of 0.5 to 0.7 cun. Then Zhaohai (K 6) was perpendicularly punctured to a depth of 0.3 to 0.5 cun. Both were applied with the reinforcing method. The needles were retained for fifteen minutes. The second treatment was given on the following day, by selecting the same points as above. The throat was eased. On the third treatment Zhaohai (K 6) was used as the main point and Lieque (L 7), Zhongwan (Ren

12), Zusanli (S 36) and Sanyinjiao (Sp 6) as the secondary ones. The throat became normal and the appetite was restored.

Case 5: Epilepsy

Name, Zhang x x; sex, male; age, 3; date of the first visit, July 10, 1979.

Complaints The child got a smallpox vaccination at the age of one and a half years. He had a high fever and convulsions, but when the fever was gone convulsions frequently attacked. In the previous months it had become aggravated, and he had several attacks a day. Other symptoms were dull-looking eyes, low intelligence, disturbed sleep, slightly dry stools, violet finger print, red tongue tip and border with white coating.

Prescription Houxi (SI 3) and Shenmai (B 62).

Treatment procedure On that day from 9 a.m. to 11 a.m. the two points were opened. The former was used as the main point and the latter as the secondary one. The reducing method was applied without retention of the needles. After the first treatment, attack of convulsions decreased. Three treatments of the same method cured convulsions. Then one treatment a week helped him recover. He goes to school and no relapse has been seen since.

Case 6: Palpitation

Name, Lu x x; sex, male; age, 50; occupation, office worker; date of the first visit, September 1984.

Complaints One year before he had had an attack of palpitation and was hospitalized. Three months later he was discharged. When he came to be consulted he had symptoms of oppressed feeling in the chest, lassitude, pale complexion, low spirits, weak voice, poor appetite, abdominal distension after meals, loose stools, scanty urine, rapid and thready pulse (140 beats per m.), dark tongue and violet lips.

Differentiation Lowered functioning of the heart and spleen, stagnation of qi and blood due to deficiency in the heart and spleen which fail to invigorate the flow of qi and blood.

Method Strengthen the function of the heart and spleen, generate qi and blood.

Prescription Neiguan (P 6), Tanzhong (Ren 17), Sanyinjiao (Sp 6).

Treatment procedure Neiguan (P 6) was perpendicularly punctured 0.2 to 0.4 cun in depth with the reinforcing method. Tanzhong (Ren 17) was obliquely needled, 0.5 to 0.7 cun in depth with the needle tip directing upward. Sanyinjiao (Sp 6) was perpendicularly punctured, 0.5 to 0.7 cun in depth. All were retained for five minutes. After the second treatment on the third day the oppressed feeling in the chest was relieved but other symptoms remained. A course of treatment for twenty days was given. On the 13th visit, palpitation, oppressed feeling and lassitude were alleviated, but there remained poor appetite, abdominal distension, loose stools, slightly rapid pulse (96 beats per m. and 3 to 4 intermittence each minute). Besides the above points Zhongwan (Ren 12) was perpendicularly punctured, 1 to 1.5 cun in depth, Tianshu (S 25) was perpendicularly punctured, 1.5 to 2 cun in depth and Zusanli (S 36) was perpendicularly punctured about one cun in depth to regulate qi. The three needles were retained for ten minutes. Then treatment was given every other day for a course. On the twenty-fourth visit the patient was able to ride a bicycle to cover about twenty miles. He began to work half a day. The oppressed feeling and palpitation were greatly removed. He had a good appetite, but bowel movements were twice a day, discharging loose stools. Thready pulse was seen, the heart beat was 90 per m. with three or four intervals. Now Xinshu (B 15) and Geshu (B 17) were perpendicularly punctured, 0.5 to 0.7 cun in depth with the reinforcing method and without needle retention. Then Neiguan (P 6), Tanzhong (Ren 17) and Yinlingquan (Sp 9) were perpendicularly punctured, 1 to 1.5 cun in depth with the reinforcing method and needle retention for ten minutes, in which manipulation is done once. Moxibustion was applied to Yinlingquan (Sp 9) for five minutes. Ten treatments consisting a course were given every other day. After that, the ECG became normal. In the following years no relapse was found.

Case 7: Spontaneous sweating

Name, Jing x x; sex, female; age, 68; date of the first visit, June, 1986.

Complaints From the spring that year she had spontaneous sweating day and night associated with an oppressed feeling in the chest, lassitude, disturbed sleep, poor appetite, soreness in the mouth, thready pulse, or slightly red tongue with white thin coating. Two 2 x 2 mm ulcers were seen on the side of the glossodesmus and the lower lip mucosa.

Differentiation Excessive fire in the heart and loss of kidney yin.

Method Remove fire from the heart and generate kidney yin.

Prescirption Yinxi (H 6) and Fuliu (K 7).

Treatment procedure Yinxi (H 6) and Fuliu (K 7) were perpendicularly needled, 0.3 to 0.5 cun and 0.5 to 0.7 cun in depth respectively. The reducing method was applied to the former and the reinforcing method to the latter. Needle retention was for ten minutes, but in the middle manipulation was conducted once. Four days later on the second visit, the patient felt relieved chest oppression and spontaneous sweating. Mouth ulcers remained as before. The pulse was still rapid. Then same treatment was given. On the third visit (two days later) she no longer had the oppressed feeling in the chest. The mouth ulcer was still there. Dicang (S 4) was obliquely and laterally punctured with the reducing method, 0.3 to 0.4 cun in depth to regulate the local qi. Yinxi (H 6) was replaced by Hegu (LI 4) to clear the excessive heat. Fuliu (K 7) was applied in the same way as before. Needles were retained for fifteen minutes. On the fourth visit she said severe pain of the sores had been relieved. No spontaneous sweating and lassitude were seen. The pulse was deep and thready and the tongue was pale red. There was no marked sign of sores on the side of the glossodesmus. The same treatment was given again. On the fifth visit (two days later) she said she only had slight sweating, the sores were completely removed. Appetite became normal. She was advised to take another treatment to strengthen the effect.

REINFORCING AND REDUCING MANIPULATIONS AND THE PROPERTIES OF THE POINTS, INVESTIGATION OF NEW POINTS AND EMPHASIS ON DIFFERENTIATION ACCORDING TO THE THEORY OF MERIDIANS AND COLLATERALS

—Gao Zhenwu's Clinical Experience

Gao Zhenwu was born in January, 1927. He followed his father, Dr. Gao Shengshui, learning traditional Chinese medicine from the age of 12. In 1947, he took up study in the Chinese Acupuncture Research Clinic under Dr. Cheng Dan'an, and in the same year, he finished his course in the Tianjin Traditional Chinese Medicine Correspondence School. He then started a private clinic the following year. In August of 1950, he was invited to work at the Xiaolin Clinic in Yuyao County. Meanwhile, he was also given a chance to take a two-year course for teachers in the Zhejiang Traditional Chinese Medicine Refresher School. From 1957, Dr. Gao began to work as a teacher.

Having done clinical work for thirty-eight years, Dr. Gao is well-experienced with many acute and severe diseases such as angina pectoris, hypertension, and acute febrile diseases. He has also successfully treated arrhythemia, dizziness, Wei Syndrome, epilepsy, deaf-mutism, facial paralysis and sciatica. In collaboration with anatomy and art teachers, he edited the *Acupuncture Anatomical Colour Atlas*, which won the excellent scientific research achievement award at the Provincial Science Conference. His research programme on acupuncture treatment of arrhythemia was the fourth class winner of the provincial best achievement on science and technology. Dr. Gao is also the editor-in-chief of *New Acupuncture*. So far, he has published more than twenty theses and papers. At present, Dr. Gao is an associate professor and dean of the Acupuncture and Massage Department of Zhejiang Traditional Chinese Medicine College; head of the Acupuncture Research Section of his college; director of the Acupuncture Department in the Affiliated Hospital of the college; and a member of the Board of Directors of the Chinese Acupuncture Society.

I. Academic Characteristics and Medical Specialities

1. Emphasis on the needling speed and technique for the reducing and reinforcing method

It is stated in *Miraculous Pivot,* "A reducing or reinforcing effect results from the needling speed," and "The appropriate needling speed is decided only after the excess or deficiency condition of the disease is investigated." Again in the same book, it says, "The pathogenic factors come violently and quickly while the nutrient qi comes gently and slowly." Dr. Gao has followed these tenets and is skillful in the reducing and reinforcing needling methods. His experience can be summarized as follows:

1) *Reinforcing method* A filiform needle of 0.28 to 0.32 mm in diameter is used. After the needle is quickly inserted into the skin, it is slowly rotated back and forth within 180°, or lifted and thrust to a depth of 0.5 cm at a frequency of one rotating or lifting-thrusting movement every eight to ten seconds. The stimulation should be mild or moderate, and the patient should feel comfortable as the qi arrives slowly and gently. On the other hand, the doctor feels a relaxed sensation under the needle. After the arrival of qi, rotation, lifting-thrusting or gentle vibration of the handle of the needle continue for 30 to 60 seconds. The needle may also be retained for 5 to 20 minutes without manipulation. After that, the needle is removed and the hole is pressed with a clean cotton ball. This method is applied for deficiency syndromes.

2) *Reducing method* A filiform needle of 0.38 to 0.45 mm in diameter is used. After the needle is thrusted deep into the point, it is quickly rotated back and forth in a range of 360° to 720°, or lifted and thrust to a depth of 1.0 cm at the frequency of one to two rotating or lifting-thrusting manipulation. The patient quickly has a heavy and uncomfortable sensation from the needles, and simultaneously, the doctor also notices a tight and heavy sensation under the needle. After the patient feels the needling sensation, manipulation continues for two or three minutes, then the needle is either retained for thirty to sixty minutes and manipulated once every five minutes during the treatment, or is retained for fifteen to thirty minutes and manipulated several times during retention. The hole of the needle remains open after the needle is removed. This method is applied for excess syndromes.

3) *Even method* A filiform needle of 0.32 to 0.38 mm in diameter is used. In the application of this method, the degree of rotation of the needle, the lifting-thrusting amplitude, the time for "the arrival of qi," the intensity of stimulation, and the doctor's feeling under the needle all fall in between those specifications for the reducing method and the reinforcing method. After the patient feels the needling sensation, the needle is continuously manipulated for one or two minutes, then retained for ten to twenty minutes, either with frequent manipulation or without manipulation. The hole of the needle is pressed for a short while with a clean cotton ball after the needle is removed. This method is applied to the condition in which neither excess symptoms nor deficiency symptoms are evident. For a deficiency syndrome complicated by excess symptoms, the reinforcing method is applied first, and then the reducing method follows. For an excess syndrome complicated by deficiency symptoms, the reducing method is applied before the reinforcing method.

According to Dr. Gao's experience, invigorating the antipathogenic factors and eliminating the pathogenic factors depend on the skill of the needling technique. In the treatment of some chronic deficiency syndromes of the internal organs, the appropriate needling method must follow the changes of the disease, and the actual condition of the patient. Cooperation and confidence on the part of the patient is of primary importance. Excessively strong stimulation in the first few treatments may consume qi and cause the patient to feel tired, or to feel an aversion to needles, thereby resulting in the interruption of treatment. Most excess syndromes are seen in the acute stage with hyperactive pathogenic factors. In that case, the symptoms should be primarily treated and the pathogenic factors be eliminated as soon as possible. If they cannot be promptly dispelled, the retention of these pathogenic factors in the body may injure the antipathogenic factors and cause future trouble.

2. The properties of the points

The points have special properties, some tending to possess reinforcing action, such as Guanyuan (Ren 4), Qihai (Ren 6), Shenshu (B 23), Mingmen (Du 4), Yaoyangguan (Du 3) and Zusanli (S 36), and some tending to have reducing action, such as the Jing-Well Points and Rong-Spring Points. Meridians and collaterals are related to each other on the basis of the interacting five elements. According to the principle of reinforcing the mother in case of deficiency, and reducing the son in case of excess, the mother point is more relevant for reinforcing action, while the son point is appropriate for reducing action.

For example, an elderly woman who had a peptic ulcer for nearly twenty years came to see Dr. Gao. She had a stomachache, frequent belching and poor appetite. These symptoms had been noted since five days before, and had occurred due to emotional disturbance and stagnant liver qi. She also had a thin, white tongue coating, and a thready, string-taut pulse. The case was diagnosed as stomachache due to liver qi affecting the stomach.

Prescription: Taichong (Liv 3), Ganshu (B 18) and Zusanli (S 36). The reducing method was applied to the first two points and the even method to the third one. Treatment was given daily. A marked improvement was achieved after the first five treatments. Another three treatments were given to consolidate these good results.

Ganshu (B 18), the Back-Shu Point of the liver, is where the liver qi is transmitted. Taichong (Liv 3) is the Yuan-Source Point of the Liver Meridian. Since the Liver Meridian passes by the stomach, related to the liver and connected with the gallbladder, the first two points can regulate rebellious qi of the liver and stomach. Zusanli (S 36) is the He-Sea Point of the Yangming Meridian of Foot. Following the tenet that He-Sea Points are indicated in disorders of fu organs, Zusanli (S 36) is used to balance and tone the stomach.

In another case, a student had a chronic cough with little sputum following a common cold. He had the condition for over three months, and also had poor appetite for nearly two months. There were accompanying symptoms of a cold appearance, cold limbs, emaciation, restlessness, occasional spontaneous sweating, a superficial, soft pulse, and a thin, white tongue coating. The diagnosis was deficiency of lung qi causing impairment of the dispersing function of the lung. The case was initially an exterior excess syndrome, but as the cough became chronic, the disease of the son affected the mother, resulting in spleen and stomach qi deficiency. Due to poor appetite, earth fails to promote metal normally, resulting in the more serious condition of deficient lung qi.

The treatment principle was to tone the spleen so as to strengthen the lung. Prescription: Pishu (B 20), Zusanli (S 36), Taiyuan (L 9), and Dingchuan (Extra 14).

The reinforcing method was applied to all of these points, and treatment was given every other day. Appetite and coughing gradually improved after four treatments. Marked improvement was obtained after eight treatments. Another four treatments were given to consolidate the curative effect.

Pishu (B 20), the Back-Shu Point of the spleen, and Zusanli (S 36), the He-Sea Point of the Stomach Meridian, were used together to strengthen the spleen and pacify the stomach. Taiyuan (L 9), the Yuan-Source Point, the Jing-River Point, as well as the earth point of the five elements, has the action of toning earth to help metal. Dingchuan (Extra 14) is an empirical point for coughing and asthma. These four points were used in combination to improve appetite and check coughing in an attempt to tone the spleen and lung.

Another case involved a male patient fifty years old, who had repeated occurrence of dizziness and distension in the head for three years. He also complained of distending pain at the vertex, redness in the eyes, blurred vision, unsteady walking, insomnia, normal urination and bowel movement, red tongue with thin, white coating, and deep, string-taut, and forceful pulse. His blood pressure was 186/112 mm Hg. This case was diagnosed as dizziness caused by upward disturbance of hyperactivity of liver yang and excessive liver fire.

Following the principle of reducing the son in case of excess, the treatment principle was to eliminate fire and check liver yang. Prescription: Xingjian (Liv 2) as the principal point and Fengchi (G 20) as the subordinate point. The reducing method was applied to both points. Treatment was given every day. The headache diminished, sleep was improved, and all the symptoms began to be relieved after four treatments.

Xingjian (Liv 2) is the Rong-Spring Point, and also the fire point of the Liver Meridian. The Liver Meridian enters the throat and nose and connects with the eyes, then emerges from the forehead and reaches the vertex to join the Du Meridian. Needling Xingjian (Liv 2) is able to reduce the son of wood. Fengchi (G 20) soothes the liver and checks the exuberance of liver yang, since the liver and gallbladder are related to each other.

3. Application of the warming needle

Dr. Gao believes that the warming needle has the advantages of both needles and moxa treatment, and so has a special effect for some chronic diseases caused by weakness of yang qi and invasion of cold, such as Wei Syndrome, Bi Syndrome, hemiplegia, impaired movement of the joints, obstruction of meridians and collaterals, heart and lung qi deficiency, deficiency and cold of the spleen and stomach, and the decline and weakness of kidney yang.

The material quality and the thickness of the needle, as well as the size and firmness of the moxa cones will have a direct influence on the warming needle. As early as the mid 1960s, Dr. Gao made laboratory experiments with the warming needle treatment. These included experiments on the temperature of the needles of different qualities and types of metal, the time for the increase and retention of temperature, the size and firmness of the moxa cones, the relation between the number of moxa cones and the needle temperature in the treatment, the relation between the warming needle and the climate temperature, the significance of the temperature on the different parts of a needle, and the blisters on the skin caused by warming needle.

These experiments revealed that needles made of different metals, and also needles of different thickness would show a difference in the temperature in the needle body, and also in the time for the increase and retention of the temperature. For instance, one moxa cone of 0.8 gram was applied to needles 38 mm in length and 0.38 mm in diameter, which were respectively made of steel, stainless steel and silver. A semi-conductor temperature examiner was used to take the temperature of the needle on the body about 10 mm from the handle when the room temperature was at 18°C. A clear difference in temperature was noticed for needles made of different metals: the stainless steel needle was 32°C, the steel needle was 34.5°C, and the silver needle was 80°C. These experiments also showed that thick needles had higher temperatures than thin needles.

Through careful observations, Dr. Gao has noted that the size and the number of moxa cones, the firmness of the cones, the method used to fix them, and the climate temperature will affect the result of the warming needle therapy. During treatment, the needle temperature should definitely be higher than the temperature in the dermal region or subcutaneous tissues where the needle is inserted. If the moxa cones are placed too distant to give adequate heat to the skin, the warming needle will be of no significance. Because of the high temperature in treatment, the silver needle, and possibly the steel or stainless steel needles, may cause blisters on the skin. Therefore, needles of different metals are chosen to treat different diseases, and the number of moxa cones should vary accordingly.

After observing 128 cases of bi syndrome due to wind, cold and dampness treated by warming needle, Dr. Gao summarized his experience and presented the opinion that a stainless steel needle or steel needle 0.32 mm in diameter should be chosen for those patients who are weak in body constitution or very sensitive to needles, and also for cases with mild symptoms and signs, short duration of the disease, or for diseases only in the superficial part of the body, but without cramping. Such a needle may also be used for a condition of mild cramping if the movement of the joints is only slightly hindered.

However, for patients with a strong body constitution and tolerance towards the needling sensation, and for severe cases with long duration, serious pain and soreness, particularly with symptoms of cold and dampness, and also for diseases located deeply in the tendons and bones and cases with cramping and severe hindrance of joint movement, the stainless steel needle of 0.45 mm or 0.32 mm in diameter is used for the warming needle treatment.

In March, 1970, a farmer fifty-four years old came to Dr. Gao for treatment. He complained of bi syndrome in the anterior part of the left shoulder for three years, and stated that he had not been properly treated before. The pain gave him sleepless nights and was aggravated by cold. His left arm when raised could only touch his left ear lobe, and when bent behind him, could only touch the lumbar region. Stainless steel needles 0.32 mm in diameter were applied to Jianyu (LI 15), Jianliao (SJ 14), Jianwaishu (SI 14), Naoshu (SI 10), Quchi (LI 11), Shousanli (LI 10), Waiguan (SJ 5), Wangu (SI 4) and Hegu (LI 4). Treatment was given every other day for the first three treatments, and moxa was added from the fourth treatment. Since little result was obtained after a course of ten treatments, Dr. Gao changed to silver needles 0.32 mm in diameter with moxibustion for the second course of treatment. Some improvement in the pain and restriction of movement was then seen after four treatments. The pain had distinctly diminished after seven treatments. His left hand could touch his right scapula from the back and the left temple from the front after the second course of treatment was completed. The third course continued after a rest of seven days. His arm could move normally at the end of the third course. Six more treatments were given to consolidate the effect.

4. Application of the Front-Mu Points, Back-Shu Points, Yuan-Source Points, Luo-Connecting Points, He-Sea Points and Xi-Cleft Points in the treatment of zang-fu diseases

All points have common and specific properties. The common properties provide great flexibility in selection of points, while the specific properties make the prescription more concise and effective.

Dr. Gao believes that acupuncture is not only limited to the treatment of common diseases, such as Wei Syndrome, hemiplegia, and painful conditions. Dr. Gao has successfully treated with acupuncture many diseases of zang-fu organs, which various kinds of medication had not helped. In the treatment of such diseases, he primarily uses Front-Mu, Back-Shu, Yuan-Source, Luo-Connecting, He-Sea, and Xi-Cleft Points. He also uses Huatuojiaji points, because Dr. Huatuo (?-208 A.D.) substituted these points for the Back-Shu Points. Back-Shu Point is the place where the qi of the zang-fu is transfused; Front-Mu Point is the place where the qi of the zang-fu converges; the qi of the zang-fu is manifested most easily on Yuan-Source Points; Luo-Connecting Points link two meridians exteriorly and interiorly; the qi meets from outside and from inside in the He-Sea Points; and Xi-Cleft Points are indicated in acute diseases. Dr. Gao has combined these points in various ways to cope with actual situations, including combinations of Front-Mu and Back-Shu Points, Yuan-Source and Luo-Connecting Points, Back-Shu and He-Sea Points, Front-Mu and He-Sea Points, Yuan-Source and He-Sea Points, Back-Shu and Yuan-Source Points, and Luo-Connecting and Xi-Cleft Points.

In March, 1981, Dr. Gao treated a young worker who had palpitation, shortness of breath, and stuffiness in the chest following an attack of acute myocarditis three months before. Drugs had not relieved these symptoms. ECG showed the heart rate was 108 beats per minute. He was subsequently given a Western diagnosis of sinus tachycardia, and a TCM diagnosis of palpitation. Dr. Gao pointed out that this case was deficiency in root but excess in symptoms due to retention of pathogenic factors. The treatment principle was to tone heart qi and eliminate the remaining pathogenic factors. Prescription: Neiguan (P 6) and Shenmen (H 7). The reinforcing method was applied primarily, with the reducing method as secondary. The needles were retained for thirty minutes and manipulated several times during the treatment, which was given once daily. The heart rate decreased to ninety-three beats per minute after the first treatment, and dropped to eighty-two beats per minute after four treatments. Another three treatments were given to consolidate the effect.

In May, 1979, Dr. Gao treated a young worker for impotence of 15 months. He wished to try acupuncture treatment after unsuccessfully attempting many other methods. Dr. Gao diagnosed the case as impotence and premature ejaculation due to deficiency of the kidney. The treatment principle was to tone the kidney and strengthen yang. Prescription: Shenshu (B 23) or Mingmen (Du 4), and Guanyuan (Ren 4). The reinforcing method and the warming needle were applied. Treatment was given daily. Ten treatments comprised a course. The patient had fully recovered after three courses of treatment.

In May 1980, a middle-aged woman worker complained of edema in the legs above the ankles for three months. Her legs became pitted on pressure, and the condition was worse in the evening. She also had puffy cheeks in the morning and occasional palpitation. The symptoms had not been relieved after treatment with medicinal drugs. She also presented with normal appetite, scanty urine, pale and flabby tongue with thin coating, and thready and soft pulse. The urine test and ECG were normal. This case was diagnosed as edema caused by excessive dampness due to deficiency of the spleen. The treatment principle was to strengthen the spleen, eliminate dampness and relieve edema. Prescription: Pishu (B 20) and Zusanli (S 36) together, or Weishu (B 21) and Yinlingquan (Sp 9) together, or Pishu (B 20) and Taibai (Sp 3) together. The reinforcing method was used. The needles were manipulated in the Back-Shu Points for one minute before being removed. The needles in the leg points were retained for fifteen minutes. Treatment was given every other day. Needles were only used for the first four treatments, and then warming needles were substituted. Edema was relieved and the patient fully recovered after twenty treatments.

5. The development of the nail root points

In his application of the Jing-Well Points, Dr. Gao has discovered the nail root points. These new points have proved effective and easily applied. Patients can also learn to use these points themselves.

1) *Location* The nail root points are located 0.1 cm posterior to the root of the fingernails on the dorsal aspect of the hand. This curved line is very sensitive to pressure. There are altogether ten points, respectively termed the thumb root, index root, middle root, ring root and small root. Usually, fingernail pressure or needles are applied to these points to treat diseases. Actually, the nail root points are an extension of the Jing-Well Points, where yin meridians and yang meridians meet. By stimulating these points, qi from both yin and yang meridians is promoted and regulated. When qi flows freely to the extremities, the disease will be cured.

2) *Indications* Common indications: Coma, fever, sunstroke, pain, infantile convulsions, hysteria, and finger numbness. Specific indications: The thumb root is indicated in sore throat, stuffiness and pain in the chest, cough, asthmatic breathing, stomachache and frontal shoulder pain. The index root is indicated in toothache, nasal obstruction, sore throat, tinnitus, frontal headache, stomachache, and shoulder pain. The middle root is indicated in stuffiness and pain in the chest, palpitation, angina pectoris, insomnia, stomachache and pain in the liver region. The ring root is indicated in tinnitus, migraine,

sore throat, shoulder pain, back pain, pain in the chest, hypochondriac region, and hepatic distending pain. The small root is indicated in stuffiness and pain in the chest, palpitation, angina pectoris, insomnia, headache, tinnitus, shoulder pain and back pain.

3) *Cases treated with the nail root points* In March, 1978, Dr. Gao treated a young woman worker who often suffered palpitation, along with stuffiness and pain in the chest, following a previous penicillin anaphylactic reaction. There was currently a recurrence of palpitation and stuffy chest due to poor sleep. After fingernail pressure was applied to her middle root for eight minutes, she felt relaxed in the chest and also noticed a relief of palpitation. She was then instructed to treat herself on the middle root and small root for eight to twelve minutes whenever she had palpitation. She subsequently reported that her symptoms were quickly relieved.

In September, 1979, a middle-aged woman worker was treated for stomachache. She had a history of peptic ulcer. Dr. Gao instructed her to press the index root with her fingernail. Ten minutes later, the pain was relieved. Later, she again felt pain during the night. After being treated with the index root and middle root for fifteen minutes, the stomach pain diminished.

A middle-aged office worker had a history of chronic hepatitis. Her liver could be felt 2 cm below the ribs. A dull pain occurred in the liver region whenever she felt tired. In July, 1985, she was treated on the middle root and ring root by the fingernail pressure. Fifteen minutes later, the distending sensation in the liver region disappeared and she felt comfortable. Since then, she often treated herself if she had discomfort, with very positive results.

6. The empirical points for hemoptysis

Dr. Gao is very eager to learn special skills from the experience of the folk doctors. In 1965, he learned from a folk doctor about the treatment of hemoptysis by needling Jingming (B 1). This had not been previously recorded in medical literature. Dr. Gao explains that Jingming (B 1) is from the Bladder Meridian, which enters the brain. Jingming (B 1) has a sedating action on the mind. When the mind becomes calm, blood will be pacified, and hemoptysis can be checked. Dr. Gao's new experience with Jingming (B 1) was included in his book *New Acupuncture*.

In October, 1979, a middle-aged worker had bronchiectasis with hemoptysis. He stated that he had the same condition ten years before, and this recurrence was due to frequent coughing from a recent cold. He also presented with a cold appearance, cold limbs, dark tongue with thin, white coating, and deep, thready and rapid pulse. The condition was diagnosed as deficiency of lung yin caused by autumn dryness leading to frequent coughing, which then injured the lung collaterals. The treatment principle was to moisten the lung, check coughing, soothe the collaterals and stop bleeding. Prescription: Jingming (B 1), Chize (L 5) and Lieque (L 7).

A thin needle 0.28 mm in diameter was quickly inserted into Jingming (B 1), and then slowly inserted to a depth of 1.4 inches, causing a slight needling sensation. The needle was retained for twenty minutes. Following this, needling with the even method was applied to Chize (L 5) and Lieque (L 7) to cause moderate stimulation. The needles were retained for twenty minutes with frequent manipulation. The hemoptysis was immediately improved after the first treatment. The patient was then treated daily and fully recovered after four treatments. Six months later, he had another relapse of hemoptysis due to another cold. The same treatment was given and the symptoms were relieved after three treatments.

7. Treatment of two hundred cases of arrhythmia by selecting points on the basis of meridian differentiation

Dr. Gao emphasizes not only the use of the regular meridians, but also application of the extra meridians. He has carefully studied the course of each meridian and its connection with specific zang or fu organs, and how each zang or fu organ is related to different meridians and collaterals.

Arrhythmia manifests as palpitation, stuffiness and pain in the chest, shortness of breath, and asthmatic breathing. These are possibly accompanied by insomnia, dizziness and restlessness. The pulse is either thready and soft, or knotted and intermittent, or slow, or thready and rapid. The tongue is pale, flabby and tender, with tooth prints on the edge. The tongue coating is red or dark.

According to TCM syndrome differentiation, arrhythmia is primarily located in the heart and pericardium and their pertaining meridians. It is classified into heart qi deficiency, heart yin deficiency, obstruction of the heart vessels and weakness of heart yang. The points to be treated are usually selected from the Heart and Pericardium Meridians and their Front-Mu and Back-Shu Points. However, zang-fu theory maintains that, in addition to the Heart and Pericardium Meridians and their exteriorly-interiorly related meridians, many other meridians are also involved. It is said that the Spleen Meridian enters the heart, the Kidney Meridian connects with the heart, the Liver Meridian passes the heart, and the Du Meridian ascends and passes the heart. This explains why the heart and spleen, the heart and kidney, or the heart and liver may be diseased simultaneously. The Du Meridian dominates the yang of the whole body. Therefore, points from the Du Meridian are often used to promote yang for heart yang deficiency after a prolonged illness. As the heart vessel ascends to the lung, heart disease may affect the lung, causing shortness of breath and asthmatic breathing.

In the treatment of arrhythmia, Dr. Gao pays special attention to meridian differentiation in selecting the points. Neiguan (P 6), Shenmen (H 7), Jueyinshu (B 14) and Xinshu (B 15) are used as the main points, but only one or two of these points are selected for each treatment. Tanzhong (Ren 17), Lieque (L 7), Pishu (B 20) and Zusanli (S 36) are added for heart qi deficiency (usually accompanied by spleen qi deficiency); Sanyinjiao (Sp 6), Taixi (K 3) and Taichong (Liv 3) are added for heart yin deficiency; Geshu (B 17), Sanyinjiao (Sp 6), Tanzhong (Ren 17) and Lieque (L 7) are added for stagnation of blood and qi in the heart and lung; and Suliao (Du 25), Dazhui (Du 14), Zusanli (S 36) and Guanyuan (Ren 4) are added for heart yang deficiency (usually accompanied by yang deficiency of the Du Meridian).

Neiguan (P 6), the Luo-Connecting Point of the Pericardium Meridian, and Shenmen (H 7), the Yuan-Source Point of the Heart Meridian, are used together to strengthen the action of regulating the heart function. Jueyinshu (B 14) and Xinshu (B 15), as the Back-Shu Points of the heart and pericardium, are good for heart disease. Tanzhong (Ren 17), the Front-Mu Point of the pericardium, tones heart qi and treats palpitation. Pishu (B 20) and Zusanli (S 36) are reinforced to promote the source of qi and blood. Lieque (L 7) is used to regulate qi of the heart and lung, which helps shortness of breath and asthmatic breathing. Taixi (K 3), and Taichong (Liv 3), the Yuan-Source Points of the kidney and liver, are combined with Sanyinjiao (Sp 6) to tone kidney yin and liver yin for deficiency of heart yin. Geshu (B 17) and Sanyinjiao (Sp 6) are needled to invigorate blood circulation. Tanzhong (Ren 17) and Lieque (L 7) conduct qi, and are therefore used to remove obstruction from the collaterals of the heart and lung. Suliao (Du 25) and Dazhui (Du 14), from the Du Meridian, are reinforced to activate heart yang in the case of heart yang deficiency. Guanyuan (Ren 4), from the Ren Meridian, has a good effect in toning qi and strengthening yang. Because a branch of the Yangming Meridian of Foot connects with the heart, Zusanli (S 36) is able to promote heart qi when needled with the reinforcing method.

Dr. Gao has used these points in the treatment of two hundred cases of arrhythmia, with an effective rate of over 80 percent.

8. Treatment of intractable insomnia by selecting the points from the Du Meridian

Points selected from the Heart, Pericardium, Kidney, Spleen and Stomach Meridians are always quite effective to treat insomnia due either to imbalance of the heart and kidney, or to imbalance of the spleen and stomach. In some intractable insomnia, however, the patient may still be unable to sleep through the night in spite of several courses of acupuncture treatment and many kinds of medicine. These patients may also present with symptoms of dizziness and aversion to cold caused by deficiency of yang qi. For these cases, Dr. Gao selects Dazhui (Du 14), Baihui (Du 20), Fengfu (Du 16) and Mingmen (Du 4), using the reinforcing method. Moxibustion is also applied. Often, a satisfactory result will be obtained with this method. Dr. Gao explains that Du Meridian ascends to connect with the heart, and enters the collaterals of the brain. It also dominates the yang of the body. Insomnia essentially results from deficiency of yin. When this becomes chronic, there will eventually be deficiency of both yin and yang. When points from the Du Meridian are needled to invigorate yang qi, the mind will be calmed and the brain quieted, thereby controlling insomnia.

II. Case Analysis

Case 1: Palpitation

Name, Yang x x; sex, female; age, 43; occupation, office worker; date of the first visit, June 15, 1981.

Complaints The patient had palpitation, along with pain and stuffiness in the chest for a year and a half. She was diagnosed as having frequent ventricular premature contractions and coronary heart disease. She had been treated by Western medicine and Chinese herbs, but with only slight improvement. Her current symptoms included poor sleep and a dry mouth. She had a normal appetite, and normal urination and bowel movement. She also had a red tongue without coating, and a short pulse. Examination revealed that her heart beat was irregular and had a rate of 106 beats per minute. ECG gave the following results: 1) ventricular proiosystole; 2) sinus tachycardia; and 3) a tendency of low voltage. This case was diagnosed as deficiency of both qi and yin, which is a complicated condition of deficiency in the root cause, but excess in the symptoms. The treatment principle was to tone qi, replenish yin, tranquilize the heart and calm the mind.

Prescription Neiguan (P 6), Shenmen (H 7) and Anmian (Extra).

Treatment procedure The reinforcing method was applied primarily, combined with a reducing method. The needles were retained for twenty minutes, and treatment was given daily. The premature contractions markedly improved and the heart beat became normal after three treatments. Treatment was then reduced to once every other day. After ten treatments, the premature contractions were under control. The patient then stated he felt well, and the ECG proved normal.

Explanation Neiguan (P 6), the Luo-Connecting Point of the Pericardium Meridian, and Shenmen (H 7), the Yuan-Source Point of the Heart Meridian, are a combination of Yuan-Source and Luo-Connecting Points. Along with Anmian (Extra), they are able to tone the heart qi and heart yin, tranquilize the heart and calm the mind. This was a complicated case of deficiency in root cause, but excess in symptom. Therefore, the reinforcing method was used primarily, but combined with the reducing method. Dr. Gao has treated fifty-two cases of proiosystole, with an effective rate of 86 percent.

Case 2: Heart Bi syndrome

Name, Xia x x; sex, male; age, 42; occupation, worker; date of the first visit, May 7, 1981.

Complaints The patient had stuffiness in the chest and shortness of breath for three years. Other symptoms included chest pain, dizziness, poor sleep, aversion to cold, edema in the ankles which was worse in the evening, dry mouth, pale and flabby tongue with tooth prints, and thready and slow pulse, or sometimes knotted and intermittent pulse. The patient had been hospitalized twice, but the treatment was not satisfactory. ECG indicated: 1) sinus bradycardia (forty-eight beats per minute); and 2) frequent atrioventricular premature beats coupled rhythm in some beats. The case was diagnosed in Western medicine as sinus bradycardia and frequent atrioventricular premature beats, and in TC as deficiency of qi and yin. The treatment principle was to tone heart qi, relieve heart Bi syndrome, and also to calm the mind and improve sleep.

Prescription Neiguan (P 6), Suliao (Du 25), and Anmian (Extra).

Treatment procedure One and a half inch stainless steel needles of 0.28 mm in diameter were used. After the reinforcing method was applied, the needles were retained for five minutes. The needle at Suliao (Du 25) was scraped at a rate of sixty times a minute. On the second treatment two days later, the patient reported an improvement in the stuffiness in the chest. Sanyinjiao (Sp 6) was then added, with the needling method described above. By the third treatment, the heart rate had increased to fifty beats per minute. Also, the knotted and intermittent pulse occurred less frequently. The same treatment was continued, and on the fourth treatment, the patient reported he could now sleep well. The heart beat had become regular at a frequency of fifty-four beats per minute, and the knotted and intermittent pulse was absent. The patient was pleased with the result. Treatment was then reduced to once every two to three days. In these treatments, Neiguan (P 6) was replaced by either Lieque (L 7) or Tanzhong (Ren 17), which were both needled with the method as described above. The needles were retained for five to fifteen minutes. After nine treatments, the subjective symptoms were gone. An ECG showed that the heart rate had increased to fifty-eight beats per minute, and the premature contractions were absent. Another four treatments were prescribed to strengthen the effect. When treatment concluded, the heart rate had become normal at a frequency of sixty-four beats per minute.

Explanation Since this condition was located in the heart and its related meridians and collaterals, the points from the corresponding meridians were chosen for treatment. Neiguan (P 6), the Luo-Connecting Point of the Pericardium Meridian, is one of the Eight Confluent Points, and connects with the Yinwei Meridian. With the action of toning heart qi, this point was able to relieve Heart Bi Syndrome. Anmian (Extra) was used to calm the mind for insomnia. The Du Meridian dominates the yang qi of the body and its branches ascend to connect with the heart. This is why Suliao (Du 25) was needled to invigorate heart qi. Sanyinjiao (Sp 6) is the crossing point of the Liver, Spleen, and Kidney Meridians, and it can also balance the heart and kidney, tranquilize the heart and calm the mind. Lieque (L 7), the Luo-Connecting Point of the Lung Meridian, relaxes the chest and conducts qi. It was used here for stuffiness in the chest and shortness of breath. Tanzhong (Ren 17), the Front-Mu Point of the pericardium, and also the Influential Point dominating qi, has a very good effect in invigorating heart qi. These latter two points were alternated with Neiguan (P 6) in order to increase the therapeutic effect. Dr. Gao has currently treated fifty-four cases of sinus bradycardia with an effective rate as high as 88 percent.

Case 3: Deaf-mutism

Name, Qing x x; sex, male; age, 5; date of the first visit, April 8, 1965.

Complaints Three months before, this boy had lost consciousness during a high fever which had lasted for five days. After taking medication, the fever subsided and consciousness was restored, but he was then unable to speak or hear. He was then treated both by Western drugs and Chinese herbs, but with little help. His appetite, urination, bowels, sleep, tongue coating and pulse were all normal. Dr. Gao determined that this case was caused by blockage of qi of the ear and tongue. The treatment principle was to remove the obstruction, conduct the qi, and normalize the auditory function.

Prescription Tinggong (SI 19), Yifeng (SJ 17), Yamen (Du 15), Lianquan (Ren 23), Waiguan (SJ 5), Zhongzhu (SJ 3), and Hegu (LI 4).

Treatment procedure Stainless steel needles 0.28 mm in diameter were used with mild stimulation. The needles were slowly manipulated for fifteen to thirty seconds in an amplitude of 90°, then removed. Treatment was given daily, then reduced to every other day after six treatments. The boy was able to hear a watch ticking after twenty treatments. On the evening of the twenty-sixth treatment, the boy's father was overjoyed to hear his son talk with his neighbour.

Explanation The deaf-mutism in this case resulted from a febrile disease. Most of the points were chosen from the Hand-Taiyang, Yangming and Shaoyang Meridians, which are all related to the ear. Yamen (Du 15) and Lianquan (Ren 23) are able to remove obstruction from the tongue. A 5-year-old child is considered to have a young body constitution in TCM. Therefore, mild stimulation and quick removal of the needles should be applied. The short duration of the disease and the timely treatment were key points why this case obtained such quick and successful results. However, the result would not have been so good if the condition had existed for over one year.

Case 4: Retention of urine

Name, Cheng x x; sex, male; age, 79; occupation, retired worker; date of the first visit, August, 1979.

Complaints The chief complaint was retention and dribbling of urine for one month, and also difficulty in passing stool. The case had been diagnosed as prostatomegaly in the urogenital department, but Western medicine had failed to relieve the symptoms. The current symptoms included unsmooth and frequent urination four to five times every night, and also a distending and bear-down sensation in the perineum. Other symptoms were tinnitus, thin, white tongue coating, and deep, string-taut pulse. Dr. Gao diagnosed this case as downward movement of dampness, causing obstruction of the meridians in the perineum. The treatment principle was to eliminate dampness and remove the obstruction from the meridians in the perineum.

Prescription Ciliao (B 32), Baihuanshu (B 30), Yaoshu (Du 2), Yinlingquan (Sp 9).

Treatment procedure The even method was used. Needles were retained for fifteen minutes. Treatment was given every day or every other day. There was less difficulty in passing urine after three treatments, and almost no difficulty in passing urine and feces after six treatments. The patient was cured after a total of twelve treatments.

Explanation Ciliao (B 32) and Baihuanshu (B 30) were chosen from the Bladder Meridian, whose branch is said to enter the anus, thereby relating to the perineum. Yaoshu (Du 2) is a point from the Du Meridian, which emerges from the perineum. Yinlingquan (Sp 9), the He-Sea Point of the spleen, has the action of relieving difficulty in urination so as to eliminate dampness. When qi moves freely in the perineum, and dampness is dispelled, urination will become normal.

Case 5: Wei syndrome

Name, Chen x x; sex, male; age, 43; occupation, farmer; date of the first visit, October 8, 1965.

Complaints The patient reported that he had suddenly fallen on the day before the treatment. He was then unable to stand or walk due to weakness of the legs, and was subsequently sent to the hospital where he was examined. Clinical manifestations included inability of voluntary movement of the legs, retention of urine, distension in the lower abdomen, anxiety and frustration, poor appetite, thin, white tongue coating, and thready, string-taut pulse. He had been catheterized three times. This case was diagnosed in Western medicine as acute myelitis, paraplegia and retention of urine, while in TCM it was considered to be dysfunction of the urinary bladder in controlling water due to deficiency of kidney yang and kidney qi. The treatment principle was to nourish the kidney, tone qi, and strengthen the function of the urinary bladder.

Prescription Mingmen (Du 4), Yaoyangguan (Du 3), Shenshu (B 23), Huatuojiaji (Extra), Guanyuan (Ren 4), Shuidao (S 28), Huantiao (G 30), Futu (S 32), Liangqiu (S 34), Zusanli (S 36), Yinlingquan (Sp 9), Fuliu (K 7) and Jiexi (S 41).

Treatment procedure The reinforcing method was used, combined with the even method. The points on the back and lumbar region were treated first. Moderate stimulation was given. After manipulation continued for one minute, the needles were then removed. Guanyuan (Ren 4) and the points in the lower limbs were then treated. Needles were retained for fifteen minutes, during which manipulation was given several times. The patient was treated twice on the first day, once in the morning and once in the afternoon eight hours later. On the second day, the patient had slight dribbling of urine. The same treatment was continued, with warming needle added on Huatuojiaji (Extra). On the third day, he could pass urine, although with some difficulty. His knees were also able to bend slightly. Treatment was then reduced to once daily, with warm needling added on Lianqiu (S 34), Zusanli (S 36) and Futu (S 32). On the fourth day, urination became normal. Guanyuan (Ren 4) and Shuidao (S 28) were then eliminated from the prescription. On the fifth day, the patient could slowly bend his knees and toes, and was able to stand by himself, if supported by an object. The bowel movement had also become normal. After nine treatments, the patient could walk slowly for a few steps around the ward. After fifteen treatments, he recovered and was discharged from the hospital.

Explanation This is a case of Wei Syndrome involving retention of urine caused by weakness of kidney yang. Mingmen (Du 4), Yaoyangguan (Du 3), Shenshu (B 23), Huatuojiaji (Extra), Guanyuan (Ren 4) and Fuliu (K 7) have the action of relieving obstruction, so urine can return to normal. Futu (S 32), Lianqiu (S 34), Zusanli (S 36), Huantiao (G 30) and Jiexi (S 41) were selected with a warming needle in order to warm and nourish the meridians and vessels in the legs so as to relieve the various symptoms.

Case 6: Mania (mental disorder)

Name, Li x x; sex, female; age, 43; occupation, office worker; date of the first visit, October 20, 1982.

Complaints It was reported that the patient had first developed the symptoms of headache, poor sleep and uttering to herself. Later, she was noticed laughing or angry without apparent reason, and sometimes she gurgled or cursed angrily. Lately, she had become more irritable, staying awake the whole night, and even smashing things. Her appetite, urination and bowel movement were normal. She had been placed in a mental hospital, and was given wintermin and diazepam. Examination showed that the patient stared ahead with an apathetic look, and only answered at random while being questioned. She also had red tongue with dry, yellow coating, and string-taut, forceful pulse. Dr. Gao believed the condition was caused by mental depression and disturbance of the mind. The treatment principle was to soothe the liver, relieve depression, tranquilize the heart and calm the mind. Mental support and comfort were also important. The patient was advised to reduce the dosage of wintermin and other Western medicine.

Prescription

1) Baihui (Du 20), Anmian (Extra), Ganshu (B 18), Shenmen (H 7) and Zusanli (S 36).

2) Baihui (Du 20), Anmian (Extra), Neiguan (P 6), Sanyinjiao (Sp 6) and Taichong (Liv 3).

Treatment procedure The even method was applied and needles were retained for twenty minutes. Treatment was given daily. Two groups of the points were used alternately. Ten treatments comprised a course. After sixteen treatments, the wintermin was stopped altogether, although diazepam was still taken. At the end of the third course, only two pills of diazepam were taken daily and all symptoms were under control.

Explanation Baihui (Du 20) is a point from the Du Meridian, which enters the brain and ascends and connects with the heart. Shenmen (H 7), the Yuan-Source Point of the Heart Meridian, and Neiguan (P 6), the Luo-Connecting Point of the Pericardium Meridian, calm the heart and ease mental strain when combined with Anmian (Extra). Ganshu (B 18) and Taichong (Liv 3) were used together to soothe the liver and relieve depression. Zusanli (S 36) or Sanyinjiao (Sp 6) were chosen to strengthen the spleen and stomach and eliminate damp and phlegm. Mental comfort helps to relax and calm the mind. Follow-up visits for four years showed that the patient was quite normal and had resumed her work.

RESEARCH ON BREAST TUMOURS

—Guo Chengjie's Clinical Experience

Guo Chengjie, a native of Fupin County, Shanxi Province, was born in 1920. At the age of seventeen, he began to study traditional Chinese medicine and acknowledged as his masters two famous Chinese physicians, Bie Jiantang and Jia Hanqin. In 1949, he began to study at the Qinling School of Traditional Chinese Medicine. In 1959, he was assigned to work at the Shanxi School of Traditional Chinese Medicine as a teacher of acupuncture after he graduated from the Teachers Training Class run by that school. Since then, he has compiled six volumes of teaching materials on acupuncture, totalling about 1,200,000 Chinese characters. He has been in charge of clinical research on acupuncture treatment of hyperplasia of the breast, which has won a first prize award for scientific research in the higher education system of Shanxi Province, and a second prize award of provincial excellent scientific article for his work. Since 1982, he has taken up research on the causative factors and mechanisms of acupuncture treatment of hyperplasia of the breast. Now he is a member of the standing committee of the China Association of Acupuncture, a member of the standing committee of Shanxi Society of Traditional Chinese Medicine, director of Shanxi Acupuncture Association and member of the Provincial Scientific Committee.

I. Academic Characteristics and Medical Specialities

Dr. Guo's knowledge and treatment of breast tumours are original.

1. Stagnation of liver qi causing failure to promote free flow of qi, blockage of the Stomach Meridian, and obstruction of the collaterals in the breast are the causative factors of breast tumours

The breast tumour in TCM corresponds to hyperplasia of the breast in modern medicine. The first description of this condition is in the book of *General Treatise on the Etiology and Symptomology of Diseases* written in the Sui Dynasty. It says, "One of the branches of the Foot Yangming Meridian runs from the supraclavicular fossa to the breast. Wind-cold, which may congeal blood into nodules, is liable to invade the meridian if it is weak... The nodule will never disappear if cold still exists." In the book *Collection of Personal Experience on Carbuncles*, written by Gao Jinting in the Qing Dynasty, there is detailed information: "Breast tumours, which are literally nodules in the breast, have the shape of a small ball, may or may not have pain when moved, involve no change in the colour of the skin, and disappear or develop along with the emotional fluctuations of joy and anger, are often caused by injury of the spleen due to excessive thinking, and injury of the liver due to excessive anger. As for its etiology, someone says of breast tumours that, "They form from invasion of the Foot-Yangming Meridian by wind-cold, which congeals qi and blood." Here is Gao Jinting's experience: Breast tumours caused by dysfunction of the spleen and liver due to emotional depression, and the size of the breast tumours and nodules always change along with emotional changes.

By a study on more than two thousand women and treatment of more than eight hundred cases, Dr. Guo has found that breast tumours are closely related to the liver and stomach (spleen), as well as to the Chong and Ren Meridians. The liver functions to promote free flow of qi and stores blood; the Liver Meridian runs through the chest and connects with the breast. The breasts pertain to the stomach, and are the place passed by the Stomach Meridian and permeated by qi and blood of the Chong and Ren Meridians. Disorders of the seven emotional factors, especially excessive thinking and anger, may cause stagnation of liver qi, dysfunction of the spleen in transportation and transformation, unsmooth circulation of qi and blood in the liver and stomach, and imbalance of the Chong and Ren Meridians. This will result in stagnation of qi and blood in the breast collaterals and manifest as tumours or nodules of the breasts. The observation of five hundred patients who received acupuncture treatment revealed that 374 of the cases, making up 74.8 percent, complained of irritability. Dr. Guo therefore believes that stagnation of liver qi and unsmooth circulation of Stomach Meridian qi, which lead to obstruction of the breast collaterals, are the main pathogenic factors of the disease.

2. Soothing the liver is essential to the treatment of breast tumours, which can be divided into four types

Breast tumours manifest as breast pain and enlarged nodules. This pain is usually aggravated and the nodules usually hardened before the menstrual period or after emotional changes or after too much stress, but is usually relieved when the menstrual period is gone. On the basis of these features, Dr. Guo advocates that treatment should be given according to the differentiation of syndromes and consideration of the patient's constitution. The disease is divided into four types:

1) *Stagnation of liver qi* In this type, distending pain and nodules of the breasts are often aggravated before the menstrual period and after anger. The pain may radiate to the axillary fossa, the shoulder and the back, accompanied by fullness in the chest, abdominal distension, poor appetite, irregular menstruation, foreign sensation in the throat, pale tongue with occasionally purple marks, and string-taut pulse.

2) *Liver fire* This type manifests as distending pain in the breasts and hypochondriac regions, which is aggravated after anger or on pressure, and is accompanied by burning sensation, palpable nodules in the breasts, restlessness, irritability, bitter taste in the mouth, dry throat, red eyes, short menstrual cycle, yellow urine, red tongue with yellow coating, and string-taut, rapid pulse.

3) *Deficiency of yin of the liver and kidney* In this condition, the breast pain and nodules may sometimes fluctuate between better and worse. Other manifestations include fullness in the chest, dull pain in the hypochondriac regions, dizziness, blurred vision, dry eyes, weakness and soreness of the lower back and knees, burning sensations in the

palms and soles, red tongue with little coating, and string-taut thready and rapid pulse.

4) *Deficiency of qi and blood* In this condition, the breast pain and nodules become worse after fatigue, which is accompanied by general weakness, lassitude, poor appetite, dizziness and blurred vision on slight exertion, palpitation and anxiety. The patient will be able to fall asleep, but will be easily startled awake. Pallor, a pale tongue and deep and thready pulse are also present.

If clinical manifestations are unable to provide a clear diagnosis, Dr. Guo advocates laboratory tests to avoid misdiagnosing breast cancer. These tests may include B-scope ultrasonic examination and cytology tests to determine the nature and size of the tumours and nodules. This will be a great aid in prescribing appropriate clinical treatment.

Dr. Guo has successfully treated with acupuncture more than eight hundred cases of breast tumours. The main principle of treatment is to soothe the liver, relieve stagnation of qi, soften tumours, disperse nodules, and promote the circulation of qi of the Yangming Meridian. Both the short and long term therapeutic results are quite satisfactory. The method has the advantages of simple needle manipulation, rapid analgesia, quick disappearance of nodules, and short duration of treatment.

Selection of points a. Group A (Chest Group): Wuyi (S 15), Tanzhong (Ren 17), and Hegu (LI 4). b. Group B (Back Group): Jianjing (G 21), Tianzong (SI 11) and Ganshu (B 18).

Additional points Yanglingquan (G 34) for stagnation of liver qi; Taichong (Liv 3) instead of Hegu (LI 4) for liver fire; Taixi (K 3) instead of Ganshu (B 18) for deficiency of yin of the liver and kidney; Pishu (B 20) and Zusanli (S 36) instead of Hegu (LI 4) for deficiency of qi and blood; and Sanyinjiao (Sp 6) for irregular menstruation.

Explanation Wuyi (S 15) is located superior to the breast, and Tanzhong (Ren 17) is located lateral to the breast. These two points are used in combination to regulate meridians qi in the breast, activate blood, eliminate stagnation and disperse nodules. Jianjing (G 21) and Ganshu (B 18) will soothe the liver, relieve depression and remove obstruction from the Liver Meridian. Hegu (LI 4) controls the circulation of qi of both the Yangming Meridians of Foot and Hand. Tianzong (SI 11) will free the meridians and collaterals, and is effective in treating disorders of the breast. Adding or eliminating these points on the basis of clinical manifestations will relieve stagnation of qi, free the circulation of the meridians, stop pain and disperse nodules.

Dr. Guo has used radiommunoassay to study the results of the treatments. Using ten cases (in which six were cured and four improved), he has measured the changes of concentration of estradiol, progesterone and testosterone before and after acupuncture treatment. He then compared these results with those of thirty healthy females to study the causative factors of the disease and the mechanism of the acupuncture treatment. The results revealed that before treatment all of the three above hormones were higher for breast tumour patients than for a healthy person. (Estradiol and progesterone: $P<0.01$; testosterone: $P<0.05$). After acupuncture treatment, the estradiol levels were reduced to normal ($P>0.05$), while the progesterone and testosterone levels were continuously raised. Observation of pathological tests of rat breast hyperplasia with high estradiol levels showed that acupuncture had a marked counter-acting effect, and that it sped up the recovery. Further studies showed that acupuncture also had a counter-acting effect on rabbit breast hyperplasia due to elevated estradiol. These studies revealed that one of the main causative factors of hyperplasia of the breast is the elevation of plasma estradiol. The positive results of acupuncture treatment for this disease are obtained by lowering the plasma estradiol level (probably including estriol).

Some doctors have advocated that surgery must be performed immediately for hyperplasia of the breast, since it has been reported that this condition may develop into cancer. Based on his experience of many years, Dr. Guo believes that acupuncture should be taken as the first method of treatment for this condition, if there are no obvious signs of cancer.

II. Case Analysis

Case 1: Hyperplasia of the breast

Name, Hu x x; sex, female; age, 31; occupation, doctor.

Complaints The patient reported that four years before she had found two 2 x 2 cm tumours in each breast. The tumours were separated from the surrounding tissues. There was no pain when they were pressed, and there was no clear relation with the menstrual period. The condition had been previously diagnosed in a hospital as hyperplasia of the breast. She had not been previously treated, however. The tumours had enlarged gradually, and in the last two or three months, the distending pain of the breasts was aggravated about ten days prior to her menstrual period, and then relieved slightly after the period. A past history of rheumatic arthritis was noted. Her first menstrual period had come at the age of fourteen, and menstruation had since been normal. The 6 x 6 x 3 cm tumours were palpable on the lateral upper quadrant and the medial upper quadrant of both breasts. The tumours were neither excessively hard or soft, and did not adhere to the surrounding tissues. There was a pain when the breasts were pressed, no fluid excreted from the nipples, and no colour changes on the skin. The tongue was red, and the pulse was string-taut.

Diagnosis Stagnation of liver qi, resulting in stagnation of blood, which caused phlegm-damp to develop into tumours of the breasts.

Principle of treatment Soothe the liver and regulate qi.

Prescription

1) Tianzong (SI 11), Ganshu (B 18).

2) Tanzhong (Ren 17), Wuyi (S 15), Zusanli (S 36).

All points were treated bilaterally.

Treatment procedure The above two groups of points were used alternately. Treatment was given daily using the even method; and eight treatments comprised a course. After four courses of treatment, the breast pain disappeared, and the tumours were markedly reduced. Two years later, the patient wrote to say that the pain had not recurred, and that tumours were now completely gone.

Explanation Dr. Guo has treated with acupuncture more than eight hundred cases of breast tumours. The curative rate is 40.4 percent to 54.3 percent, and the total effective rate is 93.5 percent to 97.3 percent. Ninety cases were followed up after one, two and five years and the results showed that the long-term effects were 81.4 percent, 92.5 percent, 92 percent respectively. Compared with various control groups (Western medicine group, injection group, Chinese herbal medicine group, and natural group), the therapeutic result of the acupuncture group was the best.

Case 2: Hyperplasia of breast

Name, Gu x x; sex, female; occupation, shop assistant.

Complaints The patient reported that two years before, tumours had been found in her breasts bilaterally. These tumours were accompanied by pain which was aggravated before her menstrual period and after anger. Chinese herbal medicine had been taken but had no effect. Examination in the hospital determined she suffered from hyperplasia of the breasts. The tumour in her left breast was comparatively large. Pathological tests during previous surgery for the breast tumour revealed hyperplasia of the breast nodule. The breast pain had not improved after the operation, and the tumours were found again a half year later. Since both Chinese and Western medicine had not helped her, she decided to try acupuncture treatment. Clinical manifestations included a rosy complexion with normal appearance, a light red tongue, a string-taut pulse, a soft abdomen and impalpable liver and spleen. The heart and lungs were normal. A 3 x 2.5 cm tumour was palpated in the lateral upper quadrant of the left breast. The tumour was movable, had a distinct border, and was neither soft nor hard. A few bean-like nodules were also scattered in the lateral upper quadrant of the right breast. Pain was evident if the breasts were pressed.

Diagnosis Stagnation of liver qi.

Principle of Treatment Soothe the liver and regulate qi.

Points and treatment procedure Two groups of points as described above were used alternately. The even method was used, needles were retained for twenty minutes, and were manipulated twice during retention. After the first course of treatment, the breast pain was alleviated, and the tumours softened. Another two courses followed, after which the distending pain was virtually gone, being only slightly present before her menstrual period or after getting angry. In a follow-up visit the next year, she reported that she had at that time been married for half a year, and had been pregnant for three months. She further reported that she had no lumps, pain, or abnormal feelings in her breasts.

Explanation Young women (eighteen to twenty-five years old) may have multiple tumours of the breasts because of an abundant discharge of estrogen. In this case, surgery may be of little help because of the great number of tumours and nodules. Especially in younger women, surgery will not eliminate the causative factors of the disease, and so the condition will easily recur after the operation. This is a further reason for treating such a condition with acupuncture, since this may regulate and restore the endocrine balance and treat the disease completely.

Case 3: Pain in the left breast

Name, Ji x x; sex, male; age, 57.

Complaints The patient came for his first visit in February of 1979. The left breast was enlarged, and a hard mass was palpable. The patient reported he had this condition along with breast pain for one month. Vitamin E had been taken but had given no improvement. The mass had grown gradually, and surgery had previously been recommended. The patient, however, wanted to determine if acupuncture might help instead. Other clinical manifestations included a prominently swollen left breast, a 2 x 2 x 0.8 cm crescent-shaped tumour palpable below the left nipple, non-adhesion of the tumour to the skin, and distinct pain upon pressure.

Diagnosis Stagnation of liver qi resulting in obstruction of qi of the Yangming Meridians.

Principle of treatment Regulate qi, activate blood, disperse tumours and stop pain.

Prescription Tanzhong (Ren 17), Hegu (LI 4), Wuyi (S 15), Ganshu (UB 18).

Treatment procedure After seven treatments with the reducing method, the pain had stopped and the tumours had softened. After fifteen treatments, the tumours had been markedly reduced to a size of about 0.5 x 0.5 cm. A follow-up visit two months after the conclusion of the treatment showed no recurrence of pain and tumours.

Explanation It is usually thought that hyperplasia of the breast in males is liable to develop into cancer. In recent years, Dr. Guo has treated more than ten such cases, the youngest being fourteen, and the oldest being sixty. Dr. Guo found that none of these cases developed into cancer. He therefore suggests that acupuncture is an appropriate first treatment for such a case. Usually two to three courses of treatment are sufficient to bring good results.

THEORY AND APPLICATION OF THE EFFECTIVE SPOTS IN ACUPUNCTURE

—Guo Xiaozong's Clinical Experience

Guo Xiaozong, a native of Huining County, Gansu Province, was born in 1924. At the age of thirteen, he began to learn acupuncture from his mother and then took Shu Guangdou, a veteran traditional medical practitioner as his teacher. He started his medical career in 1948 after passing the medical examination for a licence. In the past forty years he has devoted his efforts to acupuncture treatment, teaching and research. He served as a teacher successively in the National Training Class of the Acupuncture Experiment Institute of the Ministry of Public Health, Class for Acupuncturists of the Red Cross of the Soviet Union, Class for Doctors of Western Medicine Studying Traditional Chinese Medicine, and Acupuncture Class of TB Institute. In 1986 he visited Belgium and lectured at the European University of Traditional Chinese Medicine. He has given many presentations at national, army and international acupuncture conferences, about the theory and application of the effective spots. Research on needling benign thyroid tumours won a prize awarded by the China Academy of Traditional Chinese Medicine. Now he is a professor and director of the Manipulation Section of the Acupuncture Institute of the China Academy of Traditional Chinese Medicine.

I. Academic Characteristics and Medical Specialities

1. Classification of the effective spots

1) *Benign spots* It is stated in *Treatise of Mania, Miraculous Pivot* that when the symptoms are clear to us, a press given to a particular point or relating spot can relieve symptoms. The very spot pressed to relieve symptoms is called the benign spot. For example, pressing Sidu (SJ 9) may alleviate migraine.

2) *Positive spot* This is a spot where pain, cords and nodules are felt on pressure when a disease is getting better. Besides, there are other signs such as soreness, numbness, skin hypersensitivity and papules.

3) *Negative spot* When the positive spot is found, try to find the spot according to the distribution law of the effective spots which can alleviate symptoms. This spot is called negative spot. For example, when a positive spot on the Weishu (B 21) presents in a patient with gastric pain, which can be relieved by a press to Zusanli (S 36). Then Zusanli (S 36) is known as a negative spot.

Generally speaking, benign spots, positive and negative spots can be found in the acute stage of a disease. In the remission stage negative and positive spots are usually found. In treatment the benign and negative spots are often needled.

2. Distribution of the effective spots

Although the effective spots are different from meridian points, they are helpful in identification and treatment of diseases.

1) *Distribution around the branches of the blood vessels* The book *Classic on Medical Problems* points out, "Arteries are on the twelve meridians." For instance, "arteries are on Zhongfu (L 4), Yunmen (L 2), Tianfu (L 3), Xiabai (L 4), Hegu (LI 4), Yangxi (LI 5), Jiquan (H 1)...." The above tells us that meridians are closely related to blood vessels. Guo holds that the effective spots are distributed around the arteries and veins, especially around the branches of the blood vessels, e.g. at the branches of the arteria carotis interna and arteria carotis externa.

2) *Distribution around the neuroplex and the nerve trunk* Meridians are not only related to blood vessels but also to the nervous system, which is pointed out in the ancient medical literature. The effective spots can be found around the neuroplex and the nerve-trunk, e.g. the paravertebral points.

3) *Distribution among the muscle group* The effective spots can be found among the muscle groups, e.g. around the deltoid.

4) *Symmetrical distribution at the left and right* The fourteen meridians, and eight extraordinary meridians, the twelve muscle regions and collaterals are distributed symmetrically at the left and right side of the body. The function of the Sanjiao, distribution of the Qi Street and the four reservoirs explain the connection between the left and right. When one side is in trouble, qi stagnation of the other side must be found and imbalance occurs. For this reason at the other side the effective spot which reflects and cures the problem should exist. For example, when there is a pain in the left elbow, the effective spot can be found at the right elbow.

5) *Symmetrical distribution in the upper and lower portions of the body* The upper and lower portions of the body are organized as an organic whole, because the meridians and collaterals, the extraordinary meridians, etc. are also distributed symmetrically in the upper and lower, keeping a relative equilibrium. For this reason it is possible to treat the lower part of the body while symptoms appear in the upper part, and vice versa. For instance, the effective spot can be found at the back of the knee when there is a problem at the back of the head.

6) *Crossing and symmetrical distribution* Based on the above distribution of the meridians we may draw hypothetical longitudes and latitudes over the body. The effective spots symmetrically distributed at the left and right side of the body may be found on the same latitude; those symmetrically distributed in the upper and lower portions of the body may be found on the same longitude; and the effective spots crossedly and symmetrically distributed may be found at the cross of the longitude and latitude. For example, the effective spot can be seen at the right knee joint where there is a pain in the left elbow.

7) *Distribution along the meridians* Most of the benign spots distributed along the meridians are located on its own meridian, the exterior-interior related meridian, and around the given points of its own meridian. On identification of the effective spots one should especially concern the effective ones close to the meridian points. There are about

a hundred effective spots distributed along the meridian corresponding to the meridian points.

3. The puncture technique of the effective spots

According to his own clinical experience, Guo has developed five puncture techniques for the effective spots.

1) *Horizontal puncture* The needle is slowly inserted into the skin with the left hand to press the effective spot. The lift-thrust method is used to induce the needling sensation. After arrival of qi the spot remains to be pressed by the left hand and eight or nine rotations of the needle is done. Afterwards, the needle body is scraped eight to nine times. The manipulations are repeated three to five times. The spot is then pressed by one of the left fingers and the needle is pulled out. This technique is for cases of affliction of the zang-fu organs with minor dysfunctions.

2) *Heat-removing technique* When the effective spot is chosen by the left index finger, the needle is immediately inserted to the desired depth. The lift-thrust method is used to induce arrival of qi. Then the spot remains to be pressed by the left index finger and the needle body is scraped by the right middle finger from below to above six times. The lift-thrust method is done six times too. Then the manipulations are repeated three or four times. Afterwards the needle is pulled out. This technique is for marked heat syndromes.

3) *Warming technique* The effective spot is chosen by the left hand and the needle is inserted into the desired depth to bring about the needling sensation with the lift-thrust method. The spot remains to be pressed by the left hand and the needle body is scraped by the right index finger from above to below nine times. The lift-thrust method is conducted nine times. Then the same manipulations are repeated three to nine times and the needle is pulled out. This technique is for yin syndromes.

4) *Tonifying technique* The effective spot is pressed strongly by the left index finger and the needle is inserted into the desired depth to induce the needling sensation with the lift-thrust method. The spot remains to be pressed by the left index finger, 360° twirling clockwise is given and the needle body is scraped from above to below nine times. The lift-thrust method is conducted nine times until the part where the needling reaction reaches presents tic and peristalsis. The manipulations are repeated three to five times. The spot is strongly pressed by the left index finger while the needle is pulled out. Afterwards the spot is pressed close. This technique is for syndromes of yin, cold and deficiency.

5) *Reducing technique* The effective spot is chosen by the left index finger and the needle is quickly inserted to the desired depth. The lift-thrust method is used to induce the needling sensation. Then the needle is twirled counterclockwise and upwardly. Quick lift-thrust-scrape method is conducted six times. The manipulations are repeated two to four times. This technique is for syndromes of yang, heat and excess.

The warming and toning methods bring abundant meridian qi around the needle and the patient may have a warm sensation under the needle. The heat-removing and reducing methods eliminate the pathogenic factors and disseminate meridian qi. The patient may have a cool sensation. This is the proof to tell whether the technique is successful or not. A 29-year-old male patient had lumbago for eight years due to strain of the lower back. An X-ray showed deformity of the second to the fourth sacral vertebrae. Symptoms included lumbago, aversion to cold, soreness and distension of the lower back on long standing or sitting, pale tongue with tooth prints on its border and white thin coating, thready pulse, deformity of the spinal column, "4" test (±). He was diagnosed as having lumbago (due to cold, damp and blood stasis). Points or the effective spots are selected as follows: Shenshu (B 23) (both) Dachangshu (B 25) (both), Dazhui (Du 14), Tianzhu (B 10) (both), and Weizhong (B 40) (both). The reinforcing method is applied. The reduction is given first for deformity of the spinal column, then acupuncture is followed. The patient felt a warm sensation and slight sweating at the lower back. Five treatments relieved the pain and six treatments cured the case.

II. Case Analysis

Case 1: Goiter

Name, Zhang x x; sex, female; age, 40; date of the first visit, April, 1983.

Complaints At the level of the Adam's apple there was a 3.5 x 2.5 cm hard, painless, movable and smooth swelling. Radioisotope scan showed normal left lobe of the thyroid gland and enlarged right lobe of the thyroid gland. Ultrasonic examination showed a 2.5 x 1.2 cm lower echo area in the right lobe of the thyroid gland with bigger evenly distributed light spots.

Differentiation Qi stagnation and phlegm accumulation.

Prescription Tianzhu (B 10), Dazhu (B 11), Neiguan (P 6), Qugu (Ren 2) and the swollen part.

Treatment procedure Needles of No. 32 were used. After arrival of qi, six to eight needles were inserted into the base of the swelling. Manipulations were conducted for twenty minutes respectively. Seventy-four treatments made the swelling disappear. The ultrasonic examination showed the right lobe of the thyroid gland was normal. A follow-up survey showed no relapse.

Explanation All the points used were the effective spots. Seventy-eight cases of benign thyroma were treated by this method. The current effective rate was 94.86 percent and long effective rate was 83.33 percent by palpation. The ultrasonic film showed the current effective rate was 86.54 percent and the long effective rate was 77.4 percent. After cessation of acupuncture 34.15 percent were getting better, among which 24.39 percent were nearly recovered.

Case 2: Deviated mouth and eyes

Name, Zhang x x; sex, male; age, 69; date of the first visit, April 27, 1978.

Complaints At first he had an uneasy feeling at the right side of the face and a pain behind the ear. On the following day he had deviated mouth and eyes. The right eye was not able to close and tears ran down.

Differentiation Attack of the meridians by wind and impeded flow of qi and blood.

Prescription Shangjuxu (S 37), Jiache (S 6), Yuyao (Extra 3), Sibai (S 2), Taiyang (Extra 2), Sidu (SJ 9).

Treatment procedure The horizontal puncture was applied with minor stimulation to the diseased side and strong stimulation to the healthy side. After ten treatments the right eye was able to close and other symptoms were removed.

Explanation According to his experience, local points are not used for early-stage facial paralysis. One course of treatment is enough to cure the case by selection of the distal effective spots. Most of the patients who had the problem for over three weeks could be cured by the above manipulations associated with the distal effective spots.

Case 3: Knee joint pain

Name, Wang x x; sex, female; age, 49; date of the first visit, December, 1982.

Complaints In 1973 she suffered from dislocation of the left patella due to trauma. Roentgenogram showed malacia of the patella. There was a constant pain in the left and right knee joint. In 1982 the condition deteriorated, accompanied by swollen joints, motor impairment. Physical examination showed there was no deformity of the knees, slight swelling of the joints, motor impairment, floating patella test (+), left circumference of the left knee joint, 41.5 cm, circumference of the right knee joint, 42 cm. Roentgenogram diagnosis: traumatic arthritis of the left knee joint and right bony knee joint arthritis.

Differentiation Bone bi syndrome due to cold and damp.

Prescription Heding (Extra 31), Xiyan (Extra 32), Renying (S 9), Yinmen (B 37) and Sidu (SJ 9).

Treatment procedure The warming technique was applied to Heding (Extra 31) and Xiyan (Extra 32); horizontal acupuncture was given to Renying (S 9), Yinmen (B 37) and Sidu (SJ 9). Twenty-one treatments alleviated the swollen knee joints, pain, and motor impairment, the circumference of the left and right knee joint was 38 cm and 37 cm respectively. The floating patella test was (-). The treatment ceased. A follow-up survey in September, 1985 showed no relapse.

Explanation Thirty cases of hydro-knee joint (including bone arthritis, traumatic arthritis, rheumatic and rheumatoid arthritis) were treated by selection of the effective points. The cure rate was 36.7 percent, the markedly effective rate was 43.3 percent, 20 percent improved. The total effective rate was 100 percent. A follow-up survey of eighteen cases showed no relapse.

TREATMENT WITH REN-DU ACUPOINTS, BLEEDING COLLATERALS IN RELIEVING BLOOD STAGNATION

—Xi Yongjiang's Clinical Experience

Xi Yongjiang, a native of Chuansha County, Shanghai, was born in March, 1925. Working as a medical assistant, he studied medicine from his father since his boyhood, and afterwards he specialized in medicine in the Shanghai Chinese Medical College and graduated in 1943. Since then he has been engaged in clinical and educational work. In 1958, he was transferred to the Shanghai Research Institute of Acupuncture, Moxibustion and Meridians to be in charge of research. Also he taught acupuncture and moxibustion in the Shanghai College of Traditional Chinese Medicine and the International Acupuncture Training Centre. He has published more than ten academic theses of research work. And he has worked on the textbook *Techniques of Needling and Moxibustion* as a chief editor, and he has written the teaching materials about acupuncture and moxibustion for the students in the Shanghai College of Traditional Chinese Medicine. He also helped compile the *Dictionary of Acupuncture and Moxibustion* and in designing glass human models with 14-meridian acupoints. At present he is an associate professor of the Shanghai College of Traditional Chinese Medicine.

I. Academic Characteristics and Medical Specialities

1. Common methods in clinical treatment

Dr. Xi emphasizes that it is very important to have medical knowledge in clinical practice; that being a practitioner, one has to understand the constant change in diseases and one has to be free from the previous expression and experience in syndrome-pattern diagnosis, acupoints and therapeutic methods in order to find the correct differentiation of syndromes and to seek the corresponding therapy.

In the treatment of rheumatoid arthritis, he always takes local acupoints in predomination. He thinks that this disease is deficiency in constitution and excess in symptoms, it is necessary to support the constitution systematically by using acupoints of the Du Meridian and the Back-Shu points of the Bladder Meridian; also this disease is due to invasion of pathogenic wind, cold and dampness which cause stagnation of qi and blood, therefore "the painful spots are taken as acupoints" which can be inserted by the techniques of "Lateral, Joint, Trigger and Collateral Punctures," which are mentioned in *Miraculous Pivot*, in cooperation of auricular seed-embedding therapy, seven-star needling technique and cupping therapy for obtaining satisfactory results.

In 1956, Dr. Xi pioneered in the application of the acupoint-injection therapy, i.e.

to inject a small dosage of drugs into acupoints, which is indicated in insomnia, neurasthenia and injuries of soft tissues for effectiveness. Dr. Xi thinks it is necessary to choose proper acupuncture therapies in the estimation of their effectiveness. In the treatment of certain diseases, single needling therapy, or single moxibustion, or the acumoxatherapy in coordination of drugs, neither needling therapy nor moxibustion would be the choice separately and accordingly in the different stages of the disease.

2. Palpation of meridians

Dr. Xi thinks that there is a close relationship between meridians, acupoints and treatment by differentiation of syndromes. Therefore, it is necessary to have inspection by the way of palpation on the body surface. For instance, in the treatment of zang-fu disease it is important to detect the sensitive and painful spots on the corresponding Back-shu points, Front-mu points and Huatuojiaji points, and also to notice painful spots and other abnormal manifestations on the corresponding Yuan-Source, Xi-Cleft and Luo-Connecting points on the four limbs. Just as the following expression in *Miraculous Pivot*, that says that if it needs to know acupoints, they are just where the pain can be relieved by pressure. When five zang organs are diseased, the manifestations would appear on the twelve Yuan-Source points which are related to their respective internal organs, therefore the manifestations can be used as reference for estimating the conditions of five zang organs. These painful and sensitive spots, subcutaneous nodes, tuberosity and depression of soft tissues, and other abnormal manifestations found in palpation can be used as reference for diagnosis and also used as basic for acupoint selection. For example, in the treatment of diseases in five zang organs, Huatuojiaji points can be chosen when painful spots are detected on them, or the Back-shu points can be used if pain appears on them by palpation.

3. Back-shu points and acupoints of Ren and Du Meridians

In the treatment of zang-fu diseases and miscellaneous conditions, Dr. Xi often prefers to use the Front-mu points of the Ren Meridian in coordination with the corresponding Back-shu points and acupoints of the Du Meridian. For instance, he chooses Dazhui (Du 14), Shenzhu (Du 12), Shendao (Du 11), Zhiyang (Du 9), Feishu (B 13), Jueyinshu (B 14), Xinshu (B 15), Tanzhong (Ren 17), Jiuwei (Ren 15) primarily for the diseases in the Upper Jiao; and he uses Zhiyang (Du 9), Jinsuo (Du 8), Jizhong (Du 6), Geshu (B 17), Ganshu (B 18), Pishu (B 20), Zhongwan (Ren 12) and Xiawan (Ren 10) mainly for the diseases in the Middle Jiao; and Mingmen (Du 4), Yaoyangguan (Du 3), Shenshu (B 23), Dachangshu (B 25), Xiaochangshu (B 27), Pangguangshu (B 28), Qihai (Ren 6), Guanyuan (Ren 4) and Zhongji (Ren 3) in prominence for the diseases in the Lower Jiao. In acute conditions the corresponding Huatuojiaji (Extra) points would be added, and in deficient conditions Gaohuang (B 43) and Zhishi (B 25) would be done with the toning technique. Dr. Xi thinks that the extraordinary meridians have the composing and governing function for the whole meridian system, and among the eight extra meridians, the Ren and Du Meridians are the main part and their acupoints are very extensive in the indications. The combination of points from the Ren and Du Meridians together with the Back-shu points where the qi of the zang-fu organs flows into, and the Front-mu points where qi accumulates in chest and abdomen, can not only regulate the functions of organs but also treat diseases of the five sense organs which are respectively related to zang-fu organs. Clinically special and surprising therapeutic effectiveness often can be obtained.

4. Bleeding collaterals in relieving blood stagnation

Dr. Xi prefers this bleeding technique. He thinks that all the obstructions in meridians, local swelling, congestion, heat and painful symptoms must be treated with bleeding techniques and afterwards with cupping therapy according to the therapeutic principle of reducing excess and removing the accumulated pathogens. For example, in the treatment of acute eryspelas, the therapeutic result is very significant when the bleeding technique with a three-edge needle and cupping therapy are applied, for expelling heat, diminishing swelling and relieving pain. Also in rheumatoid arthritis, local swelling and pain will subside rapidly if the bleeding technique and cupping are applied on swollen joints. In the treatment of finger rigidity, it is able to promote movement of fingers if Sifeng (Extra) is punctured with a three-edge needle to squeeze out fluid. Dr. Xi says that the bleeding technique and the squeezing method are able to activate blood and disperse stagnation, and able to treat local inflammation.

II. Case Analysis

Case 1: Mumps (acute parotitis)

Name, Xu x x; sex, female; age, 18; occupation, student.

Complaints The patient had pain and swelling on the left auricular base for two days, accompanied with fever (T 38.5°C). The patient had been treated by Western medications without any effect. Therefore, acupuncture treatment was tried. The patient was found out to be ill with obvious congestion and swelling on the left auricular base, together with tenderness, enlargement of the lymph nodes on the lower jaw, and superficial rapid pulse and thin white tongue coating. It was differentiated as upward disturbance of wind and heat. It was treated to expel wind and clarify heat.

Prescription Jiaosun (SJ 20) (left), Yifeng (SJ 17), Quchi (LI 11).

Treatment procedure Ignite a match and blow it out, and then swiftly touch and leave Jiaosun (SJ 20); and afterwards puncture Yifeng (SJ 17) (needle tip towards the affected area) and Quchi (LI 11) with reducing method by slow and rapid manipulation, and retain needles for twenty minutes, during which the needles are remanipulated every ten minutes. On the next visit, fever disappeared and local distending pain also decreased. Yifeng (SJ 17) and Jiache (S 6) (penetrated towards Daying (S 5)) were selected to consolidate the therapeutic effect. The disease was cured after three treatments.

Explanation Direct moxibustion with a matchstick evolved from folk "oil-lamp moxibustion." It is simple to use and rapid in effectiveness. It is able to clarify heat and diminish swelling in acute inflammations.

Case 2: Erysipelas

Name, Fan x x; sex, male; age, 45; occupation, teacher; date of the first visit, May 6, 1979.

Complaints The patient had erysipelas on the left leg for five years, with two to three recurrences every year. Previously, the patient was only treated with antibiotics. On the first visit, the inner side of the left calf was found to have obvious congestion, swelling, heat and pain, accompanied with fever, aversion to cold, 38.5°C body temperature, poor appetite, yellow-thin tongue coating, string-taut, rapid pulse, 14,000/mm^3 WBC and 84 percent neutrophil. It was differentiated as the accumulation of heat toxin in the muscle and skin. It was treated with the principle of clarifying heat, relieving toxin, dissolving dampness and cooling blood.

Prescription Diji (Sp 8), Xuehai (Sp 10), Sanyinjiao (Sp 6), Fenglong (S 40), Taichong (Liv 3) (all punctured on the left side).

Treatment procedure The reducing method was done with twisting, rotating, lifting and thrusting manipulations, as well as swift and slow manipulations. The needles were retained for twenty minutes and were remanipulated once in between. Then the bleeding technique was done with a three-edged needle on the local congested area and afterwards the cupping therapy was used. The treatment was given once every day. After three treatments, congestion and swelling on the left leg decreased obviously and body temperature became 37.1°C, WBC reduced to 9,100/mm^3 and neutrophil, to 74 percent. Then Diji (Sp 8), Xuehai (Sp 10), Zusanli (S 36) and Shangqiu (Sp 5) were punctured instead. After five treatments, congestion, swelling and pain on the affected leg nearly disappeared, the body temperature remained normal, WBC became 7,500/mm^3 and neutrophil, 68 percent. For further treatment, Yinlingquan (Sp 9), Zusanli (S 36) and Sanyinjiao (Sp 6) (all on the affected side) were punctured with even manipulation and the needles were retained for twenty minutes. Later the treatment was given twice every week, and after one month the treatment was given once a week, and three months later the treatment was given once every two weeks to consolidate the therapeutic effect. There was no recurrence in follow-up visit one year later.

Explanation Erysipelas tends to occur on the lower leg as well as the face and head, with a high recurrence. Since 1979, twenty cases of acute erysipelas were treated by acupuncture with good results. According to the principles of reducing the excess and removing the accumulated pathogens, the main acupoints were chosen from the Spleen Meridian of Foot-Taiyin and assisted by the acupoints from the Stomach Meridian of Foot-Yangming. Acupoints from the Liver Meridian of Foot-Jueyin must be added in case of blood heat to enhance the functions of cooling blood and clarifying heat. And acupoints of the Large Intestine Meridian of Hand-Yangming should be added for the disease on the head and face. By clinical observation, acupuncture treatment is able to control inflammation and to relieve symptoms and signs rapidly in the acute period of erysipelas, and able to restore the blood condition to a normal level gradually in two or three days.

Case 3: Jaundice (acute infectious hepatitis)

Name, Ji x x; sex, male; age, 32; occupation, worker; date of the first visit, September 4, 1961.

Complaints The patient had lassitude, nausea, anorexia, pain in the liver area and black tea coloured urine for one week. His sleeping and bowel movement were all right, and he had been in contact with people who had hepatitis. Examination showed that there was a slight yellow colour in sclera and skin, heart and lung (-), soft and flat abdomen, soft liver 3 cm below the rib with tenderness and percussive pain, unpalpable spleen below the rib, thin and yellow tongue coating, string-taut and slightly rapid pulse. Blood test showed that SGPT was 320u, bilirubin was 4.2 mg, TTT was <8, and ZnTT was <12. It was differentiated as dampness and heat in liver and gallbladder. It was suitable to be treated with the principle of clarifying heat and promoting liver and gallbladder.

Prescription Dazhui (Du 14), Zhiyang (Du 9), Ganshu (B 18), Pishu (B 20), Danshu (B 19).

Treatment procedure Do one treatment per day with the reducing method by the slow and swift manipulation, and by inserting the needle against the direction of the meridian, and to give 30 grams of Artemisia Capillaris orally per day additionally. The clinical manifestations decreased after seven days. SGPT reduced to 116u, bilirubin was 2.2 mg. Zusanli (S 36) and Yanglingquan (G 34) were added with the above method in the second course of treatments. Acupuncture treatment was given once every other day. After twelve continuous treatments, SGPT decreased to less than 40u, bilirubin was 0.8 mg. Symptoms were relieved mostly and the patient was discharged from the hospital with recovery after consolidation.

Explanation In traditional Chinese medicine, acute infectious hepatitis is classified into the category of acute jaundice and intercostal pain. The problem is caused by accumulation of dampness and heat, therefore it is necessary to clarify heat and promote the liver and gallbladder emphatically. Previously a hundred cases of acute infectious hepatitis were treated with acupuncture, and among those forty-eight cases recovered, forty-five cases improved and seven cases failed. The results were satisfactory.

Case 4: pulmonary tuberculosis

Name, Zhang x x; sex, male; age, 47; date of the first visit, February of 1959.

Complaints In a physical examination in 1956, the patient was found to have infiltrating pulmonary tuberculosis on the right lung, pulmonary cavity, hemoptysis, cough and chest pain. There was no obvious improvement with two-year chemotherapy. Afterwards acupuncture treatment was added. Isoniazid as well as P.A.S. were still prescribed because of sputum culture being (+).

Prescription First group: Feishu (B 13), Gaohuang (B 43). Second group: Geshu (B 17), Danshu (B 19). Third group: Dazhui (Du 14), Shenzhu (Du 12). The above three groups of acupoints were used alternately with moxibustion (three to five wheat-grain cones), two treatments were given per week.

Treatment procedure With forty-nine treatments, tomography showed that pulmonary cavity disappeared, pulmonary focus calcified. The spontaneous symptoms disappeared. And (-) appeared in several sputum cultures.

Case 5: Bi syndrome (rheumatoid arthritis)

Name, Zhu x x; sex, female; age, 34; occupation, medical worker; date of the first visit, January 16, 1985.

Complaints For four years, the patient had a symmetric pain in the joints of the limbs, especially worse in shoulders and knees with motor impairment. Pain increased with cold. Joints became obviously stiff and painful on getting-up. DXM had been used since six months after the onset of the disease. In clinic, it was found out that there was swelling and distension in both knees, obvious tenderness in shoulders, motor impairment, slight swelling and a distending pain in the wrist, ankle and finger joints, thin and white tongue coating, soft pulse. Blood test showed that rheumatoid factor was positive, ESR was 26 mm/hour, mucin was 6.2 mg, IgG was 1,200 mg% and IgM, 180 mg%. It was differentiated as the bi syndrome of cold and dampness.

Prescription 1) Holistic treatment: Dazhui (Du 14), Shenzhu (Du 12), Shendao (Du 11), Zhiyang (Du 9), Jinsuo (Du 8), Pishu (B 20), Shenshu (B 23), Xiaochangshu (B 27), Weizhong (B 40), Yanglingquan (G 34), Zusanli (S 36), Taixi (K 3), Tianzong (SI 11), Zhibian (B 54). These acupoints were done with the toning method by shallow insertion and a slight twist. Tianzong (SI 11) was done with Hegu Puncture, making the needling sensation radiate to the shoulders. Zhibian (B 54) was done with Shu-Point Puncture, making the needling sensation go to the lower limbs. 2) Local treatment: The bleeding technique was used on swelling and distension of the wrist, ankle and knee joints and on stagnation of collaterals, afterwards the cupping therapy followed. For motor impairment of finger joints, a three-edge needle was used on Sifeng (Extra) to squeeze out yellow fluid. 3) Auricular therapy: In every treatment, two to three auricular points corresponding to the painful area were detected to look for tenderness and then afterwards Semen Vaccariae were stuck on these points with plaster to fix them. 4) Seven-star needle technique and cupping therapy: A seven-star needle was used to tap slightly along both sides of the Du Meridian till bleeding, and then the cupping therapy was added.

Treatment procedure The treatments were given twice per week, ten treatments as one course. The treatments were suspended for two weeks between the courses. The symptoms improved obviously after one course of treatments and dexamethasone decreased to half a tablet per day. Examination after a two-week rest showed that the rheumatoid factor became negative, ESR was 27 mm/hour, mucin was 5.0 mg. After a further two courses of treatments all the hormones stopped, and most joint pain disappeared except slight soreness in shoulders and in the knees on walking. Blood tests showed that the rheumatoid factor was negative, ESR was 18 mg/hour, mucin was 2.5 mg%, IgG was 1,250 mg%, IgA was 130 mg% and IgM, 100 mg%. One year later, the condition was stable and blood showed normal level.

Explanation Since November of 1984, fifty cases of rheumatoid arthritis had been treated, in which the disease was classified into two types of damp heat and cold damp. Acupoints and techniques were chosen emphatically to support body resistance by holistic treatment, and results were satisfactory. Among fifty cases, fifteen cases improved obviously, thirty-one cases were effective, four cases failed. The total effective rate was 92 percent. It had been observed clinically that with acupuncture treatments, thirteen cases in which symptoms were only controlled by hormone drugs stopped medication and symptoms were basically stable. It indicated that acupuncture has the prominent regulation to immunological system. Local Collateral Puncture, cupping therapy and fluid-squeezing technique are able to activate blood and remove stagnation and able to improve local inflammation.

Case 6: Edema (Chronic nephritis)

Name, Zhu x x; sex, male; age, 45; occupation, technician; date of the first visit, January 8, 1981.

Complaints The patient presented with lumbar pain and edema in lower limbs for three years, and the patient was hospitalized with the diagnosis of acute nephritis complicated by common cold, fever, sore throat, slightly edema in limbs, protein (++++) and RBC (+++) in urine test in April of 1978. By the application of prednisone and cyclophosphamide for two months, and of indomethacin for three months, the condition did not improve. When Chinese herbal medicine was added in treatment, the improvement of symptoms and signs was not obvious too. Acupuncture treatment was sought. Symptoms were lumbar soreness, lassitude, distension and numbness in the lower limbs, accompanied with slight edema, 134/96 mmHg of blood pressure, urinary protein (+++) with granular casts, RBC (++). The total volume of urinary protein in twenty-four hours was 2.92 g. Tongue body was slightly red in colour with tooth prints on the margin, tongue coating was thin and white, pulse showed thready quality. It was differentiated as yang deficiency in both spleen and kidney. Therapy is to support and tone the liver, spleen and kidney principally, with the combination of acupoints from the Du Meridian and the Ren Meridian for regulating yin and yang.

Prescription 1) Ganshu (B 18), Pishu (B 20), Shenshu (B 23), Zhishi (B 52), Feiyang (B 58), Fuliu (K 7). 2) Shufu (K 27), Tanzhong (Ren 17), Bulang (K 22), Jiuwei (Ren 15), Qihai (Ren 6), Sanyinjiao (Sp 6), Taixi (K 3).

Treatment procedure Ganshu (B 18), Pishu (B 20), Zhishi (B 52), Shufu (K 27), Tanzhong (Ren 17), Bulang (K 22) and Jiuwei (Ren 15) were punctured superficially with slight toning. All the others were inserted by even manipulation. The two groups of acupoints were used alternately with two treatments per week and thirty minutes of needle retention. Additional moxibustion was done on Dazhui (Du 14), Mingmen (Du 4) and Guanyuan (Ren 4) alternately (wheat-grain moxa cones, once per week, three cones every time). After one-year treatments, symptoms decreased and blood pressure was reduced to a normal level with protein (+-++) and RBC 0-5. After one and a half years of treatment, the total volume of urinary protein in twenty-four hours decreased to 0.54 g. And renal functions were restored to normal. Urinary protein was between 1 to 10. Afterwards the treatments were reduced to once a week for consolidation of the results.

Explanation Chronic nephritis mostly belongs to the deficient syndromes and is classified as yin deficiency and yang deficiency. Clinically most cases attribute to yang deficiency. In the treatments, it is used accordingly the techniques of Quintuple Puncture introduced in *Internal Classic* and of Shallow Puncture in *Classic on Medical Problems* and of slight toning and superficial insertion. Prominently, acupoints from the Kidney, Liver and Spleen Meridians, as well as the Back-shu points are chosen with the combination of Tanzhong (Ren 17) and Qihai (Ren 6) in the Ren Meridian for supporting body resistance and expelling pathogenic factors. Only when the kidney essence is able to be supported and kept, can the condition be cured.

FOUR NEEDLING METHODS AND EYE DISORDER DIFFERENTIATION

—Huang Shengyuan's Clinical Experience

Huang Shengyuan was born in Jianwei County, Sichuan Province, in 1913. He was a student in 1938 at the Specialized Acupuncture Training Course run by Rao Tianming, a renowned acupuncturist then in the city of Chengdu. Having accomplished his study there, he started his own acupuncture practice at Guangming Lane, Chengdu. In 1951, he received further training at the Acupuncture Seminar sponsored by the Chengdu Public Health Society. He was the director of the United Clinic in the Western District of Chengdu in April, 1956. In the same year, he became a faculty member at the Sichuan Medical College (present-day Western China University of Medicine).

Dr. Huang has concentrated on needling techniques and eye problems. He summed up a set of four needling methods based on yin-yang, reinforcing and reducing. Because of his studies of these methods and his success in such studies, he won the third class award for achievement in medical science and technology of Sichuan Province (1984), and the fourth class award for great achievement in science and technology approved by the Sichuan Provincial Government (1985).

Dr. Huang is very experienced in treating patients for eye disorders. Such experience over his decades of acupuncture practice has been implemented in the HSY-86 Computer-aided Niagnotherapeutic Programme for Treating Eye Disorders. The system was awarded the third class award for the best achievement in technological research in medicine in Sichuan Province (1986). He has published a number of academic papers. Now, he is an associate professor at the Western China University of Medicine, and the board member and advisor of the Sichuan Acupuncture Society.

I. Academic Characteristics and Medical Specialities

1. Reinforcing and Reducing and the Theory of Yin-yang

The quintessence of acupuncture manipulation, according to Dr. Huang, fuses chiefly in the changes in motion, quietness, gentleness and heaviness. Gentleness and heaviness express the degree of motion and stasis; while motion and quietness stand for the two extremes of gentleness and heaviness. *The Illustrated Supplementary to the Classified Canon* states, "Motion pertains to yang, while quietness pertains to yin. Motion gives rise to yang, while quietness gives rise to yin. Motion produces yang at its beginning, yet yin at its extreme. On the other hand, quietness produces gentleness at its beginning, heaviness at its extreme." Therefore, he advanced that: 1) A small amplitude of lifting, thrusting and rotating with a gentle manipulation, known as the vibrating needling retention, manifests yang activating at the beginning of motion. Such a yang reinforcing method is applicable to yang deficiency syndrome; 2) A frequent lifting, thrusting and rotating of needle in a big amplitude, known as sparrow-pecking needling retention, manifests yin activating at the extreme of motion. Such a yang reducing method is applicable to hyperactive yang syndrome; 3) A moderate needling manipulation between the above two, known as intermittent needling retention, which strengthens yin and reduces the hyperactive yang, is applicable to the excess yin syndrome; and 4) A gentle stimulation with the retained needles, known as static needling retention, manifests gentleness producing at the beginning of quietness. Such a yin nourishing method is applicable to yin deficiency syndrome.

The operation of these four acupuncture methods, all with 1.0 to 1.5-inch needles, is described as follows:

1) *The sparrow-pecking needling retention* After the needle is inserted at a certain depth to gain the arrival of qi, withdraw the inserted part of the needle by 2/3. This is then followed by a frequent lifting, thrusting of the needle as if a sparrow is pecking the grain. Each time, the needle is lifted and thrust seven times before a transient stop, which is repeated for three turns before withdrawal of the needle. The needling manipulation here needs to be handled appropriately regarding the patient's constitution because such a stimulation is relatively strong.

2) *The intermittent needling retention* After the needle is inserted at a certain depth to gain the arrival of qi, retain it for three minutes before the inserted part of the needle is withdrawn by 1/2. Each time, the needle is lifted, thrust and rotate for nine minutes before a transient stop for three minutes. This is then followed by repeating the above manipulation, until the patient nearly sweats or has slight sweating. In general, the needles are taken out when three complete manipulating processes are finished.

3) *The vibrating needling retention* After the needle is inserted at a certain depth to gain the arrival of qi, retain it for one minute and withdraw the inserted part of the needle by 1/3. This is then followed by a gentle lifting, thrusting and rotating with a slight vibration of the needle nine times. Repeat the above manipulation between every three or five minutes for three complete turns before withdrawal of the needle.

4) *The static needling retention* After the needle is inserted to gain the arrival of qi, retain it for thirty minutes before withdrawal.

Since these four needling methods embody the combination of motion and quietness, as well as gentleness and heaviness, they are appropriate for the changing mechanism and etiology of the various syndromes. Especially for some difficult and severe conditions with excess and deficiency factors, different reinforcing or reducing methods can be used according to the actual condition of yin-yang, excess or deficiency of a patient.

Infantile hydrocephalus, for example, is the consequence of upward invasion of pathogenic damp and fluid into the cranial cavity due to deficiency of the spleen and kidney. In the acute stage, Fengchi (G 20), Renzhong (Du 26) and Zhigou (SJ 6) are needled with the sparrow-pecking method to drain the cranial water and reduce the cranial distension, whereas Hegu (LI 4), Zusanli (S 36), Sanyinjiao (Sp 6), Xuanzhong (G 39) and Fuliu (K 7) are needled with either the vibrating or static retention method to reinforce spleen and kidney. However, the static retention method is more often used for patients with chronic ailments or poor constitution in order to reinforce both yin and yang, strengthen spleen and kidney, and remove damp and fluid.

Dr. Huang values highly the application of the static needling retention—a reinforcing approach characterized by gentle manipulation and static retention of needles. This method is exactly the same as what *Miraculous Pivot* states, i.e. "Insert the needle slowly and gently with longer time for needling retention. The antipathogenic factor is thus reinforced while the pathogenic factor is dispelled. The withdrawal of the needle in this manner serves to reinforce the body energy." *Miraculous Pivot* also states that the static needling retention not only reinforces the deficient qi and builds up the antipathogenic factor, but also regulates either cold or heat conditions in the body. In fact, the static needling retention directs qi in an orderly circulation, preserves the vital energy, nourishes yin and reduces hyperactive yang. The reducing effect is also accomplished by a predominant reinforcing process.

The static needling retention is extensively used in the clinic. Infantile acute poliomylitis or its sequela, for example, is often treated by using such a method. Due to the fact that poliomylitis is a deficiency syndrome mixed with some excessive factors, static needling retention is applied for ten to twenty minutes during treatment. Dr. Huang has treated 144 cases of poliomylitis with 96 percent effectiveness being achieved.

The static needling retention can be used to treat optic nerve disorders caused by deficiency of kidney, liver, spleen, stomach and gallbladder, or due to deficiency of qi and blood, or due to deficiency of both yin and yang. However, there are some exceptions. For instance, in a small number of acute inflammations of the eye, the sparrow-pecking needling method is used for dispersing heat; and the intermittent needling retention is used for dispelling cold and strengthening yang in the case of the eye disorder involving pathogenic cold. Dr. Huang pointed out many times that static needling retention will work if the doctor intends to reinforce yin, or both yin and yang, or to obtain the reducing effect in the overall reinforcing.

2. Eye Disorder Differentiation

Eye disorder differentiation mainly includes the following four aspects:

1) *Differentiation based on meridians and collaterals* This is to make the differentiation, determine the needling method and select points for treatment according to the meridians and collaterals distributed in the eye region, and the etiology associated with the eye disorders. Specifically, the three yang meridians of the Foot, Yinqiao and Yangqiao Meridians merge at the inner canthus. A branch of the Small Intestine Meridian also distributes in the inner canthus. In the outer canthus, there distributes the Sanjiao, Gallbladder and Small Intestine Meridians. In the superior eye region, there are the distributions of Shaoyang Meridians of Foot and Hand, Yangming and Yangwei Meridians. In the inferior eye region, there are distributions of the Ren and Yangqiao Meridians. The Stomach Meridian starts from the inferior orbit. The Liver and Heart Meridians connect with the eye. The eyeball connects with the brain through the eye system. The brain is situated in the head which is the merging place of all yang meridians. The Bladder and Gallbladder Meridians communicate with the Du Meridian and connect with the brain. According to such meridian connections in the eye region and the etiology of the eye disorders, points can be selected for treatment on the basis of the meridian

differentiation.

Cortical blindness, for example, is mostly encountered in general disease such as high fever with convulsions, in which the blindness is due to the impairment of qi and blood, and stagnation of yang qi. The brain is primarily infected. So, the treatment principle is to activate the circulation of yang qi and brighten the eye by needling points mainly from the Liver, Large Intestine and Stomach Meridians.

A 4-month-old boy was blind for fifty-six days due to repeated high fever with convulsions. He was diagnosed as having cortical blindness and meningitis due to bacteri colli in a Western medicine hospital. According to the above principle of meridian differentiation, Tongziliao (G 1), Zanzhu (B 2), Fengchi (G 20), Dazhui (Du 14), Waiguan (SJ 5), Hegu (LI 4), Zusanli (S 36), Guangming (G 37) and Taichong (Liv 3) were needled with mild stimulation. When five treatments were finished, the little boy regained his vision, which was quite normal after twenty treatments within twenty-three days. Follow-up visit one year later showed normal vision.

Another 19-year-old boy had double vision in his left eye and non-abducted eyeballs for seventeen years. The Western medicine diagnosis was the paralysis of nervus abducens. According to traditional Chinese medicine, his non-abducted eyeballs were due to qi of the Shaoyang Meridians which was too weak to make the eyeballs abduct. The treatment principle was to reinforce qi of the Shaoyang Meridians. Left side Tongziliao (G 1), Fengchi (G 20), Sizhukong (SJ 23) and bilateral Waiguan (SJ 5), Zhongzhu (SJ 3) and Hegu (LI 4) were needled with the vibrating retention method. His eye recovered after eighty treatments.

2) *Differentiation based on zang-fu theory* All of the zang-fu organs have close relations with the eye. The inner eye can be observed according to the zang-fu theory, as well as the interacting relations of the five elements. Specifically, choroid belongs to the heart; sclera, cilliary body, retina and optic nerve belong to the liver; yellow spot belongs to the spleen, yet is closely related to the liver. Acqueous humour belongs to the gallbladder. The crystalline lens belong to the kidney, and the vitreous body belongs to the lung. In treating the inner eye and optic nerve disorders, differentiation and treatment are often made on the basis of the interrelationship of the five elements and the specific zang or fu organ to which a given part of the inner eye pertains.

a. For eyeground disorders, the treatment principle is to reinforce the liver and kidney. The stomach is the sea for digesting food, while the spleen and stomach jointly form the source for producing the acquired qi and blood. Only when the spleen and stomach are duely reinforced, can the five zang and six fu organs be supplied with enough energy to nourish the eye, keeping a normal vision. Therefore, consideration is also given to the spleen, stomach, gallbladder and bladder, for these organs are the outer organs to the liver and kidney. Here are two examples:

A 24-year-old student had blurring of vision in both eyes for two years. The ophthamological examination showed that his vision was 0.4 (left) and 0.5 (right). He had redness with dark spots in the central field of vision, accompanied by pterygium in the right eye. The eyeground on either side appeared normal. The Western medicine diagnosis was bilateral retrobular neuritis, and genine pterygium (right). The diagnosis in TCM was deficiency of liver and kidney, and heat retention in the large intestine.

Quchi (LI 11), Hegu (LI 4), Fuliu (K 7), Xiaxi (G 43), Zhaohai (K 6), Sanyinjiao (Sp 6) were needled with static retention method. When fourteen treatments were finished, the clinical symptoms and signs disappeared. The pterygium in the right eye was diminished, and the vision improved respectively to 1.0 and 1.2. The dark spot in the central field of vision also disappeared without any abnormal change in the eyeground.

Madam Yang, aged fifty-six, saw red as white for more than half a year. The accompanying symptoms included lumbar soreness, blurring of vision, weak "chi" pulse, and string-taut "cun" and "guan" pulse. Ophthamological examination showed no pathological change in her eyeground, nor in the external eye. The diagnosis was colour amblyopia. According to TCM differentiation, the condition was due to hyperactivity of lung qi and deficiency of heart qi, viz, the metal counteracted on the fire. Hegu (LI 4), Lieque (L 7), Zhaohai (K 6) were needled with the static retention method to reinforce the kidney, regulate the lung and activate the yang qi circulation in the meridians and collaterals. She recovered within ten treatments.

b. Cataract affects the crystalline lens, which results from poor eye metabolism due to deficiency of the kidney and stomach, and poor nourishment of the liver and gallbladder. So, the treatment principle is to reinforce the kidney and stomach, and to regulate the function of the liver and gallbladder. For example, Mr. Du, aged sixty-four, had blurring of vision in both eyes for half a year. His vision was 0.2+1 (right) and 0.3+2 (left) with phacosclerosis in both eyes. The Western medicine diagnosis was senile cataract. He had loose stool ever since he got the cataract. The pulse was thready and soft. According to the above treatment principle, Zanzhu (B 2), Fengchi (G 20), Hegu (LI 4), Zusanli (S 36), Fuliu (K 7); and Tongziliao (G 1), Waiguan (SJ 5), Zusanli (S 36), Guangming (G 37), Taichong (Liv 3), Taixi (K 3) were applied alternately with the static retention method for thirty minutes. Beginning from the fourth treatment, nine moxa cones were added at Zusanli (S 36). His appetite increased after eight treatments, which was followed by an improved energy, and normal stool. His vision was improved respectively to 0.7 (right) and 0.8 (left). This was then followed by another twenty treatments when the treatment was finally stopped with the vision being improved to 1.0 on both sides.

3) *Differentiation based on the yin-yang theory* According to either hyperactive or hypoactive condition of yin-yang, points are selected to reinforce the deficiency and reduce the excess, and harmonize yin and yang, also in consideration of the functional activities of zang-fu organs. Here are two sample cases for comprehension:

Ametropia, according to TCM, is due to deficiency of yang qi and excess of yin qi. The treatment principle is to reinforce qi of the three yang meridians, particularly the Shaoyang Meridian. For example, Miss Xu, aged twenty, had blurring of vision for nine years. Her vision was only 0.1. According to the above treatment principle, Zanzhu (B 2), Hegu (LI 4), Fengchi (G 20), Tongziliao (G 1), Waiguan (SJ 5) and Guangming (G 37) were needled with vibrating retention method for thirty minutes. Her vision improved to 0.4 after twenty treatments. She was then given another seventy treatments on the basis of the above prescription plus Zusanli (S 36). Her vision was improved to 1.0 when the treatment was stopped. Follow-up two years later showed stable vision.

Thyrotoxic or pituitary exophthalmos causes a distending pain in the eye which is accompanied by dizziness, insomnia and irritability. The condition is primarily due to yin deficiency. The treatment principle is to reinforce yin and reduce hyperactive yang. For example, Mrs. Gao, aged thirty-four, had II thyroid enlargement, exophthalmos and distending pain accompanied by symptoms of thyroidism. The diagnosis was thyrotoxic exophthalmos. According to the above treatment principle, Zanzhu (B 2), Fengchi (G 20), Hegu (LI 4), Fuliu (K 7), Sanyinjiao (Sp 6), Taichong (Liv 3), Tongziliao (G 1), Neiguan (P 6), Ququan (Liv 8), Zusanli (S 36), Taixi (K 3) and Zhaohai (K 6) were needled with the static retention method. Altogether, 120 treatments were given to her before her complete recovery from the thyroid enlargement and exophthalmos.

4) *Differentiation according to the five zones and eight directions* Eye disorders here are analysed on the basis of the different eye zones related to the specific zang-fu organs. Points are thus selected from the respective meridians to deal with the eye disorders in combination with appropriate needling or moxibustion methods. The five zones are briefly described as follows:

The upper and lower eyelids, known as the muscle zone, belong to the spleen and stomach. The inner and outer canthuses, known as the blood zone, belong to the heart and small intestine. The white part of the eyeball, known as the qi zone, belongs to the lung and large intestine. The black part of the eyeball, known as the wind zone, belongs to the liver and gallbladder. And the pupil, known as the water zone, belongs to the kidney and bladder. Although the five zones pertain theoretically to different zang-fu organs, they are closely related to the kidney and bladder. In particular, the black part and pupil of the eye which are located in the center of the eye, coincide with the fact that most vision defects are related to ill-conditioned liver and kidney.

The eight directions constitute another major approach in observing eye disorders. Specifically, east belongs to the liver; southeast to the gallbladder; south to the heart and small intestine; southeast to the stomach; west to the lung and sanjiao; northwest to the large intestine; north to the kidney and bladder; and northeast to the pericardium. Differentiation is thus made to find out the specific meridians involved in the eye disorders according to their pathological changes.

There was one patient who had blurring of vision in the inferior 1/3 of the both eyes at noon or from 5-9 p.m. every day for half a year. Various examinations excluded any intracranial organic changes. The ophthalmological diagnosis was optic nerve neurosis. Approaching from the eight directions, the inferior portion of the eye pertains to the kidney and bladder. On either side of this portion, the eye is connected with the large intestine and pericardium. Noon is the heart time, which is replacable by pericardium time, while 5-9 p.m. belongs to the time range of the kidney and pericardium. The liver has its opening into the eye. Both the liver and pericardium pertain to the Jueyin Meridian. The large intestine belongs to metal, while the bladder and kidney belong to water. Therefore, such an optic nerve neurosis is actually an impairment of yin affecting the yang, and imbalance of the qi mechanism due to water failing to nourish wood. The principle of treatment was to reinforce the large intestine, kidney, pericardium, and regulate the liver and gallbladder. Chengqi (S 1), Fengchi (G 20), Hegu (LI 4), Fuliu (K 7), Sanyinjiao (Sp 6), Taichong (Liv 3), Tongziliao (G 1), Neiguan (P 6), Ququan (Liv 8), Taixi (K 3) and Zhaohai (K 6) were needled with the static retention method for thirty minutes. The patient's vision became normal after nineteen treatments.

The above-mentioned summarizes the main part of Dr. Huang's experience in syndrome differentiation in regard to eye disorders. The meridian and zang-fu differentiations are to determine the affected part of the eye and to select the possible points. Yin-yang differentiation is to determine the nature of the disease so as to work out the prescription and needling methods. Differentiation according to the five zones and eight directions embodies the application of the zang-fu theory and that of the five elements in TCM ophthalmology.

II. Case Analysis

Case 1: Cortical blindness

Name, Yang x x; sex, female; age, 7; date of the first visit, April 16, 1978

Complaints Nine days before, the patient caught epidemic encephalitis, accompanied by high fever and convulsions. She had been in a coma for eight days. After being treated, she regained her consciousness, but became blind. She had poor energy, and thin white coating. Ophthalmological examination showed that her pupils were the same size, approximately 3 mm, with contralateral reflexes though her eyegrounds remained normal. The diagnosis was cortical blindness due to collapse of yang and consumption of qi and yin. The treatment principle was to strengthen yang qi and brighten the eyes.

Prescription A Zanzhu (B 2), Tongziliao (G 1), Fengchi (G 20), Hegu (LI 4), Waiguan (SJ 5), Zusanli (S 36).

Prescription B Baihui (Du 20), Dazhui (Du 14), Zhigou (SJ 6), Zhongzhu (SJ 3), Guangming (G 37) and Taichong (Liv 3).

Treatment procedure The treatment was given daily by using the two prescriptions of points alternately with retention of needles for twenty to thirty minutes. After three treatments, she could see again, and walk within one meter's distance by following her mother. She could count her fingers after thirteen treatments. When she was given sixteen treatments within eighteen days, she could quickly pick up small pieces of paper on the floor. Seven months later, her vision turned to 1.2 (right), and $1.0^{-0.3}$ (left).

Explanation Cortical blindness is mostly caused by high fever with convulsions in epidemic encephalitis, viral meningitis, bacterial meningitis, newly-born baby tetanus and the sequelae of congenital growth retardation. The affected part of the body primarily involves the brain. Following the above treatment principle, fifteen such cases were treated. The follow-up observation showed that, after one or two months of treatment, two were completely cured, nine were obviously improved, and four with some effect. Patients with one month duration of disease often had satisfactory effects. Therefore, an earlier acupuncture treatment will bring a better therapeutic effect.

Case 2: Sequelae of meningitis

Name, Yan x x; sex, male; age, 7; case No. 43755

Complaints Fourteen days before, the patient caught a high fever and was in a coma for half a day with intermittent convulsions. After being admitted into the emergency department, he was diagnosed as having meningitis caused by meningococci. He was treated with Western medicine for ten days, which helped him relieve the high fever and regain a clear mental state. The cerebrospinal fluid turned normal. But his facial expression appeared dull with indifferent vision. He could not chew, nor swallow food. When doctors from the acupuncture department were invited to make the consultation, the boy was pale with dull vision and poor energy, enlarged pupil and blind eyes, lying in bed with neck rigidity. Pathological reaction appeared positive. Food was supplied by nasal feeding.

Differentiation Blindness due to impairment of qi and blood after the febrile disease. The treatment principle was to regulate and reinforce yang qi, clear the mind, regain vision by strengthening qi and blood and nourishing the liver and kidney.

Prescription A Baihui (Du 20), Renzhong (Du 26), Yamen (Du 15), Dazhui (Du 14), Fengchi (G 20), Hegu (LI 4), Zusanli (S 36) and Taichong (Liv 3). These points were needled with the sparrow-pecking retention method for ten minutes.

Prescription B Bilateral Shenshu (B 23), Ganshu (B 18), Jingming (B 1), Waiguan (SJ 5), Zhongzhu (SJ 3), Zusanli (S 36), Guangming (G 37), Fuliu (K 7) and Taichong (Liv 3). These points were needled with the static retention method for twenty minutes.

Treatment procedure After prescription A was applied for two treatments, the rigid neck became released. The sparrow-pecking retention method was changed into the static retention method. Another four treatments were given, and the patient could eat by himself. Auditory function also improved. At that time, he could eat porridge, cake, and knew to refuse more by shaking his head when his stomach was full. He could also say, "mami." The remaining problems were blindness and listlessness. Therefore, prescription B was followed for six treatments. His vision, speech and energy of the four limbs all improved, especially the auditory function which already had become normal. His vision was then 0.4 on both sides. Prescription C was now followed for nine treatments when his vision was improved to 1.0. Speech, intelligence and movement all recovered considerably, thus the treatment was stopped. He was treated altogether thirty-three times within one and a half months. The follow-up visit seven years later at his school showed normal eyeground and 1.0 vision on both sides.

Explanation The sequela of meningitis in this case included the dullness, deaf, mute, blind eyes and paralysis. *Miraculous Pivot* states, "Disharmony of the five zang organs leads to the obstruction of the sense organs." Therefore, the treatment principle was to regain the normal function of the sense organs by strengthening yang qi, blood, and clearing the mind. This is because only when there is harmony among the zang-fu organs, qi and blood, can there be a normal function of eyes and ears, and a clear mental state. Dr. Huang has treated three such patients whose basic functions all recovered within one and a half to four months of treatment. Only one patient got mild hemiplegia of the left leg due to traumatic injury.

Case 3: Optic nerve atrophy

Name, Wang x x; sex, male; age, 19; case No. 98964

Complaints For one year or so, his vision declined. In recent months, the vision was even worse than before. The impaired vision was accompanied by aversion to light, therefore difficulty in walking and bumping into other people. He often felt lumbar pain radiating to the chest and back which was accompanied by dizziness, insomnia, urinating six to ten times at night and two dry bowel movements a day. His pulse was thready and rapid. Ophthalmological examination showed that the vision was 0.3 (right) and 0.4 (left). The papillate on both eyegrounds appeared wax-yellow, yet with clear margins. The bilateral peripherial vision was diminished toward the center of the eye by 20°- 40°. There was a peared 25° white dark center spot in the central field vision. The Western medicine diagnosis was bilateral optic nerve atrophy.

Prescription A Fengchi (G 20), Ganshu (B 18), Shenshu (B 23), Hegu (LI 4), Taiyuan (L 9), Feiyang (B 58), Taixi (K 3).

Prescription B Hegu (LI 4), Zusanli (S 36), Sanyinjiao (Sp 6), Fuliu (K 7), Taichong (Liv 3). Points in both groups were needled with the static retention method equally for thirty minutes.

Treatment procedure Prescription A was followed for eight treatments when the patient's vision improved to 0.8, and the papilla turned slightly red; and when the bilateral peripherial vision was basically recovered. The dark spot in the center of the eye was diminished to 10°. Meanwhile, dizziness, insomnia, night urination were obviously improved. Then, prescription B was also followed for eight treatments, when all the clinical symptoms and signs disappeared. The vision on both sides were improved to 1.2. Bilateral peripherial field vision became normal. The dark spots in the eyes merged away. The eyeground became normal. Follow-up visit three months later showed both the eyeground and vision normal.

Explanation This is an example of eyeground disorder. By applying the zang-fu differentiation, the treatment principle was to focus on differentiation of the liver and kidney. This was because kidney deficiency led to the lung deficiency. Prescription A regulates the kidney, liver and lung. In prescription B, Hegu (LI 4), Zusanli (S 36) and Sanyinjiao (Sp 6) strengthen both the spleen and stomach, the source for acquired energy. Fuliu (K 7) as a secondary point reinforces the kidney water, and Taichong (Liv 3) reinforces the liver. This is to let the liver blood go up to nourish the eyes. A good therapeutic effect was achieved even though points around the eye were not needled.

Case 4: Blindness

Name, Li x x; sex, female; age, 2.5; case No. 2435

Complaints Two days before, the patient had vomiting due to the injection of 11 ml of quinine, which was followed by a coma for twenty-four hours. She became blind when she recovered from the coma. Ophthalmological examination showed: both pupils in 9 mm diametre, disappeared contralateral reflex, pale retina on the eyeground, diminished vessels, yellow spot edema, and no abnormal muscular movement in the external eye. The differentiation was stagnation of qi due to impairment of the liver and kidney. The treatment principle was to reinforce the liver and kidney.

Prescription Fengchi (G 20), Zanzhu (B 2), Tongziliao (G 1), Quchi (LI 11), Hegu (LI 4), Fuliu (K 7), and Taichong (Liv 3). Needles at these points were retained for ten minutes. Then, Feishu (B 13), Ganshu (B 18), Shenshu (B 23) were pricked without retention. Huatuojiaji points were applied with plum-blossom needles.

Treatment procedure After seven treatments, both pupils diminished to 6 mm in diameter. The contralateral reflex in the pupil appeared again after ten treatments. The blood vessels in the eyeground grew bigger. The retina edema was improved. She could move her eyeballs to follow the doctor's examination. After sixteen treatments, she could pick up small needles within 1/3 of a meter's distance. The vision was recovered. Follow-up visits in the following eleven years showed normal vision.

Explanation In Western medicine, her blind eyes were diagnosed as due to quinine injection which poisoned her nerve ganlia cells, and caused the artery spasm of the retina. Angiectasis medicines can often in this case hopefully help the patient restore the central vision but leave permanent damage to the peripherial vision. By reinforcing the liver and kidney, and activating the circulation of qi and blood to restore the vision, Dr. Huang treated four such cases. These patients not only had their central vision recovered, but also the peripherial one.

Case 5: Deaf due to overdose of streptomycin

Name, Wu x x; age, four and a half months; sex, male; case No. 663582

Complaints More than twenty days before, due to an attack of bronchitis, the boy received overdose of streptomycin injection. Five days later, he lost his hearing in both ears. For these twenty days, he had poor appetite, listlessness, disturbed sleep at night, and urinated four to five times at night. Accompanying symptoms included a yellowish dark complexion, emaciated figure, dull expression, pale tongue proper, white sticky tongue coating, slightly purplish nail-fold and cold limbs. The differentiation was the stagnation of qi of the Shaoyang Meridians, deficiency of kidney qi. The treatment principle was to relieve pathogenic qi by regulating the function of the sanjiao, and reinforce the kidney qi to restore the auditory ability.

Prescription A Fengchi (G 20), Quchi (LI 11), Zhigou (SJ 6), Hegu (LI 4), Zusanli (S 36), Fuliu (K 7) and Taixi (K 3). These points were needled by a gentle insertion and rapid withdrawal, plus plum-blossom needle tapping on Huatuojiaji Points.

Prescription B Yifeng (SJ 17), Tinggong (SI 19), Zhigou (SJ 6), Zhongzhu (SJ 3), Xuanzhong (G 39) and Fuliu (K 7). These points were needled with the static retention method for thirty minutes.

Prescription C was formed on the basis of prescription B, plus Baihui (Du 20), Fengfu (Du 16), Yamen (Du 15) and herbal thread moxa at Sanyinjiao (Sp 6) and Guanyuan (Ren 4) equally for ninety times.

Treatment procedure . After prescription A and B were jointly applied for about two months, the boy's energy recovered. He could shout when he was excited, and could also hear the sound of a locking door. But still, it was difficult to call him directly. There was yet excessive urine at night nd cold limbs. Then, prescription C was used plus herbal thread moxa. Two days later, he could hear the radio sound, and turn his head towards the person who called him. His sleep was better. Following prescription C, another nine treatments were given. After the total sixty treatments within three months, he assumed a red complexion again, together with an active response and warm limbs. His auditory function turned normal. A follow-up visit in the following one and a half years showed a normal growth, good speech and intelligence.

Explanation This is a case of deafness resulting from stagnated qi in meridians and collaterals due to drug poisoning, in which kidney qi fails to nourish the ears. At first, the treatment principle was to regulate the function of the sanjiao, dispel poisoning and reinforce kidney essence. This was then followed by moxibustion to help ascend yang qi and achieve the cure.

Case 6: Infantile hydrocephalus

Name, Xie x x; age, one year old; sex, male; case No. 472189

Complaints The boy's head grew abnormally big when he was three months old. The accompanying symptoms and signs included a full fontanel, restlessness, poor sleep, fear, excessive sweating over the head, which was aggravated since last September, with retarded growth and movement. He had a dull expression and weak, emaciated legs. The head measurement was 50.7 cm (5 cm bigger than normal). There was a distended prominence (5 x 5 cm) at the fontanel, increased cranial creases, narrowed external ear cavity, and positive resonance like the sound of a pot breaking. The cerebral ultrasonic examination showed that the distance from either ventricular wave to the middle wave was 2 cm. X-ray showed an external cranial cavity. A CT scan showed that the third and fourth ventriculars were slightly expanded. But there was no sign of pressure on the ventriculars. The Western medicine diagnosis was communicating hydrocephalus. Differentiation in TCM was emptiness of the brain due to congenital deficiency. The treatment principle was to regulate the Ren and Du Meridians in function.

Prescription A Tounao (Extra), Renzhong (Du 26), Zhigou (SJ 6), Hegu (LI 4), Shuifen (Ren 9), Yinjiao (Ren 7), Shuidao (S 25), Zhongji (Ren 3), Zusanli (S 36) and Sanyinjiao (Sp 6).

Prescription B Fengfu (Du 16), Fengchi (G 20), Dazhui (Du 14), Mingmen (Du 4), Yaoshu (Du 2), Yinmen (B 39), Weizhong (B 40), Chengshan (B 57), Xuanzhong (G 39) and Fuliu (K 7).

Prescription C The plum-blossom needle tapping over Huatuojiaji Points to cause local redness. Treatment was given daily, with the plum-blossom needle tapping being applied first. Then, one group of points was applied with rapid insertion. The sparrow-pecking method was applied to Fengfu (Du 16), Fengchi (G 20) and Zusanli (S 36) without needle retention. In the treatments which were given later, needles at points on the four limbs were retained for thirty minutes.

Treatment procedure Following the above treatment principle, he was given a hundred treatments in a five-month period. The boy graudally became active, spoke a few words and walked by himself. The prominence in the fontanel diminished. Herbal thread moxibustion was then used for Shuifen (Ren 9) and Yinjiao (Ren 7) ninety times during treatment. One year later, his skeleton, intelligence and growth all appeared normal. The frontal fontanel was closed. Ultrasonic examination showed no obvious increasing of the ventricular waves. X-ray did not show any abnormal change in the skull except the expanded arteria meningea on the left side.

Explanation Over the last two decades, Dr. Huang has used acupuncture in treating nearly a hundred cases of infantile hydrocephalus in collaboration with neurosurgens at the teaching hospital of the Western China University of Medicine. About 84 percent cases turned out effective. Most of these patients now have normal intelligence growth. However, Dr. Huang's experience also proved that the prognosis for obstructive hydrocephalus is far from promising. Therefore, it is not recommended for acupuncture treatment.

CONCISE SELECTION OF ACUPOINTS AND SEEKING QI ARRIVAL BY MANIPULATING THE NEEDLES

—Huang Xianming's Clinical Experience

Huang Xianming, a native of Wuxi, Jiangsu Province, was born in October of 1920. He studied in the Shanghai College of Traditional Chinese Medicine in the 1930s, and then he apprenticed to Bao Shisheng to study internal medicine. Early in the 1950s, he was the director of Acupuncture Department in the First Public Hospital of Traditional Chinese Medicine in Shanghai (the eleventh People's Hospital of Shanghai Municipality), and the director of the Acupuncture Department of the Shanghai First People's Hospital. Dr. Huang is good at treating gastric ulcer, duodenal ulcer and diabetic bladder diseases. Early in 1985, in cooperation with the Western medical doctors, he performed a tonsillectomy with his experience of acupuncture analgesia instead of drug anaesthesia, and initiated the induction of manipulating needles before an operation, which was successfully applied in subtotal thyroidectomy and ophthalmic operations. He tested the diagnosis and the treatment of ear acupuncture. In the 1970s, he manufactured a glass model of meridians and points with a field magnetic light which won a second prize of the scientific achievement awarded by the Ministry of Light. His works include *Essential of Chinese Acupuncture, Chinese Acupuncture and Moxibustion, Hanging Chart of Anatomy of Points of 14 Meridians, Tomographic Anatomic Illustrations of Points*, etc. Now he is a professor in the Shanghai College of Traditional Chinese Medicine, the director of the Shanghai International Acupuncture Training Center, a committee member of the Acupuncture and Moxibustion Speciality in Medical Scientific Commission of the Ministry of Public Health, and a member of the standing committee of the China Association of Acupuncture and Moxibustion.

I. Academic Characteristics and Medical Specialities

1. Combination of the points according to the treating principle

Huang thinks that without the correct differentiation of cold, heat, deficiency and excess, the treating principles for warming, cooling, reinforcing and reducing cannot be properly selected. Selection of points should be based on the treating principles, especially when a disease is complicated. He held that the etiology should be carefully analyzed and one or two points are selected as the main points according to the main causative factors of the disease. For example, dizziness and vertigo caused by deficiency of liver and kidney should be treated by needling Fuliu (K 7) or Ququan (Liv 8) in accordance with the principle of reinforcing the mother in case of deficiency in order to help the main points reinforce the liver and kidney. The combination of points is very important for miscellaneous cases. The points Fengchi (G 20), Shenting (Du 24), or Yintang (Extra) for dizziness and vertigo can be used if necessary. For another example, insomnia resulting from heart fire due to imbalance between heart and kidney should be treated on the basis of reinforcing and reducing at the same time. Shenmen (H 7), the Yuan-primary point, is punctured with the reducing method, in combination with Zhaohai (K 6) or Taixi (Liv 3) to nourish the kidney yin in order to control its yang. Or the moxa cones may be used on Guanyuan (Ren 4) to conduct the fire back to its origin.

2. Selecting fewer and concise points

Huang often says, "A commander who is good at commanding chooses his soldiers concisely not numerously; an acupuncturist who is good at acupuncture selects less points but effectively." The points must be chosen exactly on the basis of differentiation and treating principles. The points along the meridian are different but have the same functions. The doctor should take into consideration main points and which ones are the secondary choice, especially for the treatment of chronic diseases. In case the points are used by turns, they can take a rest to function more effectively. When there is preparation, the effects will be better. But patients are usually impatient. They think the more points the better. If the doctor doesn't persist in the selective principle, and chooses points blindly and shoots one hundred arrows and only one hits the target, it will not do any good. Puncturing blindly will disturb the qi circulation which leads to dysfunction. He puts forward that an odd point can be used for simple disease. For instance, acute tonsilitis is usually caused by fire flaring up, so clearing fire is the treating principle, and bloodletting at Shaoshang (L 11) or needling Hegu (LI 4) will be effective. The empirical points should be taken into consideration too, e.g. the early acute lumbar sprain responds to the empirical point very well. For the miscellaneous diseases, the points should also be selected concisely. Huang is adept at the application of the five shu points and the points related to the meridians according to the differentiation.

3. The nature of points is not the same as that of herbs

From his long-term clinical practice, he has understood that the nature of points is completely different from that of herbs. The herbs are of sweet flavour and warm in nature; sweet flavour and cold in nature; pungent flavour and warm in property; or pungent flavour and cool in property, while the point is the place where the meridian qi converges. The therapeutic effect must result from the stimulation by acupuncture or by moxibustion. For example, Zusanli (S 36) is thought a toning point, reducing cannot be applied at this point for shi syndrome of Yangming. Guanyuan (Ren 4) is thought a toning point, reducing cannot be used for difficulty in urination resulting from shi heat of the small intestine. The functions of acupuncture in regulating the organs and tissues are excited through the internal conduction of points and along the meridians, which is different from the four natures and five flavours of the herbs. The point cannot directly replenish any substances to the human body. However, this function may be completed indirectly by regulating the functions of a certain zang or fu organ through acupuncture and moxibustion. Therefore, the nature of herbs is not the same as that of points.

4. Needle insertion and manipulating qi at five fingers

When Huang treats his patients, he concentrates his attention on his needles in rythm with the patient's respiration. When he selects the points he manipulates qi at his fingers and is absorbed in waiting for qi. As soon as the meridian qi comes, lift the needle slightly and then apply reinforcing or reducing. He holds that reinforcing and reducing are performed by lifting, thrusting or rotating the needle, but the key point is of the patient's sensation and the doctor's manipulating force and speed. The supplementary techniques such as pressing, palpation, twirling and plucking have nothing to do with the reinforcing and reducing.

Huang combats the incautious operation of acupuncture. Some doctors do acupuncture carelessly. They insert the needles deeply and thrust blindly. Huang thinks the blind insertion and thrusting can damage the antipathogenic qi. So he treats the patients according to their individual conditions. Too strong or too mild stimulation is not suitable. He stresses the regulation of qi, functioning in removing obstructions from the meridians, keeping qi going inside to treat various bi syndromes receiving qi to promote qi circulation in the meridians, retaining qi to treat paralysis and masses in the abdomen, long-time conducting qi to relieve spasm and stop pain and puncturing collaterals to dissolve blood stasis.

5. Penetrating technique

Huang thinks that depth of insertion should be in accordance with the locations of diseases. Generally speaking, deep insertion can be applied for diseases located in the ying system, while shallow insertion is used for diseases located in the wei system. Huang is good at penetrating technique which is devided into perpendicular and horizontal penetrating. The former, named as deep penetrating too, indicates in the interior, cold and ying system syndromes. For example, Jianshi (P 5) penetrating towards Zhigou (SJ 6) treats manic disorders while the latter, also known as shallow penetrating, is indicated in the exterior, heat and wei system syndromes. For example, Yuwei (Extra) penetrating towards Yuyao (Extra) treats the red and swelling eye due to pathogenic heat, Sizhukong (SJ 23) penetrating Shuaigu (G 8) or Xuanlu (G 5) penetrating Hanyan (G 4) treats migraine due to fire of liver and gallbladder. In addition, there are penetrating the same meridian and penetrating the different meridians. As for penetrating the same meridian, Yemen (SJ 2) penetrating horizontally to Yangchi (SJ 4) is for the redness, swelling and pain of the hand and arm, Dichang (S 4) penetrating Jiache (S 6) for facial paralysis, and Huiyang (B 35) penetrating Ciliao (B 32) for retention of urine and prolapse of uterus. As for penetrating the different meridians, Yinlingquan (Sp 9) penetrating Yanglingquan (G 34) is for the pain of knee joints.

6. Moxibustion treatment of hypertension

In the summer of 1940, Huang treated a patient in a hotel located in Fuzhou Road. The room windows were all closed, and the air was turbid. It was very hot at that time, but the patient was dressed in thin cotton clothes without any hot sensation. The patient's family told Huang that the patient had a history of alcoholism for thirty years. He could drink a bottle of Brandy every day. The patient suffered from hypertension for a long time and took medication very often. He followed his doctor's advice and gave up drinking for one year already, but the blood pressure remained the same. He had aversion to cold which was aggravated day by day, normal body build, cold limbs, lassitude, preference for warmth and fearing cold, soft, thready and forceless pulse, a flabby tongue with tooth marks on the border, loss of appetite, loose stool, clear and profuse urine and frequent at night. Huang thought that it was a rare case because the patient put on cotton clothes during the summer. The disease lasted for one year and acupuncture might not achieve immediate effect. Giving up drinking may disturb the circulation of qi and blood. Alcohol was considered as balancing blood, replenishing qi, warming stomach and removing cold. The patient was ill since he gave up drinking. Why not advise him to drink appropriately in order to improve the circulation of qi and blood? Therefore, he asked the patient to drink a little every day at noon. The patient did and told Huang later that day that his cotton clothes could be taken off. He tried this way for three days, and then applied warm moxibustion on Qihai (Ren 6), Guanyuan (Ren 4) and Zusanli (S 36). The patient recovered after one month, and the blood pressure was almost normal.

7. Example of treating fever by cutting heat method

In May, 1983, Huang came back from Bulgaria via Moscow. On his way back in the Soviet Union, he was invited to treat a patient who was admitted to the hospital and had a fever for more than ten days. It was very difficult to diagnose the case. Antibiotics were applied but didn't help. Huang was told that the patient had a fever around 40°C every afternoon at 2 o'clock, and was gradually reduced with profuse sweating in the evening. It seemed to be the fever of malaria, but there was no malarial parasite found. The patient was big and tall, his body was hot like a charcoal fire, accompanied by flushed face, fullness in the chest, dry mouth, preference for drinks, yellow and scanty urine, dry and hard stool, yellow sticky tongue coating, full, rapid and forceful pulse. Huang thought that the antibiotics were helpless, thus it might be the attack of viruses. On the following day, he treated the patient before attack of the fever with the method of cutting heat. He used the reducing method by rapid insertion on Dazhui (Du 14), Taodao (Du 3), Quchi (LI 11), Hegu (LI 4), Zusanli (S 36) and Fengchi (G 20). In total, 2000 ml of fluid infusion was applied at the request of the patient's family. When Huang saw the patient for the third time, the patient was somewhat better. His temperature was 38°C. From the fourth day, the patient was prescribed to take two bottles of indomethacin daily for three days, and acupuncture was still given daily. Three days later, the fever was gone.

8. Regulating stomach first for receiving food

In March, 1961, a steel worker was admitted to the First People's Hospital because he was seriously burnt by molten steel. A rescue group with the combination of Western and Chinese medicine was immediately set up and Huang was one of the members in the group. According to Western medicine, nourishment should be replenished because of his critical exhaustion. Fluid food with enough heat must be given to the patient, who failed to eat because of frequent nausea and vomiting. Huang held that although the burn did not indicate the use of acupuncture, nausea and vomiting responded to acupuncture well. The burned area was up to 90 percent. Huang only punctured Neiguan (P 6) on both sides with the reducing method, and retained and manipulated the needles several times. The nausea was immediately stopped. The favourable conditions were created by taking Chinese herbs. But the patient could not take the fluid food orally. Without restoration of the body resistance, healing the burn would be delayed. He asked the patient, "Why did you refuse to have milk and food?" The patient answered, "Generally, I don't drink milk. If necessary, I will take it as medicine." "Generally, what kind of food do you eat?" "Pancake, deep-fried twisted dough sticks and rice." Therefore, Huang put forward a proposal in the discussion meeting, "Everyone has food preferences. If a person doesn't like the food, even if it's delicacies from the sea, the stomach will refuse them. But in the case that he likes the food, the stomach will digest it, even if it is plain tea or simple food. This is the saying that preference is the best. We can stop the fluid food for a while and try to stimulate appetite." The doctors consented to the suggestion. The patient was allowed to eat what he preferred. His appetite gradually increased three days later. Stimulating the appetite for reinforcing the body resistence was effective as expected.

ELABORATION OF ACUPUNCTURE ESSENTIALS AND EYE NEEDLING THERAPY

—Peng Jingshan's Clinical Experience

Peng Jingshan was born in Kaiyuan County, Liaoning Province, in 1909. He began to devote himself to the study of traditional Chinese medicine when he was sixteen. He learned the essential knowledge from Professor Ma Erqin, a famous TCM physician, and Dr. Tang Yunge, a well-known acupuncturist. Later on, he studied Western medicine for one year in the Manzhou Medical University. Now, it is fifty-six years since he hung out his shingle at the age of twenty-two. He has written twelve books and more than fifty articles, of which *Simplified Acupuncture Therapy*, published in 1954, played an active role in popularizing acupuncture. In 1971, the Hong Kong Yimei Publishing House reprinted this book, and in 1986, another reprint in the American Acupuncture Journal aroused the interest of acupuncturists in Europe and America. His application of acupuncture to the ophthalmic micro-system won the third prize award of the Important Scientific Outcomes and Creations in Liaoning Province. Presently, he is a professor and director of the Research Section of Meridians and Collaterals and the Research section of Ophthalmic Diseases in the Liaoning College of Traditional Chinese Medicine, a member of the directors of Liaoning Association of Traditional Chinese Medicine, and a member of Liaoning Association of Acupuncture.

I. Academic Characteristics and Medical Specialities

Academically, Professor Peng stresses diligent study of the ancients' wisdom. He devotes much time to the study of *Internal Classic*, *Systematic Classic of Acupuncture*, *Compendium of Acupuncture* and other acupuncture literatures in past dynasties, trying to grasp their essentials. In clinic, he emphasizes the correct differentiation of syndromes, accurate selection of points and skillful manipulations.

1. Creating three methods to improve the needling techniques

1) *Exercise of the arms and hands* The success of acupuncture treatment depends not only on the doctor's expertise in TCM theory, but also on proficient needling skills. Exercising the arms and hands is one of the basic ways to perfect needling skills before treating patients with acupuncture. In this exercise, one should stand firmly "like a stone pillar, with the distance between the feet equal to that between the shoulders. Extend and flex the arm levelly and concentrate the mind on the Dantian area." "Extending and flexing the arm levelly" includes: a) First, extend the arms forward level with the shoulders. Then flex the forearms with the palms facing downward to keep the fingers

closed. Curve the hands inward and outward thirty-two times. b) Abduct the arms with the palms facing downward to make curve from exterior to interior for thirty-two times. c) Extend the arms forward with the wrists and fingers shaking to make counterclockwise circles sixteen times and clockwise circles sixteen times.

2) *Practising needling on water surface* Professor Peng thinks that there have been many needling methods since ancient times. The pricking, superficial and deep insertion describe the depth of needling; perpendicular, oblique, sideways and horizontal insertion relate to the angle of needling; whereas inserting the needle along or against the course of the meridians, using many or a few points and forceful insertion determine the function of the needling. Among these various techniques, gentle insertion is the most difficult one to perform. Peng advises beginners to perfect this technique since it is the most difficult one to apply.

Professor Peng created the method of practising needling on water surface with four steps. Firstly, let a small, round, flat Chinese chess float on the water. Insert the needle into the wood chess without upsetting its floating position. Secondly, place a soft plastic bottle cover on the water and needle again as described above. The needling technique is considered proficient if the cover does not tilt, although the water rocks it slightly. The third step is to needle into a sponge, which is free from movement, but with a slight quivering when the needle is inserted. For the fourth step, needle into a piece of floating fruit without grazing the skin or moving it. Practise each step with the right and then the left hand alternately. Following the proper sequence of steps will insure progress. Then the doctor will be able to perform gentle and slow insertion without causing pain.

3) *The skill of holding the needle properly and painless insertion* Professor Peng stresses that the shape of the dragon eye or phoenix eye should be formed between the thumb and the index finger during insertion and withdrawal of the needle. The principle is to concentrate one's attention on the needle, manipulate it with the thumb and the index finger forming the shape of a dragon's eye and insert it forming the shape of the eye of a phoenix.

Painless insertion is based on accurate location of the points, avoiding skin pores and rapid insertion of the needle. The key point to locate the points is that prefer to puncture a non-point rather than to deviate from the meridian. In addition, tender spots, palpable nodules, cysts or cords can be used as points. By needling the tender spots, which usually appear at skin pores, rapid insertion between skin pores will kill the pain.

2. Eight methods for selecting points along the meridians

1) *Selecting points along the meridians according to differentiation of syndromes* When treating a disease, first trace the cause by analyzing the symptoms and then determine the treatment principle. For example, insomnia may be caused by several factors. With correct analysis of the causative factors and selection of points along the meridian, satisfactory therapeutic results may be obtained. Insomnia due to emotional stimulation is considered as a disease of the heart, and Shenmen (H 7) from the Heart Meridian is selected. Xingjian (Liv 2) is used to treat insomnia caused by injury of the liver due to anger; Sanyinjiao (Sp 6) is selected for insomnia due to injury of the spleen

due to over thinking: Lieque (L 7) is for insomnia due to injury of the lung due to grief; Taixi (K 3) is for insomnia due to injury of the kidney due to frightening or invasion of cold or due to excessive sexual activities. On July 14, 1974, Professor Peng treated a 13-year-old girl student, who complained of insomnia for the past four months with difficulty in falling asleep and being awakened easily every night. Sedative drugs or Chinese herbs for calming the mind and toning the heart and blood did not help her. On examination she manifested sallow complexion, emaciation and deep, string-taut pulse, especially at the left "Guan" region. From her mother, Professor Peng knew that the patient had a quick temper and insomnia was usually aggravated after anger. Diagnosis: Insomnia due to hyperactivity of liver yang. Treatment: The reducing method was applied because it was an excess condition. Xingjian (Liv 2), a Rong-Spring Point, was selected instead of Dadun (Liv 1), a Jing-Well Point, since the special needling technique was impossible to apply at Dadun (Liv 1). Therapeutic result: Treat once a day. After four treatments, the girl could sleep eight hours every night.

2) *Selecting either the starting point or the end point of the meridian* Puncture the end point when the disease is located at the starting point of the meridian and vice versa. Here, the starting point means the first point of the meridian, and the end point means the final point of the meridian. The method is effective for local pain, paralysis, and extremely good for furuncles which often occur at the locations of the points on the face, lips, hand and foot. The main symptoms are pain, fever, chills, restlessness and nausea. Sometimes, red streaks appear at the side of furuncle. Pricking with a three-edged needle is applied at the end of the streaks. For example, a 16-year-old girl first visited on October 20, 1974. Her chief complaints were sudden onset of swelling and pain of the right cheek, a blister at the side of nose, vomiting once, restlessness, a dry and red tongue, and deep and rapid pulse, especially at right "guan" region. Blood test: WBC 15400/mm^3, Neutrophils 90 percent, LYM 10 percent. Analyzed in terms of the pulse picture, it was caused by stomach heat manifesting on the face. The blister was located just on Sibai (S 2) point. Diagnosis: Facial furuncle. Treatment: According to the method of selecting an end point of the meridian to treat a disease at the starting point of the meridian, Lidui (S 45), the Jing-Well Point, was selected. It was pricked rapidly and heavily with a 0.5 inch needle of gauge 28. Puncturing the Jing-Well Point with strong stimulation is considered as the reducing method. After the needle was retained for twenty minutes, restlessness was relieved. The blood test after the first treatment showed: WBC 8100/mm^3, Neutrophils 70 percent. By the next day, the facial furuncle and symptoms disappeared except a slight swelling on the cheek.

3) *Selecting point from both sides of the meridian* The points from both sides of the meridian are often selected when a disease is diagnosed as being a disorder of this meridian. Needle the starting point and the end point of the meridian by two operators simultaneously. The same as the manipulation and withdrawal. Considering hypochondriac pain as an example, Qiaoyin (G 44) and Tongziliao (G 1) may be punctured for pain occurring on the hypochondriac region traversed by the Gallbladder Meridian. This method is effective for disorders in which the main symptom is pain, such as painful bi syndrome, epigastric pain, and limitation of walking or raising the arm due to a motor dysfunction. For example, a 34-year-old worker came for the first visit on January 31,

1975. He had been suffering for half a month from numbness on the left arm and shoulder with a dull sensation of the fourth finger and difficulty in raising the arm to touch the head. Clinical manifestations: lassitude, sallow complexion, moist tongue, scanty urine, slight edema of the lower extremities, deep and thready pulse. Differentiation: Dysfunction of Sanjiao in transporting body fluids resulting in scanty urine and slight edema, with obstruction of the Sanjiao Meridian on the left side leading to deficiency of qi and blood which resulted in numbness. Diagnosis and treatment: Muscular bi syndrome. Guanchong (SJ 1) and Sizhukong (SJ 23), two points from the both sides of the Sanjiao Meridian on the left side were selected. After the first treatment, the patient could raise his arm and numbness was less. After the second treatment, the numbness disappeared. After the third treatment, all the symptoms were relieved and there was no relapse.

4) *Selecting the distal points along the meridians* This method is different from the method of selecting the starting point or the end point along the meridian in which the points are applied only from one meridian. This method may select the starting points of the three yin meridians of the hand and the ending points of the three yang meridians of the hand, or the adjacent points.

Case example: Wang, female, 19 years old, farmer. The first visit was on October 30, 1975. Chief complaint: Finger spasm several times a day due to invasion of cold lasting more than one month. In the last three days, the fingers were clenched due to the contracture, and pain occurred if she tried to extend the fingers. Drugs and acupuncture treatments failed to help her. Clinical manifestations: No clear change of the body build, pale complexion, cold and rigidity of the fingers, a moist tongue without coating, and a deep, slow pulse. Differentiation: Stagnation of blood due to invasion of cold, which resulted in obstruction of the meridians and collaterals. Diagnosis: Chicken claw wind (spasm of fingers). Local points: Baxie (Extra), Sanjian (LI 3) and Daling (P 7) were tried without success. Adjacent points of Quchi (LI 11), Shousanli (LI 10) and Tianjing (SJ 10) were also not effective. Later, the most distal point of each of the six hand meridians was selected. This was either an ending point or starting point, being selected according to the direction of the meridian. The thumb extended when Zhongfu (L 1) was punctured. The index finger moved when Yingxiang (LI 20) was needled. The middle finger relaxed when Tianchi (P 1) was treated. Needling Sizhukong (SJ 23) made the ring finger free. Piquan (H 1) or Qinling (H 2) could be used if there was difficulty in raising the arm and exposing the axillary fossa, which was effective for extending the little finger, which pertains to the Heart Meridian and connects with the Small Intestine Meridian. Here, puncturing one meridian effected two meridians. All the symptoms disappeared after the treatment.

5) *Selecting points from the externally and internally related meridians* Meridians and collaterals connecting with the internal organs, are classified as paired meridians because they are externally-internally related with zang-fu organs. Treating a disorder of an external yang meridian by puncturing points of the paired internal yin meridian, and vice versa, is considered the method of selecting points from the externally and internally-related meridians, which is, of course, based on differentiation of syndromes.

Case example: Jia, male, 46 years old, worker. The first visit was on September 9,

1975.

Chief complaints: Epigastric pain since 1966, accompanied by loose stool, cold limbs, lassitude and emaciation. Neither drugs nor acupuncture treatment had helped him.

Clinical Manifestations: Sallow complexion, emaciation, cold limbs, a moist tongue with tooth prints but free of coating, and a deep and slow pulse, especially at the right "guan" region.

Differentiation: Since the stomach is in charge of receiving food, while the spleen takes care of transportation and transformation, deficiency of the spleen caused failure of transportation and transformation, resulting in loose stool, cold limbs and emaciation. The deep and slow pulse is the sign of internal cold.

Diagnosis: Epigastric pain due to deficiency-cold. The causative factor was related to the spleen, although the pain appeared in the stomach.

Treatment procedure: The deficiency-cold syndrome should be treated by direct moxibustion with small cones the size of a wheat kernal. Gongsun (Sp 4), the Luo-(Connecting) Point of the Spleen Meridian was treated by this method. For each treatment, ten cones were applied successively, i.e. the burning cones were taken away when the patient felt a hot sensation and replaced by new ones. The pain was relieved after the first treatment. After twelve treatments, his hands and feet regained their normal warmth. The bowel movement returned to normal and the emaciation disappeared, the muscle was thicker and epigastric pain was checked. The follow-up one year later showed no recurrence.

6) *Selecting the Yuan-(Source) and Luo-(Connecting) Point from the meridian* Select the diseased meridian on the basis of differentiation of the syndrome.

Case example: Yang x x, male, 35 years old. The first visit was on July 6, 1976.

Chief complaints: Unable to blink with the upper eyelid, aching of the eye when using the eyes for a comparatively long time, and occasional headache. The condition worsened gradually and no medicine helped him.

Examination: Healthy body build, lassitude, optimistic attitude, rosy face but a distorted facial appearance due to the disorder of the eyelid. There was no coating on the tongue. The pulse was deep and slow. In the book *Miraculous Pivot,* it says, "Taiyang Meridian passes through the upper eyelid; and the Yangming Meridian runs through the lower eyelid." For this case, the Bladder Meridian is selected because the disease has already lasted for a few years. In addition, the Spleen Meridian which controls the whole eyelids was also selected.

Diagnosis: Paralysis of the upper eyelid.

Prescription: Jinggu (B 64), the Yuan-(Source) Point of the Bladder Meridian, and Dazhong (K 4), the Luo (Connecting) Point of the Kidney Meridian which is externally-internally related to the Bladder Meridian. Moxibustion was applied on Pishu (B 20).

After fifteen treatments, the patient could blink without any pain. After twenty treatments, his eyelid recovered to normal.

7) *Combination of the Front-Mu Point of the diseased meridians* Why is combination of points mentioned here, while the above six methods are called selecting points from the meridians? That is because the therapeutic result of treating a chronic disease is obtained only upon combination of the Front-Mu Points with the points from the

corresponding diseased meridian, based on selecting common points from the corresponding diseased meridian.

Case example: Wang x x, male, 67 years old. The first visit was on October 3, 1976.

Chief complaint: Cough and asthma with profuse sputum for many years. At first it was better in summer and worse in winter. Later, it occurred year-round. He always suffered from the symptoms, but they intensified during an attack. There was no relief with various kinds of medical treatment.

Clinical manifestation: Lassitude, pale complexion, shortness of breath with gurgling sound in the throat (coarse breathing), a yellow tongue coating and rapid pulse.

Differentiation: Shortness of breath and asthma with gurgling sound in the throat and the rapid pulse indicated lung heat. The lassitude was caused by deficiency due to the long duration of the illness.

Diagnosis: Asthma with phlegm accumulation.

Treatment procedure: Zhongfu (L 1), the Front-Mu Point of the Lung Meridian, was selected as the main point. Tiantu (Ren 22) was added for the gurgling sound in the throat, Tanzhong (Ren 17) for shortness of breath and asthma, and Fenglong (S 40) for resolving phlegm.

After nine treatments, all the symptoms disappeared. Later, he had a few relapses, but the duration between attacks was longer, and the symptoms were milder. Treated with the above-mentioned method, it was effective for each treatment, but with no radical cure.

8) *Combination of the Xi-(Cleft) Point of the diseased meridian* Whereas Front-Mu Points treat chronic diseases, Xi-(Cleft) Points are selected for acute diseases. This is the principle of combination of points in acupuncture.

Case example: Ding x x, male, 16 years old.

Chief complaint: The patient often had sudden attacks of epistaxis in the spring time. On the day when he came to hospital, he had a sudden onset of massive bleeding. The blood even spurted from his mouth when he blocked his nose with cotton. Nothing could stop the bleeding.

During examination, he lay on the table and plugged his nose with cotton. Blood was still flowing from his mouth. Accompanying symptoms included lassitude, pale complexion and lips, low voice with shortness of breath, dizziness, palpitation and hollow pulse. The tongue was purple without coating and looked like a peeled pig kidney.

Diagnosis: Deficiency of the lung and blood.

Treatment procedure: The first priority of the treatment was to stop the bleeding to prevent shock. Some thread was twisted around the middle fingers (bilaterally) at the transverse creases of the inter-phalangeal joints. Then immediately Yingxiang (LI 20) (bilaterally) was punctured, and then Kongzui (L 6) bilaterally with the reinforcing method. The bleeding subsided when Yingxiang (LI 20) was inserted, and stopped immediately when Kongzui (L 6), the Xi-(Cleft) Point of the Lung Meridian, was punctured. The Xi-(Cleft) Points were always effective for acute condition.

Twisting the middle finger with thread was the first-aid to check bleeding. Stimulating Yingxiang (LI 20) caused the local vessels to contract. Using Xi-(Cleft) Point in an acute disease may tone the lung by stimulating the meridian. Thus the bleeding was stopped quickly.

3. Seven prescriptions and ten potencies in acupuncture and moxibustion

1) *Seven prescriptions are the forms of combining the points* a. Heavy prescription: A large number of points are punctured by thick needles with heavy manipulation. This is effective for acute, severe, excess syndrome and for patients who have a strong body build. b. Minor prescription: A small number of points are needled with thin needles with gentle manipulation. This is suitable for acute, mild and childrens' diseases, and patients with poor health. c. Slow-acting prescription: Fewer points are selected with short retention and longer intervals. It is effective for either chronic or mild diseases, such as neurasthenia and habitual constipation. d. Quick-acting prescription: The points are easily located and manipulated with quick effects. It is often used in emergency cases, such as car sickness, sea sickness, acute gastroen teritis, epileptic convulsion and infantile convulsion. e. Odd-numbered prescription: Only one point is needed, which may relieve the symptoms immediately. Or for each treatment select only one point until the patient recovers. For example, select Yifeng (SJ 17) for toothache, Taichong (Liv 3) for epilepsy and Xingjian (Liv 2) for insomnia. f. Even-number prescription: Needle points bilaterally or choose an equal number of points on both sides of the body. This is good for systematic diseases and regulates the balance of qi and blood in the meridians, collaterals and the whole body. g. Compound prescription: It includes the combination of points which have the same functions. For instance, select Fengchi (G 20) in combination with Tianzhu (B 10) to treat stiffness and pain of the neck; combination of syndromes and complications are treated simultaneously. For instance, a patient who has knee arthritis and indigestion is treated by needling Xiyan (Extra) to treat arthritis and Zhongwan (Ren 12) to treat indigestion. Then Zusanli (S 36) could be used to strengthen the effects of both Xiyan (Extra) and Zhongwan (Ren 12); combination of points which are selected for different diseases. For instance, a patient who had facial paralysis later developed urticaria, and Jiache (S 6), Dicang (S 4) and Sibai (S 2) may be selected to treat facial paralysis, and Quchi (LI 11) and Binao (LI 14) may be selected for urticaria.

2) *Ten potencies refer the ten functions of combining points* a. Tonic potency will reinforce poor health, e.g. Dazhui (Du 14) and Taodao (Du 13) will strengthen a weak condition caused by yang deficiency; moxibustion at Gaohuangshu (B 43) treats a lung deficiency, and Zusanli (S 36) strengthens the functions of the spleen and stomach. b. Heavy potency may check perversion, e.g. Neiguan (P 6) and Tanzhong (Ren 17) will stop hiccups. c. Mild potency eliminates excess, e.g. an embedding needle in Geshu (B 17) may treat dizziness and vertigo. d. Dispersing potency resolves phlegm, e.g. pressing Tiantu (Ren 22) with a finger can eliminate phlegm and relieve dyspnea. e. Promoting potency will remove stagnation, e.g. applying reducing method on Shimen (Ren 5) and Tianshu (S 25) treats stagnation. f. Astringing potency lifts prolapsed organs, e.g. puncture Changqiang (Du 1) and moxibustion on Baihui (Du 20) will treat prolapse of the anus. g. Lubricating potency helps discharge accumulations, e.g. puncturing Sifeng (Extra) treats infantile indigestion. h. Purgative potency stimulates the bowels, e.g. puncturing Sanyinjiao (Sp 6) with a reducing method based on respiration, or embedding

intradermal needle in left Fujie (Sp 14) can treat constipation. i. Moistening potency overcomes dryness, e.g. puncturing Tanzhong (Ren 17) and Geshu (B 17) circulates qi and activates blood for disorders of dryness. j. Desiccating potency resolves dampness, e.g. puncturing Yinlingquan (Sp 9) and Sanyinjiao (Sp 6) eliminates dampness and treats edema. In addition, there are another two potencies, cooling potency and heating potency. For example, Shenshu (B 23), Guanyuan (Ren 4) and Qihai (Ren 6) are often used to eliminate cold, while Dazhui (Du 14), Taodao (Du 13) and Hegu (LI 4) are selected to reduce heat.

4. Ten methods for lowering blood pressure

1) *Puncturing the carotid sinus near Renying (S 9)* The location of Renying (S 9) is just above the external carotid artery sinus. Ask the patient to take a supine position with the head lower than the body. Stabilize the artery in a fixed position with the left hand, and insert a 1.5-inch needle into the wall of the artery with the right hand, with the needle handle quivering. Acupuncture is forbidden if a patient feels dizzy. Retain the needle for ten seconds or more but not over two minutes. The method is mainly applied for primary hypertension, bronchial asthma, cholilthiasis and gastric spasm.

2) *Embedding intradermal needle in Geshu (B 17)* Embed an intradermal needle in Geshu (B 17) bilaterally and retain it for seven days. This method is helpful for patients who are fat or needle-shy. Although this method is simple, the points must be located accurately.

3) *Puncturing the retroauricular groove for reducing blood pressure* Prick the veins posterior to the ear which are opposite to the upper one third of the antihelix to cause bleeding. This is effective for an acute case of hypertension.

These first three methods may lower the blood pressure ten seconds after needling.

4) *Puncturing the artery near Taiyuan (L 9)* Puncture the radial artery under the location of Taiyuan (L 9) with a two-inch needle and slight shaking of the needle handle. The needle may be regulated by lifting the needle slightly in case of absence of shaking.

5) *Lowering the blood pressure with ophthalmic acupuncture* The heart and liver areas.

6) *Lowering the blood pressure with nose acupuncture* Yintang (Extra) and Suliao (Du 25) are punctured obliquely with a 45° angle by using a 0.5-inch needle.

The above three methods may lower the blood pressure within five minutes after needling.

7) *Reducing Taichong (Liv 3)* Puncture Taichong (Liv 3) with the reducing method by lifting and thrusting manipulations, which is good for hypertension due to hyperactivity of liver yang accompanied by severe dizziness and vertigo.

8) *Penetrating Hegu (LI 4) towards Houxi (SI 3)* Penetrate Hegu (LI 4) with a three-inch needle. When the needling sensation arrives, manipulate the needle with the reducing method of rotation, or even better by applying the method of Toutianliang (cooling the sky). It is suitable for hypertension accompanied by signs of interior heat, such as constipation, dark yellow urine, dry mouth and tongue and poor appetite.

9) *Lowering the blood pressure by puncturing Zusanli (S 36)* Puncture Zusanli (S

36) with the reinforcing method for hypertension accompanied by weak body condition and gastrointestinal disorders.

10) *Lowering the blood pressure by puncturing Shimen (Ren 5)* This method is often used for women who have hypertension accompanied by an excess of the Ren Meridian, manifesting fullness of the chest and abdomen, amenorrhea and leukorrhea.

Treatments for accompanying symptoms of hypertension: Select Xiaxi (G 43) and Shanglian (LI 9) for dizziness and vertigo; Xingjian (Liv 2), Shenmen (H 7) and Ganshu (B 18) for insomnia; Taichong (Liv 3) penetrating towards Yongquan, (K 1) and Huangshu (K 16) for headache; Taixi (K 3) and Shenshu (B 23) for deficiency of kidney yin; moxibustion on Guanyuan (Ren 4), Qihai (Ren 6) and Mingmen (Du 4) for deficiency of yang.

5. Ten methods for treating facial paralysis

1) *Twisting the muscle fibers* Insert a five-inch needle into Jiache (S 6) on the affected side until the tip of the needle reaches the angle of the mouth. Next, rotate the needle in one direction a few circles and pull the needle suddenly and forcefully, while the left hand presses the skin half an inch lateral from where the tip of the needle reaches. The needle will twist some muscle fibers and wrinkle the skin. Do the same manipulation five to ten times, then withdraw the needle. The therapeutic result will be better if the tip of the needle is bent twisted by the muscle fibers after a few forceful rotations, the patient can be asked to hold the twisted needle with a slight pulling action towards the ear for twenty minutes.

2) *Three needling techniques for an affected eyelid* a. Insert a 1.5-inch needle into a tender spot between Wangu (G 12) and Yifeng (SJ 17) one inch deep and towards the pupil. If the point is located accurately and the angle of insertion is correct, the eye will close immediately. b. Press the upper eyelid down securely with the left hand: With the right hand, hold the needle with an angle of 15 degrees and prick the outside surface of the eyelid with a pecking motion. This method could be used for mild paralysis of the upper eyelid. Deep insertion is forbidden to prevent bleeding. Usually, the eyelid returns to normal after one treatment. c. Insert a 1.5-inch needle (Gauge 30 or 32) into the inner surface of the upper eyelid to treat lingering paralysis and spasm of the upper eyelid. Retain the needle for five minutes, then withdraw it slowly to avoid bleeding. After the treatment, the eyelid usually feels relaxed and he can close the eye slightly. Since this method requires a skillful technique, it is only applied in cases which have not been cured by other methods.

3) *Pricking the lips* This treats lingering deviation of the mouth, difficulty in chewing, retention of food in the mouth and excess salivation. While stretching the affected side of the lip (either lip can be treated) with one hand, prick the lip with the other hand by using a small three-edged needle to cause a little bleeding.

4) *Bloodletting in the mouth* For the patient whose eyelid has recovered, but the mouth remains deviated, prick the oral mucous membrane superficially with a three-edge needle to cause bleeding. Then press and squeeze the needling holes to let more blood ooze out. Afterwards, simply have the patient spit out the blood, it is not necessary to

clean the mouth with water.

5) *Two points and four lines* For a severe case which has not improved after a few courses of treatments, two points on the affected side, Sibai (S 2) and Yifeng (SJ 17) may be punctured with the reinforcing method. Then insert a needle from Dicang (S 4) on the affected side towards Renzhong (Du 26). From Renzhong (Du 26), insert another needle towards Dicang (S 4) on the healthy side. From there, insert the needle towards Chengjiang (Ren 24). Finally, insert a needle from Chengjiang (Ren 24) towards Dicang (S 4) on the affected side. Thus, four lines are formed around the mouth. The method is especially effective for deviation of the mouth.

6) *Ophthalmic acupuncture* Puncture the upper jiao area of the orbital region with a 0.5-inch needle (Gauge 30). Retain the needle for five minutes. This method is effective for acute onset of facial paralysis and infantile facial paralysis.

7) *Crossing puncture* For lingering facial paralysis, select three to four points between the eye and mouth at the healthy side of the face and puncture them with the reducing method.

8) *Tapping with a seven-star needle* Tap the affected side with the routine technique once every other day. This method is mainly applied for the patient who has a dull sensation on the affected side of the face and no success with the standard acupuncture treatment.

9) *Selecting points from the corresponding meridians* For the paralysis mainly occurring on the area traversed by the Bladder Meridian and Gallbladder Meridian, Shenmai (B 62), Jingmen (B 63), Guangming (G 37), Diwuhui (G 42) can be selected. For the condition mainly occurring on the area of the Large Intestine, Stomach and Small Intestine Meridians, Jiache (S 6), Dicang (S 4), Taichong (Liv 3), Quanliao (SI 18), Daying (S 5), Yanggu (SI 5) and Xiaxi (G 43) should be selected.

10) *Regulating the meridians and collaterals* First see whether the right or left meridians and collaterals are deficient or excessive. This is determined by testing the relative tolerance of indirect heat applied to the nails beside Jing-Well Points of the twelve regular meridians, or to the Yuan-(Source) Points of the twelve regular meridians. Then, secure embedded needles in the Back-Shu Points of the deficient side (the side more tolerant of heat) or puncture points of the diseased meridians. This method is applicable for cases which have not improved after a period of treatment.

6. Ten methods for treating bi syndrome

1) *Four essential point* Jianyu (LI 15), Quchi (LI 11), Huantiao (G 30) and Yanglingquan (G 34) are the key points for the bi syndrome of the for limbs due to invasion of pathogenic wind, damp, cold and heat. The points may be used independently or in combination. Either the routine manipulation or deep insertion with a long needle may be applied.

Case example: Yang x x, male, 55 years old. He had left shoulder pain for more than one month. He could not extend the arm freely or raise it higher than the shoulder. Penetrate Jianyu (LI 15) towards Quchi (LI 11) with a long needle without retaining. The patient could extend the arm after the first treatment and raise the arm after the second treatment. All of the symptoms disappeared after the third treatment.

2) *Crossing puncture* The method is good for the severe pain of the Bi syndrome. Needle a point on the healthy side which is within one centimeter around the pain on the diseased side. This approach may also be applied by selecting a corresponding point from the front of the body to treat a disease on the back of the body and vice versa. Finally, one may select a corresponding point from the upper part of the body to treat a disease on the lower extremities and vice versa.

Case example: Xue x x, female, 39 years old, worker. The movement of the right arm was extremely limited because the arm was exposed to a draft while sleeping at night. There was an obvious tenderness on the upper part of scapula. A corresponding point of identical location was punctured on the left scapula. Only one treatment was needed to relieve her pain.

3) *The intradermal needle* For wandering bi syndrome due to invasion of wind, embed an intradermal needle in the most painful point or the Back-Shu Point. For knee pain, embed the intradermal needle in a point which feels painful two cun above the knee. The therapeutic result of this method is usually good.

4) *Ophthalmic acupuncture* Immediate results are obtained after puncturing the orbital areas of the upper, middle and lower jiao and other points around the eye according to differentiation.

Case example: Cai x x, male, 25 years old, teacher. He had a history of rheumatoid arthritis and usually had numbness in the legs after sitting for a long time. He had a sudden onset of sharp pain in the left knee joint which gradually increased when he rode his bicycle to school that morning. He was not able to extend the left leg when he arrived at school, and had difficulty in walking up the stairs when he came to the hospital. The pulse was deep and slow. The colour and shape of the capillaries in the orbital areas of the lower jiao on both eyes had changed obviously—the colour was pale. Which indicated a cold syndrome of deficiency type. The pain was relieved immediately after the orbital areas of lower jiao on both eyes were punctured. All the clinical manifestations disappeared five minutes afterwards.

5) *Puncturing along the border of the scapula to treat difficulty in raising the shoulder* Actually, the needle is inserted under the scapula and above the pleura. Ask the patient to sit with the chest stuck out to expose the medial border of the scapula for locating tenderness. Then, insert a needle perpendicularly 0.5 inch deep into the tender area along the border of the scapula. Next, flatten the needle and insert it horizontally towards the centre of the scapula. For example, there was a patient who had suffered from pain on the medial border of the left scapula for a few months, disturbing the movement of the shoulder. Recently, the pain was aggravated although he had received many treatments. Two tender areas were punctured as above. The pain disappeared immediately when the needle was withdrawn.

6) *Puncturing Tiaokou (S 38) for raising the arm* For limitation of arm movement due to the bi syndrome of cold and damp, Tiaokou (S 38) on the affected side can be punctured or penetrated towards Chengshan (B 57) with heavy stimulation. The therapeutic result is usually excellent.

7) *Puncturing Xuanzhong(G 39) for raising of the shoulder* It is applied for the

same cases mentioned as above. The therapeutic result of many cases was successful.

8) *Pricking the finger joints* Pricking the finger joints to cause little bleeding for heat bi syndrome due to invasion of wind and damp which is manifested by swelling of the finger joints and limited movement or rigidity of the finger joints.

9) *Application of the angled-needle* This method is effective for limited movement occurring only in one finger or toe without any other symptoms.

Case example: Wang x x, male, 63 years old, doctor.

Chief complaint: Rigidity and limitation of movement of the right thumb.

Treatment: An angled-needle was fixed on the joint of the thumb with an adhesive plaster. The needle was taken away after one week and the symptoms disappeared.

10) *Selecting points along the meridian* Select starting points, ending points, the points on both sides and the distal points along the meridians according to the location of the disease.

7. Application of ophthalmic acupuncture

Based on the theory, all qi and blood of the twelve regular meridians and 365 collaterals run upward to the face and brain, and their condition is manifested in the eyes, the orbital area can be divided into sections and the diseases can be differentiated according to the Eight Diagrammes in the seventh volume of *Treatment Standards* written by Wang Kengtang. Professor Peng has created his new ophthalmic acupuncture therapy by combining these classics with his clinical experience.

1) Division of the orbital areas With the eyes looking straight ahead, make an imaginary horizontal line from the inner canthus to outer canthus, passing through the centre of the pupil, and then make a vertical line from the upper orbit to the lower orbit, passing through the center of the pupil. In this way, the eye is divided into four quadrants. Each quadrant is subdivided into two equal areas, totaling eight equal-sized sections, which are considered as the eight orbital areas.

The book *Plain Questions* says, "Left and right sides of the body are the passages of yin and yang." The ancient physician Yang Shangshan was quoted, "Yin runs along the right side and yang runs along the left side." The left eye pertains to yang, which is promoted from yin. The order of the eight areas of the left eye is arranged clockwise, while the right eye pertains to yin which is promoted from yang, the arrangement of the eight areas is counterclockwise. But zang-fu organs, the area each represents, are the same on both sides.

Area 1. Lung and Large Intestine
Area 2. Kidney and Bladder
Area 3. Upper Jiao
Area 4. Liver and Gallbladder
Area 5. Middle Jiao
Area 6. Heart and Small Intestine
Area 7. Spleen and Stomach
Area 8. Lower Jiao

In order to describe the location of the eight orbital areas, we compare them to a

Distribution of the points around the eyes (13 points in 8 regions)

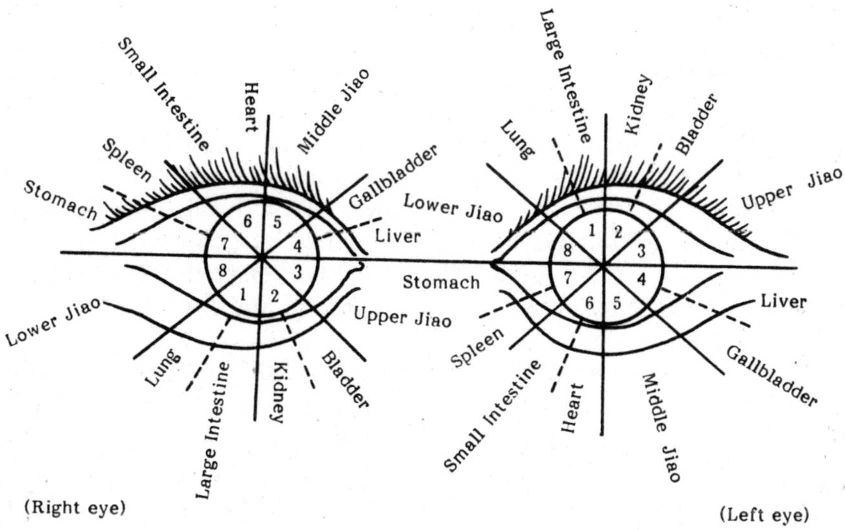

clock and the twelve hours. Ninety minutes represent the size of each orbital area, i.e. one-eighth of twelve hours.

For instance, Area 1 of the left eye is from 10:30-12:30 while Area 1 of the right eye is computed from 7:30-6:00.

There are altogether thirteen points in the eight orbital areas. In Area 1, 2, 4, 6 and 7 each area contains two organs, one zang and one fu i.e. lung, large intestine, kidney, bladder, liver, gallbladder, heart, small intestine, spleen and stomach, each occupying one half of each orbital area respectively. Areas 3, 5 and 8 represent the upper, middle and lower jiao respectively. The thirteen points are located around the orbit, one finger's width away from the pupil, i.e. between the lower edge of the eyebrow and a line 0.2 cun inferior to the lower border of the orbit. The eight areas and the thirteen points are called orbital areas and points.

2) Diagnosis by observing the eye Diagnosing a disease is performed by observing the changes of the shape and colour of the sclera and its capillaries. Capillaries with thick roots indicate a stubborn disease; tortuous and curving capillaries a severe disease; elongated capillaries, which may even affect the pupil or other areas, show that the disease has been transformed into another disease, or that more than two diseases or complications have occurred simultaneously; crisscrossing capillaries with many branches are the signs of emotional depression; protuberance of the capillaries are often seen in the disorders of the six fu organs; blurred or flaked capillaries mainly appear in disorders of the liver and gallbladder; and protuberance of capillaries in the stomach area indicates ascariasis or stagnation of blood if it also appears in other areas.

Fresh red colour indicates acute disease of excess type; a purple colour indicates excessive heat; a dark-red colour is considered as a severe disease; while a dark-purple colour is a sign that a recent disease has turned into heat. A mixture of red and yellow sclera or eye shows that the disease is a mild case. A light yellow shows improvement of the disease. A light red indicates a syndrome of the deficiency type or cold syndromes. A dark grey colour is a sign of chronic disease.

3) Principle for selecting points a. Selecting points according to the symptoms. Select the points in the area in which the changes of capillaries correspond to the symptoms. b. Selecting points by observing the eye. Just select the points in the area in which changes of capillaries are most obvious regardless of the symptoms. c. Selecting points from the areas of three jiao. This method is also named as selecting the points according to location of the diseases. For disorders of the head, upper extremities and chest, the upper jiao area could be used. For disorders of the epigastric region, back and corresponding organs, the middle jiao area may be selected. For disorders of the lumbar-sacral region, lower abdomen, urogenital system and disorders of lower extremities, the lower jiao area is used.

4) Method for locating the points a. Apply even, gentle pressure on the orbital areas and points with a detecting stick or the handle of three-edged needle. Any sensation of soreness, numbness, distension, heaviness, heat, coolness, slight pain or comfort is an indication of a point location. Then, press that particular point with more force to make a small pit as the marking of the point. Sometimes, just puncture the pit which appears spontaneously after pressing in case the patient reports absence of any particular sensation. b. Locating the point with the help of a meridian instrument. The spot which registers the highest reading on the meter is the location of the point. c. Puncture along the dividing line between areas. First divide the orbital area accurately with the pupil as the centre. Then insert the needle subcutaneously, horizontally or longitudinally along the dividing line between two areas.

5) Needling method First, press the eyeball and tighten the intraorbital skin with the left fingers, and then insert a 0.5-inch needle (32 gauge) with the right hand gently into the point. Usually a horizontal or oblique insertion is applied and the tip of the needle never goes beyond the selected area. Perpendicular insertion can be applied sometimes but never with manipulation. The needle should be lifted slightly and inserted towards another direction if there is no sensation of electrical shock, soreness, numbness, heat, coolness or comfort. The therapeutic result will be satisfactory for the patient who feels the needling sensation quickly, but unsatisfactory for the patient who has no sensation after needling. Inserting the needles into the orbital areas in the order of their numbering is considered as a reinforcing method, whereas inserting the needle against the order of the number arrangement is considered as a reducing method. Observation of a thousand cases with a double blind test showed that the results of 626 cases conformed to this rule, constituting 62.6 percent. The total conforming rate was above 99 percent. In clinical observation of 188 cases of hemiplegia due to apoplexy, the immediate therapeutic effect of ophthalmic acupuncture in restoring motor function was successful. Using the pre- and immediately post-treatment measurements of the straight leg elevation test in centimeters, 85.66 percent of the patients improved more than 5 cm. Forty-one cases (18.55 percent) could walk immediately after the treatment. In another study, 442 cases of six frequently seen pain syndromes were observed. The rate of effectiveness for leg pain was 97.6 percent, that for shoulder pain was 96.8 percent, that for lumbar pain was 96.8 percent, that for headache was 87.4 percent, and that for gastric and hypochondriac pain was 82.6 percent. The combined rate of effectiveness was 92.17 percent. In a clinically controlled study of the effect of this method on regulating blood pressure (103 cases), the statistics showed that there were marked improvements.

II. Case Analysis

Case 1: Windstroke (cerebral thrombosis)

Name, Lu x x; sex, female; age, 43.

Complaints During the night of September 10, 1979, she suddenly had hemiplegia on the left side of the body and was quickly admitted to the hospital. On examination, she was in a clear state of mind, had a slightly flushed face, heavy body-build and a deep and slow pulse. The myodynamia of the right side was 0 degree. The observation of the orbital area showed that the capillaries in the areas of upper and lower jiao of both eyes were thick and dark-red in colour. The diagnosis was stirring of liver wind.

Prescription Bilateral upper and lower jiao orbital areas.

Treatment procedure Immediately after insertion, the patient could raise her right leg and move her right arm. Then she was asked to walk around with the needles in place, while someone carried the intravenous perfusion bottle for her. She found with astonishment that she could walk as normally as a healthy person. She was discharged from hospital the next day and walked home unassisted. In all, five treatments were given. She returned to work two weeks later and has been healthy since then.

Case 2: Dizziness and vertigo (hypertension)

Name, Zhen x x; sex, male; age, 50; date of the first visit, October 8, 1976.

Complaints The patient had a past history of hypertension and often felt dizziness, blurred vision, dry eye and leukoma of the left eye (a thin white film over the eye). Upon examination, he was in a clear state of mind accompanied by a flushed face, red tongue with little coating, and a string-taut pulse, especially in the left Guan region. Blood pressure was 170/100 mmHg.

Prescription The radial artery near Taiyuan (L 9), liver orbital area.

Treatment procedure Puncture the radial artery near Taiyuan (L 9). The body of the needle quivered slightly after needling. The blood pressure was 156/90 mmHg after the needle was removed. It was 160/100 mmHg before receiving the second treatment, in which the ophthalmic liver areas were needled bilaterally. The needles were retained for ten minutes and the blood pressure dropped to 150/98 mmHg. All the symptoms were alleviated and the patient felt comfortable. The blood pressure was 120/80 mmHg before the third treatment. The liver areas (bilaterally) were punctured again in the third treatment, and the blood pressure remained stable. Before the fourth treatment, the patient had no uncomfortable feelings although the blood pressure had risen to 150/90 mmHg, which was considered normal for his age. The same points were repeated in the fifth treatment and the blood pressure dropped to 130/90 mmHg.

Case 3: Erysipelas

Name, Li x x; sex, female; age, 19; date of the first visit, June 10, 1977.

Complaints The patient was usually healthy. Erythema, about the size of her palm, suddenly appeared on her leg, accompanied by a fever of 39°C at night.

Injections of penicillin and streptomycin did not help her. On examination, her mind was clear. She had a fat body-build, a flushed face, a dry tongue and a superficial and rapid pulse. In the lung areas of the eyes, tortuous, dark-red capillaries could be seen. WBC was 15,300 mm^3, Neut. were 85 percent, and LYM were 26 percent. It was diagnosed as lung heat.

Prescription Lung orbital areas.

Results after treatment: The blood test showed that WBC was 10,000 mm^3, Neut. were 61 percent, and LYM were 39 percent twenty minutes after treatment.

Case 4: Lumbago

Name, Tian x x; sex, male; age, 47; date of the first visit, October 4, 1976.

Complaints The main symptom was lumbago due to lumbar sprain, accompanied by pain and numbness of the left leg and limitation of movement. The X-ray showed obvious protrusion of the third and fourth intervertebral disc. Examination by a surgeon revealed an injury of the pirifrom muscle. All the symptoms remained even though massage was applied and drugs were taken. He could not walk, turn the body or go upstairs, because he could only elevate the left leg 50 cm and the right leg 45 cm (above the surface of the bed). The pulse was deep and slow, with a weak quality in the Chi region. Marked changes, such as thin pale-coloured capillaries, were seen in both the ophthalmic middle and lower jiao areas. The diagnosis was deficiency of yang qi due to injury of the Du Meridian.

Prescription Middle and lower jiao orbital areas (bilaterally).

Treatment procedure After the first treatment, the left leg could be elevated 67 cm and the right leg 63 cm. After the second treatment, he could walk a little with the help of others, since the pain was diminished greatly. After the third treatment, he could walk slowly without anyone's help, since the pain and numbness were getting better. Altogether five treatments were given. Then he could raise both of his legs 74 cm above the surface of bed.

Case 5: Hysteria

Name, Wang x x; sex, male; age, 14; date of the first visit, April 30, 1974.

Complaints Three months before, the boy's head was hit powerfully by his playmate. Since then, he often suffered from headaches, dizziness, vertigo and poor appetite, which became so bad that he was unable to eat. During the previous two weeks, he suffered often from anorexia, and his only nourishment was sugar water. He had to lie in bed all day. Neither herbal medicine nor drugs helped him. All the laboratory tests were normal, excluding any organic disorders. Clinical manifestations were emaciation, lassitude, no desire to open the eyes, sallow complexion, a dry tongue without coating, rigidity of the limbs, and a deep and thready pulse. The diagnosis was deficiency of qi and blood, resulting in exhaustion of stomach yang.

Prescription Sifeng (Extra) was punctured first and much white mucus spurted out. Then he took a decoction for toning yang and strengthening the stomach, created by Li Donghen, an ancient physician.

Treatment procedure After five treatments, the boy began to feel better and could walk with help. The pulse was stronger, but the anorexia had failed to improve. Any food intake made him suffer with stomach distension. Thus, retention of food in the stomach was confirmed, according to the saying, "people who have a stomach disorder dislike food." When questioned about his daily food intake, it was reported that he ate steamed bread or wheat flour bread and cooked sorghum. Then, he was asked to take a mixture of charred and ground steam bread and cooked sorghum, 100 gm of each were taken with brown sugar water. In the meantime, Sifeng (Extra), Zhongwan (Ren 12), and Chengshan (B 57) were needled. Three days later, he could eat a little. He continued the treatment for one week and his anorexia was relieved. Thirteen days later his appetite was better than before. After the eighth treatment, he was cured completely and had an active spirit and strong body-build.

Deficiency of stomach yang, manifesting in anorexia with a duration of more than two weeks, is rarely seen in the clinic. The reason for this recovery includes three aspects as follows:

1) Puncturing Sifeng (Extra) may restore the functions of the six hand meridians so as to maintain the normal function of their corresponding internal organs.

2) The decoction for toning yang and strengthening the stomach may rescue the stomach yang from deteriorating into exhaustion. Therefore, the appetite returned to normal.

3) Mixing brown sugar with a charred form of the food which caused the disease is a folk prescription for retention of food. It is always effective whenever it is used.

TREATMENT BASED ON DIFFERENTIATION OF SYNDROMES, HERBS AND ACUPUNCTURE BEING OF THE SAME SOURCE

—Cheng Xinnong's Clinical Experience

Cheng Xinnong, a native of Huaiyin County, Jiangsu Province, was born in August 1921. He began to learn traditional Chinese medicine from his father in 1930 and took Lu Muhan, a famous practitioner in his hometown as his teacher in 1936. He started his medical career in 1939 and in 1947 he got his medical licence. Just after 1949 he was admitted to the class for advanced studies of Chinese medicine in Qingjiang, Jiangsu Province and Jiangsu College for the Advanced Study of Traditional Chinese Medicine. In 1957 he began to work in the Acupuncture Teaching Section, Beijing College of Traditional Chinese Medicine. At first he chiefly treated internal and gynecological problems, especially acute febrile diseases. Later, he practised acupuncture. His works include *Annotations on Classic on Medical Problems, Explanation of Classic on Medical Problems, Essentials of Chinese Acupuncture,* etc. Now he is an acupuncture professor at the Acupuncture Institute, the China Academy of Traditional Chinese Medicine, the deputy-director of the China Beijing International Acupuncture Training Center, Adviser of the Beijing Acupuncture Society and Vice-president of the Chinese Acupuncture Association.

I. Academic Characteristics and Medical Specialities

1. Giving acupuncture before disease arises

Giving treatment before disease arises is one of the principal concepts in *Internal Classics.* It is stated in *Classic on Medical Problems* that, "while treating the liver disease it is necessary to reinforce the spleen before it is involved, because the liver and spleen are closely related to each other." Cheng believes when a diseased organ is being treated, measures must be taken to prevent its complication in other related organs. For example, in treating exuberance of yang of the liver, Sanyinjiao (Sp 6) or Zusanli (S 36) are often punctured to prevent complication in the spleen. When heat in the lung is being eliminated, acupuncture is applied to Qimen (Liv 14) or Yanglingquan (G 34) to prevent complications in the liver. Here is an example. A 51-year-old Mr. Zhou had had hemiplegia of the right side four months before, accompanied by nausea, vomiting and loss of consciousness. He was diagnosed as having cerebral hemorrhage, and hospitalized for about twenty days. He recovered movement of the left arm. When he came for treatment, he felt weakness of the left arm, numb fingers and motion impairment of the left leg. Other symptoms included a bitter taste in the mouth, a sensation of head distension, dream-disturbed sleep, night sweat, puffy, dark red tongue with yellow greasy coating, and a deep and slippery pulse. This was a case of exuberance of yang of the liver and obstruction of the meridians by phlegm. The following points were selected. They were Baihui (Du 20), Dazhui (Du 14), Fengchi (G 20), Taiyang (Extra 2), Taichong (Liv 3), Fenglong (S 40), Sanyinjiao (Sp 6) and Hegu (LI 4), on both sides, and Jianyu (LI 15), Quchi (LI 11), Waiguan (SJ 5), Baxie (Extra 28), Yanglingquan (G 34) and Xuanzhong (G 39) on the left side. They were used to subdue exuberance of yang of the liver, dispel phlegm to remove obstruction. However, there was no response after a week's treatment. Then Cheng pointed out although there was no deficiency in the spleen it was necessary to invigorate the spleen and prevent complications of the spleen due to liver disorders. Zusanli (S 36) was added with the reinforcing method. Two treatments cured the night sweat and nine treatments cured numbness of the finger and motion impairment. The patient recovered in sixteen treatments and began to do a half day's work.

2. Treatment based on the patient's condition

Treatment based on the patient's condition is one of the treating principles in traditional Chinese medicine. Diseases of the same cause, symptoms and pathogenesis may be treated differently because of different ages, constitution and sex. Shallow needling with minor stimulation is usually used by Cheng for women, the elderly and thin patients. For children he gives mild stimulation without needle retention. For strong patients he gives strong stimulations. Furthermore, in acupuncture therapy he takes psychological factors into consideration. Minor stimulation is given to those who are afraid of acupuncture and the first visitors. Shallow puncture is applied with less points selected to avoid fear and restlessness.

Different methods are used for various conditions. For example, acupuncture and moxibustion are often applied to syndromes of wind, cold, damp and numbness. Acupuncture is given to the diseased part and moxibustion to the healthy part for facial paralysis. For patients of muscular spasm the reinforcing method is applied to the diseased part and the reducing method to the healthy part. Distal points are selected first to alleviate pain, afterwards the local points are used. Acupuncture is given to the tender spot for acute lumbar sprain with needle retention of ten to twenty minutes, during which manipulations are done two to three times. Cheng had treated two cases of facial paralysis due to obstruction of the meridians by pathogenic wind on the second day of the attack. Both Dazhui (Du 14), Fengchi (G 20), Taichong (Liv 3), Hegu (LI 4), Xiaguan (S 7), Jiache (S 6), Dicang (S 4) and Quanliao (SI 18) were selected with the even movement method and needle retention for twenty minutes. Two weeks later, a middle-aged woman patient of strong constitution was better but a 58-year-old thin male patient did not improve. Based on the difference of constitution, shallow puncture and minor stimulation were given first to the healthy part and then to the diseased part to promote the flow of meridian qi. Afterwards Zusanli (S 36) was needled to improve the function of the acquired material basis. Invigorated function of the spleen and stomach could help to expel the pathogenic factors. After thirty-six treatments the man recovered. Thus it is important to treat patients and select points based on different conditions.

3. Combination of points

The number of points to be selected in treatment is not fixed or unchangeable. It is said in *Elementary of Medicine* that "one needling is enough for a disease, four needlings are at most. It is bad to give so many needlings." Cheng thinks that the number of points selected is decided by the manifestations of the case. Sometimes he uses one or two points or fifteen to thirty points for one treatment. For instance, Mr. Wang had suffered from a pain of the left arm for a month. Pain ceased after acupuncture was applied to Yangxi (L 25) and Ashi for four times. Another, 48-year-old Mr. Zhao had exuberance of yang of the liver, stirring up internal wind. Symptoms included vomiting, dizziness and numbness of the left side. Acupuncture was given to Baihui (Du 20), Fengchi (G 20), Dicang (S 4), Jiache (S 6), Hegu (LI 4), Sanjian (LI 3), Waiguan (SJ 5), Houxi (SI 3), Huantiao (G 30), Yanglingquan (G 34), Chengshan (B 57) and Taichong (Liv 3) (some points only to be used on one side) to check liver yang and wind. On the following day the blood pressure turned to normal. Twenty-five treatments in total relieved the symptoms. Cheng usually selects three to five points in one treatment, e.g. Baihui (Du 20), Hegu (LI 4), Taichong (Liv 3) for apoplexy; Jianyu (LI 15), Quchi (LI 11), Huantiao (G 30) and Yanglingquan (G 34) for hemiplegia; Jiache (S 6) and Dicang (S 4) for facial paralysis. The other points are the secondary points.

In the final analysis, a disease means the confrontation between the anti-pathogenic and pathogenic factors, its development is a process from quantitative change to qualitative change. The change of a chronic disease is more prolonged and the appearance of the curative effect is slower too. A doctor must be clear-headed. When he believes he knows what the syndrome is, he has to stick to the prescription, never using this point today and that point tomorrow. For example, a 38-year-old Ms Li was diagnosed as having rheumatic heart disease due to insufficient heart qi and blood stasis in the meridians. She was treated by puncturing Neiguan (P 6), Tanzhong (Ren 17), Xinshu (B 15), Feishu (B 13) and Sanyinjiao (Sp 6). Forty-eight treatments in three months finally cured the case without any changes of points. This is evidence showing the importance to stick to the same prescription when the syndrome is decided. Frequent change of the prescription may have bad result.

4. Stress on manipulation

Cheng emphasizes the importance of manipulations, but he maintains that some manipulations that cannot be repeated by others should be abandoned. Light, quick and correct puncture is the feature of his manipulations. He often punctures a point without pain in one or two seconds.

How to use finger force is thought to be the basic skill in acupuncture. That is why Cheng often stresses the finger force in manipulations. He can cure a case with the same points which were used by others with failure because of his manipulations. For example, a patient had suffered from facial paralysis for a month and there was no response to any treatment including acupuncture. He came to Cheng for help. Jingming (B 1), Juliao (S 3) and Sibai (S 2) were needled. The condition was markedly improved in 13 treatments, and 24 treatments cured the case.

5. Theory guiding compatibility of herbs and points

Cheng points out that same theory guiding compatibility of herbs and points, and subjects for treatment. For instance, in treating a case due to breakdown of the normal physiological coordination between the heart and kidney *Rhizoma Coptidis* and *Cortex Cinnamomi* are administered to restore the normal balance between the heart and kidney. In acupuncture Taixi (K 3), the Yuan-(source) point of the Kidney Meridian and Shenmen (H 7), the Yuan-(source) point of the Heart Meridian are used to reach the same purpose. "Decoction for Reinforcing the Stomach and Replenishing Qi" is prescribed for cases due to deficiency in the spleen and stomach, and sinking of qi of the spleen. For these cases Cheng often uses Baihui (Du 20), Qihai (Ren 6) or Guanyuan (Ren 4), Sanyinjiao (Sp 6), Yanglingquan (G 34), Zusanli (S 36) and Quchi (LI 11). He believes that Qihai (Ren 6), or Guanyuan (Ren 4) may invigorate yang of the stomach and spleen, functioning as that of *Radix Astragali* and *Radix Codonopsis Pilosula.* Baihui (Du 20) may bring yang upward, having the same function as *Rhizoma Cimicifugae.* Zusanli (S 36), Sanyinjiao (Sp 6) have the same effect as *Rhizoma Atractylodis Macrocephalae, Radix Glycyrrhizae* and *Radix Angelicae Sinensis* in regulating qi and blood, and replenishing yin. Quchi (LI 11) has the same function as *Rhizoma Zingiberis* and *Fructus Ziziphi Jujubae* in dispelling wind and regulating qi and blood. For example, 52-year-old Ms Zeng complained she had had weak, numb left hand three years before. Then she had speech disturbance, difficulty in writing with the right hand and weak legs. She was diagnosed as having Parkinson's disease. Because she was allergic to artane she came to ask for help. On the first visit, she was found to have shortness of breath, slow action, difficulty in swallowing, dizziness, stuffiness of the chest, dry cough, poor appetite, dry stools, weak thin legs, a pale red tongue with thin white coating, string-taut and thready pulse. This was a case due to deficiency of qi and blood, malnutrition of muscles and tendons and obstruction of meridians by pathogenic wind. Points used were Guanyuan (Ren 4) (with moxibustion), Baihui (Du 20), Zusanli (S 36), Sanyinjiao (Sp 6), Yanglingquan (G 34), Quchi (LI 11), Fengchi (G 20), Hegu (LI 4) and Taichong (Liv 3). After ten treatments the case was markedly improved. Then Lianquan (Ren 23), Shenshu (B 23) and Ganshu (B 18) were added. Another thirteen treatments cured the case. Qi deficiency was the main problem of the case and it resulted in blood deficiency. Deficiency of qi and blood was thought to be the root cause and obstruction of meridians by pathogenic wind the secondary cause. For this reason, Guanyuan (Ren 4), Baihui (Du 20), Zusanli (S 36), Sanyinjiao (Sp 6), Yanglingquan (G 34), Quchi (LI 11) were applied to invigorate qi and benefit the spleen and stomach. Taichong (Liv 3), Fengchi (G 20) and Hegu (LI 4) were selected to remove obstruction. The Shenshu (B 23), Ganshu (B 18) were added to replenish yin and blood. The effect of this prescription is similar to that of herbs.

6. Puncture of four pass points to regulate qi and blood

Normal physiological activity cannot be separated from qi and blood and disturbance of qi and blood brings about disease. Acupuncture therapy is an approach to regulate qi and blood by puncturing points. In terms of qi and blood, the former serves as the leading role and dynamic force of blood flow. Therefore, regulation of qi is most important. Any disease due to deficiency of yin, yang, qi or blood is often accompanied by the unsmooth flow of qi. For example, cases of hemiplegia due to apoplexy, numbness of limbs, flaccid paralysis of limbs or obstruction of meridians are usually associated with stagnation of qi. In treatment Taichong (Liv 3), the Yuan-(source) point of Liver Meridian, Hegu (LI 4), the Yuan-(source) points of the Large Intestine Meridian, are selected to regulate qi flow. The Yuan-(source) points are closely related to the Sanjiao which not only generates qi but also distributes qi and blood. From the above we can see the Yuan-(source) points are so important in regulation of qi and blood. Taichong (Liv 3) and Hegu (LI 4) are known as four pass points, which are believed to be the most important points in regulation of qi and blood of the zang-fu organs. Through his long clinical practice Cheng understands the four pass points may promote the smooth flow of qi and blood and shorten the treatment course. Once he treated a 56-year-old male patient, who had suffered from cerebral thrombosis with symptoms of dizziness, insomnia, lassitude, motion impairment of the left arm and leg, deep, thready pulse and pale tongue. This was a case due to deficiency of qi and blood, malnutrition of blood vessels. Baihui (Du 20), Guanyuan (Ren 4) (with moxibustion), Jianyu (LI 15), Quchi (LI 11), Waiguan (SJ 5), Huantiao (G 30), Weizhong (B 40), Zusanli (S 36), Yanglingquan (G 34), Taixi (K 3) and Baxie (Extra 28) were applied for three months without much success. Then Taichong (Liv 3) and Hegu (LI 4) were added. Another one month treatment nearly cured the case. The patient could walk around and took care of himself.

Taichong (liv 3) and Hegu (LI 4) were punctured with the even movement method to induce and regulate smooth flow of qi.

II. Case Analysis

Case 1: Five retardations—retarded in standing, walking, hair-growing, tooth formation and speaking.

Name, Cheng Kuangbo; sex, male; age, 2; date of the first visit, August 31, 1985.

Complaints He was a premature infant, born two months earlier than normal. Five months after his birth, he was found to be underdeveloped and was diagnosed by a local hospital as having calcium deficiency. Treatment was given without success. When he was one year old he was diagnosed at the Taiyuan Hospital, Shanxi Province as having cerebral paralysis. He started to get his teeth at fourteen months. When he came for treatment, the baby could not speak, stand, walk or eat properly. He has a dull expression and general paralysis. His tongue was pale red with thin white coating and the superficial veins of his fingers were light red.

Differentiation Deficiency in the liver and kidney, insufficient qi and blood.

Method Tone the liver and kidney, regulate qi and blood, strengthen the function of the brain.

Prescription Baihui (Du 20), Ganshu (B 18), Shenshu (B 23), Guanyuan (Ren 4), Taixi (K 3), Sishencong (Extra 6), Lianquan (Ren 23), Tianquan (P 2), Fengchi (G 20), Dazhui (Du 14), Neiguan (P 6), Hegu (LI 4), Taichong (Liv 3), Zusanli (S 36), Yanglingquan (G 34), Xuanzhong (G 39) and Sanyinjiao (Sp 6).

Treatment procedure The reinforcing method was applied and the needle was immediately withdrawn after appearance of the needling reaction. After treatments for four months, symptoms were markedly relieved. He could stand and walk a little with the help of his parents and have a soft diet. Treatment was given continuously once a day for four months and the case was cured.

Explanation This is a premature infant, suffering from innate insufficiency, deficiency in the liver and kidney and postnatal malnutrition, leading to underdevelopment. Ganshu (B 18), Shenshu (B 23), Guanyuan (Ren 4) and Taixi (K 3) were needled to tone the liver and kidney. The secondary points were Sanyinjiao (Sp 6), Zusanli (S 36) used to strengthen the function of the spleen and stomach, the acquired material basis. Sishencong (Extra 6) and Dazhui (Du 14) were selected to improve the brain function. Lianquan (Ren 23) was for retarded speaking. Neiguan (P 6), Tianquan (P 2) and Hegu (LI 4) were for smooth flow of the meridian qi. Deficiency in the liver and kidney was the principal aspect of the case and the main points were used to solve this problem. Other points were applied for the secondary symptoms.

Case 2: Herpes zoster

Name, Zhou Zhongwen; sex, male; age, 52; date of the first visit, July 24, 1985.

Complaints Two days before the acupuncture therapy he suddenly had a patch of 4 x 4 cm red spots on the left side of the waist and a patch of 4 x 7 cm red spots above them. There was intolerable pain, a bitter taste in the mouth and brown urine. It was diagnosed as herpes zoster by a clinic and he was given herbs without success.

Differentiation Invasion of the flesh and muscles by pathogenic fire.

Method Eliminating fire and toxicity, promoting the smooth flow of qi and blood.

Prescription Both Fengchi (G 20), Daling (P 7), Weizhong (B 40) and Quchi (LI 11); and plum-blossom needling applied to Waiguan (SJ 5) and Yanglingquan (G 34).

Treatment procedure The first treatment alleviated pain. On the second visit, the red spot turned to light red. Ten treatments stopped pain and the diseased part got smaller. Fourteen treatments cured the case.

Explanation This was a case due to pathogenic fire invading the blood system and the flesh and muscles, resulting in stagnant qi and blood. Fengchi (G 20), Quchi (LI 11) were needled to dispel fire and regulate qi and blood. Weizhong (B 40) and Daling (P 7) were for eliminating fire and toxity. Waiguan (SJ 5) was selected to remove stagnancy of qi and blood. Yanglingquan (G 34) was for regulation of qi flow in the liver and gallbladder.

Case 3: Migraine

Name, Wang Yanzheng; sex, female; age, 66; date of the first visit, March 4, 1986.

Complaints She had had migraine for two months, and it became worse recently. There was a paroxysmal or persisted pain and a numb feeling at the crown, associated with left toothache. There was no response to herbs and acupuncture treatment. Symptoms included costal pain, a red crack tongue with thin white coating, string-taut and thready pulse.

Differentiation Stagnation of liver qi, yin deficiency in the liver and kidney and fire due to deficiency going upward.

Prescription Baihui (Du 20), Taiyang (Extra 2), Fengchi (G 20), Hegu (LI 4), Taixi (K 3), Waiguan (SJ 5), Taichong (Liv 3), Sanyinjiao (Sp 6); Touwei (S 8), Xiaguan (S 7), Jiache (S 6), Shuaigu (G 8) of the left side.

Treatment procedure The reducing method was applied. Two treatments cured the toothache and alleviated the headache markedly. Then the even movement method was used for eight treatments and all the symptoms disappeared.

Explanation This case was due to insufficient yin because she was over sixty. The red crack in the tongue was also from the same problem. Stagnation of the liver qi impaired yin too, resulting in fire going upward and headache. Baihui (Du 20), Taixi (K 3) were selected to replenish yin and tone the kidney. Taichong (Liv 3) was for regulation of the liver qi. Taiyang (Extra 2), Fengchi (G 20) and Hegu (LI 4) were used to eliminate fire and remove obstruction of the meridians. Touwei (S 8), Xiaguan (S 7), Jiache (S 6) and Shuaigu (G 8) were points helpful to migraine. Sanyinjiao (Sp 6) was punctured to strengthen the function of the spleen and stomach. Good compatibility of points led to successful results.

Case 4: Facial paralysis

Name, Meng Jianhua; sex, female; age, 28; date of the first visit, November 16, 1985.

Complaints She had had wry mouth for eight days, associated with failure of the right eye to close and a tight feeling on the right side of the face. Other symptoms included red tongue tip with yellow greasy coating, deep, thready and weak pulse.

Differentiation Invasion of the meridians by pathogenic wind.

Method Dispel wind and promote smooth flow of meridian qi.

Prescription Baihui (Du 20), Fengchi (G 20) and Hegu (LI 4) on the left side; Yangbai (G 14), Taiyang (Extra 2), Zanzhu (B 2), Sibai (S 2), Quanliao (SI 18), Jiache (S 6), Dicang (S 4) and Jingming (B 1) on the right side.

Treatment procedure The right eye was able to close after one treatment. Yuyao (Extra 3) was added in addition to the above points. Thirteen treatments cured the case.

Explanation The patient was a young strong woman peasant, and the disease course was short. Deep, thready and weak pulse was due to invasion of meridians by pathogenic wind, which should not be considered as a deficiency case. The chief points used were Baihui (Du 20), Fengchi (G 20), Hegu (LI 4) to dispel wind and strengthen the meridian function. The secondary points were selected to relieve other symptoms. Although the reducing method was applied, the genuine qi must not be injured because it was the basis of vital function.

Case 5: Numbness in the face

Name, Wu Chuanming; sex, male; age, 65; date of the first visit, August 30, 1984.

Complaints About forty days before he had found numbness in the left part of the face, because of working too hard and affliction of wind. He was diagnosed as having terminal nervous paralysis. VB_1, VB_6, injection of *Fructus Chaenomelis* and Bolus of *Rhizoma Gastrodiae* were given, accompanied by acupuncture treatment for thirty days without success. His tongue was red with a white coating and his pulse was string-taut.

Differentiation Invasion of meridians by pathogenic wind, unsmooth flow of qi and blood.

Method Dispelling wind and promoting smooth flow of meridian qi.

Prescription Baihui (Du 20), Hegu (LI 4), Taichong (Liv 3), Fengchi (G 20), Jiache (S 6) and Heliao (LI 19).

Treatment procedure Numbness alleviated after seven treatments with mild stimulations. Another eight treatments markedly relieved the symptoms. Nineteen treatments cured the case.

Explanation The patient said he had been treated by acupuncture with strong stimulations without success. Same points had been used except Baihui (Du 20). The patient was a 65-year-old intellectual. All day long he worked at a desk and had a weak constitution. Therefore mild stimulation was given with the appropriate reducing technique. Finally pain ceased. From this we can see the importance of treating different conditions with different methods.

ADOPTING RIGHT SECONDARY POINTS AND PUNCTURE TECHNIQUES, COMBINING ACUPUNCTURE WITH QIGONG

—Jiao Guorui's Clinical Experience

Jiao Guorui, a native of Fengren County, Hebei Province, was born in a well-known family of traditional Chinese medicine. He started practising qigong since childhood. As a graduate of the North-China School of Traditional Chinese Medicine, he has made great contributions to training domestic and foreign acupuncturists, and popularizing qigong. He has passed on his knowledge about qigong to people from about forty countries. Now he is a research fellow of the Acupuncture Institute, director of the Qigong Teaching Section, China Academy of Traditional Chinese Medicine, vice-chairman of the All China Qigong Science Association, and member of the Standing Committee of the China Qigong Science Society.

I. Academic Characteristics and Medical Specialities

1. Coordination of points selection and bodily posture

Curative effect is influenced by point selection and correct selection of points is closely related to bodily posture in acupuncture treatment. In his practice Jiao has discovered a tense posture to get special needling result in certain conditions. For example, when there is a soft tissue injury, one should try to find the most painful muscles on motion, then keep it fixed (known as the tense posture) and give acupuncture. It may greatly improve the results.

2. Giving considerations to points and point area

It is generally held that a point is only a fixed spot on the body, that is why it is sometimes called a stimulating spot. Some people believe a point extends, forming an area and any spot on the body can be needled. Jiao thinks that points are distributed on the body as spots with different depth, size and function. The size of a point is flexible, some are bigger and some are smaller. For example, Hegu (LI 4) is bigger and Yifeng (SJ 17) is smaller; Huantiao (G 30) is far bigger and Sibai (S 2) is far smaller. In addition, every point has its effective area, known as point area. Points may be round-shaped or linear-shaped. The most sensitive part of the point area is called the effective spot, which can be measured by an apparatus or finger pressure. For instance, a sensitive spot may appear at Zhiyang (Du 9) on the back and Zusanli (S 36) in patients with acute hepatitis and gastroduodenal ulcer.

3. Appropriate combination of points

Combination of points varies based on theories of meridians, organs, yin-yang and five elements, neurophysiology and anatomy. Jiao thinks that the following must be kept in mind no matter what kind of combination of points is used.

1) *Combination of the main and secondary points* This is a usual approach. For example, in treatment of the common cold, Dazhui (Du 14) and Fengchi (G 20) are the main points, Hegu (LI 4) and Zusanli (S 36) are the secondary points. In treatment of bed-wetting, the chief points are Qihai (Ren 6) and Guanyuan (Ren 4), while the secondary points are Sanyinjiao (Sp 6) and Zusanli (S 36). Besides, the combination of the chief and secondary points must be decided by symptoms. For instance, if a patient with a common cold has headache (in the upper), fever, cough and tiredness, Dazhui (Du 14), Taiyang (Extra 2) and Hegu (LI 4) are the main points and Zusanli (S 36) is the secondary point. But point selection should not only be decided by symptoms. The main points are usually used to treat the chief problem of the disease, and the secondary points help the main points and solve the minor problems.

2) *Selection of local and distal points* Any point may bring effect to the local part, vicinal part, distal part or the whole body. These are the four functions, yet they are inseparable from each other. Therefore, selection of local and distal points must be used together to supplement each other. People often attach importance to the general effect of acupuncture and pay less attention to its local function. When he joined a mobile medical team working in the countryside, Jiao often encountered patients with joint pains. He treated them by using the local points with a quick response. However, we must point out that one must never puncture points on the head when the head aches and puncture points on the foot when the foot hurts. The distal point effect must be taken into account. Based on his experience, Jiao combined the local with the distal points to treat the case and improve the effect.

3) *Number of points selected according to different individual conditions* Some people believe that using less secondary points may reduce patients' sufferings. This is not always true. The number of secondary points selected is determined by the conditions. For example, only Huantiao (G 30) is used for simple sciatica with marked results.

But for frequently seen arthritis or hemiplegia, more points are selected. Otherwise the effect is not so good. In short, the number of points used is decided by different conditions.

4) *Points selected in the diseased side and the healthy side* The diseased side and the healthy side form part of an organic whole. Both sides are related to each other physiologically and pathologically. A diseased part of the body often affects the opposite side or the part connected with the former. A correspondent tender spot and other pathological changes may be found there. This is the basis of selection of points in the diseased and healthy sides. But for a case whether to select points in the diseased side or the healthy side is decided by the particular condition. According to his experience, Jiao usually needles the points in the diseased side. If there is no marked effect, he needles

the points in the healthy side or uses points on both sides to improve effects. For instance, in treatment of facial paralysis Yangbai (G 14), Xiaguan (S 7), Dicang (S 4) and Hegu (LI 4) of the diseased side and those on the healthy side are punctured.

4. Appropriate needling technique

There are varied needling techniques according to the ancient medical classics and records of development by the later generations. Based on his own clinical experience Jiao has summarized the following aspects:

1) *Appropriate stimulation* Acupuncture is a kind of stimulation in detail in terms of modern physiology. Some works about acupuncture offer the idea that "mild stimulation is an excitation, while strong stimulation is an inhibition." But this idea cannot reflect the whole effect of acupuncture on the body. Jiao holds that the effect of acupuncture is based on the stimulating part, nature, intensity, duration and time. Under the same stimulating condition, the effect of acupuncture is decided by the patient's functional state. Therefore the effect of acupuncture is adjustment. Excitation and inhibition are actually a dual-direction adjustment induced by acupuncture. If we want to bring acupuncture therapy into full play, we must study the transforming process, and give appropriate stimulation according to the functional state and reaction capacity.

2) *Appropriate depth of puncture* Some doctors advocate deep puncture, and others advocate shallow puncture. Jiao believes the depth of puncture is not rigid. Different depth is for various points. As to a particular point the depth of puncture varies and a different effect is brought about. Generally, shallow puncture produces weak stimulation and vice versa. For example, Huantiao (G 30) is often punctured deeper to treat sciatica, but Feishu (B 13) is shallowly needled to treat lung problems.

3) *Appropriate rate of puncture of a needle* Similar to the opinions of deep and shallow puncture, there are varied opinions and some people advocate quick puncture and some advocate slow puncture. Jiao holds that the rate of insertion of a needle is decided by the case condition, the stimulation desired, and the location of the points in terms of anatomy. Generally, slow puncture is applied to points on the face and head, where the muscle is thin. Quick puncture is applied to the part where the muscle is thick. Furthermore, the speed of puncture is related to the process of acupuncture. Quick insertion of a needle into the skin is done to avoid pain at first and then it is slowly thrust to the intended depth.

4) *Duration of stimulation* It includes the time for operation and needle retention, decided by the case condition and the desirable intensity of stimulation. Generally, short effect is produced by short stimulation and vice versa. But it is not necessarily that the longer the stimulation the better. When the volume of stimulation goes beyond limitation, qualitative change occurs. When the needle is retained and the needling reaction decreases or disappears, it does not mean stimulation ceases. At this moment the stimulation is weaker than when the needle is being rotated.

5) *Appropriate manipulations* Appropriate manipulations are extremely important to an acupuncturist. In 1965 Jiao encountered a patient of metatarsal bones not due to inflammation, which affects walking. At first acupuncture was given to the painful part

or to its vicinity with strong stimulation. After a dozen treatments pain was temporarily relieved. The needling was given to Rangu (K 2) towards the little toe, 2.5 cun in depth. One treatment of moderate persistant stimulation relieved most pain and another five treatments cured the case.

6) *Appropriate stimulation* Some people think mild stimulation may produce excitation or reinforcement, strong and moderate stimulation may produce inhibition or reduction. Jiao does not agree with the idea. For example, facial paralysis is a condition of inhibition and moderate stimulation may produce better effect. But for insomnia, a condition of excitation, persisted strong stimulation does not produce inhibition, on the contrary it induces strong excitement. Therefore, it is better to give moderate stimulation. Dr. Jiao's experience tells us that mild, moderate and strong stimulations with or without needle retention may produce excitation and inhibition and different individuals have varied physiological reactions and effects.

5. Emphasis on the needling reaction

Needling reaction is closely related to effect. Generally, appropriate needling reaction brings about good effect. For instance, a patient with rheumatism in the legs was treated by Dr. Jiao. When Zusanli (S 36) was needled, the patient had a feeling of a regular flow of warm water for a long time. With every twirling of the needle, the same feeling appeared. Every three to four hours after acupuncture treatment given that day and the following day he had such a feeling. Five treatments cured the case.

6. Combining acupuncture with qigong

Through the regulation of body and mind, using breathing by qigong exercises, acupuncturists can bring the genuine qi into full play. A patient practising qigong may benefit from the regulation of qi and blood to speed up recovery. A qigong-acupuncturist can promote travel of his internal qi to the finger and toes before acupuncture treatment. Then he can improve his treatment with manipulations. The mechanism of qigong-acupuncture still has to be explored, but there is no doubt that a new way to improve the curative effect has been found.

II. Case Analysis

Case 1: Schizophrenia

A foreign child; age, 5; date of the first visit, March, 1954.

Complaints As a baby she was cared for by a nurse. Afterwards, she was found to have dull-looking eyes, an uncommunicative and eccentric disposition and a preference for hygine. She liked to bite nails and muttered to herself. She was diagnosed as having child schizophrenia by a hospital in her own country and there was no response to any treatment. When she was in China her parents asked for help from acupuncture therapy.

On the first visit, the physical examination showed she had a normal development and nutrition. There was no sign of a vegetative nervous disturbance and no trauma. She did not like to be examined. She had a pale tongue and slippery pulse.

Differentiation Internal growth of phlegm and damp leading to mind disturbance.

Prescription Baihui (Du 20), Naohu (Du 17), Yamen (Du 15), Fengchi (G 20), Renzhong (Du 26) (occasionally used), Dazhui (Du 14), Shenzhu (Du 12), Mingmen (Du 4), Shenshu (B 23), Xinshu (B 15), Quchi (LI 11), Neiguan (P 6), Hegu (LI 4), Shenmen (H 7), Daling (P 7), Zusanli (S 36), Sanyinjiao (Sp 6), Taichong (Liv 3) and Xingjian (Liv 2).

Treatment procedure Four to eight points were used ålternately with mild, short and intermittent stimulations for about a minute and without needle retention. Treatment was given once a day, twelve times constituted a course. Two weeks later treatment was given every other day. The first course did not show marked effect. During the second course, the dull-looking eyes more or less changed. Sometimes she demonstrated a child's lively state or said a few words. After four courses of treatment, she became lively and was able to sing songs along with the radio. Fifty treatments given in three months nearly cured the case.

Explanation Points of the Du Meridian and the Yang Meridians were selected with mild or moderate stimulation to invigorate yang, resulting in removal of phlegm and the case was cured.

Case 2: Paroxysmal burning pain along meridians

Name, Feng x x; sex, male; age, 57; date of the first visit, early October 1965.

Complaints He had a burning pain in the right leg to the shoulder for three years. In the spring three years before there was an occasional burning pain in the right leg. The area of pain was as big as a thumb, located at Xuanzhong (G 39). There was no lumps or swelling found. Then a paroxysmal burning pain attacked every morning. Because it was not so serious, he continued with his farm work without any treatment. Half a month later the pain radiated to the fourth toe (along the course of the Gallbladder Meridian). Another month passed and a sharper burning pain spread to the right buttock (along the course of the Gallbladder Meridian to Huantiao (G 30)). He was treated by the local hospital without any effect. Two months later pain went up to the shoulder (from Huantiao (G 30) along the Gallbladder Meridian to Jianjing (G 21)). Then a few days later the pain spread to the ear, causing ear ringing and pain, and to the right eye, causing a distending pain in the eye. The burning pain attacked every morning, lasting for about an hour. He was diagnosed as having neurosis by several hospitals and there was no response to any treatment. Physical examination showed a strong constitution, good development. Tenderness was found in the diseased part except Fengchi (G 20), Danshu (B 19), Yanglingquan (G 34) and Xuanzhong (G 39).

Prescription Jianjing (G 21), Huantiao (G 30), Xuanzhong (G 39), Yanglingquan (G 34), Danshu (B 19), Fengchi (G 20) and Zulingqi (G 4) of the diseased side.

Treatment procedure The needles were twirled continuously with the moderate stimulation to dispel the pathogenic factors from the yang meridians. After three treatments, the condition was getting better, and the upper limb pain disappeared after five treatments. Seven treatments relived the burning pain in the back. Half a month later the pain in the leg disappeared. Twenty-eight treatments in total cured the case. A 5-month follow-up study did not show any relapse.

Explanation In terms of meridians the pain occurred along three meridians—the Gallbladder, Bladder and Sanjiao Meridians. But the pain mainly was in the latter two meridians. The case was diagnosed as rarely seen paroxysmal burning pain along meridians. In treatment, points along the meridians and the tender spots were selected. But actually the tender spots were the very places of the spots. In this way qi and blood were regulated and the pain alleviated.

RESEARCH ON SCALP ACUPUNCTURE

—Jiao Shunfa's Clinical Experience

Jiao Shunfa was born in Jishan County, Shanxi Province, on December 25, 1938. In 1956, he joined the medical training class run by the Jishan People's Hospital and worked there after graduation. In 1961, he studied neurosurgery at the affiliated hospital of Shanxi Medical College. Since 1969, he has studied scalp acupuncture in treating hemiplegia. He summarized the scalp acupuncture systematically in 1971, and edited *Scalp Acupuncture Therapy and Scalp Acupuncture.* Now he is the chief of the Yuncheng District Public Health Bureau of Shanxi Province, associate professor and director of the Institute of Scalp Acupuncture of Yuncheng District.

I. Academic Characteristics and Medical Specialities

1. The theoretical basis of scalp acupuncture

Scalp acupuncture is formed on the basis of the theory of transverse connection of meridian qi in combination with anatomy and physiology of modern medicine. It is stated in the book *Miraculous Pivot* that, "Brain is the sea of marrow, its upper part is at the vertex, and the lower at Fengfu," indicating that there is a special relationship between the brain and the head, and the points for treating encephalogenic diseases are situated at the vertex.

The theory of the Front-Mu points inspired his studies on scalp acupuncture. The Front-Mu points are the place where the meridian qi of zang-fu organs is infused and each of the twelve zang-fu organs has one Front-Mu point in the chest and abdomen. The most Front-Mu points are not the Shu points of their meridians, but they are the important points in treating the diseases corresponding to the internal organs, because these Front-Mu points are distributed at the adjacent parts of the corresponding zang-fu organs. For example, the Front-Mu point of the stomach, Zhongwan (Ren 12), (4 cun above the umbilicus), is not a point of the Stomach Meridian, but a point of the Ren meridian, however, Zhongwan (Ren 12) is directy under the stomach; the Front-Mu point of the large intestine, Tianshu (S 25) (2 cun apart from the umbilicus), is not the point of the Large Intestine Meridian, but the point of the Stomach Meridian, however, it is situated at the corresponding part of the large intestine. This is the same as the Front-Mu points of the pericardium, spleen and kidney. From these facts, Dr. Jiao has realized that since all the Front-Mu points the zang-fu organs are situated at the body surface corresponding to their internal organs, the points for treating cerebral disease should be located at the place corresponding to the brain—the scalp.

2. Determination of scalp acupuncture stimulating area and its indications

In order to determine the stimulating area more conveniently, two standard lines are established on the basis of the landmarks of the head surface (Fig. 1). Antero-posterior midline: The midline connecting the glabella with the lower border of the tip of external occipital protuberance. Eyebrow-occipital line: The lateral line connecting the upper border of the midpoint of the eyebrow with the external occipital protuberance.

1) *Motor Area (Fig. 2)* Location: A line starting from a point 0.5 cm posterior to the midpoint of the anterior-posterior midline of head and stretching diagnoally across the juncture between the eyebrow-occipital line and the anterior border of the corner of the temporal hairline. Main indications: a. The upper 2/5 line: Paralysis of the lower limb of the opposite side. b. The middle 2/5 line: Paralysis of the upper limb of the opposite side. c. The lower 2/5 line: Facial paralysis of opposite side, motor aphasia, dribbling saliva, impaired speech.

2) *Sensory Area (Fig. 3)* Location: A line parallel and 1.5 cm posterior to the Motor Area. Main indications: a. The upper 1/5 line: Lower back and leg pain of the opposite side, numbness, paresthesia, occipital headache, neck pain and tinnitus; b. The middle 2/5 line: Pain, numbness or paresthesia of upper limb of the opposite side; c. The lower 2/5 line: Numbness and pain of the head and facial region of the opposite side.

3) *Chorea and Tremor Control Areas* Location (Fig. 3): A line 1.5 cm anterior and parallel with the Motor Area. Main indications: Involuntary movement and tremor of the limbs of the opposite side.

4) *Blood Vessel Dilation and Constriction Area (Fig. 3)* Location: A line 1.5 cm anterior and parallel with the Chorea-Tremor Control Area. Main indications: Primary hypertension and cortical edema.

5) *Vertigo and Hearing Area (Fig. 3)* Location: A 4-cm horizontal line, 1.5 cm directly above the apex of the auricle. Main indications: Dizziness, tinnitus, auditory vertigo, cortical hearing disturbance, auditory hallucination, etc. of the same side.

6) *Speech II Area* Location: A line from the parietal tubercle parallel with the antero-posterior midline of the head, a vertical line 2 cm posterior to the former line, 3 cm in length. Main indication: Anomic aphasia.

7) *Speech III Area* Location: A horizontal line overlaps Vertigo and Hearing Area at the midpoint and continues 4 cm posteriorly. Main indication: Sensory aphasia.

8) *Praxis Area (Fig. 3)* Location: There are three 3 cm long lines, a straight line from the parietal tubercle to the middle of mastoid process, and the other two lines anteriorly and posteriorly with a 40° angle respectively between it. Main indication: Apraxia.

9) *Foot Motor and Sensory Area (Fig. 4)* Location: From the point 1 cm posterior to the upper end of the Sensory Area, draw a line, 3 cm in length, parallel with the anterior-posterior midline of head. Main indications: Lower back and leg pain, numbness, paralysis of the opposite side. Needle this area bilaterally to treat infantile enuresis, cortical frequent urination, cortical dysuria, cortical incontinence of urine and prolapse of the rectum. Acupuncture on both sides of this area and both sides of Genital Area to treat frequency and urgency of urine caused by acute cystitis, polydipsia, overdrinking,

polyurea, impotence, seminal emission and prolapse of the uterus, etc. Needling bilaterally together with bilateral Intestinal Area to treat allergic colitis and diarrhoea. Needling bilaterally together with bilateral Thoracic Area, is effective for oliguria caused by rheumatic heart disease. Needling bilaterally together with upper 2/5 of bilateral Sensory Area is effective for cervical syndrome, lumbar vertebral degeneration contact dermatitis and neuro dermatitis.

10) *Vision Area (Fig. 5)* Location: A line 1 cm lateral and parallel to the anterior-posterior midline of the head, intersecting the horizontal line of the external occipital protuberance, draw a line 4 cm in length. Main indications: Cortical visual disturbance, cataract, etc.

11) *Balance Area (Fig. 5)* Location: 3.5 cm lateral to the external occipital protuberance, parallel with the midline of head, 4 cm in length, extending downward. Main indications: Loss of balance caused by cerebella disorders.

12) *Stomach Area* Location: Starting from the hairline directly above the pupil, parallel with the midline of head, 2 cm in length, extending posteriorly. Those who have unclear hairline can be measured from the points 6 cm directly above the glabella. Main indications: Acute and chronic gastritis, pain caused by gastro-duodenal ulcer.

13) *Liver and Gallbladder Area (Fig. 6)* Location: A line 2 cm long parallel with the anterior-posterior midline, extending anteriorly from the lower margin of the Stomach Area. Main indication: Pain due to liver and gallbladder illness.

14) *Thoracic Cavity Area (Fig. 6)* Location: Midway between and parallel with Stomach Area and midline of head, bilaterally 2 cm in length. Main indications: Allergic asthma, bronchitis, angina pectoris, rheumatic heart disease (certain effects on palpitation, shortness of breath, edema, oliguria), paradoxysmal supraventricular tachycardia.

15) *Genital Area (Fig. 6)* Location: 2 cm extending upward from the frontal corner of the head and parallel with the anterior-posterior midline. Main indication: Functional uterine bleeding. If it is used in combination with bilateral Foot Motor and Sensory Area, it is effective for frequent and urgent urination caused by acute cystitis. Polydipsia, excessive drinking, polyurea caused by diabetes, impotence, seminal emission, prolapse of the uterus, etc.

16) *Intestinal Area (Fig. 6)* Location: A 2 cm line going downward from the lower end of the Genital Area and parallel with the anterior-posterior midline. Main indication: Lower abdominal pain.

3. New exploration of scalp acupuncture

Dr. Jiao has summarized three swift needling methods, i.e. insertion, rotation and withdrawal of the needle by quick movement.

1) *Insertion* a. Flying insertion of the needle: Hold the needle body with the thumb and index finger approximately 2 cm from the needle tip. Hold the handle so that the distance between the index finger tip and the scalp is about 5 to 10 cm, with the needle aimed at the area where stimulation can be felt. Hyperflex the wrist so the needle tip is 10 to 20 cm from the scalp, then flex the wrist quickly inserting the needle tip into the subcutaneous or muscular layer. b. Rapid thrusting: Push the needle quickly to a certain

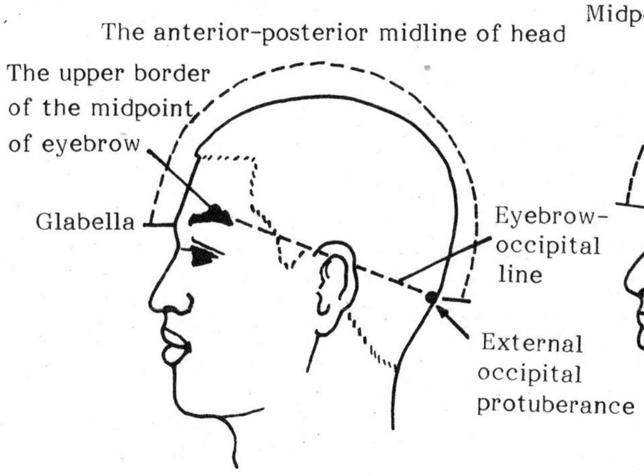

Fig. 1 Standard Line of Measurement

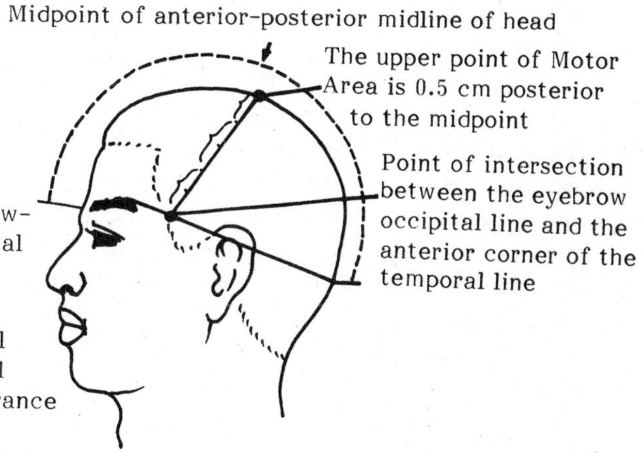

Fig. 2 Location of Motor Area

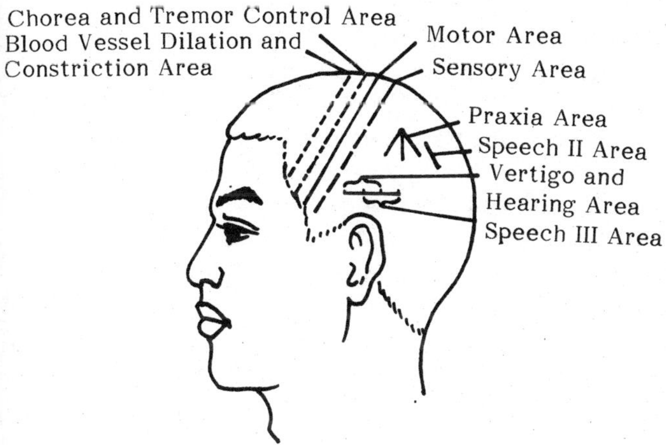

Fig. 3 Side View of the Stimulating Area

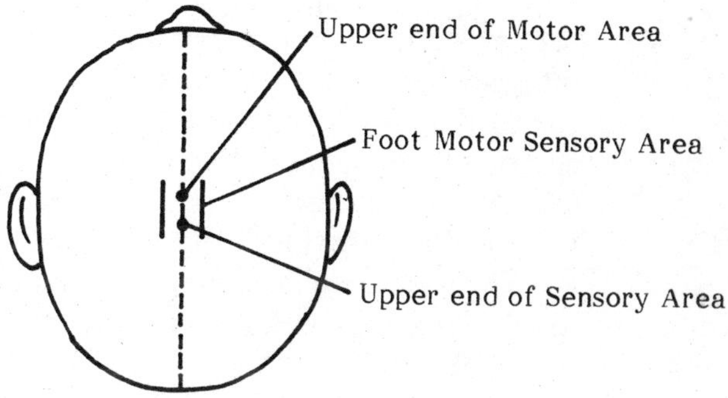

Fig. 4 Top View of the Stimulating Area

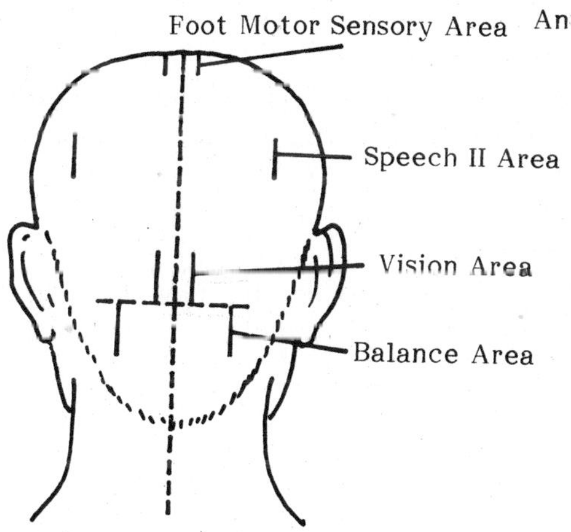

Fig. 5 Back View of the Stimulating Area

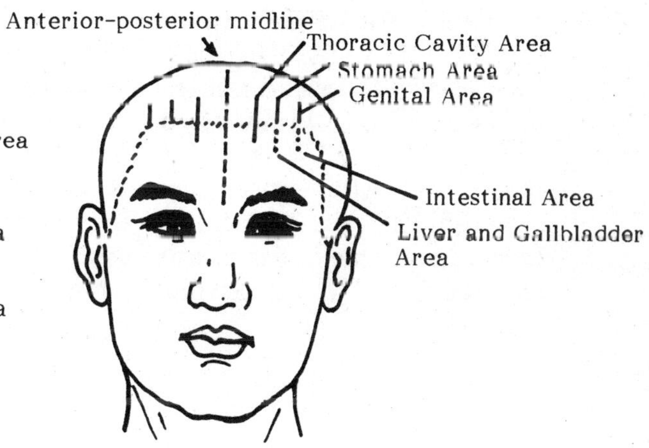

Fig. 6 Front View of the Stimulating Area

depth without rotation after the flying insertion into subcutaneous or muscular layer along the stimulating area. About 65 percent of cases took 0.2 seconds to complete this action.

2) *Manipulating the needle* a. Rotating method: This method needs fast rotation without lifting and thrusting. During rotation, it is essential to have a fixed position of the shoulder, elbow, wrist joint and the thumb in order to stabilize the needle body. After the needle body is fixed, the index finger is half flexed. Hold the needle handle with the radial aspect of the distal phalanx of the index finger and the distal phalanx of the thumb. Then the metacarpal phalangeal joint of the index finger is constantly flexed and extended, making the needle rotate rapidly. Generally the needle is rotated 200 times/min., the quickest will reach more than 400 times/min., and twisting the needle sustainedly for 0.5 to 1 minute, the symptoms usually will be alleviated or disappear within 5 to 10 minutes if there is needle sensation after twisting and rotation, so twisting and rotation should be repeated twice every 5 to 10 minutes. Then take the needle out. b. Retention of the needle: The symptoms and signs in a few patients may be alleviated evidently or disappear soon after the needle is inserted. Therefore, for these kinds of patients, no rotation is needed, only retain the needle for thirty minutes. c. Embedding needle: Some patients may have symptoms and signs relieved soon after needling. However, for up to one day, the symptoms and signs could be aggravated or reappear. This may be due to the stimulation. For this problem we adopted the embedding needle method, i.e. twisting and rotating the needle quickly and intermittently three times after insertion and then retaining the needle for five hours to three days instead of taking it out. Pay attention to strict sterilization to avoid infection and bleeding. The position of insertion should not influence sleep or movements.

3) *Withdrawal of the needle* Hold the cotton ball with one hand, aiming at the acupoint, swiftly slant down along the needle body with the middle or ring finger of the other hand. Then pinch the needle body with the thumb and index finger (or thumb, index and middle fingers) to withdraw it quickly.

The three quick needling techniques may shorten the time for insertion, reduce the patient's suffering and increase the therapeutic effects.

II. Case Analysis

Case 1: Windstroke (cerebral hemorrhage)

Name, Li x x; sex, female; age, 34.

Complaints She had headache and nausea frequently. She fell into coma following dizziness for twenty minutes on April 1, 1979 after she got up. She had complete hemiplegia on the left side after she woke up one hour later. She came to the clinic on the sixth day. After lumbar puncture, the CSF pressure was 320 mm H_2O, its colour was yellowish, RBC was 785/MM. No improvement was found after an I.V. drip seventeen times of lower molecular dextrose. She was transferred to the acupuncture department on April 19, 1979. Examination: Blood pressure 100/70 mmHg, clear consciousness, normal speech, normal cranial nerves, normal extension and flexion of right hand, grasping force 4 kg (34 kg for left hand), Hoffmann's sign (-), right upper arm could elevate to the xyphoid process, complete paralysis of the right lower limb, increasing of muscle tonicity, hyperactivity of the knee reflex, Babinski's sign (-), the temperature, pain and cortical sensation of the right side normal, the cardiac rhythm normal, heart beat 70/min., fundi: bilateral congestion of the optic disc, their margin not clear, more severe on the left side, 3 to 4 D. higher than the retina, dilatation and curvature of the vein, the artery normal, A: V=1:2, no crossing pressure of the vein by the artery, no bleeding or exudation, clear central reflex of the maculla.

Prescription Upper 3/5 of the left Motor Area and Foot Motor Sensory Area were needled once daily.

Treatment procedure She improved evidently after six treatments. Her right upper limb could elevate normally, the grasping force of the right hand was 26 kg, the movement of her right lower limb was within normal range. She could walk four to five steps. After fifteen treatments, the muscle power of her right hand recovered to normal range, her grasping force was 32 Kg. All joints of her right lower limb could move except ankle and toes.

Case 2: Craniocerebral trauma

Name, Kong x x; sex, male; age, 24.

Complaints The left frontal area was injured eleven days before, and he lost his consciousness. Seven days later, he was conscious after emergency treatment. On eleventh day, he was clear in his mind, but with motor aphasia. The right naso-labial fissure was shallow and he had complete paralysis of the right Hoffmann's sign (+), right lower limb had normal extension and flexion movement, and he could elevate the right leg 80°. He could not stand up and the left limbs were normal.

Prescription Left Motor Area and Foot Motor-Sensory Area were needled once daily.

Treatment procedure He recovered and was discharged from the hospital after nineteen treatments. A follow-up on May of 1985 showed his spirit and mental state were normal. He could speak fluently, with no headache or dizziness. The four extremities were normal and he could work sometimes.

Case 3: Sequelae of infantile craniocerebral injury

Name, Yi Pengfei; sex, male; age, 6.

Complaints He fell down from a stage five days before and lost consciousness. He had right hemiplegia after waking up on the second day. No effect was found when he was treated at the local hospital. Examination: Good body build, clear mind, no evident trauma to the head, his left limb normal, but complete hemiplegia of the right limb.

Prescription Left Motor Area and Foot Motor Sensory Area were selected.

Treatment procedure His right limb had power and he could walk by himself after the second needling. His right upper limb could be elevated normally after the eighth treatment.

Case 4: Encephalitis sequela

Name, Pan x x; sex, female; age, 2; date of the first visit, April 5, 1971.

Complaints She had a 40°C high fever suddenly, accompanied by coma and convulsion in March of 1971. She was clear in mind after half a month's treatment, but she was blind bilaterally with motor aphasia and tetraplegia. Examination: clear mind, platycoria, complete aphasia, tetraplegia, and soft neck.

Prescription Bilateral Motor Area and Vision Area were needled once daily.

Treatment procedure She could see objects clearly, and start restoration of her paralyzed limbs after five treatments. Her four limbs could move within normal range and she could stand by herself, and was gradually restored to normal after twenty treatments. As a follow-up visit, after fourteen years: Normal mentally, fluent speech, normal visual acuity and movement of the four limbs.

Case 5: Tuberculous meningitis sequela

Name, Zhang x x; sex, male; age, 4.

Complaints He had a 40°C high fever and vomiting in January of 1975. He was diagnosed as having tuberculous meningitis after lumbar puncture. He gradually improved after treatment. Ten days later, he suffered involuntary tics of the right limb, and he had right hemiplegia that night. The convulsion was controlled ten days after treatment, but the hemiplegia remained. No response was found after body acupuncture and Western drugs. Examination on June 8, 1988: Clear mind, normal speech, the muscle tonicity of his right upper limb increased, weakness of the right lower limb, failure in standing up, walking or extension of his toes.

Prescription The upper 3/5 of the left Motor Area and Foot Motor Sensory Area were needled once daily.

Treatment procedure After one treatment, he could walk with his right foot with help and extend his right hand after three treatments and could hold objects, he could walk by himself and his right hand could touch his head after the fourth treatment.

Case 6: Paralysis agitans (parkinsonism)

Name, Yao x x; sex, male; age, 70.

Complaints He had a tremor of his right limb which was aggravated gradually, then could not extend his waist, and he had difficulty in walking for eight years. Examination: clear mind, unable to extend the waist, couldn't walk or stand up by himself, prominent tremor of the right limbs, and wheel-like increase of muscle toning.

Prescription Left Chorea-Tremor Control Area was needled once daily.

Treatment procedure His right lower limb had strength and the tremor was alleviated. He could walk with straight waist, and his right hand could hold chopsticks after the fourth treatment. He could walk independently for eight miles six months later after stopping treatment.

Case 7: Nervous deafness

Name, Wang x x; sex, male; age, 40; date of the first visit, September 19, 1978.

Complaints He had tinnitus of the left ear after he got up one morning in 1966. He could not hear when spoken to face-to-face or from the telephone. His right ear could not hear the watch sound suddenly after catching cold in 1973. No response was found after taking Chinese herbs and Western medicine, and needling Tiangong (SI 19) and Ermen (SJ 21). There was no improvement in the last three years. Examination: Failure in hearing the tick of a watch and in talking face-to-face.

Prescription Bilateral Vertigo Hearing Area was selected.

Treatment procedure He was treated once daily, he could hear the watch sound and the phone with his left ear after the fifth treatment. He could listen clearly to the TV sound three meters away after the ninth treatment.

Case 8: Impotence

Name, Zhang x x; sex, male; age, 26; date of the first visit, May 23, 1978.

Complaints He had seminal emission twice half a year ago due to overwork. He was nervous and worried very much, then he had insomnia, impotence, and lost sexual desire. His wife wanted a divorce. This made him more irritable. His impotence became severe and he had retraction of the penis. No response was found after being treated with Chinese herbs and Western medication for three months.

Prescription Bilateral Foot Motor Sensory Area and Genital Area were needled once daily.

Treatment procedure He slept well and his sexual life was restored to normal after seven treatments.

Case 9: Obstinate headache

Name, Sun x x; sex, male; age, 35; date of the first visit, August 8, 1978.

Complaints He suffered tines capitis when he was fourteen years old and it was cured at the age eighteen. Since then, he had headache and cold feeling of his head. He had to wrap his head during sleep, but he still felt cold. No response was found after treatment with Chinese and Western drugs. Examination: A little hair over his vertex, and scars at the other place of the head after healing from the tinea, normal pain sensation of the head and the cranial nerves.

Prescription Bilateral upper 2/5 of the Sensory Area and Foot Motor Sensory Area were selected.

Treatment procedure Headache was alleviated and his mind was clear after the first treatment. The treatment proceeded once daily. He could take off his cap and had no more headache and cold feeling of his head after the fourth treatment. He could walk five km without symptoms and completely recovered after ten treatments.

TECHNIQUES OF DEEP INSERTION AT FENGFU POINT AND THE APPLICATION OF DIRECT MOXIBUSTION

—Xie Xiliang's Clinical Experience

Xie Xiliang was born in Bulang County, Henan Province, in September, 1926. He started learning TCM in 1948 under his brother's influence. In 1950, he apprenticed to Cheng Dan'an to learn acupuncture. Xie emphasizes the application of the theory of Ziwuliuzhu, the techniques of the deep insertion at Fengfu (Du 16) and the application of direct moxibustion. He has published the works of *Moxibustion Therapy* and *Calculating Diagram Dish of Ziwuliuzhu*, etc. He is at present associate chief doctor of the Acupuncture Department of the Xiangfen People's Hospital, Shanxi Province; permanent member of the Board of Directors of the Shanxi Branch of the All-China Traditional Chinese Medicine Association; and advisor to the Hong Kong Acupuncture Society.

I. Academic Characteristics and Medical Specialities

1. Deep insertion at Fengfu (Du 16)

This requires a skillful needling technique. The operator must prepare everything in advance including the necessary instrument and assistants, select a quiet place with proper atmospheric temperature and enough light, try to keep the patient calm in order to obtain his cooperation, and tell the patient the needling sensations promptly.

1) *The posture and method for selecting the points* Let the patient take a sitting position with something in front so that he could support himself. The patient's neck should be erect as though in a formal standing posture, his jaw raised a bit upward. In this position there may appear a depression in the centre of the posterior neck where the point is located. Too much raising of the jaw would made the depression unclear, too much bending of the head may cause the tension of the muscle. Anyway, a natural and comfortable position should be adopted for the patient with full exposure of the point. In order to get the accurate site of Fengfu (D 16), Fengchi (G 20), Yamen (Du 15) and Naohu (Du 17) should be located first, as said in *Ode to the Standard of Mystery*. "If one point is to be located from the above five, all these points should be first located, then the accurate location of each can be made." Generally, the patient is asked to hold the head with both hands with his elbows resting on a table, keeping the distance of the two elbows as wide as his shoulders. In this way the patient may feel comfortable, while the doctor locates and needles the point. Assistants are needed in the treatment of mental

disorders. The first assistant stands opposite to the patient, his left hand holds the patient's jaw, while the right hand holds the vertex to keep the patient's head erect; the second assistant fixes the patient's left arm and the left leg and the third one keeps the patient's right side. The operator needles the patient behind the patient. For the patient who is unconscious or suffers from hemiplegia with more impairment, either the lateral recumbent position or lying position may be adopted. Great attention is paid to the needling direction and depth, in general, about 2 to 2.5 inches. If the therapeutic result is not good as the deeper insertion, one more treatment is advisable. Usually, children could hardly offer any active cooperation because of their constant moving, so great care should be taken to prevent any accident when they are needled. The operator has also to pay great attention to the posture of elderly people, women or those with thin body.

2) *Method*

a. Three needle inserting steps:

Inserting the needles with the coordination of both hands. After everything is prepared and strict sterilization is made, the operator holds the needle handle with the right hand and the needle tip with the index finger and the thumb of the left hand. Place the needle at the point and insert the needle with both hands gently and forcefully into the skin about 0.1 to 0.2 inches, and then further insert the needle deeper with a small amplitude of rotation and somewhat lifting and thrusting slowly in order to find out the tiny spaces in case the needle tip is stuck underneath. It is quite safe when the needle stays in this depth. After inserting about one inch, release the right hand to see the direction of the needle handle. This is the first step. If the direction of the needle is the same as that at the beginning, insert the needle to the depth of two inches with very small amplitute of rotation; and again observe the direction of the needle handle and the patient's complexion. This is the second step. If there is nothing abnormal, go on inserting the needle to the depth of 2.5 inches without any rotation, and leave the needle there. This is the third step. Now the needle tip remains in the dangerous district, the operator must pay great attention to the finger feeling under the needle and the reactions from the patient, and keep his hands at the needle during the whole process of treatment.

b. Manipulate the needle with lifting and thrusting two or three times:

If everything is all right, the needle will be lifted 0.2 to 0.3 of an inch slowly and then gently thrust 0.2 to 0.3 inch. Repeat the same procedure two or three times in order to strengthen the needling stimulation. This method is called the lifting-thrusting manipulation. Never rotate, lift or thrust the needle violently to prevent any injury of the spinal marrow or the vessels from bleeding. The operator should concentrate his mind and hold his breath to keep the needle firm in his hand, and carefully experience the sensation under the needle and observe the patient's response. If the patient screams or trembles or complains of heaviness, the operator should immediately lift the needle 0.3 to 0.5 inch to let it stay in the safe district, and retain the needle there for a while before withdrawal. If the patient is free of needling sensation after lifting-thrusting for two or three times, the operator can do the same manipulation another two or three times. Even if there is no sensation at all, it is forbidden to insert the needle any more after manipulation for another two or three times. Instead, the needle should be withdrawn slowly and gently.

Remark Dep Insertion at Fengfu (Du 16) is sometimes dangerous, so great care should be taken and much experience is needed for the beginners.

c. Withdrawing the needle

It also takes three steps. Slowly and gently lift the needle two inches from the deep area; leave the needle there for a while and then take the needle one inch upward; leave the needles for a while, and withdraw the needle completely without rotation. The whole procedure of withdrawal of the needle should not be noticed by the patient. Afterwards, press the needling point with a piece of cotton and apply massage superficially and deeply, then turn the patient's head slowly and gently. After that, let the patient have about twenty to thirty minutes rest in either a sitting position or lying position in order to ease the patient who might be a bit nervous. For a severe case, treat once every day during the first three days and treat every other day or every two or three days later. Eight to ten treatments constitute a course, and start another course (if neceasary) after a ten to fifteen-day interval. In general, treatment at Fengfu (Du 16) is not too much. Deep puncturing at Fengfu (Du 16) may also be combined with some other points such as Dazhui (Du 14), Taodao (Du 13), Shengzhu (Du 12), which have the same effect as that of Fengfu (Du 16) but which are much safer during treatment. When those points are needled, the patient is usually asked to take a natural sitting position, with shoulders loosened and head bent forward. In this way the scapulae are separated naturally, the space between the vertebrae get larger and the site of the points becomes clearer. Method: Insert a three-inch long needle No. 28 into the skin at an angle of 45° at the depression of the superior border of the spinous process, retain there for a while, then make an angle about 20° to 30° between the needle handle and the skin surface. Then forcefully penetrate into the spinous ligament until a loose sensation undernearth the needle is felt, stay for a moment, and then adjust the direction by aiming at the vertebral canal. For an adult, generally the needle may go about 2 to 2.5 inches deep in those points. After taking a rest for a while with the needle inside the vertebral canal, the operator may lift and thrust the needle three to five times and then pull it 0.3 to 0.4 inch out. A short retaining is required. Then remove the needle completely. When a lifting-thrusting manipulation is given, the patient may feel a radiating sensation going up and down or spreading over the shoulders, which is the normal needling sensation. During treatment, if there appears a tough or tensile sensation undernearth the needle, it means the tip of the needle touches the spinous ligament. When punctured forcefully with the rotating or lifting-thrusting manipulation, the needle may easily pierce through the ligament. Afterwards a loose sensation might be felt. If, during needling, a hard sensation is felt, it means the bone is touched. The operator should withdraw the needle somewhat and change the direction in order to find a suitable space for further insertion. The needling direction should be maintained obliquely upward along the midline. Withdrawal of the needle is divided into three steps. Press the needling spots for a while after the needle is removed. Do not give a violent rotating or lifting-thrusting to those points to prevent possible injury of the spinal marrow or internal hemorrhage. Care also should be taken for sterilization and needle selection.

2. Direct moxibustion therapy (scarring and nonscarring moxibustion)

Direct moxibustion is a treatment by applying the ignited moxa cones directly at the point on the skin surface. The size of the moxa cone is only as big as a piece of wheat; and its temperature during burning is about 70°C. So there is no reason to worry about the heat since it is gone immediately when a burning sensation is just felt. Cooperation from the patient is important. Effective results can be obtained by selecting high quality and fine moxa wool with skillful techniques and a long treatment. There are two methods of moxibustion in general, scarring and nonscarring moxibustion.

1) *Scarring moxibustion*

a. Method: First, the patient's permission and cooperation should be obtained before the treatment, then sterilize the point area with a 75 percent alcohol cotton ball, and then put a piece of small moxa cone directly at the point on the skin surface. The cone is as big as a piece of wheat in a taper form with very fine moxa wool. But it is all right if the cone is a little bigger. A piece of tiny incense is used to light the moxa from its top to let it burn evenly downward. When the first cone burns to half and the patient gets a warm sensation, the operator may use either his finger or a pair of forceps to remove it and replace another cone just on the ash of the first one. The second moxa cone is then extinguished when it burns more than half and the patient feels hot. The third one should be quickly removed only when it burns nearly to its end and the patient complains of a burning pain. At the same time, the three fingers, the thumb, the index and the middle fingers are used to massage or tap gently around the point area for alleviating the pain. After the first three cones are finished, the patient will not feel much pain, then more cones are given later. The patient will just feel a hot sensation for a short while with about ten pieces of moxa cones and the hot sensation goes without any pain. The treatment is continued until there appear blisters. (Today the operator prefers to use a large number of cones doing nonscarring moxibustion with which the effect is the same as that of scarring, but more acceptable by the patient in the clinic.) Applying the scaring method at Guanyuan (Ren 4) to treat incomplete erection, seminal emission and prospermia. About two hundred to three hundred moxa cones may be used for each treatment. After the treatment, there may appear a mark of 5 x 5 cm reddened skin at the local place, and 3 x 3 cm hard tissue but 2 x 2 cm black burnt in the centre of that mark. At the beginning of the treatment there is pain and burning sensation. As the treatment is continued, there will be only a hot sensation with no more pain at all but comfort. After the first treatment, the point area becomes dark, the local tissue gets hard and scar forms there. Moxa cones can be placed on the scar for the second treatment. In the case of scar formation, one may press the pus out with the normal procedure by putting some dressing or compress over the area if the scar falls. No other treatment is necessary until the new scar forms. The suppuration under the moxibustion scar is quite different to other inflammatory symptoms of boils, sores or wounds, because it does not lead to any bad results. The treatment might be continued if the suppuration is localized. If the ulceration gets bigger with excessive pus which turns yellow or blue from thin and white; or the patient feels severe pain and has the foul smell at the inflammatory area, that means a secondary infection. Some routine treatment should be given and the ulceration may soon recover. In general, postulation after the direct moxibustion belongs to a benign stimulation which may improve the body constitution and strengthen the body resistance in order to prevent or treat a disease. So there is no reason to worry about the suppuration. Otherwise, the treatment may be delayed. The wound after the direct moxibustion usually does not need to be treated, and it will spontaneously recover within thirty days. But if pus appears or ulceration forms, dressing or some other compress should be applied to keep the area from further infection or friction with the clothes.

b. Indications: Scarring moxibustion is mainly used to treat asthma, chronic gastroentestinal disorders, weakness, maldevelopment, chronic bronchitis, pulmonary tuberculosis, impotence, seminal emission, premature ejaculation, incomplete erection and some other chronic and intractable cases. It needs a long treatment with this method for the purposes of prevention and health care.

2) *Non-scarring moxibustion*

Method: Take a piece of tiny moxa cone as big as a piece of wheat, light it after it is placed at the point on the skin surface as mentioned before. Remove the moxa cone and put out the fire immediately when a burning pain is felt. Three to five moxa cones are used at each point and stop the treatment when the skin of the local area gets pink or there appear some tiny blisters, generally, free from ulceration. Overtreating might cause severe blisters, but they can be broken with a well-sterilized needle to expel the fluid. It is quite safe to start the treatment again at the same spot. The nonscarring method is easy to apply but it needs more points and long treatment in order to obtain a good results. This method is used to treat all the diseases or disorders that can be treated by moxibustion therapy. From our clinical experience we have found that the above two methods, scarring and nonscarring moxibustion are quite similar in nature but different in intensity. Clinically, any kind will be selected according to the patient's condition.

II. Case Analysis

Case 1: Depressive psychosis

Name, Niu x x; sex, female; age, 20.

Complaints The onset started in the summer of 1957 after a quarrel about family problems. Usually she kept inside her room and avoided meeting people. She muttered to herself all the time and lost her appetite, had a sallow complexion, constipation and white tongue body, thin body and weakness.

Prescription Fengfu (Du 16), Tanzhong (Ren 17), Neiguan (P 6) and Taichong (Liv 3).

Treatment procedure Deep insertion at Fengfu (Du 16) clears and calms the mind. The needle may go as far as 2.5 inches deep. Tanzhong (Ren 17), Neiguan (P 6) and Taichong (Liv 3) are used to pacify the liver and regulate the qi circulation in the meridians. Treat once every other day. After seven to eight treatments, the patient improved and finally she recovered. Now she is quite healthy and works well at home.

Case 2: Mania (schizophrenia)

Name, Xue x x; sex, female; age, 25.

Complaints The onset occurred in the autumn of 1958 after a severe emotional disturbance. She was restless and had incoherent speech and delusions. She was treated in a mental hospital, but little result was obtained; She had string-taut and tense pulse, loss of appetite, red tongue tip with sticky and white coating; sluggish and sallow complexion with expressionless blank attitude, incorrect response, constipation, yellow scanty urine, and insomnia. The patient had average stature for her age and her constitution was all right.

Prescription Fengfu (Du 16), Daling (P 7), Taichong (Liv 3).

Treatment procedure Fengfu (Du 16) was deeply inserted about 2.7 inches in combination with Daling (P 7) and Taichong (Liv 3) which were normally inserted to clear the mind and bring back consciousness. After the first treatment, there was no improvement at all. The symptoms remained the same. The second treatment started with the same method and points, but needles were retained for forty minutes. That evening the patient had a three-hour sleep. Zusanli (S 36) was added in the third treatment, the patient had a bowel movement that afternoon, and she drank a big bottle of water as well. The first three treatments were given daily and then every other day. After nine treatments she improved. After more than a month's rest, she completely recovered. She now works normally and the follow-up examination revealed no recurrence of the disease.

Case 3: Epilepsy

Name, Nian x x; sex, male; age, 30.

Complaints The disease occurred after he had had an emotional disturbance about family problems. Three years before epilepsy occurred abruptly, a grand mal happened once a month or about every twenty days, accompanied with a sudden loss of consciousness, convulsion, foaming mouth and incontinence of urine. Each attack usually lasted ten minutes. The patient recovered from the epileptic attack after a sound sleep. He had an average stature of his age and looked strong and heavy but with no sick expression. He also complained of excessive sputum.

Prescription Fengfu (Du 16), Dazhui (Du 14), Shenzhu (Du 12), Taichong (Liv 3), Fenglong (S 40).

Treatment procedure Deep insertion at Fengfu (Du 16), Dazhui (Du 14), and Shenzhu (Du 12) was applied, but mainly at the first point. The patient was also prescribed the herbal decoction of the Decoction for Eliminating Sputum, which was noted in the book *Prescriptions Based on the Combination of TCM and Western Medicine*. This decoction may promote the bowel movement, and the patient had excessive mucous stool after having taken it. He was treated all together twelve times in one month. After that no attack occurred again.

Remarks Deep insertion at Fengfu (Du 16) is used not only for the treatment of severe mental diseases, but also for treating epilepsy, headache, high fever, convulsion, windstroke and paralysis.

Case 4: Hepatitis

Name, Zhang x x; sex, female; age, 37.

Complaints General lassitude, poor appetite with nausea for about three months. Examination of the blood test: Transaminase: 145; TTT: 9; TFT: (++) and other items normal. She was diagnosed as having hepatitis, and then treated by various kinds of methods including forty to fifty herbal decoctions, VB 6, VB 1, yeast, multienzyme, glucuronolactone, and hepatic glucoside, but little result was obtained. The next blood examination showed that Transaminase was 200. The patient continued to take both Western medicine and Chinese herbs and her blood was continuously examined once a month. The transaminase count of her last test before she came to take acupuncture treatment reached 210 and she had dizziness, distension of the head, insomnia, weakness of the lower limbs, loss of appetite and nausea, sallow complexion, dry hairs, no hepatosplenomegaly, no yellow sclea, clear mind, emaciation, red tongue with white and thin coating, slightly string-taut pulse, dry mouth, normal feces and urine.

Prescription Ganshu (B 18), Zusanli (S 36).

Treatment procedure The patient was asked to stop medication, but treated by direct moxibustion with small moxa cones. Treatment was given daily with about five to seven pieces to each point, and then treatment was given every other day after the first ten days. Her blood was examined monthly and the result on November 3, 1983 was: Transaminase, 100 and other items normal. The patient's appetite was much improved after one month's treatment. She had more energy and there was pink colour on the face. The treatment was continued and the examination on December 12, 1983 showed transaminase under 100. The above mentioned symptoms were relieved completely. The follow-up visit four months later in April of 1984 showed a healthy condition.

Case 5: Chronic hepatitis

Name, Ma x x; sex, male; age, 41.

Complaints The patient used to be quite healthy and looked strong. About half a year ago, he got jaundice with the symptoms of poor appetite, nausea, and aversion to oily food. He was diagnosed as having hepatitis after a liver function test. In a hospital the patient was treated about four months with different methods including eighty and more herbal decoctions and some Western medications. Most of the symptoms seemed to improve, but the patient still felt general lassitude. His transaminase was around 180-220, TFT, (++), and TTT, 8.

Prescription Ganshu (B 18), Zusanli (S 36).

Treatment procedure The direct moxibustion was used at the above two points with small moxa cones. Treatment was given daily for the first five days and then every other day. The patient was anxious to recover, so he tried to use bigger moxa cones. After ten treatments, there appeared scars at the points with white fluid undernearth. The liver function test made less than one month showed his transaminase below 100; and TFT, TTT and other items all became normal. The treatment was continued for another month. A follow-up visit one year later revealed that the patient works normally.

Remarks Dr. Xie has been applying the direct moxibustion therapy for many years. He has much experience in treating chronic hepatitis with thirty-two cases of successful results, as well as with the treatment of impotence, seminal emission, enuresis, asthma, dizziness and vertigo, lung lymph node tuberculosis, cervical lymph node tuberculosis, longstanding infantile fever, infantile maldevelopment, functional uterine bleeding, malposition of the fetus, common cold, weakness of the spleen and stomach, indigestion, chronic diarrhoea or constipation, abdominal distension, ascites and anemia.

TREATMENT METHODS VARYING WITH DIFFERENT SYMPTOMS, EFFECTS OBTAINED FROM DIFFERENT ACUPOINTS

—Lou Baiceng's Clinical Experience

Lou Baiceng was born in 1913 in Zhuji County, Zhejiang Province. In 1930, he entered the Zhejiang Special School of Traditional Chinese Medicine and graduated in 1935. In 1947 he moved to Hangzhou where he started his private practice. In 1956 he was employed by the Zhejiang Provincial Research Institute of Traditional Chinese Medicine. Dr. Lou has been engaged in traditional Chinese medicine for more than fifty years and devoting himself to the study of acupuncture and internal medicine of traditional Chinese medicine. He has especially original views of various acupuncture techniques. In 1980, he cooperated with the Zhejiang Computer Research Institute, his acupuncture clinical experience was put into the computer and then applied in clinical practice. This success has won the third prize in scientific research on the provincial level. He has published over thirty treatises and has successively held the posts of research fellow and the director of the Acupuncture Research Section of the Zhejiang Institute of Traditional Chinese Medicine and Chinese Materia Medica, is chairman of the Zhejiang Acupuncture Society, and member of the All-China Acupuncture Association and member of the Standing Committee of the Zhejiang Branch of All-China Acupuncture Association.

I. Academic Characteristics and Medical Specialities

1. The importance of acupuncture techniques

Acupuncture is an external treatment with proficient techniques. In addition to differentiation of syndromes and accurate location of acupoints, the effect is closely related to manipulations. Since the ancient acupuncturists created many needling techniques, Dr. Lou, after a thorough study of *Internal Classics* and *Classic on Medical Problems,* has summarized and analyzed the different acupuncture manipulations and then written his own views.

1) *Basic technique* Dr. Lou emphasizes the importance of coordination between the pressing hand and the puncturing hand. Press beside the acupoint with the nail of the index finger of the pressing hand, insert the needle gently into the point against the nail to avoid pain and injury of the blood vessels.

2) *Reinforcing and reducing methods* Dr. Lou holds that the reinforcing and reducing methods should be applied based on the arrival of the needling sensation. Reinforcing and reducing by lifting and thrusting the needle are mainly applied to regulate yin and yang of the nutrient and defensive systems of the body. This method is

frequently used on the points relating to zang-fu organs located on the body trunk. It is stated in *Classic on Medical Problems* that "after needling sensation appears, pressing of the needle to a deep region is known as reinforcing, while lifting of the needle to the superficial regions is known as reducing." Rapid lifting of the needle and slow thrusting is reducing, while slow lifting of the needle and rapid thrusting is reinforcing. Procedure: After the needling sensation appears, the reinforcing is performed by lifting and thrusting the needle repeatedly from superficial to deep with heavy thrusting and gentle lifting. The reducing is achieved by heavy lifting and gentle thrusting from deep to superficial. For example, a male patient aged thirty suffered from impotence shortly after his marriage for three and half years, accompanied with dizziness and dream-disturbed sleep. He had been treated for a long time in his hometown but without any effect. In March of 1963, accompanied by his wife he came to the Urology Department of the First Affiliated Hospital of Zhejiang Medical College, where he was diagnosed as impotent and then introduced to Dr. Lou's clinic for treatment. His diagnosis was deficiency of kidney qi and points Guanyuan (Ren 4), Mingmen (Du 4), Shenshu (B 23) and Sanyinjiao (Sp 6) were needled with the reinforcing method by lifting and thrusting the needle. After the first treatment, erection was possible the next morning, after three treatments voluntary erection was obtained but was not firm enough. After one course (ten times) of treatment both the erection and firmness were generally normal and the treatment finished. The follow-up visit for half a year by correspondance showed he had a normal sexual life.

Dr. Lou holds that reinforcing and reducing by twirling and rotating the needle are mainly used to regulate qi and blood of the meridians and mostly used on the points of the limbs. The reducing method is like Phoenix Spreading Wings and performed by rotating the handle of the needle with the thumb and index finger and then by setting free abruptly with the thumb and index finger parted from each other like wings spread for flying, while the reinforcing is like Hungry Horse Wagging Head and performed by rotating the handle of the needle with the thumb and index finger as a hungry horse seeking food. Procedure: After the needling sensation appears, rotating the needle heavily in a large amplitude is reducing; and on the contrary, rotating the needle gently in small amplitude is reinforcing. Here is a case example. A male patient aged twenty-eight had neurosthenia. He used to have mental depression which recently became worse after an incident. Irritability, insomnia, palpitation, spiritlessness, timid and easily frightened, dizziness, tinnitis, temporal distention, poor appetite, hypomnesia, thin white tongue coating, string-taut and thready pulse appeared. Diagnosis: Deficiency of qi of the heart and gallbladder. Shenmen (H 7), Fengchi (B 20) and Hegu (LI 4) were selected with the reinforcing method by twirling and rotating the needle. When Fengchi (G 20) was needled, the needling sensation should radiate to the forehead along the temples on both sides. Treat once a day at the beginning, and once every other day three days later. Fifteen treatments constitute one course. After the first treatment, he felt relaxed in the head and after three treatments he could sleep a little, and after five treatments he could sleep a little more. When the first course of treatment finished, he could sleep over six hours a day, the rest of the symptoms and signs all disappeared and no relapse was found in the follow-up visit.

Dr. Lou holds that the even reinforcing and even reducing are to induce the pathogenic qi to come out and to restore the antipathogenic qi. This method is suitable for cases without obvious deficiency or excess or with complication of both deficiency and excess and for cases with temporary disturbance of qi and blood in the body. It is said in *Miraculous Pivot* that "slow insertion of needle and slow withdrawal of needle should be administered which is called directing qi. Reinforcing and reducing do not have any fixed techniques here which is called protection of pure qi. Within this context, it is not like reducing the excess and reinforcing the deficiency, but rather to prevent disordered qi from offending each other." After the needling sensation appears, lift and thrust the needle evenly to limit the stimulation so that the patient is able to withstand the tolerance, then gently rotate the needle for a few minutes, and withdraw it. For example, a patient had lumbar pain due to carelessness in lifting heavy objects a week ago, associated with severe lumbar pain, difficulty in turning over and bending. He was treated in a local acupuncture clinic but without effect. Ten years ago he suffered the same symptoms and was cured by Dr. Lou with two treatments. So this time he came again. He was usually strong and healthy, his pain was worse on the right side, associated with local swelling and obvious tenderness on Shenshu (B 23). Differentiation: Injury of meridians by overloading which led to disturbance of qi circulation in meridians and stagnation of qi and blood in the local area. Bilateral Shenshu (B 23) and Weizhong (B 40) were selected. After the needling sensation appeared in Weizhong (B 40), the needle was retained and the needling sensation was continuously maintained. When the needling sensation arrived in Shenshu (B 23), the even reinforcing and even reducing methods were applied by manipulating the needle alternatively on both sides. Fifteen minutes later after the needle was removed, he felt more relaxed in the lumbar region and bending and extending were possible. The next day he repeated the same treatment and he was cured.

The comprehensive reinforcing and reducing of "setting the mountain on fire" and "penetrating-heaven coolness" are developed on the above mentioned techniques. Procedures: For setting the mountain on fire, the needle is inserted to half of the desired depth, and then rotated forward and backward nine times to wait for the arrival of qi. If a tight feeling is felt under the needle, puncture the needle to the desired depth, rapidly lift and thrust the needle three times together with the slow lifting and rapid thrusting and rotating methods, thus a warm sensation appears, while for penetrating-heaven coolness, the needle is inserted to the desired depth, and rotated six times to wait for the arrival of qi. If a tight feeling is felt under the needle, the needle is lifted to half of the depth and then rapidly thrust and lifted three times with rapid lifting and slow thrusting together with rotating, thus a cool sensation appears. For example, a female aged fifty-two suffered from right shoulder joint pain for over two years due to heavy housework and exposure to cold during sleep. The gradually aggravated pain resulted in impaired movement of the joint, and the arm could reach only the lower border of the left clavicle. In backward extension she could not reach the lower back. The pain was aggravated on cold weather, accompanied by aversion to cold all year round. Even in summer the shoulder and elbow joints should be kept warm. Because of impaired movement, severe pain was caused from time to time when wearing clothes or carrying objects. Although she was treated with herbal medicine and acupuncture in other places no obvious result was obtained. Nothing abnormal was found in examination. Differentiation: Invasion by pathogenic wind, cold and damp after overtraining leads to stagnation of qi and blood in the meridians and collaterals. Prescription: Jianyu (LI 15), Quchi (LI 17), Naoshu (SI 10), Waiguan (SJ 5) and Yunwai (Extra) (2 cun lateral to Yunmen (L 2) in line with the axillary fold). Setting the mountain on fire was applied at Jianyu (LI 15) and Quchi (LI 11) and reducing by twirling and rotating the needle applied in other points. Retain the needle for fifteen minutes. Treat once a day at first, and three days later, treat once every other day. After three treatments, the shoulder pain and aversion to cold were alleviated; after eight treatments, the pain and cold sensation disappeared, the arm could be raised to the level of ear, adduction reaching the upper border of the clavicle, and backward extension to the lumbar region. Subsequently reducing by twirling and rotating the needle was applied to all the selected points and the patient was cured after fifteen treatments.

Clinical experience has shown that the different acupuncture reinforcing and reducing methods provide special functions for various diseases.

2. Attention to "qi reaching the affected area"

Dr. Lou points out that in order to enhance the acupuncture effect, in addition to the mastery of correct differentiation of syndromes, selection of points, flexible application of reinforcing and reducing methods, the needling propagated sensation and "qi reaching to the affected area" should be taken into consideration. Dr. Lou has an excellent mastery of the technique to direct the needling sensation to the affected area and thus the wonderful effects have been obtained. For example, once when he was teaching Australian students in clinic, a patient came to him and complained of pain in the lateral aspect of the leg for over two years. In recent days, the pain was aggravated. He was treated with acupuncture in other places but with no response. Dr. Lou needled Yanglingquan (G 34) on the right side with reducing the twirling and rotating the needle to direct the needling sensation down to the ankle joint along the lateral aspect of the leg. The needle was retained for ten minutes with manipulation of the needle two or three times before withdrawing the needle. Pain disappeared and the patient left with joy. Another case was stiff neck on the left aspect with pain radiating to the head, and difficulty in turning the head due to sudden attack by cold three months ago. Dr. Lou needled Fengchi (G 20) on the left side with the even reinforcing and even reducing method by directing the needling sensation to the forehead upward along the nape. The needle was removed after being manipulated for five minutes and the pain disappeared.

Dr. Lou holds that to master the technique of the propagated sensation along meridians to the affected area, one should be very familiar with point location, needle tip direction and needling depth. Point location should be accurate. For example, Fengchi (G 20) point is located at the posterior hairline level with the ear lobe. The needle tip direction refers to the place where the propagated sensation may be accurately radiated. Fengchi (G 20) is needled with the tip directed to the lower border of the opposite zygoma (upward direction is forbidden). The needling depth here means the actually used depth in clinic. For example, Fengchi (G 20) is needled 1 to 1.5 cun deep in clinic, and 0.3 to

0.4 cun deep recorded in ancient classics, otherwise, the needling sensation could not radiate from the posterior aspect of the head to the temporal region and up the forehead. If the needle is inserted to a depth required, but without the propagation along meridians, the location of points and direction of needle tip should be considered to prevent injury by unnecessary deep needling.

3. Treatment should vary with different symptoms and signs

1) *Good and proper combination of points* Dr. Lou has accumulated rich experience on prescribing points during his long-term clinical practice. He prefers the combination of local and distal points from several meridians according to differentiation of syndromes. Points are strictly selected. For example, Guanyuan (Ren 4), Shenshu (B 23) and Sanyinjiao (Sp 6) are used for urinary and genital diseases; Shenmen (H 7), Hegu (LI 4) and Fengchi (G 20) for insomnia and headache; Zhongwan (Ren 12) and Zusanli (S 36) for gastro-intestinal diseases; and Bailao (Extra) and Xuanzhong (G 39) for neck pain. In addition, Dr. Lou pays much attention to the use of important empirical points. As a saying goes: "Diseases might be aggravated or alleviated and points might be more or less, but prescription depends on symptoms and signs and therapeutic effects vary with different points applied." Very often in a prescription, the wrong use of one point makes the result different. For example, Hegu (LI 4), the Yuan-Source points of the Large Intestine Meridian of Hand-Yangming, characterized by ascending, descending, opening and closing, is an important point for regulating qi and blood; if combined with Quchi (LI 11), it is good for diseases of the chest, lung, arm, head and face; if combined with Fuliu (K 7), it is an important way for arresting abnormal sweating and causing diaphoresis; if combined with Sanyinjiao (Sp 6), it is an excellent formula for regulating menstrual blood in gynecological disorders; and if combined with Taichong (Liv 3), it is able to tranquilize the blood pressure and an empirical formula for hypertension due to hyperactivity of liver yang.

2) *Combining acupuncture with drugs* Dr. Lou holds that each therapy has its own strong and weak points. Acupuncture is good at removing obstructions from the meridians and collaterals and regulating qi and blood, while Chinese herbs are good at regulating the functions of zang-fu organs and eliminating the pathogenic factors by strengthening the antipathogenic factors. For asthma, acupuncture can control it in a temporary period, but it is difficult to cure. The application of moxibustion might completely cure it; for jaundice, acupuncture is able to strengthen the spleen and promote digestion but difficult to eliminate heat damp quickly, while "Decoction of Artemisia Scorparia" (Yinchenhao Tang) will do so. Therefore, acupuncture, moxibustion and herbal medicine can be used independently or in combination.

II. Case Analysis

Case 1: Nocturnal enuresis

Name, Hu x x; sex, male; age, 12.

Complaints Since very young, he has had enuresis. He had been treated for many years but no effect. He wet the bed two to three times a night and sometimes even during a nap, it was difficult to awake him during sleep. When he was awaked, he wanted to pass urine and his mind was not clear.

Differentiation Insufficiency of kidney qi leading to dysfunction of kidney in dominating water metabolism.

Prescription Guanyuan (Ren 4), Shenshu (B 23) and Sanyinjiao (Sp 6).

Treatment procedure Reinforcing and reducing method by lifting and thrusting the needle was applied once a day, and once every other day three days later. After the first treatment, the bed-wetting disappeared. After six treatments, acupuncture was stopped on the patient's request. The follow-up visit one year later found no relapse.

Explanation Guanyuan (Ren 4), Shenshu (B 23) and Sanyinjiao (Sp 6) were used to strengthen the kidney qi, warm and tone the kidney yang to restore the kidney functions, then the enuresis was cured.

Case 2: Chronic diarrhoea

Name, Zhang x x; sex, female; age, 42.

Complaints Loose stool for one year due to irregular intake of food, two to three times a day with indigestion and recently accompanied by abdominal distension, lassitude, anorexia, tender tongue, white coating, soft and thready pulse.

Differentiation Weakness of the spleen and stomach leading to dysfunction of the spleen in transportation and transformation.

The principle of treatment is to strengthen the spleen and pacify the stomach.

Prescription Pishu (B 20), Tianshu (S 25), Zusanli (S 36).

Treatment procedure Reinforcing by lifting and thrusting the needle was applied. After three treatments, the stool turned somewhat solid and after six treatments it was normal. Then the treatment stopped. The next year she came for treatment of headache and said that her stool remained normal without any recurrence.

Explanation The Back-Shu points are the points on the back where the qi of the respective zang-fu organs is infused, while the Front-Mu points are the points in the chest and abdomen where the qi of the respective zang-fu organs is infused. Pishu (S 20), the Back-Shu point of the spleen, Tianshu (S 25), the Front-Mu point of the large intestine and Zusanli (S 36), the He-Sea point of the stomach are used in combination to regulate the qi of the stomach and intestine and to promote the recovery of the gastro-intestinal functions.

Case 3: Habitual constipation

Name, Du x x; sex, female; age, 50.

Complaints Constipation for over two years, stool movement once every three to five days, but in recent months once every seven to eight days, accompanied with anorexia, abdominal distension, yellow tongue coating and slippery pulse. She was treated by taking honey to lubricate the intestines and to promote the bowel movement, but with no significant effect.

Differentiation Stagnation of qi in the intestine and stomach leading to dysfunction of transportation and transformation.

Prescription Dachangshu (B 25), Daheng (Sp 15), Zhigou (SJ 6).

Treatment procedure Reducing by lifting and thrusting the needle was applied once a day. She had stool movement in small amount one hour later after each treatment, but difficulty at other times. The treatment was continued and after ten treatments, the bowel movement was basically normal.

Explanation Dachangshu (B 25) is used to remove stagnation of qi in the large intestine, Daheng (Sp 15) used to promote the transportation function of the spleen to facilitate bowel movements, and Zhigou (SJ 6) to activate qi activity of sanjiao. Modern medicine ascribes this condition to the impaired intestinal movement. Therefore, reducing by lifting and thrusting the needle with mild stimulation is applied to promote intestinal peristalsis and to facilitate bowel movements.

Case 4: Chronic rhinitis

Name, Gong x x; sex, male; age, 30.

Complaints Frequent nasal obstruction for more than four years (especially in the left nostril), sneezing in the morning or on sudden cold weather, dark red swollen nasal mucosa, and hyposmia.

Differentiation Impaired dispersing function of the lung and ascending of the pathogenic factors leading to stagnation of the nose.

Prescription Shangyingxiang (Extra), Tongtian (B 7) and Fengchi (G 20).

Treatment procedure Reducing by twirling and rotating the needle was applied. After being treated for three days, sneezing in the morning was greatly reduced, dark red swollen nasal mucosa was relieved; after six treatments mucous secretion was reduced, breathing of the left nostril improved, no appearance of sneezing on sudden cold weather; and after eleven treatments, nasal obstruction was removed and the sense of smell turned normal and other symptoms disappeared.

Explanation Shangyingxiang (Extra) is an important point for nasal disorders. Needling of this point may result in immediate sneezing. The combination with Fengchi (G 20) and Tongtian (B 7) may dispel wind and benefit the orifices.

Case 5: Goiter

Name, Ding x x; sex, female; age, 45.

Complaints Two years ago her husband died and she was depressed all the time. Later an enlargement about 3 x 3 cm of moderate hardness was found on the right side of the neck since about one year. It was diagnosed in one hospital as goiter and an operation was suggested. Since the patient was afraid of operations, she was introduced by her friends to Dr. Lou's clinic. Examination: String-taut rolling pulse, thin and clear tongue coating.

Differentiation Stagnation of qi and phlegm due to mental depression.

Prescription Shuitu (S 10), Tianding (LI 17) and Tiantu (Ren 22) on the affected side.

Treatment procedure After the needling sensation appeared, the even reinforcing and even reducing methods were applied for one or two minutes and then the needles were withdrawn. Treat once a day. Ten treatments constitute one course. The second course started after a one-week interval. At the end of the first course the enlargement was reduced to two thirds of the original size, and at the end of the second course it disappeared.

Explanation Shuitu (S 10), Tianding (LI 17) and Tiantu (Ren 22) located in the neck were needled to remove stagnation of qi in the related meridians and to promote the circulation of qi and blood. Since the case was not obvious in deficiency and excess, the even reinforcing-reducing method was applied.

Case 6: Mental disorder (schizophrenia)

Name, Zhang x x; sex, female; age, 24.

Complaints Her sleep had never been sound before. Two weeks ago some emotional factors provoked a mental depression, accompanied by insomnia and restlessness. In the last four or five days, she appeared apathetic, dully sitting all day long, murmuring, poor appetite and with the absence of the sense of hygiene. It was diagnosed as schizophrenia in one hospital and treated there without any effect. Then she came for acupuncture treatment.

Differentiation Misting the heart by the phlegm produced by depression of qi due to overthinking.

Prescription Shenmen (H 7), Jianshi (P 5), Ganshu (B 18) and Pishu (B 20).

Treatment procedure Even movement was applied by manipulating the needles for one or two minutes. After the first treatment her sleep was improved, and the next morning the murmuring was reduced. After the third treatment she became clear-minded and later treatments were given once every other day. Ten treatments cured the case.

Explanation Ganshu (B 18) and Pishu (B 20) were used to pacify the liver and strengthen the spleen to resolve the phlegm; Shenmen (H 7) and Jianshi (P 5) were used to remove stagnation of qi from the Heart and Pericardium Meridians to clear up the heart.

Case 7: Dysmenorrhea

Name, Luo x x; sex, female; age, 32.

Complaints Her menarche started at the age of thirteen with regular periods. When she reached the age of fifteen, lower abdominal distending pain and dizziness appeared on the first day of the menstruation but was not serious; later they became aggravated year after year. Since the age of twenty, due to emotional frustration, in addition to menstrual abdominal pain, there appeared lumbar soreness and breast distension five or six days before the menstrual period started. These symptoms became aggravated by drinking cold beverages in summer during the period at age twenty-two. Severe abdominal pain even stopped her from walking. She had to take pain killers and had a dark purplish menstrual flow, scanty in amount with clots; pain was relieved when the clots were released. She came for acupuncture treatment after medication failed. She was thin and pale, tongue coating thin and white, pulse string-taut and thready. Differentiation: Stagnation of liver qi and retention of cold in the uterus

Prescription Guilai (S 29) and Zhongji (Ren 3).

Treatment procedure Even movement was applied. The treatment started one week before the arrival of the period. Treat once a day until the end of the period. After the treatments before and during the first period, all the symptoms and signs were relieved and abdominal pain occurred only once without medication. After the treatment of the second period, the menstrual flow was normal, abdominal pain and other symptoms disappeared. In order to consolidate the therapeutic effect, another treatment was given in the third period. The follow-up visit for two years found no relapse.

Explanation Guilai (S 29) was used to warm and remove stagnation of qi and blood, and Zhongji (Ren 3) used to regulate the qi of Chong and Ren Meridians. The even method was applied because of asthenia, insufficiency of qi and blood and a small amount of menses, and a case of both excess and deficiency.

Case 8: Chronic rheumatic arthritis

Name, Fan x x; sex, male; age, 40.

Complaints Soreness and pain appeared in the bilateral elbow and knee joints due to dwelling in cold fields and wading in water during the war ten years ago. The symptoms became aggravated with weather changes. At present, there are intolerable cold and pain in the elbow and knee joints which should be kept warm even in hot summer. Medication of both Chinese herbs and Western drugs was tried, but failed to achieve the effect.

Differentiation Failing to protect the skin surface due to weakness of defensive qi and invasion by pathogenic wind, cold and damp obstructing the meridians and collaterals.

Prescription Quchi (LI 11), Dubi (S 35), Xiyangguan (G 33), Yanglingquan (G 34) and Liangqiu (S 34).

Treatment procedure Setting the mountain on fire method was applied at Quchi (LI 11) and Dubi (S 35) points. Reducing by twirling and rotating the needle at Xiyangguan (G 33) and Yanglingquan (G 34) points. After two treatments, cold and pain in the elbow and knee joints were alleviated, and after eight treatments, cold and pain in the elbow joints disappeared. Although cold and pain in the knee joints were alleviated continuously, radical elimination was impossible. At the fourteenth treatment the former four points were not used, but Liangqiu (S 34) was selected. Cold and pain in the knee joints were nearly eliminated at the night of the same day and after another two treatments the case was cured.

Explanation Local points are used to remove stagnation and obstruction of qi and blood from the meridians and collaterals and to regulate the nutrient and defensive systems to dispel the pathogenic wind, cold and damp, thus cold pain was alleviated. Although cold pain in the elbow joints was cured only by needling one point Quchi (LI 11), and needling of Dubi (S 35), Xiyangguan (G 33) and Yanglingquan (G 34) points relieved cold pain only a little in the knee joints, needling of Liangqiu (S 34) was employed instead and completely cured the case after three treatments. Liangqiu (S 34) is a Xi-Cleft point of the Stomach Meridian of Foot-Yangming. The Xi-Cleft point is the place where the qi of the meridians converges. For this case the pathogenic wind, cold and damp invaded a deep portion of the body and none other than these points can eliminate them.

Case 9: Bronchial asthma

Name, Lou x x; sex, male; age, 13.

Complaints Asthmatic cough with profuse sputum occurred after the measles at age five, initially attacked two or three times every year, but more frequent in recent years, and evoked by cold invasion. A gurgling sound was heard in the throat and suffocation appeared in the chest during attacks. In severe cases, breathing with the mouth widely open and shoulders raised, cyanosis of the complexion, emaciation, pallor, pale tongue with thin coating, thready and weak pulse.

Differentiation Retention of phlegm leading to impaired dispersing and descending function of the lung, and invasion of wind-cold causing stagnation of qi and accumulation of phlegm. The repeated attacks injured the lung qi, diseased mother affecting the son, so the kidney was involved. Deficiency of both lungs and the kidney worsened the case. The principle of treatment was to treat the root case. Moxibustion with ginger was employed to benefit the lung and kidney qi, promote qi circulation and resolve phlegm.

Prescription 1) Feishu (B 13), Lingtai (Du 10); 2) Shenshu (B 23); 3) Tiantu (Ren 22), Tanzhong (Ren 17).

Treatment procedure The above three groups of points are used alternately with moxibustion with ginger. Put the half-date sized ignited moxa cones on the points with slices of ginger in between. One group of points is applied each day, five to seven cones on each point. Nine treatments constitute one course (three groups of points used alternately three times).

Explanation Acupuncture and moxibustion are well indicated in this case. During acute attacks, puncturing Hegu (LI 4), Lieque (L 7) and Dingchuan (Extra) (0.5 to 1 cun lateral to Dazhui) with reducing by twirling and rotating the needles, which are retained for ten to fifteen minutes, then asthma can be relieved promptly. At chronic stage the above mentioned moxibustion method is applied on the three groups of points (usually in summer) to eliminate the root cause. Feishu (B 13) is used to nourish lung qi, Shenshu (B 23) is used to reinforce the kidney qi, in combination with Tanzhong (Ren 17) to promote the circulation of qi, Lingtai (Du 10) to stop asthma, Tiantu (Ren 22) to facilitate the throat and resolve phlegm, thus asthma is cured. If applied in child cases, this therapy would be especially effective. After being treated for one course, the follow-up visits during five years showed the stable therapeutic effect and the absence of relapse.

APPLICATION OF QI INDUCING METHOD AND MAKING A HERBAL FUMIGATOR

—Yan Youzhai's Clinical Experience

Yan Youzhai, born in Guilin, Guangxi Province, in 1916, began to learn medicine in his family from his childhood. He graduated from Wuxi China Acupuncture Training Centre, Jiangsu Province, in 1934, and became a teacher of the Acupuncture Training Course run by Guangxi Autonomous Regional Bureau of Public Health in 1954, where he lectured *New Acupuncture Therapy* written by Dr. Zhu Lian; and spread the needle insertion technique with the help of tube. He is now an assistant doctor-in-chief of the Acupuncture Department of Nanxishan Hospital, Guangxi Province, vice-chairman of the Committee of Guangxi Regional Acupuncture and Moxibustion Association, chairman of the Committee of Guilin Acupuncture and Moxibustion Society, and advisor to the Hong Kong-China Acupuncture Association.

I. Academic Characteristics and Medical Specialities

1. Applying qigong to induce qi arrival

It is said in *Ode to the Standard of Mystery* that "The immediate therapeutic effect results from the fast arrival of qi (needling sensation); otherwise, the diseases could be hardly treated," indicating the close relation between the arrival of qi and the therapeutic result. If a loose sensation is felt under the needle and the qi fails to arrive even after the auxiliary manipulations are applied to induce the qi, Yan will release the external qi from Dantian to the puncturing hand to rotate, lift and thrust the needle to treat a disease. Soon after the fingers of the puncturing hand feel the smooth flow of the meridian qi, either the reinforcing or reducing method may be manipulated in accordance with the pathological conditions. This method is suitable for deficiency cases. Yan once treated a middle-aged woman who had suffered from chronic epilepsy accompanied by in continence of urine. Three treatments were given in all and the symptoms of epilepsy and incontinence of urine disappeared. Such a method is also effective in the treatment of chronic gastroptosis.

In general, applying qigong to induce qi arrival may only be done three times a day.

2. Possibility of insertion to the forbidden points

The forbidden points collected in the *Compendium of Acupuncture* are: Naohu (Du 17), Xinhui (Du 22), Shentin (Du 24), Yuzhen (B 9), Luoque (B 8), Chengling (G 18), Jimen (Sp 11), Luxi (SJ 19), Jiaosun (SJ 20), Shendao (Du 11), Lingtai (Du 10),

Tanzhong (Ren 17), Shuifen (Ren 9), Shenque (Ren 8), Huiyin (Ren 1), Henggu (K 11), Qichong (S 30), Chengjin (B 56), Wuli (LI 13), Sanyangluo (SJ 8) and Qingling (H 2), etc., which are the clinical experiences recorded by the ancient physicians. In fact, there are no important internal organs under these points except Naohu (Du 17), Shenque (Ren 8) and Qichong (S 20). They are considered as the forbidden points in ancient times, as Yan estimated, because at that time needles were rough and thick and there might be some accidents when those points were needled. Hence they were noted as the forbidden points. This idea could be confirmed from the other records of some other medical classics, as plenty of those points were used to treat certain diseases. For instance, *Acupuncture Prescriptions,* Vol. 6 says, "Tanzhong (Ren 17) and Juque (Ren 14) may be used to stop phrenalgia and promote appetite." "Needling Xinhui (Du 22) and Yuzhen (B 9) together treats headache due to exogenous wind invasion." Here in this book that Tanzhong (Ren 17), Xinhui (Du 22) and Yuzhen (B 9) are all noted able to be needled. Yan once used Shenting (Du 24) to treat nasal disorders with very good results. All these enlightened him to use modern anatomy knowledge to study those forbidden points. He thinks that the needles may be certainly inserted to those points according to the pathological conditions if there are no important zang or fu organs under the points. For instance, Shangxing (Du 23) is only 0.5 cun superior and posterior to Shenting (Du 24), and there is not any important organ there. Shangxing (Du 23) can be needled, as so might be Shenting (Du 24). Shendao (Du 11) and Lingtai (Du 10) are found as the reaction spots of gastric disorders in clinical treatment. Thus, needling these two points may stop gastric pain: The combination of Tanzhong (Ren 17) with Shaoze (SI 1) for treating lactation deficiency has already been applied all over the country. Sanyangluo (SJ 8) is used to treat arm pain; Shuifen (Ren 9) helps urination; Luxi (SJ 19) may treat ear disorders; Huiyin (Ren 1) is always used as an emergency point for loss of consciousness due to drowning. Yan emphasizes that these forbidden points are from the records of the ancients' experience, and there is surely some validity for their observations. However, we should carefully study the application of the forbidden points, but not take chances.

3. Reforming the herbal fumigator on the basis of the ancient techniques

In order to overcome the shortcomings of the old fumigation therapy consuming the medicine but with low effect, Yan has designed a new fumigator for steaming purposes. Through seven years of clinical practice, he has found it effective in treating rheumatic arthritis, sciatica and chronic facial paralysis, among which it is especially good for treating painful joints with a swelling and hot sensation. Only two or three treatments might alleviate the swelling and stop the pain, and the curative rate was above 90 percent by observing eight cases.

Prescription for fuming herbs:

Notopterygium 10 g.
Radix Angelicae Pubescentis 10 g.
Chinese mugwort leaves 8 g.

Schematic drawing for drug smoker

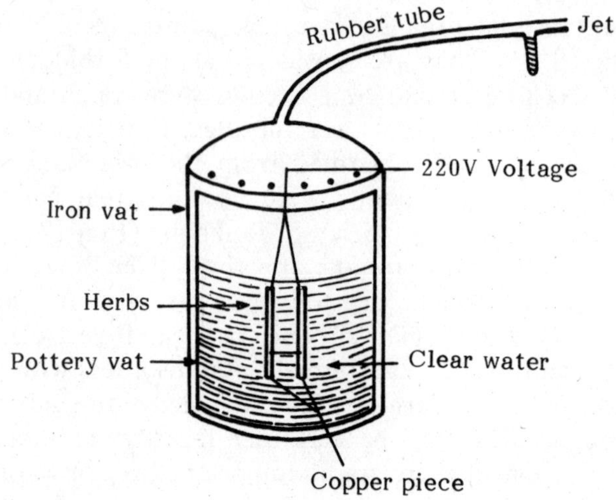

Radix Ledebouriellae 8 g.
Herba Schizonepetae 6 g.
Radix Angelicae Dahuricae 10 g.

II. Case Analysis

Case 1: Gastroptosis

Name, Yan x x; sex, male; age, 45.

Complaints The patient developed gradually epigastric pain and distension for three years, as he had generally worked very hard and had a weak constitution. He preferred acidic or pungent food. He was treated with both herbal medicine and Western drugs, but with little help. At present he had fullness at the epigastric region which became aggravated after a meal, poor digestion, borborygmus without gas, loose stool with about five to eight bowel movements each day. Examination: Poor nourishment, sallow complexion, general lassitude, unformed stool for two years, poor appetite, deep, thready and forceless pulse; red tongue body with thin and white coating. The patient preferred smoking and drinking. The barium meal examination with X ray showed 9 cm. down of the stomach—the gastroptosis.

Differentiation Dysfunction in transportation and transformation. Treatment principle is to strengthen the yang and body resistance, regulate the function of the spleen and stomach.

Prescription Pishu (B 20), Weishu (B 21), Zusanli (S 36), Shangwan (Ren 13), Zhongwan (Ren 12), Xiawan (Ren 10), Lingtai (Du 10), Zhiyang (Du 9) and Baihui (Du 20).

Treatment procedure Only one of the three points, Shangwan (Ren 13), Zhongwan (Ren 12) and Xiawan (Ren 10) was needled in each treatment and so was Lingtai (Du 10) and Zhiyang (Du 9), just select one of them each time. Pishu (B 20) and Weishu (B 21) were used alternately with the fumigator. The other points were reinforced with either lifting-thrusting rotating techniques or the breathing technique. Moxibustion was applied at Baihui (Du 20). The distension was somewhat alleviated after three treatments, and his appetite also improved. He had gas, formed stool with two bowel movements daily, but no more lassitude. His pulse became forceful after the fifth treatment. The epigastric distension was totally gone and stool was well formed with only one bowel movement daily; his spirit became good. The barium X-ray showed the stomach ascend 8 cm. The patterned medicine Buzhong Yiqi Wan (pills for reinforcing spleen and stomach and replenishing the vital energy) was prescribed to him for consolidating the result when acupuncture treatment stopped. A 3-year follow-up visit revealed no recurrence of the disease.

Explanation Ptosis of the internal organs pertains to deficiency of qi, which falls into the category of yang and blood pertains to yin. Du Meridian governs the yang of the body. Moxibustion at Baihui (Du 20) may raise up yang. Lingtai (Du 10) is considered as a reaction and tender of gastric disorders and is one of the forbidden points, but it is found all right to be needled throughout Yan's clinical practice, as needling this point may stop the pain at once. Puncturing Zhiyang (Du 9) strengthens yang qi as well. Shangwan (Ren 13), Zhongwan (Ren 12) and Xiawan (Ren 10) in combination with the points from the Du Meridian may regulate both yin and yang to promote the circulation of qi and blood.

Case 2: Constipation

Name, Xie x x; sex, male; age, 38.

Complaints The patient had about twenty years chronic constipation with five to ten days a bowel movement. And he could hardly have a bowel movement in two weeks if he stopped taking any cathartics. He had no pain or distension in the abdomen, but he felt dryness in mouth; or at times he had swelling and pain of the gum which might go away after bowel movement. His appetite was all right. The patient looked strong, but he had foul breath, a rolling rapid pulse, rough and dry tongue coating. It was a complete excess condition.

Principle of treatment To eliminate the heat from the large intestine and Sanjiao.

Prescription Dachangshu (B 28), Zhigou (SJ 6).

Treatment procedure The above two points were needled with reducing method by applying lifting-thrusting and rotating techniques. Treatment was given daily. Three days later the patient had a bowel movement with extremly dry stool. After that the treatment was given every other day another five times. The patient had a bowel movement each day; dryness of mouth was alleviated and there was no swelling and pain of the gum. The heat was dispelled from the large intestine which became normal. The treatment was stopped. A follow-up visit 2 years later revealed that the bowel movement remained normal and occurred once daily or every other day.

Explanation Reducing method given at Dachangshu (B 28) has great effect in the treatment of habitual constipation according to Yan's experience.

Case 3: Bi syndrome of the tendons

Name, Huang Lanzhen; sex, female; age, 61.

Complaints The patient had three years of pain at the lower back and knee with frequent attacks which worsened when the weather changed. Examination showed that her right knee was swollen and red; hot sensation on superficial skin when palpated. She could hardly extend her leg or walk, and she was carried into the clinic for acupuncture treatment. The patient had no other complaints except the right knee problem. Her pulse was rapid, tongue was slightly yellow but sticky.

Differentiation Bi syndrome of the tendons due to the invasion by the exogenous wind, cold, and damp which stagnated the circulation of qi and blood.

Treatment principle To eliminate damp and heat from the blood.

Prescription Neixiyan (Extra), Dubi (S 35) were needled on the diseased side; and Xuehai (Sp 10) was needled bilaterally.

Treatment procedure Reducing method was applied with rotating, lifting and thrusting techniques. The fumigator was used at the local area. The pain and swelling were much alleviated after the first treatment. About 2/3 alleviation of the swelling was obtained when the second treatment finished; and the hot sensation at the local area was also released. She could extend her right leg. After the third treatment there was no any pain or swelling, and she could walk slowly. The patient recovered after the fourth treatment. A follow-up visit three years later revealed no recurrence of the disease.

Explanation Needling Dubi (S 35) and Neixiyan (Extra) may eliminate the damp from the knee joint. Puncturing Xuehai (Sp 10) dispels the heat from the blood. A fumigator was then added to disperse wind and damp, remove the stagnation and promote the circulation of qi and blood in the meridians and collaterals in order to strengthen the therapeutic result.

Case 4: Blindness

Name, Deng Xialian; sex, female; age, 52.

Complaints Several months before the patient had received five to six injections of penicillin and streptomycin after an illness. Then she developed a reaction to the drugs with symptoms of blindness of both eyes and tinnitus, dizziness and vertigo. The patient usually had soreness of the lower back and weakness of the knee, dream-disturbed sleep, and difficulty falling asleep. After having the adverse reaction she got edema on the face and on the lower extremities, difficulty in urination, spontaneous sweating or night sweating, aversion to wind even in hot days; poor appetite, loose stool, dry mouth, palpitation and insomnia, severe dizziness. She was treated over one month in the county hospital, but with little help. She was subsequently diagnosed as having sequela of streptomycin poisoning.

Examination Edema on the face below the two eyes and on the legs below the knee; sallow complexion, lassitude, weak voice, deep, thready and forceless pulse, especially at "Chi" region, flabby tongue body edged with tooth prints, slightly yellow and sticky tongue coating. Since the liver and kidney were involved, the points of the Liver and

Kidney Meridians should be primarily selected in combination with some other points.

Prescriptions Three groups of points for the first course of treatment: 1) Ganshu (B 18), Shenshu (B 23), Mingmen (Du 4), Fengchi (G 20), Guangming (G 37); 2) Zanzhu (B 2), Jingming (B 1), Yifeng (SJ 17), Xingjian (Liv 2); and 3) Ganshu (B 18), Shenshu (B 23), Yuzhen (B 9), Sanyinjiao (Sp 6).

Three groups of points for the second course of treatment: 1) Qiuhou (Extra), Zanzhu (B 2), Guangming (G 37), Fengyan (Extra); 2) Shenshu (B 23), Mingmen (Du 4), Taixi (K 3), Yuzhen (B 9); and 3) Shenshu (B 23), Taichong (Liv 3), Qiuhou (Extra), Zanzhu (B 2).

Three groups of points for the third course of the treatment: 1) Sibai (S 2), Shangjingming (Extra), Yuzhen (B 9), Sanyinjiao (Sp 6); 2) Qiuhou (Extra), Yuyao (Extra), Taixi (K 3), Fengyan (Extra); and 3) Jingming (B 1), Sibai (S 2), Zhongzhu (SJ 3), Mingmen (Du 4).

Treatment procedure Ten treatment constituted a course and treatment was given daily during the first course with each group of points for one treatment alternately. Guangming (G 37) and Ganshu (B 18) were needled with the reducing method first and the reinforcing method afterward by rotating, lifting and thrusting techniques. The other points were needled with the reinforcing method only and the breathing reinforcing technique in addition. Treatment was given every other day during the second course. Guangming (G 37) and Taichong (Liv 3) were needled with the reducing method first and the reinforcing method applied afterward; the rest points were all needled with the reinforcing method. Treatment was given also every other day during the third course and all the points were needled with the reinforcing method. When the first course finished, the patient could see a little light on both eyes, and she also could walk at home; her tinnitus was somewhat alleviated, her hearing was improved and dizziness and vertigo were relieved. Treatments of the first course were repeated again. In the middle of the second course the visual acuity became 0.4 and the other symptoms improved. When the third course finished, the dizziness and tinnitus were much alleviated, hearing became normal, and she also could walk normally. Visual acuity was 0.6. Acupuncture treatment then stopped, but the patient was prescribed some herbal medicine for regulating yin and yang in order to consolidate the acupuncture therapeutic result. Half a year later the patient wrote a letter saying that she had been working normally. A 3-year follow-up visit revealed no recurrence of the disease.

Explanation Streptomycin poisoning is usually characterized by damage of the acoustic nerve. But in this case, the patient previously suffered long-term kidney qi deficiency. Pupil pertains to the kidney, so the eyes may also be involved. The principle of treatment should regulate the qi circulation of both the kidney and liver; and puncture some local points to enhance the therapeutic result.

SIMULTANEOUS NEEDLING OF TWO ACUPOINTS AND SELECTION OF SPECIFIC POINTS

—Wei Fengpo's Clinical Experience

Wei Fengpo was born on December 25, 1928 in Yingkou of Liaoning Province. He studied in the China Medical University from 1948 to 1952. After graduation he was assigned to work in the Xiehe Hospital which was affiliated to the South China Tongji Medical College. In 1957, he started working with Zhu Shimo, a well-known traditional Chinese medical doctor in the TCM Department of the hospital. During the period between 1962 to 1965, he studied Traditional Chinese Medicine in a course offered to Western doctors in the Hubei College of Traditional Chinese Medicine. After finishing the course, he started his practice in the Acupuncture Department of the Affiliated Hospital of Hubei College of TCM. In 1973, he received one year's further training in the Brain Department and the Department of Neurology of Tianjin Medical College. Between 1974 and 1976, as a member of a medical team aiding foreign countries, Dr. Wei worked in the acupuncture department of a hospital in Algeria.

He has accumulated experience in simultaneous needling of two points and selection of specific points in the treatment of disease. He has published more than ten papers and compiled *Acupuncture and Moxibustion,* which is a part of the book called *New Compilation of Clinical Traditional Chinese Medicine.*

Dr. Wei is now the deputy director of the Acupuncture Department of the Hubei College of Traditional Chinese Medicine and associate professor.

I. Academic Characteristics and Medical Specialities

1. Insertion and manipulation of two needles with both hands at the same time

Two needles are held with the operator's left and right hands and inserted into two points at the same time; meanwhile, lifting, thrusting and rotation techniques as well as reinforcing and reducing by needling along and against the running course of the meridians respectively are manipulated in order to obtain arrival of qi, propagated sensation along the meridians and the reinforcing and reducing requirements. Repeat the above-mentioned procedure once or twice every ten minutes.

1) *Simultaneous insertion and manipulation of two needles at two points from the same meridian or from the nearby two meridians* An even number of the points two to six is selected from the same meridian or from the nearby two meridians, and two points are needled and manipulated at the same time. This method is applicable to such diseases as the bi syndrome, hemiplegia, sciatica and sequelae of infantile paralysis. In the treatment of sciatica, for example, Zhibian (B 54), Huantiao (G 30), Chengfu (B 36) and Yinmen (B 37) are needled two times, two points each, and at the same time, insertion

and manipulation are performed. Since these four points are located either on or close to the course of the sciatic nerve, deep insertion may ensure a 100 percent success rate of radiating the needling sensation down to the dorsum of the foot or toes. Simultaneous needling of the two points greatly enhances the needling sensation, thus dredging the meridians, circulating qi and blood and eliminating wind and cold.

In March, 1969, a middle aged male patient complained of severe pain in the left lower extremity for one week, which was aggravated at night. Before the attack he used to sit in a damp place while working.

He had difficulty in walking, and his left lower limb was under compulsive position. Examination: Tenderness along the course of the sciatic nerve; (+) straight leg raising test: 30 degrees; Absence of tenderness or percussion pain around the lumbar vertebrae. Cough was not present.

The disease was diagnosed as primary sciatica.

The above mentioned four points were needled four times. The disease was cured after one week.

2) *Simultaneous needling of the two points from the meridians of the same name or from the two meridians of yin and yang* This includes the selection of the points from the meridians on the upper and lower extremities with the same name or from the meridians of yin and yang.

In the treatment of hemiplegia due to windstroke, for example, Jianyu (LI 15), Quchi (LI 11), Hegu (LI 4), Zusanli (S 36), Fenglong (S 40) and Jiexi (S 41) are selected; Huantiao (G 30), Yanglingquan (G 34) and Xuanzhong (G 39) are also applicable; and Xuehai (Sp 10), Sanyinjiao (Sp 6), Xingjian (Liv 2) and Taichong (Liv 3) can also be used.

Simultaneous needling may invigorate the Yangming Meridian which has ample qi and blood. The circulation of qi leads to free circulation of blood, thus resulting in spontaneous elimination of wind. The combination of the points from the yin meridians is aimed at nourishing yin, suppressing yang, pacifying the liver to stop wind, balancing yin and yang, dredging the meridians and promoting the circulation of qi and blood.

Simultaneous needling of the symmetrical points on both sides from the meridians with the same name is applicable to such diseases as swelling and pain of the throat, myasthnia laryngitis, hoarse voice and hyperthyroidism. Renying (S 9), Shuitu (S 10), Qishe (S 11), Hegu (LI 4) and Zhaohai (K 6) are needled bilaterally, which have the functions to circulate qi, reinforce qi, nourish yin and resolve masses in the local area.

A hundred and sixty-five cases of throat problems, including myasthenia larynx, hoarse voice, vocal nodules, polyp of vocal cord, hematocele of vocal cord, acute and chronic laryngitis, were treated with satisfactory results, especially for myasthenia laryngitis and hoarse voice.

3) *Simultaneous deep needling of the Back-Shu points and Baliao points on both sides* This means that each of these points on both sides is needled deeply at the same time, deeper than that described in general acupuncture books. Simultaneous deep needling at Feishu (B 13) on both sides, for example, is very effective for bronchial asthma. In May 1982, this needling technique was demonstrated in the advanced course for Japancsc acupuncturists hcld in thc Norman Bcthunc IIospital in Changchun. The

Japanese students made comparisons between respiratory sounds and wheezing sounds before and after needling by recording them on auscultation stethoscope. The wheezing sound was improved or even disappeared soon after needling, as did the other symptoms and signs.

Baliao includes Shangliao (B 31), Ciliao (B 32), Zhongliao (B 33) and Xialiao (B 34).

Ciliao (B 32) can be needled as deep as three or four inches. Simultaneous needling of the point on both sides generally effects downward radiation of the needling sensation to the perineum and external genitalia. This method is applicable to many diseases such as infantile enuresis, retention of urine, constipation, incontinence of urine and feces, impotence, nocturnal emission and diseases of the uterus, appendix and pelvic cavity. Satisfactory results can be expected generally, and some patients will notice marked improvement after the first treatment.

In July, 1968, a middle aged male patient came to the acupuncture clinic for the treatment of arthritis. The case history showed that seventeen years before he was hospitalized for six months due to traumatic paraplegia, which was gradually resolved later, but he still couldn't control urine and feces effectively. For this he had consulted many doctors in different hospitals, but in vain.

Ciliao (B 32) was needled deeply on both sides at the same time, and the needling sensation was referred to the penis. The patient noted marked improvement after the first treatment, as the urine could be basically controlled. He didn't continue the treatment until early September, when another two treatments were given. The disease was almost cured after these treatments.

4) *Shallow penetration of a few points from different meridians with a long needle, and deep penetration of points* Shallow penetration of a few points with a long needle is usually applied to the points on the head and face, while deep penetration of points is applied to the points from opposite yin and yang meridians in the four limbs.

Examples of shallow penetration include Touwei (S 8) towards Shuaigu (G 8), Jiache (S 6) towards Dicang (S 4), Dicang (S 4) towards Yingxiang (LI 20), Yingxiang (LI 20) towards Jingming (B 1), Dicang (S 4) towards Sibai (S 2) or Chengqi (S 1), and Baihui (Du 20) towards Qubin (G 7), etc. In the treatment of migraine, for example, Touwei (S 8) is penetrated towards Shuaigu (G 8). For deviation of the mouth and eye, Dicang (S 4) is penetrated towards Yingxiang (LI 20) or Sibai (S 2) or Chengqi (S 1). Some of the pair points can be penetrated in either way for example Jiache (S 6) and Dicang (S 4).

Deep penetration of points is applicable to such diseases as deeply located bi syndromes and sprain of the joints. Examples of deep penetration include Quchi (LI 11) towards Shaohai (H 3), Zhigou (SJ 6) towards Jianshi (P 5), Yanglingquan (G 34) towards Yinlingquan (Sp 9), Xuanzhong (G 39) towards Sanyinjiao (Sp 6), Qiuxu (G 40) towards Zhaohai (K 6), and Taichong (Liv 3) towards Yongquan (K 1), etc.

Penetrating Quchi (LI 11) towards Shaohai (H 3) has proved effective for pregnancy hypertension and preeclampsia. Thirty cases of such diseases were treated in this way in the Gynecological Department of the hospital with satisfactory results. This method prevents the harmful influence of drugs on the fetus. Taichong (Liv 3) penetrating towards Yongquan (K 1) in combination with Zusanli (S 36) will lower the blood pressure by 20 to 30 mmHg of systolic pressure and 10 mmHg of diastolic pressure after treatment.

Penetrating Qiuxu (G 40) towards Zhaohai (K 6) is effective for acute sprain of the ankle joint. In autumn of 1970, a 50-year-old male patient was carried into the acupuncture clinic for the treatment. Qiuxu (G 40) was penetrated towards Zhaohai (K 6) and the needle was retained for twenty minutes after qi arrived. The reducing method was applied when the needle was withdrawn. The patient could walk home after the treatment.

2. Selection of specific points

Specific points refer to those having proved effective in the treatment of certain diseases. The following is a preliminary generalization of specific points according to their indications and locations:

1) *The four points related to wind on the posterior aspect of the head and neck are Fengfu (Du 16), Fengchi (G 20), Yifeng (SJ 17) and Fengmen (B 12).*

a. Fengfu (Du 16): A meeting point of the Du Meridian and the Yangwei Meridian. The Du Meridian dominates yang of the whole body, functioning to adjust all the yang meridians. Fengfu (Du 16) is able to eliminate wind and cold, clear heat and fire, and calm the mind. The book *Plain Questions* explains the relation between this point and wind, when it says: "The pathogenic wind enters Fengfu (Du 16), goes upward to the brain along the meridian, thus causing headache." The point is located midway between Fengchi (G 20) and Yifeng (SJ 17), thus commanding all the wind points. This point is also indicated in any phlegm diseases related to wind.

b. Fengchi (G 20): A meeting point of the Gallbladder Meridian, Yangqiao Meridian and Yangwei Meridian. The Yangwei Meridian is in communication with all the yang meridians, and dominates the exterior of the body. Fengchi (G 20) functions to relieve exterior syndromes, eliminate pathogenic wind, reduce damp and heat, promote the function of the liver and gallbladder, pacify the Shaoyang Meridian and relieve pain. Since the point eliminates both external and internal wind, it is regarded as a key point in the treatment of wind diseases. Its extensive indications include febrile diseases due to cold, headache, disorders of the eye, ear and nose, and neurasthenia. In cases of common cold with the symptoms of aversion to cold, fever and headache, Fengchi (G 20) is combined with Fengfu (Du 16). Fengchi (G 20) is absolutely essential in the treatment of central or peripheral facial paralysis. It is also often selected in the treatment of migraine, headache, dizziness and headache resulting from cerebral concussion as well as diseases of the eyes.

Sixty cases of myopia of senior middle school graduates were treated before the college entrance examination in 1965. Eyesight improved by 0.2 to 0.3 on the average after six to twelve treatments. Some students recovered after a short period of time. Fengchi (G 20) is dispensable in the treatment of diseases of eye fungus. Ten cases of such diseases, different in nature and severity, were treated successfully by needling the point on both sides at the same time. The needles were directed towards the eye or zygoma on the other side 1.2 to 1.5 inches deep. Lifting, thrusting and rotation were performed, radiating the needling sensation to the forehead or eye region along the occipital and parietal regions of the head. As said in *Ode to the Standard of Mystery*, "reducing is applied in cases of excess syndromes with pain, while reinforcing is applied in cases of deficiency syndromes with itchiness and numbness."

c. Yifeng (SJ 17): A meeting point of Shaoyang Meridians of Hand and Foot, which is indicated in wind diseases and ear disorders. Its action is to circulate qi and blood, remove blood stasis, suppress fire and relieve pain. Clinical use over the past eight years has proved its effectiveness in the treatment of vascular and nervous headache, especially of migraine. Fifty cases of migraine of different types were successfully treated by needling this point three to five times. Some cases even responded markedly to the first treatment.

In early July, 1986, a female staff member of the college, aged thirty, had neurovascular migraine for many years which was characterized by periodic onsets with marked symptoms and signs of the vegetative nervous system, accompanied by headache, blurred vision, dizziness, pallor, sweating, nausea and vomiting. She had to rest in bed during the attack. Neither Western drugs nor Chinese herbs could relieve the pain.

In order to observe the specific therapeutic properties of Yifeng (SJ 17), the patient was asked to take rheoencephalography before and after needling. Its amplitude increased and exceeded the width of the rheoencephalogram paper before needling. The amplitude turned normal along with the disappearance of the symptoms and signs after three daily treatments. She had another treatment in early September for prevention. The disease never occurred again from then on.

Another female patient of fifty years old with migraine came to the clinic from Sichuan Province. She also took rheoencephology during the first treatment. Yifeng (SJ 17) was needled 2 to 2.5 inches deep with the needle directing towards the mastoid process on the other side. The needling sensation was radiated to the throat or to the root of the tongue with the technique, heavy thrusting and slow lifting. During her second visit the following day, she told the doctor that she had slept well after the first treatment, and when she woke up, she felt as vigorous as when she was young.

d. Fengmen (B 12): A meeting point of the Du Meridian and Bladder Meridian. As residence of heat is its another name, it is indicated in various heat syndromes. The point is also the gateway through which pathogenic wind invades the body, so it is also a frequently used point for wind diseases. The point is able to dispel the wind and cold, and produce sweating. When it is used in the treatment of the common cold, flu and cough, the point on both sides is needled at the same time with the reducing method (thrusting the needle once slowly followed by lifting the needle three times heavily while rotating the needle). Moxibustion is applicable if there are cold signs. Since deep needling adjusts the vegetative nerve ganglion, it is used for either profuse sweating or absence of sweating.

Among all the four points related to wind, Fengmen (B 12) is mainly for external wind, Yifeng (SJ 17) for internal wind and Fengchi (G 20) and Fengfu (Du 16) for both.

2) *Hypnotic points, analgesic points, tranquilizing points and spasmolytic points on the head, hand and foot*

a. Hypnotic point—Anmian (Extra):

Anmian (Extra), a new point discovered by Dr. Wei in recent years, is located in the middle of the line connecting Yifeng (SJ 17) and Fengchi (G 20). Since the three wind points of Yifeng (SJ 17), Fengchi (G 20) and Fengfu (Du 16) have the tranquilizing, analgesic and hypnotic effects, Anmian (Extra), which is level with the above three points and close to the brain, must have the same effects. Clinical practice has confirmed Dr. Wei's inference. Some patients with insomnia respond to the point even more effectively.

In May, 1968, a forty-year old armyman was admitted to the hospital due to severe insomnia. He couldn't sleep well for one month and couldn't fall asleep at all over the past week. The daily oral administration of Chinese herbs and large dose of Western hypnagogue didn't help him. At 11 o'clock one night, Dr. Wei was asked to treat the patient with acupuncture for the first time. The patient looked indifferent with a drawn countenance. He didn't speak a lot, yet he was very anxious about the disease. He also showed a poor appetite, a pale tongue with white coating and a slow pulse.

Anmian (Extra) on both sides was needled at the same time with the even lifting, thrusting and rotation technique. The needles were retained for twenty minutes and manipulated twice, two minutes each time. The patient fell asleep soon after the withdrawal of the needles. He slept for five hours and was in much better spirits the next day. The same treatment was continued six times until he was discharged from the hospital.

Since then, Anmian (Extra) has become a point of choice for insomnia. Five cases of insomnia were treated with this point and all of them received satisfactory results.

b. Analgesic point—Hegu (LI 4):

As the Yuan (Source) Point of the Large Intestine Meridian of Hand-Yangming, which has ample qi and blood, Hegu (LI 4) is an important point for regulating qi and blood of the body, functioning to clear the meridians, circulate qi and blood, relieve the exterior syndrome, eliminate wind, clear heat and regulate the stomach and intestines. According to Dr. Wei's experience, Hegu (LI 4) is also an important analgesic point like Yifeng (SJ 17).

In 1968, an elderly patient wanted a tooth extracted. But he was sensitive to anaesthetics. Acupuncture anaesthesia was decided. Dr. Wei punctured Hegu (LI 4) on both sides at the same time with both hands. A few minutes after qi was obtained, the tooth was extracted smoothly with little bleeding.

Female doctors and nurses of the hospital often asked Dr. Wei for help when they had dysmenorrhea. Most got relief from pain after needling Hegu (LI 4) on both sides at the same time.

Hegu (LI 4) is more often selected in the treatment of headache, facial pain, toothache and sore throat, either as a main point or as an additional one. It was so effective in the treatment of disease that medical scholars of all ages listed it as one of the four main points in the rhymes of acupuncture.

c. Tranquilizing points—Shenmen (H 7) and Neiguan (P 6):

Shenmen (H 7) is the Shu-Stream and Yuan (Source) Point of the Heart Meridian of Hand-Shaoyin. It calms the mind by nourishing and soothing the heart. Once the mind is calmed, pain will be relieved. The indication of Shenmen (H 7) is closely related to the heart and mind including cardiac pain, palpitation, restlessness, fear, fright, anxiety, poor memory, mental cloudiness and epilepsy.

In the treatment of neurasthenia with the symptoms of insomnia, Shenmen (H 7) is needled towards Tongli (H 5), or Shenmen (H 7) is tapped with a plum-blossom needle dozens of times.

In July, 1986, a middle-aged female teacher came to the clinic, complaining of neurasthenia for five years. She had nervousness, palpitation and emaciation. She weighed forty-five kilograms.

The above treatment was adopted. Treatment was given twice a week. She noted the improvement after the second treatment. After the fourth treatment, palpitation disappeared, nervousness was relieved and she could sleep better. The treatment was discontinued in August, as Dr. Wei went away on his business trip. Another two treatments were administered in September. All the symptoms and signs were basically relieved. Her weight was increased by five kilograms. In order to consolidate the therapeutic results, the patient was asked to go on with the treatment once a week. She fully recovered later.

Neiguan (P 6) is the Luo (Connecting) Point of the Pericardium Meridian of Hand-Jueyin, connecting with the Sanjiao Meridian of Hand-Shaoyang. It is also the Confluent Point of Eight Extra Meridians communicating with the Yinwei Meridian. It functions to clear the meridian, dredge sanjiao, relax the chest, regulate qi, pacify the stomach, conduct the rebellious qi downward, calm the mind and relieve pain. It is indicated in diseases of the stomach, heart and chest. Both clinical practice and experimental observation have confirmed its effectiveness in dealing with angina pectoris of coronary heart disease and arrhythmia. Dr. Wei also uses this point to treat cardiovascular neurosis, gastrointestinal neurosis, neurasthenia and menopause syndromes.

Nervous vomiting manifests as vomiting without nausea or pain. Neiguan (P 6) on both sides is needled at the same time with both hands. If the patient is afraid of needling, try to divert his or her attention and insert the needle rapidly. The needle is rotated gently and retained shallowly. In this way, good results will be obtained immediately.

d. Spasmolytic point—Taichong (Liv 3):

Taichong (Liv 3) is the Yuan (Source) point of the Liver Meridian of Foot-Jueyin. Yongquan (K 1) is on its opposite side.

Taichong (Liv 3) is able to promote the liver function in maintaining the free flow of qi, circulate blood, suppress liver yang, relieve spasm, eliminate wind and clear heat and fire. It is indicated in diseases due to liver yang rising, flaring up of liver fire and stirring up of liver wind, epilepsy due to fright, diseases due to wind, and eye diseases.

In winter, 1968, a forty-year-old armyman came to the clinic, complaining of hypertension for ten years. His blood pressure was as high as 220/125 mmHg. The accompanying symptoms and signs included headache, dizziness, vertigo, red lips, red eyes, insomnia, dream-disturbed sleep, lumbar soreness, numbness of the trunks and limbs, spasm of m. gastrocnemius, constipation, scanty and deep yellow urine, a red tongue with yellow coating and string-taut, rapid pulse.

The blood pressure dropped a little after Western and Chinese medication, but the accompanying symptoms and signs remained unchanged.

Taichong (Liv 3) was needled towards Yongquan (K 1) on both sides with the reducing method. This was aimed at nourishing yin, suppressing fire, checking the liver, relieving spasm and eliminating wind. Treatment was given twice a week. The patient noted improvement after each treatment, and marked improvement after the sixth treatment. As the hypertensive drugs he had been taking had harmful side effects for his stomach and intestines, he gave up medication completely and continued acupuncture treatment for more than two months. The blood pressure dropped to 180/100 mmHg with other symptoms and signs basically relieved.

These hypnotic, analgesic, tranquilizing and spasmolytic points can be combined according to pathological conditions. The combination of Hegu (LI 4) and Taichong (Liv 3) is known as the Four-Gate Point, which has extensive indications.

3) *Back-Shu Points* Located on the first lateral line of the Bladder Meridian on the back, the Back-Shu Points are closely related to the twelve zang-fu organs. These points are places where the qi of the respective zang-fu organs is deeply infused. When any of the zang-fu organs malfunctions, an abnormal reaction such as tenderness will occur at the corresponding Back-Shu Points. Pressure of the tenderness with the hand will relieve the uncomfortable feeling of the diseased zang-fu organs. The book *Miraculous Pivot* says: "In order to see if the Back-Shu Point is located with accuracy, one may press the region to see if the patient feels sore or if the patient's original soreness is relieved, in which case, the point has been located with accuracy." As the qi is deeply infused in these points, deep needling regulates qi and produces immediate effects.

4) *Baliao* Baliao refers to four pairs of Shangliao (B 31), Ciliao (B 32), Zhongliao (B 33) and Xialiao (B 34). At the level of Xiaochangshu (B 27), Shangliao (B 31) connects the Bladder Meridian and Gallbladder Meridian. At the level of Pangguangshu (B 28), Ciliao (B 32) connects the Bladder Meridian and the Spleen Meridian. At the level of Zhonglushu (B 29), Zhongliao (B 33) is a meeting point of the Liver Meridian and Gallbladder Meridian. At the level of Baihuanshu (B 30), Xialiao (B 34) connects the Bladder Meridian, Liver Meridian and Gallbladder Meridian. Dr. Wei thinks that there is an internal relationship between these four pairs of points and their connected meridians and the points at the same level. That is why they produce specific therapeutic results in the treatment of many diseases, such as lumbago, dysmenorrhea, irregular menstruation, leukorrhea, impotence, nocturnal emission, prolapse of the rectum, dysuria, constipation and incontinence of urine and feces.

In the spring of 1980, a 20-year-old male patient came to the clinic, complaining of nocturnal enuresis since childhood. He still wet his bed once or twice a night. He consulted many doctors in different places, but in vain. Therefore, he was very worried. He looked healthy with a normal complexion. Then pulse and tongue coating were also normal. Ciliao (B 32) on both sides was needled at the same time with both hands. As he was big, the needles went four inches deep. As soon as the needles entered the sacral foremen, numbness like electrical shock radiated to the perineum and penis. The needles were retained for twenty minutes and manipulated once or twice. Another manipulation was done before the withdrawal of the needles. He didn't wet the bed that night. Ten daily treatments cured the disease.

In November of 1985, a young man complained of impotence one year after marriage. As the disease didn't respond to herbal treatment, he decided to try acupuncture. The patient looked strong and big. Appetite, urination and defecation were all normal. Examination showed slow pulse and pale tongue with thin coating.

Ciliao (B 32) on both sides was needled four inches deep. The above method of needling was adopted. The patient's sexual life returned to normal.

II. Case Analysis

Case 1: Asthma

Name, Li x x; sex, female; age, 20; occupation, student; date, May, 1968.

Complaints Paroxysmal dyspnea of four years' duration.

Over the past two weeks, the patient noted acute onsets of dyspnea with cough due to common cold. Each attack was relieved with Western medication. Owing to the side effects induced by long-term oral administration of hormone and sensitivity to Western drugs, she decided to receive acupuncture treatment for the recent attack.

The patient looked acutely ill with a drawn countenance. She had to keep the mouth open and the shoulder raised to assist respiration. She couldn't lie flat and a gurgling sound with sputum could be heard. She also had a blue purple complexion, a slightly red tongue with a thin, white coating and a superficial and tense pulse. Auscultation revealed wheezing in both lungs.

The disease was diagnosed as asthma of the excess type.

The method of treatment was to promote the lung's function in dispersing, soothe asthma and conduct the rebellious qi downward.

Prescription Dingchuan (Extra), Feishu (B 13), Hegu (LI 4).

Treatment procedure The reducing method was applied. The main symptoms and signs started improving a few minutes later, and disappeared twenty minutes later. The wheezing in the lungs also disappeared basically. She received over ten treatments in all until the disease was resolved.

Explanation Asthma is often of excess types during the acute stage. Feishu (B 13) eliminates pathogenic factors from the lung and conducts the rebellious qi downward. If there are signs of invasion by either wind-cold or wind-heat, Fengmen (B 12) should also be selected for the purpose of circulating qi of the Taiyang Meridian of Foot. This is based on the understanding that the lung dominates the skin and bodily hair, while Taiyang dominates the exterior of the entire body. The elimination of pathogenic factors from the exterior of the body results in smooth circulation and descending of the lung qi. The two points should be deeply needled as long as the pleura is not hit (usually two or three inches deep). By doing so, marked relief or complete disappearance of the symptoms and signs will be expected.

Dingchuan (Extra) was needled one or two inches. This point is both effective and safe.

Hegu (LI 4) is the Yuan (Source) Point of the Large Intestine Meridian of Hand-Yangming, which is externally-internally related to the Lung Meridian. Clinical practice has confirmed its effectiveness in the treatment of the lung diseases such as asthma of the excess type. When this patient had mild attacks, Hegu (LI 4) on both sides was needled. The symptoms and signs were also relieved immediately after needling.

Case 2: Taiyang headache (occipital neuralgia)

Name, Ling x x; sex, female; age, 56; date, March, 1975.

Complaints Three weeks before, the patient noted occipital pain accompanied by hyperesthesia in the painful area due to a cold. The pain was continuous but tolerable in spite of intermittent aggravation. Over the past two or three days, she felt very tired after a day's hard work. However, she couldn't fall asleep due to occipital pain. She worked hard again this morning and as a result, the pain became worse and intolerable.

The patient looked chronically ill with a drawn countenance. She showed extreme tiredness, low spirits, pale complexion, slightly red tongue, slightly white coating and string-taut, forceful pulse. Physical examination showed that blood pressure, heart, lungs, liver and spleen all normal. A tenderness was present around Fengchi (G 20) on the left side, which radiated along the occipital nerve.

Differentiation The disease was due to injury of qi after overstrain and stress complicated with invasion of the Taiyang Meridian by the seasonal pathogenic factor, which blocked the meridian.

The method of treatment was to circulate the qi of meridian.

Prescription Tianzhu (B 10), Yuzhen (B 9), Houxi (SI 3), Fuyang (B 59).

Treatment procedure The pain was relieved a few minutes after needling. The patient fell asleep soon and slept for three hours. When she woke up, she was free of symptoms. She did evening work until 11 o'clock without pain.

Explanation The occipital headache is due to the involvement of the Taiyang Meridian. The distal and local points combine to circulate the qi of the meridian. Houxi (SI 3) is the Confluent Point of the Eight Extra Meridians communicating with the Du Meridian, which passes through the occipital area. As the Xi (Cleft) Point of the Yangqiao Meridian, Fuyang (B 59) is indicated in acute pain at the posterior aspect of the head and neck.

Case 3: Migraine

Name, Jia x x; sex, male; age, 42; date, December 3, 1974.

Complaints Periodic paroxysmal migraine.

Over the past ten years, migraine occurred with a frequency of once every three weeks. The patient had to rest in bed for two or three days when migraine was present. He noted premonitory symptoms before each attack such as lassitude, general weakness, poor appetite, nausea and vomiting. As the recent attack occurred when he suffered from a cold with fever, the migraine was more severe than before. He was referred to our medical team after the treatments of the local hospital failed.

The patient looked acutely ill with drawn countenance. He presented with lassitude, mental depression, pale complexion, closed eyes, dislike of noise, 39°C of body temperature, 110/70 mmHg of blood pressure, nasal obstruction, congested throat, slightly red tongue, thin white tongue coating and superficial, rapid and string-taut pulse. The heart and lungs revealed normal, abdomen soft, the liver and spleen not palpable, and urination and defecation normal.

Differentiation The recent attack of migraine was induced by invasion of the yang meridians by pathogenic wind, which affected the head and brain, and contended with the anti-pathogenic qi of the body; hence the occurrence of high fever and a severe migraine. The symptoms should be treated first in acute conditions. Therefore the method of treatment was to relieve exterior syndromes, clear heat and relieve pain.

Prescription Fengchi (G 20), Waiguan (SJ 5), Hegu (LI 4), Yifeng (SJ 17), Sizhukong (SJ 23) towards Shuaigu (G 8).

Treatment procedure A reducing method was applied to all the points. Twenty minutes after needling, migraine markedly improved. However, the body temperature remained high, Western medication was administered, which resulted in subsidence of fever. During his second and third visits, only acupuncture was applied, which made the migraine disapprear. For fear that migraine might occur again, he received another ten treatments with a frequency of three times a week for prevention. The migraine didn't come back during the next cycle. When the medical team was about to return to China two and half years later, he was visited by the doctor. He had been free of migraine since the acupuncture treatment.

Explanation The disease was diagnosed as migraine by neurologists in the Federal Republic of Germany and Italy. However, the treatment he received in those countries was not successful. An acupuncture rhyme called *Song of the Jade Dragon* says: "In the treatment of intractable diseases of headache and migraine, Sizhukong (SJ 23) is applicable; needling Sizhukong (SJ 23) towards Shuaigu (G 8) is even more effective." It also says: "There are two types of migraine. Fengchi (G 20) is needled if the disease is caused by phlegm and retained fluid; and Hegu (LI 4) is needled, if there are no signs of phlegm of retained fluid."

Fengchi (G 20) and Waiguan (SJ 5) eliminate wind and relieve exterior syndromes. Hegu (LI 4) clears heat from the Yangming Meridians of Hand and Foot. The underlying causes of the disease should be treated, following the relief of pain and subsidence of fever. The main points include Sizhukong (SJ 23) or Touwei (S 8) towards Shuaigu (G 8), and Yifeng (SJ 17). The points of Yifeng (SJ 17), Sizhukong (SJ 23) and Shuaigu (G 8) circulate the qi of the Shaoyang Meridians of Hand and Foot. Touwei (S 8) is the meeting point of the Yangming Meridian of Foot, Shaoyang Meridian of Foot and Yangwei Meridian, functioning to circulate the qi of the meridians on the forehead. Yifeng (SJ 17) should be needled two inches deep in the direction of mastoid process on the other side.

Case 4: Jaundice (chronic icteric hepatitis)

Name, Zhao x x; sex, female; age, 26; occupation, nurse; date, September, 1968.

Complaints It was more than ten months since she noted jaundice, poor appetite, nausea, emaciation and lassitude. The examination before admission to the hospital showed 2 cm. liver enlargement and six hundred units of glutamic pyruvic transaminase (GPT). The disease was diagnosed as chronic hepatitis.

During her six months' hospitalization, she was administered both Chinese herbs and Western drugs, including a hormone and intravenous drip of glucose and a small dosage of insulin for improving appetite and protecting the liver. However, neither the symptoms nor the GPT level improved. So he was referred to the acupuncture department.

The patient looked chronically ill, emaciated, low spirited and sallow in complexion. Examination showed mild yellow sclera on both sides, a two cm. enlargement of the liver which was medium in consistency, the spleen not palpable, the heart and lungs normal. Blood test showed twenty-six units of icteric index and 640 units of GPT. The tongue coating was yellow and sticky; the pulse string-taut and rapid; and the urine scanty and dark yellow.

Differentiation The disease was due to accumulation of damp-heat in the middle jiao, which affected the gallbladder and prevented the bile from circulating by its normal route. Damp turned into fire and heat over a long time. The heat of the gallbladder and damp combined to impair the spleen's function in transportation and transformation.

The method of treatment was to clear accumulated heat from the liver and gallbladder, invigorate the spleen and resolve damp.

Prescription Ganshu (B 18), Pishu (B 20), Danshu (B 19), Taichong (Liv 3), Zusanli (S 36), Zhangmen (Liv 13), Qimen (Liv 14) and Zhiyang (Du 9).

Treatment procedure These points were used in turn with two to three points for each daily treatment. The reducing method was applied, and moxibustion was not used. After three weeks' acupuncture treatment, GPT turned normal, the appetite markedly improved and the patient was in better spirits. However, the icteric index dropped to eighteen units only. After another seven weeks' treatment, she was discharged from the hospital, free from any symptoms and signs.

Explanation A hundred and twenty-five cases of acute icteric hepatitis were admitted into the hospital and treated in this way. Most of them improved. In the group of adults, jaundice subsided within twenty-one days in fifty-nine cases, constituting 67.8 percent; and it took 17.9 days on the average to drop the icteric index to the normal level. In the group of children, Jaundice subsided within fourteen days in thirty-three cases, constituting 86.7 percent; and it took 11.4 days on average to drop icteric index to the normal level. GPT turned normal within forty days in most of the cases, and within eighy days in a few cases. Along with the improvement of the symptoms and signs, the enlarged liver was markedly reduced in size. All this shows that needling improves the liver's function and reduces the hepatomegaly.

Case 5: Hysteric aphasia

Name, Li x x; sex, female; age, 22; occupation, peasant; date, March, 1977.

Complaints Half a month ago, aphasia suddenly occured to her due to mental irritation. She looked anxious, but couldn't speak when spoken to. She was in low spirits when she was left alone. As neither Western drugs nor Chinese herbs could help her, she decided to receive acupuncture treatment.

The patient was mentally clear, being able to understand all the questions asked by the doctor. However, she couldn't express herself with words. So she looked very anxious. She was normally healthy without any history of chronic diseases. Aphasia was her only complaint. The pulse was string-taut and forceful, and the tongue coating thin and white.

Differentiation The disease fell into the category of depression, which was due to drastic emotional changes. Obstruction of qi turned into fire and blocked the clear cavity.

The method of treatment was to promote the liver's function in maintaining free flow of qi and relieve aphasia.

Prescription Taichong (Liv 3), Tiantu (Ren 22), Hegu (LI 4).

Treatment procedure Taichong (Liv 3) and Tiantu (Ren 22) were needled in a regular way. Hegu (LI 4) was needled vigorously, while conversation between the doctor and the patient was tried. Two minutes later, the patient was able to answer the doctor clearly. Soon she could speak freely.

Explanation Hysteric aphasia is due to mental depression, which leads to stagnation of qi. To promote smooth circulation of qi is the key method of treatment. Meanwhile certain explanatory work should be done in order to cheer up the patient. In the acupuncture treatment, strong stimulation should be given, while the patient is asked about the needling sensation of soreness, numbness and distention. The conversation may also cover such topics as people or what the patient is most concerned about. All this is aimed at encouraging the patient to speak.

INDEX

A

B

C

D

E

F

G

H

I

N

O

P

T

当代中国针灸临证精要
陈佑邦　邓良月主编
*
外文出版社出版
（中国北京百万庄路24号）
外文印刷厂印刷
中国国际图书贸易总公司
（中国国际书店）发行
北京399信箱
1989年（16开）第一版
（英）
ISBN 7－119－01042－5／R·29（外）
07000
14－E－2435 S